Solved Papers

Orthopedics

for PG Students

A must for MS and DNB

Solved Papers

Orthopedics

for PG Students

A must for MS and DNB

Editor

Abdul Ghani

MBBS MS(Orthopedics) (AIIMS New Delhi) MRCS(Edinburgh)

Professor and Head of Unit
Department of Orthopedics
Government Medical College
Jammu, Jammu and Kashmir, India

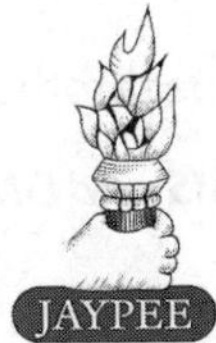

JAYPEE BROTHERS MEDICAL PUBLISHERS

The Health Sciences Publisher

New Delhi | London

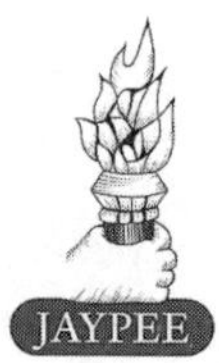

Jaypee Brothers Medical Publishers (P) Ltd

Headquarters
EMCA House, 23/23-B
Ansari Road, Daryaganj
New Delhi 110 002, India
Landline: +91-11-23272143, +91-11-23272703
+91-11-23282021, +91-11-23245672
e-mail: jaypee@jaypeebrothers.com

Corporate Office
4838/24, Ansari Road, Daryaganj
New Delhi 110 002, India
Phone: +91-11-43574357
Fax: +91-11-43574314
e-mail: jaypee@jaypeebrothers.com

Overseas Office
JP Medical Ltd.
83, Victoria Street, London
SW1H 0HW (UK)
Phone: +44-20 3170 8910
e-mail: info@jpmedpub.com

EU GPSR Authorised Representative
Logos Europe, 9 rue Nicolas Poussin
17000, La Rochelle, France
Phone: +33 (0) 6 67 93 73 78
e-mail: contact@logoseurope.eu

Website: www.jaypeebrothers.com
Website: www.jaypeedigital.com

Inquiries for bulk sales may be solicited at: jaypee@jaypeebrothers.com

Solved Papers Orthopedics for PG Students: A must for MS and DNB / Abdul Ghani

First Edition: **2026**

ISBN: 978-93-6616-292-8

Printed at: Samrat Offset Pvt. Ltd.

Dedicated To

My Family

For their unwavering love, patience, and encouragement, your sacrifices have made this journey possible.

Every Orthopedic Postgraduate

Preparing day and night for exams and striving to become a competent, compassionate surgeon—*this book is for you*.

Contributors

Aakash Deep MBBS MS(Orthopedics)
Senior Resident
Department of Orthopedics, ASCOMS
Jammu, Jammu and Kashmir, India

Aasim Maqbool MBBS MS(Orthopedics)
PG Scholar 2nd year
Department of Orthopedics
SKIMS Medical College and Hospital
Srinagar, Jammu and Kashmir, India

Abdul Maajid Bhat MBBS MS(Orthopedics)
Senior Resident
Department of Orthopedics
Government Medical College and Hospital
Jammu, Jammu and Kashmir, India

Abhai Singh Bhadwal MBBS MS(Orthopedics)
Postgraduate Resident
Department of Orthopedics
Government Medical College and Hospital
Jammu, Jammu and Kashmir, India

Abhimanu Kaith MBBS
Postgraduate Resident
Department of Orthopedics
Government Medical College and Hospital
Jammu, Jammu and Kashmir, India

Abhishek Bral MBBS MS(Orthopedics)
Senior Resident
Department of Orthopedics
ASCOMS Hospital
Jammu, Jammu and Kashmir, India

Abhishek Mahajan MBBS MS(Orthopedics)
Senior Resident
Department of Orthopedics
AIIMS Vijaypur
Jammu, Jammu and Kashmir, India

Aditya Chaubey MBBS
Postgraduate Resident
Department of Orthopedics
Government Medical College and Hospital
Jammu, Jammu and Kashmir, India

Agnivesh Tikoo MBBS MS(Orthopedics) FNB(Spine Surgery)
Senior Consultant Spine Surgeon
Department of Orthopedics
Apollo Hospitals
Navi Mumbai, Maharashtra, India

Akash Narangyal MBBS MS
Senior Resident, SMVDIME
Department of Orthopedics
Attending Consultant, SMVD, Narayana Hospital
Jammu, Jammu and Kashmir, India

Amandeep Singh Bakshi MBBS MS
Professor
Department of Orthopedics
Government Medical College and Rajindra Hospital
Patiala, Punjab, India

Aman Koul MBBS MS(Orthopedics)
Registrar, Department of Orthopedics
Government Medical College
Jammu, Jammu and Kashmir, India

Amit Kumar MBBS MS(Orthopedics)
Consultant
Department of Orthopedics
ESIC Hospital Bari Brahmana
Jammu, Jammu and Kashmir, India

Ankita Khajuria MBBS MS(Orthopedics)
Senior Resident
Department of Orthopedics
St Stephen's Hospital
Tis Hazari, New Delhi, India

Anoop Kumar MBBS MS(Orthopedics)
Professor
Department of Orthopedics
Government Medical College
Jammu, Jammu and Kashmir, India

Arun K Sharma MBBS MS(Orthopedics)
Professor and Head of Unit
Department of Orthopedics
SMS Medical College and Attached Hospital
Jaipur, Rajasthan, India

Ashish Gulia MBBS MS(Orthopedics) Fellowship-Orthopedic Oncology(HBNI) Mch-Surgical Oncology FACS EPGDHA(TISS) Diploma in Tissue Banking
Professor, Orthopedic Oncology
Department of Surgical Oncology
Homi Bhabha Cancer Hospital and Research Centre, New Chandigarh
Mohali, Punjab, India

Ashish Jaiman MBBS MS(Orthopedics)
Director Professor
Department of Orthopedics
Central Institute of Orthopedics
Safdarjung Hospital and Vardhman Mahavir Medical College
New Delhi, India

Ashish Nehru MBBS MS(Orthopedics)
Senior Resident
Department of Orthopedics
Pt BD Sharma PGIMS
Rohtak, Haryana, India

Asif Nazir Baba MBBS MS(Orthopedics)
Associate Professor
Department of Orthopedics
Government Medical College
Srinagar, Jammu and Kashmir, India

Azhar Ud Din MBBS MS(Orthopedics)
Consultant
Department of Orthopedics
District Hospital Kargil
Union Territory of Ladakh, India

Barkat Anwar Shah MBBS MS(Orthopedics)
Senior Resident
Department of Orthopedics
Government Medical College and Hospital
Jammu, Jammu and Kashmir, India

Bhaarath KS MBBS MS(Orthopedics)
Postgraduate Resident
Department of Orthopedics
Government Medical College and Hospital
Jammu, Jammu and Kashmir, India

Bhat Jameel Mohd Jabbar MBBS MS(Orthopedics)
Senior Resident
Department of Orthopedics
Government Medical College and Hospital
Jammu, Jammu and Kashmir, India

Biswajit Sahu MBBS MS(Orthopedics)
Professor
Department of Orthopedics
Medical Superintendent
PGIMER and Capital Hospital
Bhubaneswar, Odisha, India

Deepali Gupta BPT MPT(Sports) MIAP
Physiotherapist
Government Medical College and Hospital
Jammu, Jammu and Kashmir, India

Dev Kant Meena MBBS MS(Orthopedics)
Professor
Department of Orthopedics
SMS Medical College
Jaipur, Rajasthan, India

Farid Hussain MBBS MS(Orthopedics)
Assistant Professor
Department of Orthopedics
Government Medical College and Hospital
Jammu, Jammu and Kashmir, India

Harsh Chauhan MBBS
Postgraduate Resident
Department of Orthopedics
Government Medical College and Hospital
Jammu, Jammu and Kashmir, India

Heemanshu Bhat MBBS
Postgraduate Resident
Department of Orthopedics
Government Medical College and Hospital
Jammu, Jammu and Kashmir, India

Iram Mir MBBS MD(Anesthesia)
Specialist Anesthesia
Rashid Hospital
Dubai Health Corporation
Dubai, United Arab Emirates

Irfan Ahmed Poswal MBBS
Postgraduate Resident
Department of Orthopedics
Government Medical College and Hospital
Jammu, Jammu and Kashmir, India

Irfan Andleeb Gul MBBS MS(Orthopedics)
Assistant Professor
Department of Orthopedics
Hamdard Institute of Medical Sciences and Research (HIMSR)
New Delhi, India

Jujhar Singh MBBS MS(Orthopedics) DNB MNAMS FACS(USA)
Assistant Professor
Department of Orthopedics
Sports Injury Centre, VMMC and Safdarjung Hospital
New Delhi, India

Kamal Ji Pandit MBBS MS(Orthopedics) DNB(Orthopedics) D.Ortho FAA
Senior Resident
Department of Orthopedics
Hamdard Institute of Medical Sciences and Research (HIMSR)
New Delhi, India

Kanav Mahajan MBBS D.Ortho DNB
Consultant
Department of Orthopedics
Umang Healthcare and Diagnostics
Jammu, Jammu and Kashmir, India

Khalid Muzzafar MBBS MS(Orthopedics) DNB(Orthopedics)
Associate Professor
Department of Orthopedics
Government Medical College
Doda, Jammu and Kashmir, India

Kushagra Pathak MBBS MS(Orthopedics)
Senior Orthopedics
Department of Orthopedics
AIIMS
New Delhi, India

Manish Singh MBBS MS(Orthopedics) Fellowship in Sports Medicine
Consultant Knee Surgery
Department of Orthopedics
Government Medical College and Hospital
Jammu, Jammu and Kashmir, India

MD Maaz MBBS MS(Orthopedics) Fellow in Arthroscopy and Sports Medicine(ISAKOS)
Assistant Professor
Department of Orthopedics
Sri Atal Bihari Vajpayee Medical College and Research Institute
Bengaluru, Karnataka, India

Meganath Pawar MBBS MS(Orthopedics)
Professor and Unit 2 Incharge
Department of Orthopedic Surgery
AIIMS Bhubaneswar
Bhubaneswar, Odisha, India

Mohamad Waseem Dar MBBS MS(Orthopedics)
Senior Resident
Department of Orthopedics
Government Medical College
Doda, Jammu and Kashmir, India

Mohammed Farooq Butt MBBS MS(Orthopedics)
Associate Professor
Department of Orthopedics
Government Medical College and Hospital
Jammu, Jammu and Kashmir, India

Mozam Hamid Wani MBBS
Postgraduate Resident
Department of Orthopedics
Government Medical College and Hospital
Jammu, Jammu and Kashmir, India

Naresh V MBBS MS(Orthopedics)
Postgraduate Resident
Department of Orthopedics
Government Medical College and Hospital
Jammu, Jammu and Kashmir, India

Niaz Ahmed MBBS MS(Orthopedics)
Senior Resident
Department of Orthopedics
Government Medical College
Rajouri, Jammu and Kashmir, India

Nikhil Gupta MBBS MS(Orthopedics)
Senior Resident
Department of Orthopedics
Government Medical College
Udhampur, Jammu and Kashmir, India

Nusrat Jabeen MBBS MS
Professor, Department of Anatomy
Government Medical College and Hospital
Jammu, Jammu and Kashmir, India

Nitin Choudhary MBBS MS(Orthopedics)
Senior Resident
Department of Orthopedics
Government Medical College and Hospital
Udhampur, Jammu and Kashmir, India

Omeshwar Singh MBBS MS(Orthopedics)
Associate Professor
Department of Orthopedics
Government Medical College
Udhampur, Jammu and Kashmir, India

Pankaj Spolia MBBS MS(Orthopedics)
Assistant Professor
Department of Orthopedics
Maharishi Markandeshwar Institute of Medical Sciences and Research (MMIMSR)
Ambala, Haryana, India

Pankaj Vir Singh MBBS MS(Orthopedics)
Senior Resident
Department of Orthopedics
Government Medical College and Hospital
Jammu, Jammu and Kashmir, India

Pardeep Singh MBBS MS(Orthopedics)
Assistant Professor
Department of Orthopedics
Maharishi Markandeshwar Institute of Medical Sciences and Research (MMIMSR)
Ambala, Haryana, India

Priti Ranjan Sinha MBBS DNB(Orthopedics) MNAMS
Associate Professor
Department of Orthopedics
Teerthanker Mahaveer Medical College
Moradabad, Uttar Pradesh, India

Qazi Manaan Masood MS FRCS(Trauma and Orthopedics)
Specialty Doctor in Trauma and Orthopedics
Medway Maritime NHS Foundation Trust
UK

Rajesh Kapila MBBS MS(Orthopedics)
Professor and Head
Department of Orthopedics
Government Medical College and Hospital
Amritsar, Punjab, India

Rashid Anjum MBBS MS(Orthopedics) DNB(Orthopedics) MNAMS FIPO FAA(Austria)
Associate Professor
Department of Orthopedics
AIIMS Vijaypur
Jammu, Jammu and Kashmir, India

Rohit Rambani MBBS MS MRCSEng FIMSA FRCSOrth PhD
Professor and Clinical Director
Department of Orthopedics
Lincoln Medical School and United Lincolnshire Teaching Hospital NHS Trust
UK

Rifaaqat Ghani MBBS(Student)
VMMC and Safdarjung Hospital
New Delhi, India

Sachin Kudyar MBBS MS(Orthopedics)
Senior Resident
Department of Orthopedics
Government Medical College and Hospital
Jammu, Jammu and Kashmir, India

Sajad Ahmad Wani MBBS MS(Orthopedics)
Senior Resident
Department of Orthopedics
Adesh Medical College and Hospital
Mohri, Haryana, India

Sajal Maingi MBBS MS(Orthopedics) DNB MNAMS
Assistant Professor
Department of Orthopedics
Dayanand Medical College and Hospital (DMCH)
Ludhiana, Punjab, India

Sakib Arfee MBBS MS(Orthopedics)
Consultant, Department of Orthopedics
Medcard Multispeciality Hospital
Amritsar, Punjab, India

Samarth Mittal MBBS MS(Orthopedics) DNB FACS
Additional Professor
Department of Orthopedics
Jai Prakash Narayan Apex Trauma Center
AIIMS
New Delhi, India

Sanjeev Gupta MBBS MS(Orthopedics)
Professor and Head
Department of Orthopedics
Government Medical College and Hospital
Jammu, Jammu and Kashmir, India

Saransh Bahl MBBS MS(Orthopedics)
Senior Resident
Department of Orthopedics
AIIMS Vijaypur
Jammu, Jammu and Kashmir, India

Saroj Sharma MBBS MS PhD
Professor, Department of Anatomy
Amrita School of Medicine
Faridabad, Haryana, India

Shamim Ahmad Bhat MBBS MS(Orthopedics) DNB(Orthopedics) Dip SICOT
Assistant Professor
Department of Orthopedics
Government Medical College
Srinagar, Jammu and Kashmir, India

Shubam Surmal MBBS MS(Orthopedics)
Fellow Arthroplasty and Arthroscopy
Department of Orthopedics
Fortis Hospital, Shalimar Bagh
New Delhi, India

Shubham Pandoh MBBS MS(Orthopedics)
Senior Resident
Department of Orthopedics
Government Medical College and Hospital
Jammu, Jammu and Kashmir, India

Shubhranshu Choudhary MBBS MS(Orthopedics)
Senior Resident
Department of Orthopedics
IMS and SUM Hospital
Bhubaneswar, Odisha, India

Shyam Singh MS(General Surgery) MCh(CVTS)
Head
Department of Cardiovascular and Thoracic Surgery, Government Medical College and Hospital
Jammu, Jammu and Kashmir, India

Simranpreet Singh MS(Orthopedics) FNB(Arthroplasty)
Registrar
Department of Orthopedics
Acharya Shri Chander College of Medical Sciences and Hospital (ASCOMS)
Jammu, Jammu and Kashmir, India

Sparsh Dagoria MBBS MS(Orthopedics)
Postgraduate Resident
Department of Orthopedics
Government Medical College and Hospital
Jammu, Jammu and Kashmir, India

Subqat Farooq MBBS MS(Orthopedics)
Senior Resident
Department of Orthopedics
Government Medical College
Srinagar, Jammu and Kashmir, India

Sukhil Raina MBBS MS(Orthopedics)
Senior Resident
Department of Orthopedics
Government Medical College and Hospital
Jammu, Jammu and Kashmir, India

Sumeet Singh Charak MBBS MS(Orthopedics)
Associate Professor
Department of Orthopedics
Acharya Shri Chander College of Medical Sciences and Hospital (ASCOMS)
Jammu, Jammu and Kashmir, India

Sumit Banerjee MBBS MS(Orthopedics) MCh(Orthopedics) FACS
Professor
Department of Orthopedics
AIIMS Jodhpur
Jodhpur, Rajasthan, India

Suraydev Aman Singh MBBS MS(Orthopedics)
Senior Resident
Department of Orthopedics
Government Medical College and Hospital
Jammu, Jammu and Kashmir, India

Tahir Afzal MBBS MS(Orthopedics) PDCC(Rheumatology)
Assistant Professor
Department of Orthopedics
Government Medical College and Hospital
Jammu, Jammu and Kashmir, India

Tarkik Thami MBBS MS(Orthopedics) DNB(Orthopedics) MNAMS
Assistant Professor
Department of Orthopedics, Dayanand Medical College and Hospital (DMCH)
Ludhiana, Punjab, India

Tejpal Singh MBBS MS(Orthopedics)
Senior Resident
Department of Orthopedics
Government Medical College
Udhampur, Jammu and Kashmir, India

Varun Gupta MBBS
Postgraduate Resident
Department of Orthopedics
Government Medical College and Hospital
Jammu, Jammu and Kashmir, India

Vedant Bajaj MBBS MS(Orthopedics)
Senior Resident
Department of Orthopedics
Dr Baba Saheb Ambedkar Medical College and Hospital
New Delhi, India

Vijay Kumar MBBS MS(Orthopedics) (AIIMS), FRCS(Glasgow) FACS FICS FIMSA MAMS Diploma in Tissue Banking(Singapore) Commonwealth Fellow in Arthroplasty(Oxford, UK) Fellow in Sports Medicine(Singapore) Fellow in Orthopedics and Traumatology(Germany) Fellow in Arthroplasty(AIIMS) IOS-UK Fellow IOA Inland Fellow
Professor
Department of Orthopedics
AIIMS
New Delhi, India

Vineet Aggarwal MBBS MS(Orthopedics) DNB(Orthopedics) FNB(Pediatric Orthopedics)
Professor and Head
Department of Orthopedics
Indira Gandhi Medical College
Shimla, Himachal Pradesh, India

Vipin Sharma MBBS DNB(Orthopedics) D.Ortho MNAMS
Professor and Head
Department of Orthopedics
Dr Rajendra Prasad Government Medical College
Kangra, Himachal Pradesh, India

Waseem Ahmad Sheikh MBBS MS(Orthopedics)
Senior Resident
Department of Orthopedics
Adesh Medical College and Hospital
Mohri, Haryana, India

Younis Kamal MBBS MS(Orthopedics) DNB(Orthopedics) MNMS(Orthopedics)
Post DOC Fellowship in Spine Surgery (Ganga Hospital)
Associate Professor, Department of Orthopedics and Spine Surgery
Government Medical College
Anantnag, Jammu and Kashmir, India

Zubair Ahmad Lone MBBS MS(Orthopedics)
Assistant Professor
Department of Orthopedics
Government Medical College
Rajouri, Jammu and Kashmir, India

Preface

The journey through postgraduate orthopedics is both demanding and exhilarating. With an ever-expanding syllabus, exhaustive clinical exposure, and pressure to master intricate theoretical concepts, focused preparation becomes crucial—especially as the final examinations approach.

This book, "*Solved Paper Orthopedics for PG students—A must for MS and DNB*", is born out of the collective efforts of committed orthopedic academicians and residents. It presents a well-structured, chapter-wise compilation of the most frequently asked questions in MS and DNB Orthopedic theory examinations. Each answer has been crafted to be *crisp, clinically relevant, and exam-oriented*, making it ideal for rapid revision and last-minute study.

Our objective was clear: *To help postgraduates revise smartly*. The content reflects the latest examination trends while sticking to standard references and practical knowledge. Whether it is basic sciences, trauma principles, pediatric orthopedics, regional pathologies, or recent advances, this book provides *easy-to-digest yet thorough answers* to help students build confidence and clarity.

We hope this guide serves as your ready reckoner in the critical final stretch of your preparation and ultimately supports your success in the examinations. Wishing you all the very best.

Abdul Ghani

Acknowledgments

I express my deepest gratitude to the "Almighty" who has given me and all of us this wonderful opportunity to create a much-needed knowledge resource.

My sincere thanks go to Jaypee Brothers Medical Publishers Pvt Ltd, especially Mr Ankit Vij (Managing Director), Mr Sabyasachi Hazra [Director (PG and PNR Content)], and Mr Ashish Kumar (Senior Business Development Manager) for providing me this opportunity to be the editor of this book. Also, I extend my special thanks to Mr Priyansh Saxena (Development Editor) for excellent work in shaping up this project.

Thanks go to all the esteemed contributors whose expertise, dedication, and collaborative spirit have shaped this comprehensive book *"Solved Questions in Orthopedics—A must for MS and DNB"*.

I am grateful to the postgraduate students, residents, and young orthopedic surgeons, whose curiosity and quest for clarity in learning have been the primary motivation for this endeavor. It is my hope that this book serves as a reliable companion in their exam preparation and clinical practice.

Special thanks and appreciation go to my family (my wife, Dr Nusrat; my son, Rifaaqat; and my parents) and colleagues for their unwavering support, patience, and belief in me.

Finally, I am grateful to all those whose direct or indirect support made the compilation of this volume possible (Mr Vikram Khullar, Ms Meenakshi, Mr Latif Khan, Mr Akhlesh Khajuria, Ms Sadaf Hanief, and many others). This book stands as a testament to the collective effort of advancing orthopedic education.

Abdul Ghani

Contents

How to Use This Book Effectively

This book has been designed as a *strategic and high-yield revision tool* to help MS and DNB orthopedic postgraduates prepare for their final examinations in a focused and efficient manner. Here is how you can use it smartly to your advantage:

- **Use it Alongside Standard Textbooks**

  This book is not meant to replace core textbooks like Apley, Campbell, or Turek, but to *complement them*. For each topic, first understand the concept from standard references and then use this book to revise and consolidate the content in an exam-ready format.

- **Focus on Questions Asked in the Exam**

  Each section and chapter have been curated based on *repeated university exam trends*. Prioritize your revision by going through these questions, most of which recur with slight variations across institutions.

- **Revise Chapter-wise or Paper-wise**
  - Use the *Table of Contents* to navigate through the subject as per your own study plan—either *chapter-wise* (e.g., shoulder, spine, pediatrics) or *paper-wise* (e.g., trauma, general ortho, recent advances).
  - During early preparation, go chapter by chapter.
  - Closer to exams, revise in paper-wise chunks to simulate real exam scenarios.

- **Practice Writing Answers**

  Use the answers in this book as a *template for writing practice*. Meanwhile during exam, you can always expand your answers also, especially for long answers. *Add diagrams or sketches along with these answers*. Set a timer and try to write answers from memory and then compare with the book to assess your content, structure, and presentation.

- **Group Study and Peer Discussions**

  Use this book during group studies to test each other on commonly asked questions. It helps *reinforce concepts*, correct misconceptions, and simulate viva-style questioning.

- **Last-minute Rapid Review**

  In the final days before the exam, avoid bulky textbooks and turn to this book for *crisp, to-the-point revision*. Each answer has been crafted for *quick readability, recall, and retention*.

- **Adapt Based on Your Exam Format**

  DNB students can focus more on OSCE-relevant questions and surgical techniques. MS students can emphasize theory and viva-based answers. The book covers *both formats* to a great extent.

Other Practical Advice

- *Time management*: Practice writing within time limits. Allocate time for studies, revision, as well as during writing exam.
- *Presentation*: Use diagrams, bullet points, and structured formats. Underline keywords.

By consistently integrating this book into your daily preparation schedule, you will be better equipped to tackle the vast syllabus, strengthen your recall, and, most importantly, *walk into your theory and viva exams with confidence and clarity*.

Introduction

Introduction to MS and DNB Orthopedic Theory Examinations (as per Latest NMC Guidelines)

The MS Orthopedics and DNB Orthopedics final examinations are comprehensive evaluations designed to assess a postgraduate student's understanding of the theoretical, clinical, and practical aspects of orthopedics. These exams are regulated by the National Medical Commission (NMC) and National Board of Examinations (NBE), respectively, and follow a structured pattern.

MS Orthopedics—Theory Exam Pattern (NMC Guidelines)

Structure: The theory examination is divided into *four papers*, each of 100 marks, totaling *400 marks*.

- *Paper I*: Basic sciences related to orthopedics, including anatomy, biomechanics, pathology, microbiology, imaging, and pharmacology relevant to orthopedics
- *Paper II*: General orthopedics, musculoskeletal infections, metabolic bone diseases, and inflammatory disorders
- *Paper III*: Regional orthopedics—diseases and injuries involving upper and lower limbs, spine, and pelvis
- *Paper IV*: Recent advances, surgical techniques, orthopedic implants, rehabilitation, musculoskeletal oncology, and allied specialties

Duration: 3 hours per paper

Passing criteria: A minimum of *50% aggregate* marks (i.e., 200/400) across all theory papers is required to pass. Additionally, students must pass the practical/viva component separately.

DNB Orthopedics—Theory Exam Format (NBE)

Structure:

- The DNB theory exam also consists of *4 papers*, each carrying *100 marks*, similar to MS.
- The exam includes *short answer questions (SAQs)* and *long answer questions (LAQs)*.
- *Papers generally follow the same themes*:
  - *Paper I*: Basic sciences
  - *Paper II*: General orthopedics and infections
  - *Paper III*: Trauma and regional orthopedics
  - *Paper IV*: Recent advances and surgical techniques

Scoring: *Minimum of 50%* marks is required in theory to be eligible for practicals.

Universities/Institutions: While the pattern is broadly uniform, minor variations exist in formatting across different medical universities and DNB teaching hospitals (e.g., structured long questions, essay-based questions).

Syllabus Coverage and Expectations

- *The syllabus is exhaustive and encompasses all domains*:
  - Basic sciences (bone biology, biomechanics, and imaging)
  - Trauma (adult and pediatric)
  - Nontraumatic orthopedic conditions
  - Tumors, infections, deformities, and congenital anomalies

    - Arthroplasty, arthroscopy, and spine surgery
    - Rehabilitation, implants, surgical approaches, and recent advances
- *Examiners expect answers that are*:
    - Conceptually sound and evidence-based
    - Structured with headings and subheadings
    - Supported by diagrams and flowcharts where appropriate
    - Concise but comprehensive

Other Aspects of the MS and DNB Final Examinations

In addition to theory exams, both MS and DNB orthopedic programs include comprehensive assessments through *practical, clinical*, *viva voce*, and *logbook evaluations*.

- *Practical and clinical examination:*
    - *Content*: Short cases, long cases, spotters (X-rays, instruments, implants), surgical techniques, and orthotic/prosthetic applications
    - *Expectation*: Demonstrate clinical reasoning, diagnosis, examination techniques, surgical planning, and communication skills
    - *Tips*: Practice short case presentations, history taking, identifying common deformities and gait abnormalities, and describing X-ray findings fluently
- *Viva voce:*
    - *Structure*: Usually conducted in multiple stations or by different examiners
    - *Topics*: Instruments, implants, operative techniques, orthopedic pathology specimens, radiology, orthoses/prostheses, recent advances
    - *Suggestions*: Keep answers concise, revise operative steps and common implants, and stay updated with guidelines and new technologies.
- *Logbook and thesis evaluation (MS only):*
    - Students must maintain a *logbook* documenting their surgical exposure, academic participation, seminars, and teaching activities.
    - A *thesis* is evaluated before or during final exams and forms an essential eligibility criterion.
- *OSCE (DNB Specific):*
    - Many DNB centers conduct *Objective Structured Clinical Examinations (OSCE).*
    - OSCE includes clinical scenarios, radiograph interpretation, diagnosis, procedural steps, and MCQ-style stations.
    - *Advice*: Practice simulated OSCE stations and review DNB-specific recall questions.

This book is tailored precisely to meet these exam demands (*theory as well as viva*), providing a chapter-wise collection of solved theory questions written in a crisp, easy-to-remember manner. *It is a valuable resource for smart revision and confident performance in both MS and DNB orthopedics exams.*

CHAPTER 1

Basic Applied Orthopedic Sciences

Samarth Mittal, Nusrat Jabeen, Saroj Sharma

Q1. Describe the structure and composition of bone.

(AIIMS New Delhi 2017)

1. *Gross structure of bone*:
   - **Bone** is a specialized connective tissue providing mechanical support and metabolic functions.
   - It consists of:
     - *Cortical bone (compact bone)*: Dense outer layer, ~80% of skeletal mass.
     - *Cancellous bone (trabecular bone)*: Porous inner structure, ~20% of skeletal mass.
2. *Composition of bone*:
   - *Inorganic component (65–70%)*:
     - Predominantly hydroxyapatite crystals [$Ca_{10}(PO_4)_6(OH)_2$].
     - Provides hardness and compressive strength.
   - *Organic component (30–35%)*:
     - Type I collagen (~90% of organic matrix) – provides tensile strength.
     - Non-collagenous proteins (osteocalcin, osteonectin, osteopontin) – involved in mineralization, remodeling.
     - Proteoglycans – contribute to viscoelastic properties.
   - *Water (10–20%)*: Contributes to resilience and nutrient transport.

Types of Bone Cells and Their Functions

Cell type	*Origin*	*Function*
Osteoblasts	Mesenchymal stem cells	Bone formation; synthesize osteoid (organic matrix)
Osteocytes	Matured osteoblasts trapped in matrix	Mechanosensors; regulate mineral content
Osteoclasts	Hematopoietic stem cells (monocyte-macrophage lineage)	Bone resorption; secrete acids and proteolytic enzymes
Bone lining cells	Inactive osteoblasts	Cover resting bone surfaces; regulate calcium flux

Microanatomy of Cortical versus Cancellous Bone

Feature	*Cortical bone*	*Cancellous bone*
Density	High (~90%)	Low (~15-25%)
Structure	Osteons (Haversian systems)	Trabeculae (network of rods and plates)
Blood supply	Volkmann and Haversian canals	Diffusion through bone marrow spaces
Strength	High compressive strength	Adaptable to mechanical stress (Wolff's law)
Turnover	Slow	Rapid
Significance	Provides rigidity and support; protects organs	Metabolic activity (e.g., calcium homeostasis); shock absorption

Clinical Relevance

- Cancellous bone is **more active** metabolically → faster healing.
- Cortical bone fractures (e.g., shaft fractures) take longer to heal than metaphyseal cancellous fractures.

FLOWCHART: Overview of bone composition and structure

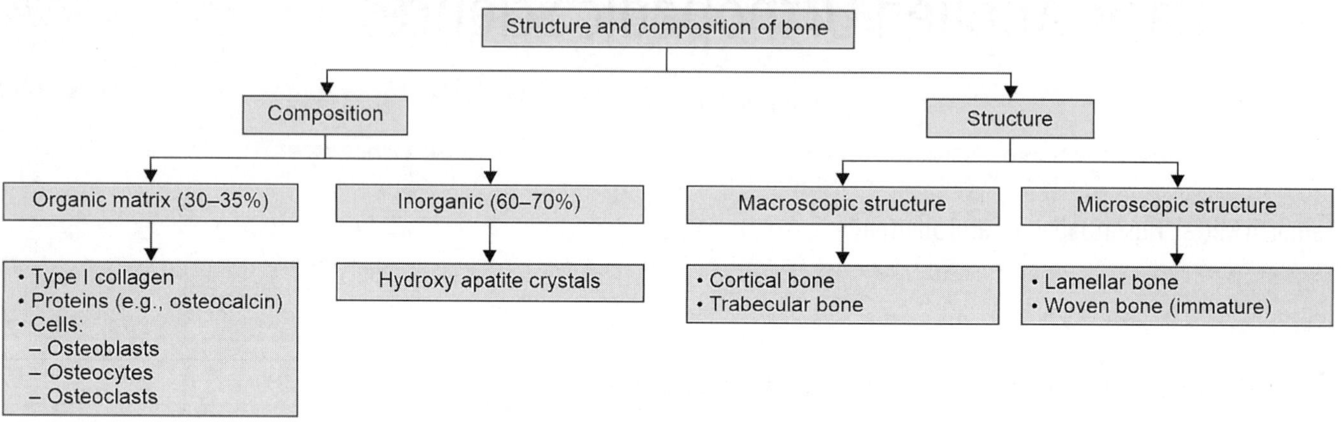

Q2. Note on bone matrix composition and role in fracture healing.

(PGIMER Chandigarh 2021)

Bone Matrix

- *Organic matrix (osteoid)*:
  - Initially laid down by osteoblasts.
  - Composed mainly of **type I collagen** and ground substance.
- *Mineralization*:
  - Occurs by deposition of hydroxyapatite into the osteoid.
  - Facilitated by alkaline phosphatase from osteoblasts.

Role in Fracture Healing

- *Inflammatory phase*:
  - Hematoma forms; cytokines recruit osteoprogenitor cells.
- *Repair phase*:
  - Osteoblasts lay down osteoid → soft callus → mineralized into hard callus.
- *Remodeling phase*:
  - Woven bone remodeled into lamellar bone based on mechanical stresses.
- Matrix proteins like **osteopontin and bone sialoprotein** regulate attachment of cells during healing.

Clinical Importance

- Adequate matrix production is critical for callus formation and bone strength.
- Delayed or impaired matrix formation → **delayed union or nonunion**.

Q3. Describe fracture healing—primary versus secondary healing.

Definition

Fracture healing is the biological process by which bone repairs itself after a break, restoring continuity, strength, and structure.

Types of Fracture Healing

Feature	Primary healing (direct)	Secondary healing (indirect)
Mechanism	Intramembranous ossification	Endochondral ossification
Requirement	Absolute stability (e.g., compression plating)	Relative stability (e.g., cast, external fixator)
Gap size	< 0.01 mm	Larger gaps allowed
Callus formation	Absent	Prominent callus formation
Process	Cutting cones with osteoclasts followed by osteoblasts	Inflammatory response → soft callus → hard callus → remodeling
Examples	Rigid internal fixation with lag screws, plates	Conservatively treated fractures, IM nailing with micromotion

Key Point

Primary healing mimics normal bone remodeling, while secondary healing recapitulates embryonic bone development.

FLOWCHART: Types of bone healing

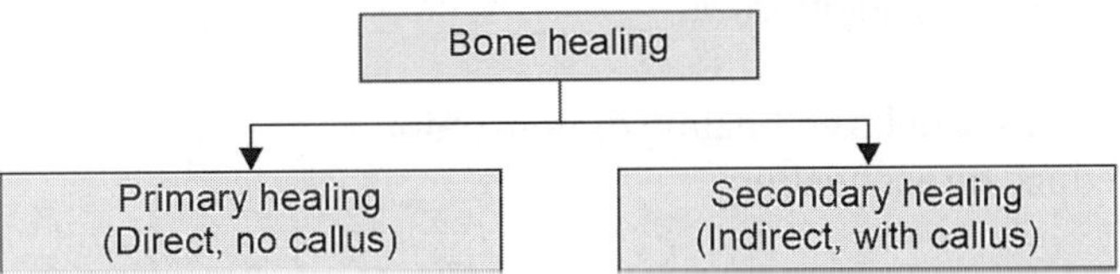

Comparison Table

Feature	Primary healing	Secondary healing
Stability	Absolute	Relative
Callus formation	Absent	Present
Gap tolerance	Minimal (<0.1 mm)	Larger gaps tolerated
Example	Rigid plate fixation	Cast, IM nail
Healing mechanism	Cutting cones	Callus + remodeling

Q4. Stages/phases of secondary fracture healing (with histology).

1. *Inflammatory phase (days 1–7)*:
    - *Histology*: Hematoma at fracture site with fibrin meshwork.
    - *Cells*: Neutrophils → macrophages → mesenchymal stem cells.
    - *Cytokines*: IL-1, IL-6, TNF-α promote cell recruitment.
    - *Purpose*: Initiates angiogenesis and matrix deposition.
2. *Soft callus formation (weeks 1–3)*:
    - *Histology*: Granulation tissue → fibrocartilaginous callus.
    - *Cells*: Fibroblasts, chondroblasts.
    - *Key process*: Chondrogenesis and early collagen type II deposition.
3. *Hard callus formation (weeks 3–6)*:
    - *Histology*: Woven bone replaces cartilage.
    - *Cells*: Osteoblasts deposit osteoid, which mineralizes.
    - *Key process*: Endochondral ossification.
4. *Remodeling phase (months to years)*:
    - *Histology*: Replacement of woven bone with lamellar bone.
    - *Cells*: Coordinated action of osteoclasts (resorption) and osteoblasts (formation).
    - *Purpose*: Restoration of bone structure along lines of mechanical stress (Wolff's law).

FLOWCHART: Phases of fracture healing

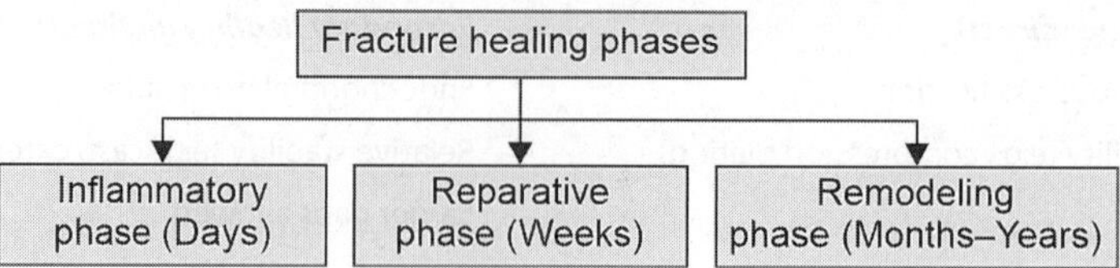

Q5. Factors affecting fracture healing.

1. *Biological factors*:
    - *Age*: Slower healing in the elderly
    - *Nutrition*: Calcium, vitamin D, and protein are essential
    - *Osteogenic potential*: Affected in osteoporosis
2. *Mechanical factors*:
    - *Stability*: Excess motion causes delayed healing or non-union
    - *Gap size*: Larger gaps reduce direct healing
3. *Local factors*:
    - *Blood supply*: Crucial for healing
    - *Infection*: Disrupts normal repair
    - *Soft tissue damage*: Impairs vascularity
4. *Systemic factors*:
    - *Medications*: NSAIDs, steroids delay healing
    - *Diseases*: Diabetes, rheumatoid arthritis
    - *Smoking and alcohol*: Reduce blood flow and cell activity
5. *Patient-related factors*:
    - Genetics
    - Compliance with treatment
    - Immune status

Summary Table

Factor type	*Examples*
Biological	Age, nutrition, stem cell health
Mechanical	Stability, load-sharing
Local	Blood supply, infection
Systemic	Drugs, comorbidities
Patient	

FLOWCHART: Factors influencing bone healing

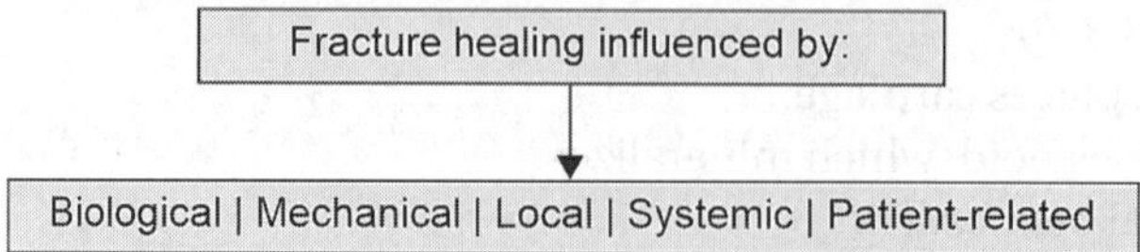

Bonus Quick Tip

Mnemonic for secondary healing stages: "*I*nflame, *S*often, *H*arden, *R*eshape" (Inflammation → Soft callus → Hard callus → Remodeling)

Q6. Molecular and cellular mechanisms in fracture repair.

1. *Inflammatory phase*:
    - **Hematoma** forms → release of cytokines **(IL-1, IL-6, TNF-α)**
    - **Recruitment of immune cells** and **MSCs**
    - **VEGF** initiates **angiogenesis**
2. *Repair phase*:
    - MSCs differentiate into:
        - **Chondroblasts** → soft callus
        - **Osteoblasts** → hard callus
    - **Endochondral ossification** transitions cartilage to woven bone
    - **BMPs, Wnt/β-catenin, TGF-β** pathways regulate osteogenesis
3. *Remodeling phase*:
    - **Woven bone** replaced by **lamellar bone**
    - Involves **osteoclast-mediated resorption** and **osteoblast-driven formation**
    - Bone architecture and strength restored

Key Molecules and Their Roles

Molecule/Factor	*Function*
BMP-2, BMP-7	Osteogenic differentiation
VEGF	Angiogenesis
Wnt/β-catenin	Promotes osteoblast proliferation
Runx2, Osterix	Osteoblast gene transcription
RANKL/OPG	Regulate osteoclastogenesis

FLOWCHART: Fracture repair mechanisms

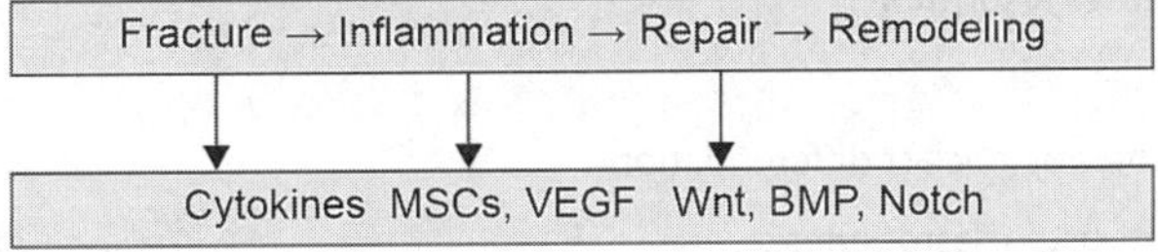

Q7. Role of angiogenesis in bone healing.

FLOWCHART: Angiogenesis in bone repair

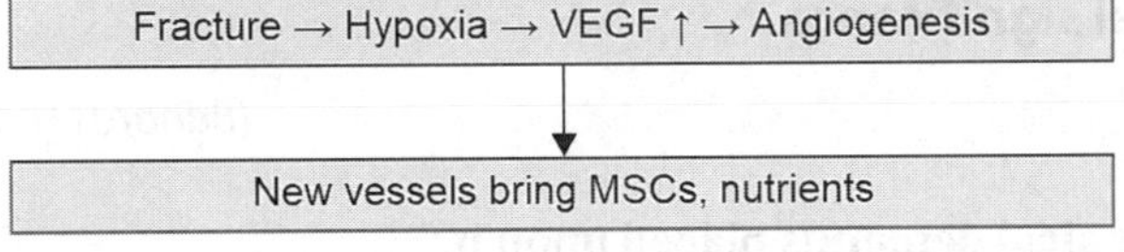

Importance of Angiogenesis

- **New blood vessels** are essential for:
    - Delivering **oxygen, nutrients**, and **progenitor cells**
    - Removing **waste products**
- Required for **cartilage resorption** and **bone formation** in callus

Key Mediators

- *Vascular endothelial growth factor (VEGF)*: Critical for vessel formation
- *Fibroblast growth factor 2 (FGF-2)*: Enhances endothelial proliferation
- *PDGF, angiopoietin*: Support vessel stability

Clinical Relevance

- Impaired angiogenesis (e.g., **diabetes, smoking, radiation**) delays healing
- Promoting angiogenesis improves **non-union** management

Q8. Describe bone remodeling and its regulation.

(NEIGRIHMS Shillong 2023)

Definition

Bone remodeling is a **lifelong, dynamic process** where mature bone tissue is **resorbed** and **new bone tissue** is formed, maintaining skeletal strength and mineral homeostasis.

Phases of Bone Remodeling

1. *Activation*: Pre-osteoclasts are recruited and differentiate into mature osteoclasts.
2. *Resorption*: Osteoclasts attach to bone surface → create sealed resorption pits (Howship's lacunae) → secrete acids and proteases to dissolve mineral and matrix.
3. *Reversal*: Mononuclear cells prepare the surface for new bone deposition.
4. *Formation*: Osteoblasts synthesize new osteoid (organic matrix) → mineralizes into new bone.
5. *Quiescence*: Bone surface becomes inactive and lined by bone lining cells.

Regulation of Bone Remodeling

Regulator	***Effect***	***Mechanism***
Mechanical stress	Stimulates bone formation	Via mechanosensing by osteocytes
Hormones		
• Parathyroid hormone (PTH)	Stimulates resorption (continuous); anabolic effect (intermittent)	Activates osteoblasts/osteoclasts
• Calcitonin	Inhibits osteoclasts	Direct inhibition
• Estrogen	Decreases resorption	Reduces osteoclast lifespan
Cytokines		
• RANKL	Promotes osteoclast differentiation	RANK-RANKL-OPG system
• Osteoprotegerin (OPG)	Inhibits osteoclastogenesis	Acts as decoy receptor
Local factors	BMPs, TGF-β stimulate osteoblast differentiation	Growth factor-mediated

Clinical Correlation

Osteoporosis results from imbalance—increased resorption or decreased formation.

Q9. Wolff's law and clinical significance.

[Banaras Hindu University (BHU) Varanasi 2024]

Wolff's Law

"Bone adapts itself to the mechanical demands placed upon it."

- Bone deposition occurs where stress is high.
- Bone resorption occurs where stress is low.
- Remodeling aligns trabeculae along lines of mechanical stress.

Mechanism

- **Osteocytes** act as mechanosensors.
- Mechanical load triggers biochemical signals (e.g., prostaglandins, nitric oxide).
- Stimulates osteoblast activity and suppresses osteoclasts in loaded regions.

Clinical Significance

Application	Example
Fracture healing	Early weight bearing enhances callus maturation (secondary healing)
Orthopedic implants	Stress shielding leads to bone resorption around prosthesis (e.g., hip arthroplasty)
Orthodontics	Tooth movement utilizes pressure-tension response (bone resorption/compression side, formation/tension side)
Physical therapy	Controlled mechanical loading (e.g., after ACL surgery) improves bone quality
Bone atrophy	Immobilization or microgravity (astronauts) causes bone loss

Q10. Explain the role of osteoblasts, osteoclasts, and osteocytes in bone remodeling.

Osteoblasts

- Derived from **mesenchymal stem cells**
- *Responsible for*:
    - Synthesis of **osteoid (type I collagen + proteins)**
    - **Mineralization** of matrix
- Secrete **RANKL**, which activates osteoclasts
- Some osteoblasts become **osteocytes** or **bone lining cells**

Osteoclasts

- Multinucleated cells from **monocyte-macrophage lineage**
- *Function*: **Resorb bone** via release of **acid and proteolytic enzymes**
- Activated by **RANKL**, inhibited by **osteoprotegerin (OPG)**
- Create **resorption pits (Howship's lacunae)**

Osteocytes

- Mature osteoblasts embedded in mineralized bone
- Located in **lacunae**, connected via **canaliculi**
- *Act as mechanosensors*: Detect mechanical load
- Regulate remodeling via **sclerostin**, which inhibits osteoblast activity

FLOWCHART: Roles of bone cells in remodeling

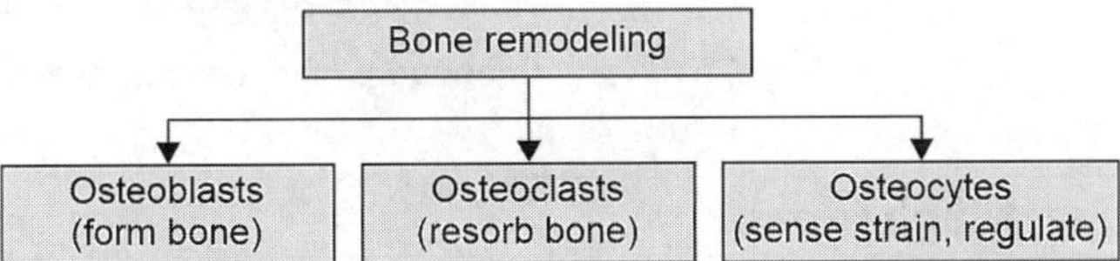

Q11. Cartilage biology and degeneration.

Structure of Articular Cartilage

Articular cartilage is a specialized **hyaline cartilage** that covers joint surfaces, providing **smooth, frictionless movement** and **shock absorption**.

Histological Zones (Superficial to Deep)

Zone	Features	Function
Superficial (tangential) zone	Flattened chondrocytes; collagen fibers parallel to surface	Resists shear stress
Middle (transitional) zone	Round chondrocytes; randomly oriented collagen fibers	Absorbs compressive forces

Continued

Continued

Zone	Features	Function
Deep (radial) zone	Columns of chondrocytes; collagen fibers perpendicular to surface	Resists compressive loads
Calcified zone	Mineralized matrix; tidemark separates it from deep zone	Anchors cartilage to subchondral bone

Matrix Composition

- *Collagen (mainly type II)*: ~60–70% of dry weight
- *Proteoglycans (aggrecan)*: Contribute to compressive resistance
- *Water*: ~70–80% of wet weight (critical for load-bearing)
- *Other molecules*: For example, lubricin (surface lubrication)

Nutrition of Articular Cartilage

- **Avascular** → receives nutrients via **diffusion** from:
  - Synovial fluid
  - Subchondral bone (minimal contribution in adults)
- Movement enhances fluid diffusion → "**pumping mechanism**" through load/unload cycles.

Healing of Articular Cartilage

- *Intrinsic healing capacity*:
  - Very **limited** due to:
    - Lack of blood vessels
    - Sparse chondrocyte proliferation
    - Poor migration of repair cells
- **Defects limited to cartilage** → poor healing.
- **Full-thickness defects** reaching subchondral bone → better healing (fibrocartilage formation, not hyaline cartilage).

Q12. Why cartilage healing is poor?

Factor	Reason
Avascularity	No direct blood supply to deliver repair cells
Low cell density	Chondrocytes are sparse and poorly mitotic
Matrix complexity	Dense extracellular matrix hinders cell migration
Lack of progenitor cells	Limited stem cell reservoirs within cartilage
Mechanical stress	Continuous load hampers healing

Q13. Methods to enhance cartilage repair.

Method	Principle
Microfracture	Perforate subchondral bone to stimulate marrow stem cells
Osteochondral autograft/allograft transplantation (OATS)	Transfer healthy cartilage-bone plugs
Autologous chondrocyte implantation (ACI)	Harvest, culture, and reimplant chondrocytes
Matrix-assisted chondrocyte implantation (MACI)	Scaffold-based cell delivery
Growth factors (e.g., BMPs, TGF-β)	Stimulate chondrogenesis
Gene therapy	Experimental—introduce genes promoting matrix production

Q14. Chondrocytes and their metabolic activity.

Chondrocytes

- Sole cell type in cartilage
- Originate from **mesenchymal stem cells**
- Maintain ECM by balancing **synthesis and degradation**

Metabolic Activity

- *Anabolic*: Synthesis of **type II collagen, proteoglycans**
- *Catabolic*: Express **MMPs, aggrecanases** under stress/inflammation
- *Sensitive to*:
    - Mechanical stimuli
    - Hypoxia
    - Cytokines (e.g., IL-1, TNF-α)

Note: Cartilage is avascular, so chondrocytes rely on diffusion and operate in low oxygen environments using anaerobic metabolism.

Q15. Role of cytokines and inflammatory mediators in cartilage degeneration.

Key Cytokines

- **IL-1β, TNF-α, IL-6**
- Stimulate **MMPs, NO, PGE2**
- Inhibit synthesis of **proteoglycans** and **collagen**

Pathogenic Mechanism

1. Cytokine release by damaged chondrocytes or synovium
2. ↑ Catabolic enzyme activity → ECM breakdown
3. ↓ ECM synthesis
4. Chondrocyte apoptosis → progression of OA

Therapeutic Insight

Biologic agents targeting TNF-α and IL-1 are under evaluation in OA management

Q16. Synovial fluid—composition and function.

- *Composition*: Hyaluronic acid, lubricin, albumin, electrolytes
- *Function*:
    - Lubrication (boundary and fluid-film)
    - Nutrient supply to avascular cartilage
    - Shock absorption

Synovium: Histology and Function

- *Layers*: Intimal (type A/B synoviocytes), subintimal (fibrovascular tissue)
- *Function*:
    - Produces synovial fluid
    - Regulates the intra-articular environment

Q17. Biochemical composition of synovial fluid and joint lubrication.

(KMC Manipal Karnataka 2021)

Composition

- **Ultrafiltrate of plasma** + secretions from synoviocytes
- *Key components*:
    - *Hyaluronic acid (HA)*: Viscosity, lubrication
    - *Lubricin*: Boundary lubrication
    - **Water, glucose, electrolytes**
    - *Enzymes*: MMPs, proteases

Role in Lubrication

- **Hydrodynamic lubrication** during movement (HA dominant)
- **Boundary lubrication** under compression (Lubricin dominant)
- Reduces **friction** and **wear** at cartilage surfaces

Q18. Role of lubricin in joint mechanics.

Lubricin (PRG4)

- *A glycoprotein secreted by*:
  - Synoviocytes
  - Superficial zone chondrocytes

Functions

- **Boundary lubrication** between articular surfaces
- Reduces **friction** and **adhesion**
- Protects cartilage from **wear-induced damage**
- Contributes to **joint homeostasis**

Deficiency

Leads to **cartilage erosion**, as seen in **CACP (camptodactyly-arthropathy-coxa vara-pericarditis) syndrome**

Q19. Effects of mechanical loading on articular cartilage health.

Positive Effects (Physiological Loading)

- Stimulates chondrocyte activity and ECM synthesis
- Enhances **diffusion of nutrients**
- Maintains cartilage thickness and integrity

Negative Effects (Abnormal Loading)

- Overloading → chondrocyte apoptosis
- **Underloading** → ECM thinning
- **Repetitive trauma** → microdamage, degeneration
- Leads to **OA-like changes** over time

Summary Table

Loading type	*Effect on cartilage*
Physiological	Promotes ECM synthesis, healthy cartilage
Excessive	Cell death, degeneration
No loading	Atrophy, ECM loss

Q20. Describe tendon and ligament healing.

Phases of Tendon Healing — Biological Processes

Healing of tendons proceeds through **three overlapping phases**

Phase	*Timeline*	*Biological process*
1. Inflammatory phase	0–7 days	• Hematoma forms • Neutrophils, macrophages infiltrate • Cytokine release (IL-1, TNF-α) → recruit fibroblasts

Continued

Continued

Phase	Timeline	Biological process
2. Proliferative (repair) phase	1–6 weeks	• Fibroblasts produce type III collagen • Angiogenesis occurs • Granulation tissue bridges the gap
3. Remodeling (maturation) phase	6 weeks to months	• Type III collagen is replaced by type I collagen • Collagen fibers align along the stress lines • Gradual increase in tensile strength

Key Points for Exams

- Early tendon healing is **scar-mediated** rather than regeneration.
- **Intrinsic healing** (from tendon cells) and **extrinsic healing** (from surrounding sheath/blood supply) both contribute.

Q21. Differences between tendon and ligament healing.

Feature	Tendon healing	Ligament healing
Vascularity	Poorer (especially flexor tendons)	Better (especially extra-articular ligaments)
Cell type	Tenocytes	Fibroblasts
Mechanical demands	High tensile load, gliding motion needed	Stability to joints against complex loads
Healing outcome	Adhesions common (especially in zone II flexor tendons)	Often heals with some laxity and scar formation
Intrinsic versus extrinsic healing	More dependent on extrinsic mechanisms early	Intrinsic healing more dominant in some ligaments
Surgical considerations	Early passive mobilization improves healing	Often immobilized initially; progressive loading later

Q22. Enhancement techniques in tendon repair.

Several methods are being explored to **optimize tendon healing** and minimize complications like adhesions:

Technique	Mechanism
Growth factors (e.g., PDGF, TGF-β, IGF-1)	Stimulate fibroblast proliferation and collagen synthesis
Gene therapy	Introduction of genes coding for anabolic factors (e.g., VEGF, BMPs)
Platelet-rich plasma (PRP)	Concentrated growth factors to enhance healing response
Scaffolds/Biomaterials	Provide a matrix for cell ingrowth and guide organized healing
Cell-based therapies (e.g., stem cells)	Deliver progenitor cells to promote regenerative healing rather than scar formation
Mechanical loading (rehabilitation protocols)	Early controlled mobilization aligns collagen fibers and strengthens repair

Important for Exams

- PRP and TGF-β are heavily studied for tendon repair enhancement.
- Too early or too aggressive loading → risk of rerupture.

Clinical Relevance Examples

- *Flexor tendon repair (Zone II)*: Early passive motion protocols (e.g., Kleinert, Duran) are critical.
- *ACL reconstruction*: Graft (ligament) healing involves a "ligamentization" process over months.
- *Rotator cuff tears*: PRP injections explored as adjuncts to surgical repair.

Quick Mnemonics

- *Tendon healing phases*: **"I PRomise to Remodel"**
  - **I**nflammatory → **P**roliferative → **R**emodeling

- *Growth factors for tendon healing*: "**PIG-T**"
  - **P**DGF, **I**GF-1, **G**F, **T**GF-β

Q23. Molecular basis of tendon healing.

Phases and Molecular Events

- *Inflammatory phase*:
  - ↑ IL-1, TNF-α, TGF-β
  - Immune cell infiltration
- *Proliferative phase*:
  - Fibroblast proliferation
  - Collagen type III deposition
- *Remodeling phase*:
  - Collagen III → Collagen I
  - Matrix reorganization

Key Molecules

- **TGF-β, PDGF, VEGF, FGF**
- Regulate fibroblast activity, angiogenesis, ECM synthesis

Q24. Phases of tendon healing and influencing factors.

Phases of Tendon Healing

- *Inflammatory (0–7 days)*
  - Hematoma, inflammatory cytokines
- *Proliferative (1–3 weeks)*
  - Fibroblasts deposit type III collagen
- *Remodeling (weeks to months)*
  - Gradual collagen I replacement
  - Realignment along stress lines

Factors Affecting Healing

- *Biological*: Age, nutrition, comorbidities
- *Mechanical*: Immobilization versus early loading
- *Surgical technique*: Minimal trauma improves outcomes
- *Systemic*: Diabetes, smoking, NSAIDs delay healing

Q25. Role of growth factors in tendon and ligament healing.

Key Growth Factors

Factor	*Role*
TGF-β	Stimulates fibroblast proliferation, ECM synthesis
PDGF	Cell recruitment, angiogenesis
FGF	Enhances collagen synthesis
IGF-1	Promotes matrix production and remodeling
VEGF	Induces angiogenesis

Functions

- Stimulate **cell proliferation**, **collagen synthesis**, and **angiogenesis**
- Modulate inflammation
- Can be delivered via **biologics, scaffolds, or PRP**

Muscle

Q26. Structure and types of muscle and their physiology.

- *Types*:
  - Skeletal: Striated, voluntary
  - Cardiac: Striated, involuntary, intercalated discs
  - Smooth: Non-striated, involuntary
- *Structure*: Myofibrils → Sarcomeres → Actin and Myosin filaments

Excitation-contraction Coupling
- Nerve impulse → ACh release → Depolarizes sarcolemma
- T-tubules transmit signal → Ca^{2+} release from sarcoplasmic reticulum
- Ca^{2+} binds troponin → exposes actin
- Myosin cross-bridges attach → contraction

Q27. Muscle healing and response to injury.

- *Phases*:
  - Inflammatory
  - Regeneration (satellite cells)
  - Remodeling
- Scar tissue impairs contractility; early mobilization aids healing

Q28. Myopathies—classification and diagnosis.

Type	*Examples*	*Diagnosis*
Congenital	Duchenne, Becker	Genetic testing, EMG, biopsy
Inflammatory	Polymyositis, dermatomyositis	CK levels, biopsy, EMG
Metabolic	McArdle's, mitochondrial myopathies	Enzyme assay, muscle biopsy

Q29. Histology and physiology of skeletal muscle.

Histology
- **Multinucleated, striated fibers** arranged in bundles (fascicles)
- Surrounded by:
  - Endomysium—around individual fibers
  - Perimysium—around fascicles
  - Epimysium—around entire muscle
- Each fiber contains **myofibrils**, made of:
  - **Actin (thin)** and **myosin (thick)** filaments
  - Sarcomere = Contractile unit (Z-line to Z-line)

Physiology
- Stimulated by **α-motor neurons**
- **Depolarization** triggers calcium release from the **sarcoplasmic reticulum**
- ATP-dependent **cross-bridge cycling** enables contraction
- Muscle returns to the resting state via **calcium reuptake**

Q30. Sliding filament theory of muscle contraction.

Key Points

- **Actin and myosin** slide past each other → **sarcomere shortens**
- ATP is required for:
  - Cross-bridge detachment
  - Re-cocking the myosin head
- *Relaxation*: Ca^{2+} reabsorbed into SR → Tropomyosin blocks myosin-binding sites

FLOWCHART: Mechanism

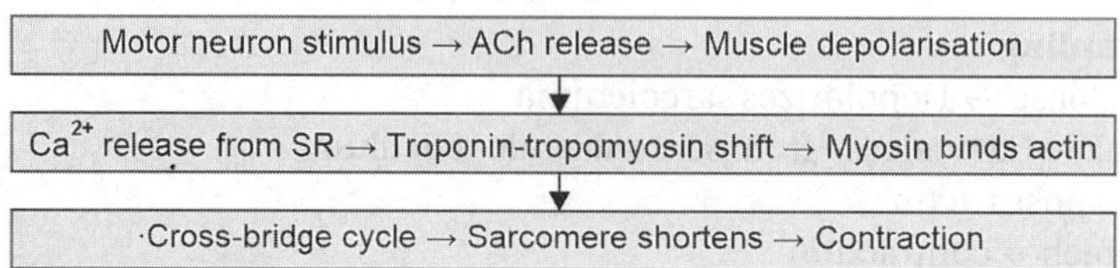

Q31. Classification and characteristics of muscle fiber types.

Fiber type	*Type I (slow twitch)*	*Type IIa (fast oxidative)*	*Type IIb (fast glycolytic)*
Contraction	Slow	Intermediate	Fast
Fatigue	Resistant	Moderately resistant	Rapid fatigue
Metabolism	Oxidative (aerobic)	Mixed	Glycolytic (anaerobic)
Myoglobin	High	Moderate	Low
Function	Postural/Endurance	Mixed activity	Power/Sprint

Q32. Muscle atrophy and hypertrophy.

Atrophy

- Reduction in muscle **mass and strength**
- *Causes*:
  - Disuse, immobilization
  - Denervation
  - Cachexia, aging
- *Molecular basis*:
  - ↑ **Myostatin, ubiquitin-proteasome** pathway
  - ↓ IGF-1 signaling

Hypertrophy

- Increase in **fiber size**, not number
- Stimulated by **mechanical overload** and **resistance training**
- *Mediated by*:
- ↑ **IGF-1/PI3K/Akt pathway**
- Satellite cell activation and protein synthesis

Q33. Effect of immobilization on muscle and tendon physiology.

(Dr DY Patil Vidyapeeth Pune 2016)

On Muscle

- Rapid **atrophy** (within days)
- ↓ protein synthesis, ↑ proteolysis

- Fiber-type shift: **Type I → Type II**
- ↓ Neuromuscular efficiency

On Tendon
- ↓ Collagen synthesis and organization
- Disrupted collagen fibril alignment
- ↓ Tensile strength and stiffness
- Delayed remodeling

Clinical Insight
Early controlled mobilization improves healing and function

Q34. Structure and function of peripheral nerves.

Structure
- Composed of **axons, Schwann cells, connective tissue layers**:
  - **Endoneurium**—around individual axons
  - **Perineurium**—surrounds fascicles
  - **Epineurium**—outermost layer, encloses entire nerve
- **Myelinated** and **unmyelinated** fibers

Function
- *Motor*: Conduct impulses to muscles
- *Sensory*: Relay input from skin, joints
- *Autonomic*: Regulate glands, smooth muscle

Summary Table

Component	*Function*
Axons	Conduct electrical impulses
Schwann cells	Myelinate axons, support regeneration
CT layers	Mechanical support, protect fascicles

Q35. Process of wallerian degeneration.

FLOWCHART: Wallerian degeneration

Nerve injury → Distal axon degeneration → Myelin clearance → Schwann cell activation

↓

Macrophage infiltration → Regeneration environment established

Key Events
- **Axonal and myelin degeneration** distal to injury
- **Schwann cells dedifferentiate**, proliferate
- **Macrophages** clear debris
- **Bands of Büngner** guide axon regrowth
- **Axon sprouting** from the proximal stump occurs

Q36. Nerve and neuromuscular physiology.

Classification of Nerve Injuries
- *Seddon*:
  - Neuropraxia (conduction block)
  - Axonotmesis (axon damage, intact sheath)
  - Neurotmesis (complete transection)
- *Sunderland*: 5-grade classification (I = neuropraxia, V = complete transection)

Reflex Arc and Neuromuscular Transmission

- *Reflex arc*: Receptor → Afferent nerve → Integration center → Efferent nerve → Effector
- *Neuromuscular transmission*: ACh release → binds receptors → Na^+ influx → muscle action potential

Q37. Explain the process of endochondral and intramembranous ossification.

(KEM Hospital Mumbai Maharashtra 2022)

A. Endochondral Ossification

- *Definition*: Formation of bone through a cartilage intermediate. Occurs in long bones (femur, tibia).
- *Steps*:
  1. **Mesenchymal condensation** → differentiation into **chondrocytes**
  2. Cartilage model formation
  3. **Chondrocyte hypertrophy**, matrix calcification, and apoptosis
  4. **Vascular invasion** brings osteoprogenitor cells
  5. **Primary ossification center** forms in diaphysis
  6. **Secondary ossification centers** appear in epiphyses
  7. **Growth plate** (physis) remains between epiphysis and diaphysis

B. Intramembranous Ossification

- *Definition*: Direct bone formation without a cartilage model. Occurs in flat bones (skull, clavicle).
- *Steps*:
  1. **Mesenchymal cells** differentiate directly into **osteoblasts**
  2. Osteoblasts secrete **osteoid**, which mineralizes
  3. Formation of **woven bone**
  4. Remodeling into **lamellar bone**

Key Differences

Feature	*Endochondral*	*Intramembranous*
Template	Cartilage	None
Bone type	Long bones	Flat bones
Cell transition	MSC → Chondrocytes → Osteoblasts	MSC → Osteoblasts
Ossification centers	Primary and secondary	No distinct centers

FLOWCHART: Types of ossification

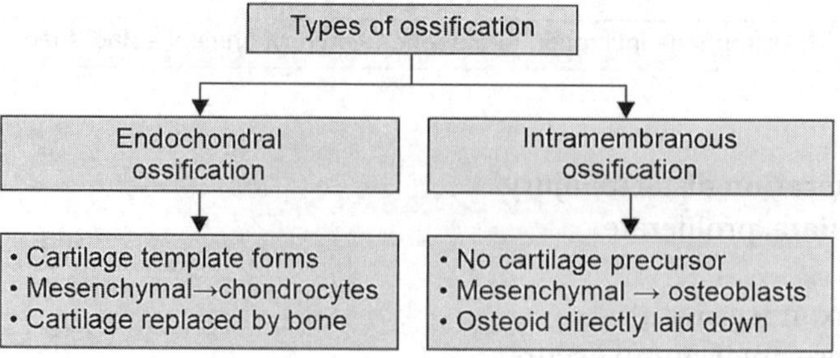

Q38. Collagen in Orthopedics.

Definition

Primary structural protein in connective tissues.

Types and Distribution

Type	Location	Role
I	Bone, tendon, ligament	Tensile strength
II	Articular cartilage	Resistance to compression
III	Skin, vessels (reticular fibers)	Wound healing, flexibility
IV	Basement membrane	Filtration and support

Role in Healing

- Scaffold for cell migration
- Stimulates matrix production
- Forms granulation tissue in early repair

Clinical Uses

- Collagen sheets in burns
- Bone graft composites
- Injectable collagen in regenerative therapy

Role of Collagen and Elastin

- *Collagen*: Type I (tendon/ligament), type II (cartilage)
- Provides tensile strength
- *Elastin*: Elastic recoil (ligaments like ligamentum flavum)

Q39. Bone turnover markers (BTMs) and clinical utility.

Types

1. *Bone formation markers*:
   - Serum bone-specific alkaline phosphatase (BSAP)
   - Osteocalcin
   - Procollagen Type I N-terminal propeptide (P1NP)
2. *Bone resorption markers*:
   - C-terminal telopeptide of type I collagen (CTX)
   - N-terminal telopeptide (NTX)
   - Tartrate-resistant acid phosphatase (TRAP)

Clinical Utility of Bone Turnover Markers

Application	Details
Diagnosis	Help identify metabolic bone diseases (e.g., osteoporosis, Paget's disease)
Monitoring therapy	Track response to anti-resorptive therapy (e.g., bisphosphonates) earlier than BMD changes
Predicting fracture risk	High turnover indicates higher future fracture risk
Research	Useful in clinical trials for studying bone disease progression or drug efficacy

Important Note

BTMs are affected by circadian rhythm, food intake, renal function—hence standardization of sampling (usually morning fasting sample) is crucial.

Quick Revision Mnemonics

- *BTMs formation*: "**BOP**" → Bone-specific ALP, Osteocalcin, P1NP.
- *BTMS resorption*: "**CAT**" → CTX, NTX, TRAP.

Q40. Short note—role of bone morphogenetic proteins (BMPs) in bone healing.

(Jammu University 2023)

Definition

BMPs are **growth factors** belonging to the **TGF-β superfamily**, crucial in bone formation and repair.

Functions in Bone Healing

- **Induce mesenchymal stem cells (MSCs)** to differentiate into **osteoblasts** and **chondroblasts**
- Promote **osteogenesis and chondrogenesis**
- Enhance **callus formation and mineralization**
- Stimulate **angiogenesis**

Key BMPs in Clinical Use

- *BMP-2 and BMP-7 (OP-1)*:
  - Used in **spinal fusions, non-unions**, and **bone graft substitutes**
  - Delivered via **collagen carriers or scaffolds**

Mechanism of Action

BMPs bind to specific receptors → activate **SMAD signaling pathway** → upregulate transcription factors like **Runx2** and **Osterix**

Q41. Short note: Role of mesenchymal stem cells (MSCs) in bone regeneration.

Definition

MSCs are **multipotent stromal cells** found in bone marrow, periosteum, adipose tissue, and synovium. They can differentiate into bone, cartilage, muscle, and fat cells.

Role in Bone Regeneration

- Differentiate into **osteoblasts and chondrocytes**
- *Contribute to*:
  - Callus formation
  - Bone remodeling
  - **Tissue engineering** and **scaffold-based bone grafts**
- Modulate immune response and secrete **growth factors** (VEGF, BMPs)

Mechanism

- Guided by local microenvironment and signaling molecules:
  - **BMPs, TGF-β, FGF**, and **Wnt pathway**
- Aid in both **endochondral and intramembranous** ossification

Clinical Use

- *MSCs are used in*:
  - Non-union fractures
  - Osteonecrosis
  - Bone graft substitutes

Q42. Force transmission in weight-bearing joints.

(Kashmir University 2024)

Principles

- Load transferred from **joint surfaces to bones** via:
  - Articular cartilage
  - Subchondral bone
  - Ligaments and muscles

Examples

- *Hip*: Force transmitted from femoral head → acetabulum → pelvis
- *Knee*: Femoral condyles → menisci → tibial plateau

Factors Influencing Transmission

- **Alignment**, **joint congruity**, **muscle force vectors**, and **surface area**

Q43. Stress-strain curve.

- *Elastic region*: Bone returns to shape
- *Yield point*: Start of plastic deformation
- *Ultimate strength*: Max load
- *Failure point*: Fracture
- *Significance*: Predicts behavior under load

Q44. Mechanical properties of bone and implants.

Property	*Bone*	*Implants (Steel/Titanium)*
Strength	Strong in compression	High tensile strength
Elastic modulus	Lower (stress shielding risk)	Higher (especially stainless steel)
Fatigue failure	Possible under repeated load	Important for implant longevity

Q45. Static versus dynamic stabilizers of joints.

Type	*Examples*	*Function*
Static stabilizers	Capsule, labrum, ligaments	Maintain passive stability
Dynamic stabilizers	Muscles, tendons	Provide active joint control

CHAPTER 2

Investigations and Diagnosis in Orthopedics

Vineet Aggarwal, Barkat Anwar Shah, Varun Gupta

Clinical Evaluation in Orthopedics

Q1. Principles and systematic approach to clinical examination in orthopedics.

(Asked in AIIMS Delhi 2021, MUHS Maharashtra 2022)

Introduction

Clinical evaluation is the cornerstone for diagnosis and management in Orthopedics. A systematic and reproducible method ensures accurate assessment, minimizes missed findings, and aids communication among healthcare professionals.

Principles of Orthopedic Examination

- *Look*: Inspection of deformity, swelling, scars, muscle wasting, discoloration.
- *Feel*: Palpation for tenderness, warmth, crepitus, abnormal movement.
- *Move*: Assessment of range of motion (ROM) – active and passive.
- *Measure*: Limb length discrepancy, muscle girth, joint angles.
- *Function*: Functional tests specific to joints or limbs.
- *Special tests*: Joint-specific or condition-specific tests to refine diagnosis.
- *Neurological examination*: Sensory, motor, reflex assessments when indicated.
- *Vascular examination*: Pulses, capillary refill, limb perfusion.

Systematic Approach

1. *History taking*:
   - Chief complaint
   - History of presenting illness
   - Past medical, surgical, trauma history
   - Family and occupational history
2. *General examination:*
   - Vital signs
   - Examination for systemic illness (e.g., rheumatoid arthritis)
3. *Local examination*:
   - Inspection, palpation, movement, special tests.
   - Examination above and below the involved joint.
4. *Neurovascular status*:
   - Always assess and document.

Q2. Outline a general orthopedic case history and examination format.

(Asked in JIPMER Puducherry 2022)

Orthopedic Case History Format

- *Demographic data*: Name, age, sex, occupation, hand dominance.
- *Chief complaints*: Pain, swelling, deformity, weakness, instability, limping.
- *History of present illness*:
  - Onset (acute, chronic)
  - Duration
  - Progression
  - Relieving/aggravating factors
- *Past history*:
  - Similar complaints in past
  - Previous surgeries, trauma, infections
- *Personal history*: Smoking, alcohol, physical activity level
- *Family history*: Genetic diseases (e.g., osteogenesis imperfecta)
- *Socioeconomic history*: Work type (labor-intensive vs. desk job)

Orthopedic Examination Format

- *General physical examination*: Vital signs, anemia, jaundice, clubbing, lymphadenopathy.
- *Local examination*:
  - *Inspection*: Deformity, swelling, skin changes.
  - *Palpation*: Tenderness, temperature, anatomical landmarks.
  - *Range of motion (ROM)*: Active, passive.
  - *Measurement*:
    - Limb length
    - Muscle bulk
    - Joint angles
  - *Special tests*: Specific to suspected pathology.
  - *Neurovascular examination*: Sensory, motor, vascular status.

Q3. Principles and systematic approach to clinical examination.

Goals of Clinical Evaluation

- Identify patient problems.
- Localize anatomical pathology.
- Determine severity and functional impairment.
- Formulate differential diagnoses.

Steps (Always Systematic)

Step	***Key points***
History	Chief complaint, HOPI (history of present illness), past history, personal history, family history
Inspection	Look for deformities, swelling, scars, muscle wasting, skin changes
Palpation	Tenderness, warmth, gap, crepitus, fluctuance
Range of motion (ROM)	Active and passive movements; compare bilaterally
Special tests	Joint-specific or pathology-specific tests
Neurovascular assessment	Sensation, motor power, pulses
Measurement	Limb length discrepancy, girth, alignment
Functional evaluation	Gait, ability to perform daily activities

Golden Rule for Exams: "Look, Feel, Move, Measure, Special Tests"

Mnemonic: "HIP ROMeS"
- *H*istory
- *I*nspection
- *P*alpation
- *R*ange of motion
- *M*easurements
- *S*pecial tests

Q4. Approach to a patient with an undiagnosed musculoskeletal disorder.

History
- Onset, duration, and progression
- Pain characteristics (location, severity, radiation)
- Associated symptoms (fever, weight loss, morning stiffness)
- Trauma history, occupation, systemic illness, family history

Physical Examination
- Inspection, palpation, ROM
- Neurological and vascular status
- Gait and posture analysis

Investigations
- *Blood tests*: CBC, ESR, CRP, RA factor, HLA-B27, uric acid
- *Imaging*: X-ray, MRI, CT
- *Special tests*: Bone scan, synovial fluid analysis, biopsy

Referral

Rheumatology, oncology, infectious disease as needed

Q5. Role of functional assessment in orthopedic patients.

Purpose

Assess disability, monitor progress, plan rehabilitation

Tools Used
- *Scores*: Harris hip score, DASH (Disabilities of Arm, Shoulder, Hand), WOMAC for knee
- **Gait analysis**
- **Timed up and go test**, 6-minute walk test

Benefits
- Quantifies functional limitations
- Helps in treatment planning and outcome evaluation

Basic Radiology

Q6. Systematic approach to interpretation of orthopedic X-rays.

(Asked in PGI Chandigarh 2021, TNMGR Chennai 2021)

Introduction

X-ray interpretation in Orthopedics requires a **structured and methodical approach** to avoid missing injuries and to ensure accurate diagnosis.

Systematic Steps for Interpretation

1. *Check patient details*: Name, age, side (right/left), date, view (AP, lateral, oblique).
2. *Assess image quality*: Adequate exposure, correct positioning, appropriate views.
3. *General survey*:
   - Compare with opposite limb if available.
   - Look for obvious fractures, deformities, or dislocations.
4. *Bone examination*:
   - *Continuity*: Breaks, cracks, cortical disruption.
   - *Density*: Osteopenia, sclerosis.
   - *Alignment*: Anatomical relationship between bones.
5. *Joint assessment*:
   - *Joint spaces*: Narrowing, widening.
   - *Articular surface*: Smoothness, step-offs, irregularities.
   - Subluxation or dislocation.
6. *Soft tissue evaluation*: Swelling, fat pad signs, gas (open fractures), foreign bodies.
7. *Special attention*:
   - Growth plates in children (Salter–Harris injuries).
   - Presence of implants or previous surgeries.

Mnemonic: "ABCS"

- *A*: Alignment
- *B*: Bone
- *C*: Cartilage (joint space)
- *S*: Soft tissue

Q7. Important radiological signs in fractures and dislocations.

(Asked in MUHS Maharashtra 2023)

Fracture Signs

- *Cortical disruption*: Break in the bony cortex.
- *Lucent lines*: Dark fracture lines in radiographs.
- *Bone angulation*: Abnormal angles at the fracture site.
- *Step deformity*: Bone fragments misaligned.
- *Bone fragmentation*: Comminuted fractures.
- *Periosteal reaction*: Healing or stress fractures.
- *Lipohemarthrosis*: Fat-fluid level in joints (seen in intra-articular fractures like tibial plateau).

Dislocation Signs

- *Loss of joint congruency*: Malalignment of articulating surfaces.
- *Empty socket sign*: Dislocated humeral head (shoulder).
- *Posterior shoulder dislocation*: "Light bulb sign" — rounded appearance of humeral head.
- *Hip dislocation*: Femoral head displaced superiorly (posterior dislocation most common).
- *Ankle dislocation*: Talus out of mortise.

Special Radiological Clues

- *Shenton's line*: Disrupted in hip dislocations or neck of femur fractures.
- *Anterior humeral line*: Not intersecting middle third of capitellum in supracondylar fractures.

Q8. Principles of radiographic imaging in orthopedics.

Basic Principle

- Based on **X-ray attenuation** through tissues of varying density:
  - Dense tissues (bone): **White (radiopaque)**

- Soft tissues: **Gray**
- Air: **Black (radiolucent)**

Key Concepts
- *Two views (orthogonal) are essential*: AP + lateral, **two joints**, one above and one below
- Uses **ionizing radiation**
- *Common uses*: Fracture diagnosis, alignment, implants, arthritis

Limitations
- Poor soft tissue contrast
- Radiation exposure

Q9. Short note on fat pad signs in elbow injuries.

(Asked in JIPMER Puducherry 2022)

Introduction

Fat pad signs are important **indirect indicators** of elbow fractures, especially **occult fractures**.

Normal Anatomy
- Elbow joint has anterior and posterior fat pads.
- In normal X-ray, **anterior fat pad** may be slightly visible; **posterior fat pad** is not visible.

Pathological Fat Pad Signs
1. *Sail sign (anterior fat pad)*:
    - Anterior fat pad becomes **elevated and prominent**.
    - Seen in supracondylar fractures in children.
2. *Posterior fat pad sign*:
    - **Always pathological.**
    - Indicates hemarthrosis due to intra-articular fracture.

Clinical Relevance
- Presence of fat pad sign → Strong suspicion of an underlying fracture even if fracture line not visible.
- *Commonly associated injuries*:
    - *Children*: Supracondylar fractures.
    - *Adults*: Radial head fractures.

Mnemonic to Remember

"Sail flies high (anterior); Posterior is a danger sign!"

Pro Tips for Theory Exam
- Always start short topics like "fat pad sign" with a **brief anatomy** overview.
- **Underline key terms** like *sail sign, posterior fat pad* in your answer sheet.
- If time permits, **draw a small diagram** of the normal versus abnormal fat pad appearance.

Q10. What is digital subtraction angiography (DSA)? What are its indications in orthopedics?

Definition

DSA is an imaging technique used to visualize blood vessels by subtracting pre-contrast ("mask") images from post-contrast images, improving vessel visibility by eliminating surrounding bone and soft tissue details.

Principle
- Based on **contrast-enhanced radiography**
- Utilizes computer algorithms to enhance vascular structures

Indications in Orthopedics
- **Vascular injury assessment** in trauma (e.g., popliteal or brachial artery)
- **Tumor evaluation** (e.g., preoperative embolization in bone tumors like ABC or GCT)
- Planning for **limb salvage surgery**
- Diagnosis of **AV malformations or aneurysms**

Advantages
- High spatial resolution
- Real-time vascular imaging
- Can guide **interventional radiology** procedures

Q11. Role of CT scan in orthopedic trauma.

(Asked in RGUHS Karnataka 2022, MUHS Maharashtra 2022)

Introduction

Computed tomography (CT) provides **cross-sectional imaging** with high resolution of bone structures, aiding in the diagnosis, surgical planning, and assessment of complex fractures.

Role in Orthopedic Trauma
1. *Fracture Evaluation*:
   - Detection of **occult fractures** not seen on X-ray (e.g., scaphoid, tibial plateau).
   - Detailed assessment of **comminuted fractures.**
2. *Preoperative planning*: Helps in understanding **fracture geometry** for surgical fixation (e.g., acetabular fractures, pelvic injuries).
3. *Postoperative assessment*: Evaluation of **implant positioning** and **fracture healing**.
4. *Intra-articular injuries*: Accurate mapping of **articular surface involvement** (e.g., distal radius fractures).
5. *Spinal trauma*: Essential for detecting **vertebral fractures**, canal compromise, and retropulsed fragments.

Special CT Techniques
- *3D reconstruction*: For better visualization of complex fractures.
- *CT angiography*: In vascular injury associated with trauma.

Advantages of CT
- Rapid acquisition.
- Superior bone detail compared to MRI.
- Helps guide surgical decision-making.

Q12. CT Scan in evaluating bone tumors (short note).

Role
- Offers **high-resolution, 3D bone detail**
- *Assesses*:
  - **Cortical destruction**
  - **Matrix mineralization**
  - **Extent of bone involvement**
- Helps guide **biopsy** and plan resection

Advantages
- Fast, widely available
- Better for calcifications than MRI

Q13. Indications of MRI in orthopedics.

(Asked in AIIMS Delhi 2022)

Introduction

Magnetic resonance imaging (MRI) uses **magnetic fields and radiofrequency waves** to produce detailed images of **soft tissues** and **bone marrow** without radiation exposure.

Indications in Orthopedics

- *Soft tissue injuries*:
  - Ligament tears (e.g., ACL, PCL)
  - Meniscal injuries
  - Tendon ruptures
- *Bone pathologies*:
  - Stress fractures
  - Osteomyelitis (early detection)
- *Spinal disorders*:
  - Disc herniations
  - Spinal cord tumors
  - Degenerative disc disease
- *Tumor evaluation*: Bone and soft tissue tumors (size, extent, marrow involvement).
- *Avascular necrosis (AVN)*: Earliest modality to detect AVN (especially femoral head).
- *Peripheral nerve disorders*: Brachial plexus injuries, sciatic nerve compression.

Q14. Advantages and limitations of MRI in orthopedic diagnosis.

Advantages

- Excellent **soft tissue contrast**
- Non-ionizing, safe for repeated use
- *Ideal for*:
  - Disc herniations
  - Ligament/tendon injuries
  - Bone marrow pathology (tumors, infections)

Limitations

- Expensive
- Time-consuming
- Contraindicated in some implants (pacemakers)
- Motion artifacts reduce clarity

Q15. Compare and contrast MRI with CT in orthopedics.

Feature	*CT scan*	*MRI*
Modality	X-ray based	Magnetic field and radio waves
Best for	Bone detail, fractures, implants	Soft tissue (ligaments, menisci, disc)
Radiation	Yes	No
Time required	Shorter (few minutes)	Longer (~30–60 minutes)
Metal artifacts	More pronounced	Less with advanced sequences

Orthopedic Uses of CT

- Complex **intra-articular fractures**
- 3D reconstruction for pre-operative planning
- Bone tumors, spinal stenosis

Orthopedic Uses of MRI

- **Disc herniations**, ligament and meniscal injuries
- Osteomyelitis and marrow edema
- AVN of femoral head
- Tumor extension into soft tissues

Q16. Applications of musculoskeletal ultrasound in orthopedics.

(Asked in JIPMER Puducherry 2023, MUHS Maharashtra 2023)

Introduction

Musculoskeletal ultrasound (MSK USG) is a **real-time, non-invasive imaging technique** that provides dynamic evaluation of soft tissue and superficial bone structures without radiation.

Applications in Orthopedics

1. *Tendon and ligament injuries*:
    - Detects tendon tears, ruptures (e.g., rotator cuff, Achilles tendon).
    - Dynamic assessment of ligament instability.
2. *Muscle injuries*: Muscle strains, hematomas, and contusions.
3. *Joint effusion and synovitis*: Detection of joint fluid, synovial hypertrophy, and guiding joint aspirations or injections.
4. *Soft tissue masses*: Differentiates between cystic and solid masses (e.g., ganglion cysts, lipomas).
5. *Fracture detection*: Useful in detecting occult fractures, especially in children (e.g., clavicle, ribs).
6. *Nerve entrapments*: Identifies peripheral nerve injuries (e.g., carpal tunnel syndrome).
7. *Procedural guidance*: Assists in accurate placement for interventions like biopsies, aspirations, and injections.
8. *Pediatric orthopedics*: Developmental dysplasia of hip (DDH) screening using Graf method.

Special Mention

High-frequency probes (7.5–15 MHz) are typically used for superficial structures.

Q17. Advantages and limitations of ultrasound in tendon injuries.

(Asked in TNMGR Chennai 2022)

Advantages

- *Dynamic imaging*: Can assess tendons during active/passive movement (helps detect subtle tears).
- *Real-time guidance*: For therapeutic procedures like tendon sheath injections.
- *High-resolution for superficial tendons*: Excellent detail for structures like the rotator cuff, Achilles tendon, patellar tendon.
- *Cost-effective and portable*:
    - Cheaper and more accessible compared to MRI.
    - Bedside and outpatient setting friendly.
- *No radiation exposure*: Safe for all age groups including pregnant women.

Limitations

- *Operator-dependent*: Requires significant expertise and experience.
- *Limited penetration*: Cannot image deep-seated tendons accurately (e.g., around hip joint).
- *Poor visualization in certain conditions*:
    - Difficult if excessive edema or in obese patients.
    - Bone, gas, and calcifications can cause acoustic shadowing.
- *Cannot replace MRI in complex injuries*: MRI still superior for detailed evaluation of intra-articular and complex soft tissue injuries.

Mnemonic for Advantages: "DRIP"

- *D*ynamic imaging
- *R*eal-time procedures

- *I*nexpensive
- *P*ortable

Exam Writing Tip

- Always present **both advantages and limitations** when asked.
- Keep examples ready (e.g., Rotator cuff tears → USG highly sensitive).
- Simple labeled sketches of ultrasound images (like transverse vs. longitudinal tendon tear) can be bonus scoring.

Q18. Dynamic fluoroscopy in spine disorders.

Applications

- *Real-time X-ray video to evaluate*:
  - **Instability (spondylolisthesis)**
  - **Facet joint motion**
  - **Spinal cord impingement during movement**

Clinical Use

- *Assess dynamic compression in*:
  - **Cervical and lumbar spine disorders**
  - **Post-operative instability**

Advantages

- Immediate feedback
- Useful in interventional procedures (epidural, facet injections)

Q19. Advancements in AI in radiology.

Applications

- *Automated image analysis*: Detects fractures, tumors
- **Pattern recognition** in MRI/CT scans
- Assists in:
  - **Triage and prioritization**
  - **Quantitative analysis** (e.g., cartilage thickness)

Benefits

- Reduces human error
- Increases diagnostic speed
- Enhances workflow efficiency

Challenges

- Requires large datasets for training
- Needs clinical validation

Q20. Principles and uses of bone scintigraphy in orthopedics.

(Asked in PGI Chandigarh 2022)

Introduction

Bone scintigraphy (bone scan) is a **nuclear medicine imaging technique** used to detect areas of increased or decreased bone metabolism, indicating pathology.

Principle

- Involves intravenous injection of a **radiotracer** (usually **Technetium-99m MDP**).
- The radiotracer binds to **hydroxyapatite** crystals in bone, especially in areas of increased osteoblastic activity.
- Gamma camera detects the emitted radiation to create images.

Phases of Bone Scan (Three-phase Scan)

1. *Flow phase*: Immediate blood flow image.
2. *Blood pool phase*: Shortly after injection, showing soft tissue perfusion.
3. *Delayed phase*: 2–4 hours later, showing skeletal uptake.

Uses in Orthopedics

- *Infections*: Osteomyelitis, septic arthritis.
- *Tumors*: Primary bone tumors, skeletal metastasis.
- *Fractures*: Stress fractures, occult fractures.
- *Avascular necrosis*: Early detection.
- *Prosthesis evaluation*: Loosening versus infection.
- *Paget's disease*: Increased uptake due to high bone turnover.

Special Types

SPECT-CT: Combines scintigraphy with CT for better localization.

Q21. Radioisotope scan findings in osteomyelitis and bone metastasis.

(Asked in RGUHS Karnataka 2022)

Osteomyelitis

- **Three-phase scan is crucial**.
- *Flow phase*: Increased blood flow to affected area.
- *Blood pool phase*: Hyperemia (increased pooling).
- *Delayed phase*: Focal increased tracer uptake ("hot spot").
- Early osteomyelitis can be detected **before X-ray changes appear**.

Bone Metastasis

- **Multiple hot spots** scattered throughout the skeleton.
- Preferential uptake in axial skeleton (spine, pelvis, ribs).
- *Blastic lesions (e.g., prostate cancer metastases)*: High uptake.
- *Lytic lesions (e.g., myeloma)*: May appear "cold" (low uptake) - hence, PET-CT may be better in some lytic tumors.

Mnemonic for Interpretation

"Hot in infection and metastasis, Cold in myeloma."

Q22. Advantages and disadvantages of radioisotope imaging.

(Asked in MUHS Maharashtra 2023)

Advantages

- *High sensitivity*: Detects early metabolic changes before structural changes occur.
- *Whole-body screening*: Ideal for metastatic disease survey.
- *Cost-effective compared to PET-CT*: Cheaper and more widely available.
- *Dynamic information*: Provides functional imaging (blood flow, turnover).

Disadvantages

- *Low specificity*: Cannot easily differentiate infection, tumor, fracture—further tests often needed.
- *Radiation exposure*: Though low, it is still ionizing radiation.
- *Limited spatial resolution*: Less anatomical detail compared to MRI or CT.
- *False positives*: Any cause of increased bone turnover (e.g., trauma, arthritis) can mimic serious pathology.

Tip

Always correlate bone scan findings clinically and radiologically (X-ray, MRI, CT).

Exam Pro Tip

- Always mention **Technetium-99m** when describing bone scans.
- Remember "Bone Scan is **Sensitive**, but not **Specific**" — use this line for better impression!
- Use simple diagrams (e.g., showing hot spots) if time permits.

Q23. PET Scan and SPECT in detection of bone tumors.

(Asked in PGI Chandigarh 2022)

Introduction

Positron emission tomography (PET) and single photon emission computed tomography (SPECT) are **nuclear imaging techniques** that assess **metabolic and functional activity** of tissues, valuable in oncology.

Role in Bone Tumors

1. *PET scan:*
   - *Tracer*: Most commonly uses **FDG (fluorodeoxyglucose)**.
   - *Applications*:
     - *Diagnosis*: Differentiating benign versus malignant lesions.
     - *Staging*: Detects primary and metastatic bone tumors.
     - *Treatment response*: Monitoring after chemotherapy or radiotherapy.
     - *Recurrence detection*: Early identification of tumor relapse.
   - *Examples*:
     - Osteosarcoma
     - Ewing's sarcoma
     - Metastatic bone disease
2. *SPECT scan*:
   - *Tracer*: Technetium-99m labeled agents.
   - *Applications*:
     - Detection of **skeletal metastases.**
     - Useful in **occult fractures**, **osteomyelitis**, and **avascular necrosis.**
     - Localizes small or multiple bone lesions with higher sensitivity than planar bone scan.

Advantages

- High sensitivity for detecting metabolically active lesions.
- Whole-body imaging in a single scan.
- PET-CT and SPECT-CT combine anatomical with functional imaging.

Limitations

- High cost.
- Limited availability.
- FDG uptake is non-specific (can occur in infections and inflammations also).

Bonus Tip for Exam

- For imaging questions, always include **at least two indications and two advantages**.
- For PET/SPECT, mention **specific tracers** like FDG and Tc-99m to impress the examiner.
- Short mnemonics can help in quick recall (e.g., "PET: primary, extent, treatment-response").

Q24. Role of CRP and ESR in diagnosis and monitoring of orthopedic infections.

(Asked in AIIMS Delhi 2021, MUHS Maharashtra 2023)

Introduction

C-reactive protein (CRP) and erythrocyte sedimentation rate (ESR) are important **inflammatory markers** used for early diagnosis, monitoring, and follow-up of Orthopedic infections.

C-reactive Protein
- *Produced by*: Liver in response to interleukin-6 (IL-6).
- *Rise and fall*:
  - Rises within **6–8 hours** after infection onset.
  - Peaks at **48 hours**.
  - Falls rapidly once infection resolves.

Erythrocyte Sedimentation Rate
- *Mechanism*: Measures the rate at which RBCs sediment in 1 hour.
- *Rise and fall*:
  - Rises **slowly (24–48 hours)**.
  - Stays elevated longer even after infection resolves.

Uses in Orthopedic Infections
- *Diagnosis*: Elevated CRP and ESR indicate infection (osteomyelitis, septic arthritis, prosthetic joint infections).
- *Monitoring response to treatment*:
  - Serial measurements.
  - CRP is more reliable for short-term monitoring.

Prognosis
Persistently high values suggest ongoing infection.

Normal Values
- *CRP*: <5 mg/L
- *ESR*: <20 mm/h (varies slightly with age and sex)

Q25. Compare sensitivity and specificity of ESR, CRP, and procalcitonin in septic arthritis.

(Asked in PGI Chandigarh 2022)

Comparison Table

Marker	Sensitivity (%)	Specificity (%)	Comments
CRP	90–95%	80–85%	Early rise, good for monitoring
ESR	80–90%	70–80%	Slower kinetics, less specific
Procalcitonin	60–70%	90–95%	High specificity for bacterial infections

Summary
- *CRP*: High sensitivity; best for early diagnosis.
- *ESR*: Good sensitivity but less specific; helpful when combined with CRP.
- *Procalcitonin*: Best for confirming bacterial infections; less sensitive for localized infections like septic arthritis.

Mnemonic
"CRP Catches, ESR Echoes, Procalcitonin Proves."

Q26. Blood markers used in prosthetic joint infections (PJI).

(Asked in JIPMER Puducherry 2022)

Markers Used in Diagnosis
1. *CRP and ESR*:
   - First-line screening tests.
   - CRP >10 mg/L and ESR >30 mm/h suggest infection.
2. *Procalcitonin*: More specific for bacterial PJI, but less sensitive for early detection.
3. *Synovial fluid markers (advanced but important to mention)*:
   - Synovial fluid CRP, WBC count, and neutrophil percentage.
   - Alpha-defensin assay (highly specific).

Scoring Systems
Musculoskeletal Infection Society (MSIS) criteria uses CRP and ESR in the first step of PJI diagnosis.

Monitoring After Surgery
Serial CRP monitoring is used to detect persistent or recurrent infection.

Special Note
Blood cultures are also taken if systemic infection is suspected.

Q27. Laboratory diagnosis of osteomyelitis and septic arthritis.

Test	*Osteomyelitis*	*Septic arthritis*
ESR, CRP	Elevated	Elevated
CBC	Leukocytosis	Leukocytosis
Blood culture	Positive in acute cases	May be positive
Synovial fluid analysis	NA	Turbid, high WBC, low glucose
Bone biopsy/culture	Gold standard	Joint aspirate culture
MRI	Early detection	Joint effusion, synovial changes

Q28. Diagnostic value of synovial fluid analysis in arthritis.

Parameter	*Non-inflammatory*	*Inflammatory (RA, gout)*	*Septic*
Color	Clear	Yellow	Turbid, purulent
Viscosity	High	Low	Very low
WBC count	<2,000/mm^3	2,000–75,000/mm^3	>50,000/mm^3
Gram stain/culture	Negative	Negative	Often positive
Crystals	None	Monosodium urate, CPPD	None

Q29. Serological tests for autoimmune arthritis.

- *Rheumatoid factor (RF)*: Present in 70–80% of RA; not specific
- *Anti-CCP antibodies*: Highly specific for RA
- *ANA*: Positive in SLE, Sjögren's
- *HLA-B27*: Ankylosing spondylitis, reactive arthritis
- *CRP/ESR*: Inflammatory markers
- *Complement levels*: Low in active SLE

Pro Tip for Exams
- Always **combine CRP + ESR** for initial screening.
- **Procalcitonin** is often reserved for **differentiating bacterial infections** versus non-infectious causes.
- Mention **MSIS criteria** if the question involves PJI for extra marks!

Q30. Short note on CB-NAAT and GeneXpert test.

Cartridge-based nucleic acid amplification test (CB-NAAT) and **GeneXpert** are rapid molecular diagnostic tools primarily used for the detection of ***Mycobacterium tuberculosis*** (MTB) and **rifampicin resistance** in suspected tuberculosis (TB) cases.

Principle
- Based on **real-time polymerase chain reaction** (PCR).
- Detects ***MTB DNA*** and ***rpoB*** **gene mutations** indicating rifampicin resistance.
- Results available in **<2 hours**.

Key Features

- High **sensitivity** and **specificity**.
- Can be used on **sputum**, **pus**, **tissue**, **gastric aspirate**, and **body fluids** (e.g., pleural, CSF).
- Can differentiate **rifampicin-resistant TB (RR-TB)** from drug-sensitive TB (DS-TB).
- Minimal biosafety requirement due to closed cartridge system.

Applications in Orthopedics

- Used in diagnosing **spinal TB**, **osteomyelitis**, and **tuberculous arthritis** from pus/tissue biopsy.
- Helps in early initiation of **MDR-TB** treatment.

Limitations

- Only detects rifampicin resistance (not full drug susceptibility).
- False negatives in paucibacillary samples.

WHO Endorsement

Endorsed by WHO for **early and accurate diagnosis of TB and MDR-TB**, especially in high-burden countries.

Q31. Principles of DEXA scanning for osteoporosis.

Principle

- **Dual-energy X-ray absorptiometry**
- Measures **bone mineral density (BMD)**
- Low- and high-energy X-rays differentiate bone from soft tissue

Sites Measured

- Lumbar spine (L1–L4)
- Hip (femoral neck, total hip)
- Forearm (if others not possible)

Interpretation

- **T-score ≤ –2.5** = Osteoporosis
- **Z-score** used in younger individuals

Advantages

- Low radiation
- Quick, reproducible
- Used for monitoring **therapy response**

Miscellaneous Diagnostic Approaches: Common Theory Questions with Answers

Q32. Discuss the approach to diagnosing unexplained chronic joint pain.

Possible Causes

- Inflammatory arthritis (RA, PsA)
- Infective (TB, fungal)
- Crystal arthropathy
- Early AVN
- Tumors or paraneoplastic
- Algodystrophy
- Neuropathic joint

Approach

- Detailed history (trauma, fever, morning stiffness)

- Systemic signs (rash, weight loss, skin lesions)
- *Physical exam:* Joint line tenderness, swelling, range of motion

Investigations

- CBC, ESR, CRP
- RF, anti-CCP, ANA
- Joint aspiration (if effusion)
- X-ray and **MRI** (especially early AVN, synovitis)
- Dual eneregy CT scan
- Synovial biopsy or arthroscopy if the diagnosis uncertain

Q33. Explain algodystrophy and its diagnostic challenges.

Also called: Complex regional pain syndrome (CRPS type I)

Etiology

- Unknown; follows trauma, fracture, or surgery
- Abnormal sympathetic nervous system activity

Clinical Features

- Burning pain, allodynia
- Swelling, color changes, temperature asymmetry
- Shiny skin, stiffness, osteoporosis
- Usually **out of proportion** to injury
- Clinical diagnositic criteria
- Budapest criteria

Diagnostic Challenges

- No definitive lab test
- Diagnosis of exclusion
- *Bone scan*: Increased uptake in affected area
- *X-rays*: Patchy osteopenia ("Sudeck's atrophy")

Treatment

- Early physiotherapy
- NSAIDs, gabapentin, bisphosphonates
- Sympathetic block in severe cases

Q34. Approach to investigation of a monoarticular swollen joint.

(North Eastern Indira Gandhi Regional Institute of Health and Medical Sciences 2015)

Step 1: Clinical Assessment

History

- *Onset*: Acute (hours to days) versus chronic (>6 weeks)
- *Pain*: Inflammatory versus mechanical
- *Systemic symptoms*: Fever, weight loss, malaise
- *Trauma*: Recent injury, sports
- *Associated disease*: TB, psoriasis, gout, RA, STDs

Examination

- Warmth, redness, tenderness → suggest inflammation
- Joint effusion or deformity
- *Movement restriction*: Active versus passive
- Look for skin lesions, lymphadenopathy, tophi

Step 2: Differential Diagnosis

Category	*Examples*
Infective	Septic arthritis, TB, Lyme disease
Inflammatory	Gout, pseudogout, RA (early), JIA
Traumatic	Hemarthrosis, fracture-dislocation
Neoplastic	Pigmented villonodular synovitis (PVNS), synovial sarcoma
Degenerative	Osteoarthritis (early monoarticular)

Step 3: Investigations

A. Laboratory Tests

- *CBC, ESR, CRP*: Indicators of inflammation/infection
- *Serum uric acid*: Gout
- *Rheumatoid factor, anti-CCP*: Early RA
- *ANA, HLA-B27*: Suspect autoimmune causes
- *Blood cultures*: Suspected sepsis
- *Tuberculin test/IGRA*: TB arthritis

B. Joint Aspiration (Most Important Test)

- *Gross appearance*: Clear (OA), cloudy/purulent (infection), bloody (trauma/PVNS)
- *Cell count*:
  - <2,000/mm^3 → Non-inflammatory
  - 2,000–75,000 → Inflammatory (gout, RA)
  - 50,000–100,000 → Infective
- *Gram stain and culture*: Rule out septic arthritis
- *Polarized microscopy*—Crystals:
  - Needle-shaped, negatively birefringent → Gout (MSU)
  - Rhomboid, weakly positive → Pseudogout (CPPD)
- *AFB stain, PCR*: Tuberculosis

C. Imaging

- *X-ray*: Effusion, erosions, joint space changes, calcification
  - *OA*: Joint space narrowing, osteophytes
  - *RA*: Marginal erosions
  - *Gout*: "Punched out" erosions
  - *TB*: Phemister's triad
- *Ultrasound*: Effusion, synovial thickening, guide aspiration
- *MRI*: Soft tissue involvement, early cartilage/bone marrow changes
- *CT*: Calcifications, subtle bone erosion
- *Nuclear scan (if chronic/occult)*: Bone scan for early infection

Mnemonic for Initial Workup: "ABC-Joint"

- *A*: Aspiration
- *B*: Blood tests (ESR, CRP, CBC, uric acid)
- *C*: Culture (blood and synovial fluid)
- *J*: Joint imaging (X-ray, USG, MRI)
- *O*: Other tests (RF, ANA, HLA-B27, AFB stain)
- *I*: Infective screen (HIV, TB)
- *N*: Neoplastic suspicion → Biopsy
- *T*: Trauma rule-out → X-ray, hemarthrosis

Q35. Fluoroscopy-guided procedures in orthopedics.

Applications
- Closed reduction and internal fixation
- Intra-articular injections
- Vertebroplasty/Kyphoplasty
- C-arm guided spinal and joint procedures
- Biopsy guidance

Advantages
- Real-time imaging
- Minimally invasive
- Enhanced precision and safety

Q36. Principles and clinical applications of emg and nerve conduction studies (NCS).

(Amrita Institute of Medical Sciences 2011)

Electromyography (EMG)
- Records electrical activity of muscles at rest and during contraction.
- Detects denervation, reinnervation, and myopathic changes.

Nerve Conduction Studies (NCS)
Measures speed and amplitude of electrical impulses in motor and sensory nerves.

Test	*Parameter measured*	*Key use*
EMG	Muscle electrical response	Detects denervation, myopathy
NCS	Latency, amplitude, velocity	Localizes site and type of nerve lesion

Clinical Applications
- Peripheral nerve injuries (localization, severity, prognosis)
- Neuropathies (diabetic, entrapment)
- Myopathies
- Neuromuscular junction disorders
- Radiculopathy and plexopathy

Q37. Role of electrodiagnostic studies in peripheral nerve injuries.

- **Localize lesion** (site of compression or trauma)
- **Classify injury** (neuropraxia, axonotmesis, neurotmesis)
- **Assess severity and prognosis**
- **Monitor recovery or reinnervation**

Findings
- Reduced conduction velocity in demyelination
- Absent/low CMAP/SNAP in axonal injury
- Fibrillations and positive sharp waves on EMG in axonal injury

Q38. What is wallerian degeneration? How is it detected on EMG?

- *Definition*: Degeneration of axon distal to site of injury due to axonal damage.
- *Timeline*: Begins 24–36 hours after injury; completes in 7–10 days.

- *EMG findings (after ~10–14 days)*:
  - Fibrillation potentials
  - Positive sharp waves
  - Absence of voluntary motor unit potentials in affected muscles

Q39. Differentiate between neuropraxia and axonotmesis (EMG and NCS).

(Grant Government Medical College 2013

Feature	Neuropraxia	Axonotmesis
Pathology	Demyelination	Axonal disruption
NCV	Slowed conduction, normal amplitude	↓ amplitude, ↓ velocity
CMAP/SNAP	Preserved/Normal	Decreased or absent
EMG	Normal early; no fibrillations	Fibrillation potentials (10–14 days)
Recovery	Weeks (rapid, complete)	Months (slow, incomplete)

Q40. Electrodiagnostic approach in brachial plexus injury.

- *NCS*: Helps distinguish preganglionic (root) from postganglionic (plexus/nerve) lesions
- *EMG*:
  - Denervation in corresponding myotomes
  - Paraspinal muscle EMG helps differentiate root versus plexus injury
- *Timing*: EMG after 2–3 weeks; repeat in 6–8 weeks if needed
- *Value*: Helps localize lesion, assess severity, guide prognosis/surgical planning

Q41. Short note—EMG findings in nerve injury and recovery.

- *Acute denervation (10–14 days)*:
  - Fibrillation potentials
  - Positive sharp waves
- *Chronic denervation*:
  - Large amplitude, long duration motor unit potentials (MUPs)
  - Reduced recruitment
- *Reinnervation*:
  - Polyphasic MUPs
  - Increased recruitment with time

Q42. Role of EMG/NCS in carpal tunnel syndrome (CTS).

(Madras Medical College 2018)

- *Median NCS*: Slowed conduction velocity across the wrist
- *Distal latency*: Prolonged in median motor and sensory nerves
- *EMG*: May show denervation in abductor pollicis brevis (late)
- *Severity*: Graded as mild, moderate, or severe based on findings

Q43. Electrodiagnostic approach in lumbar radiculopathy.

- *NCS*: Often normal (since lesion is proximal to DRG)
- *EMG*:
  - Fibrillations and positive sharp waves in affected myotomes
  - Reduced recruitment
  - Paraspinal muscles affected (L5, S1 roots)

Q44. Differentiate root lesion versus peripheral nerve lesion on EMG.

Feature	*Root Lesion (Radiculopathy)*	*Peripheral Nerve Lesion*
Paraspinal EMG	Abnormal	Normal
Sensory NCS	Normal (DRG spared)	Abnormal
Distribution	Myotomal	Nerve-specific
Reflex involvement	Often affected	Depends on specific nerve

Q45. Short note—repetitive nerve stimulation in myasthenia gravis.

- *Test*: Repetitive stimulation (2–5 Hz) of motor nerve
- *Finding*: >10% decrement in CMAP amplitude with repetitive stimulation
- *Use*: Diagnostic for myasthenia gravis, congenital myasthenic syndromes
- *Other tests*: Single-fiber EMG for increased jitter

Q46. EMG features in anterior horn cell disease (e.g., poliomyelitis).

(AIIMS Jodhpur 2013)

- *Denervation*: Fibrillations, positive sharp waves
- Reinnervation: Giant MUPS, increased duration, reduced recruitment
- Fasciculations may be seen
- Common in ALS, post-polio syndrome

Q47. Timing of EMG after injury.

- *<10 days*: EMG may be normal; denervation not yet evident
- *10–14 days*: Fibrillation potentials start appearing
- *4–6 weeks*: Peak denervation; useful for re-evaluation
- *Recovery*: Reinnervation potentials seen after weeks to months

Q48. Spontaneous activity on EMG.

Spontaneous activity	*Indicates*
Fibrillation potentials	Denervation of muscle fibers
Positive sharp waves	Denervation
Fasciculations	Anterior horn cell disease
Myotonic discharges	Myopathies, dystrophies

Q49. Interpret NCV Graph—conduction block versus slowing.

- *Conduction block*:
    - Abrupt drop in amplitude
    - Suggests focal demyelination (e.g., entrapment)
- *Slowing*:
    - Gradual ↓ in conduction velocity
    - Seen in generalized demyelinating neuropathy

Q50 Chronaxie (short note).

Definition

Chronaxie is the **minimum time** required to excite a muscle or nerve using **double the rheobase current.**

Basic Concept

- It reflects the **excitability** of nerve or muscle tissue.
- Measured using **strength-duration curve.**

Important Terms

- *Rheobase*: Minimum current needed to excite tissue with prolonged stimulus duration.
- *Chronaxie*: Time corresponding to stimulus of **twice the rheobase current.**

Clinical Significance

- Normal **motor nerve chronaxie**: 0.1–1.0 milliseconds.
- Increased chronaxie suggests **denervation or nerve injury.**
- Used in **electrodiagnosis** and in determining **stimulation parameters** for electrical therapy in rehab.

Applications in Orthopedics

- Differentiates between **partial and complete denervation.**
- Helps in **monitoring recovery** of injured nerves.
- Relevant in **physiotherapy planning.**

Q51. Somatosensory evoked potentials (SSEPs) (short note).

(Seth Gordhandas Sunderdas Medical College and KEM Hospital 2013)

Definition

SSEPs are **electrical signals** generated by the nervous system in response to **sensory (usually electrical) stimulation** of a peripheral nerve.

Mechanism

- Stimulus (e.g., median or tibial nerve) → Peripheral nerve → Spinal cord → Brainstem → Cerebral cortex.
- Responses are recorded from **scalp, spine, or periphery.**

Use in Orthopedics

- **Spinal cord monitoring** during scoliosis or spine surgeries.
- Assess integrity of **posterior columns** of spinal cord.
- Helps localize **cord or root level lesions.**

Advantages

- Non-invasive, reproducible.
- Useful in **intraoperative neuromonitoring.**

Limitations:

- Affected by anesthesia, hypothermia, and patient comorbidities.
- Does not assess motor pathways directly (for that, **motor evoked potentials** are used).

Q52. Three orthopedic conditions where EMG is diagnostic.

1. Carpal tunnel syndrome
2. Brachial plexus injury
3. Lumbar radiculopathy

CHAPTER 3

Infections in Orthopedics

Jujhar Singh, Vedant Bajaj, Abhimanu Kaith

Acute and Chronic Osteomyelitis

Q1. Describe acute osteomyelitis with its clinical features, diagnosis, and management.

(Asked in AIIMS Delhi 2022, PGI Chandigarh 2022)

Definition

Acute osteomyelitis is an **acute infection of bone and bone marrow**, usually caused by **hematogenous spread** of bacteria, commonly seen in children.

Common Pathogens

- *Staphylococcus aureus* (most common).
- *Streptococcus* species
- Kingella kingae (young children).
- *Salmonella* (especially in sickle cell disease).

Clinical Features

Symptoms	*Signs*
Sudden onset bone pain	Localized swelling, redness, warmth
Fever, malaise	Tenderness over bone
Refusal to bear weight or move the limb (in children)	Pseudoparalysis in infants

Diagnosis

- *Blood investigations*:
  - ↑ ESR, ↑ CRP, leukocytosis.
  - Positive blood cultures (~50% cases).
- *Radiology*:
  - Early X-ray may be normal; changes (periosteal reaction, lytic areas) appear after 10–14 days.
  - MRI is investigation of choice—shows early marrow edema.
- *Bone aspiration/biopsy*: For culture and sensitivity.

Management

Stage	*Treatment*
Early (no abscess)	IV antibiotics (empirical, later adjusted based on culture)
Abscess formation	Surgical drainage + IV antibiotics
Supportive	Analgesics, splinting for comfort and IV fluid

Important Tip

Empirical antibiotics: Cover ***Staphylococcus aureus*** + **Gram-negatives** initially (e.g., Cefazolin + Gentamicin).

Duration of Antibiotics

4–6 weeks (initial IV followed by oral course).

Q2. Write answers on chronic osteomyelitis, including sequestrum, involucrum, management principles.

(Asked in MUHS Maharashtra 2022, RGUHS Karnataka 2022)

Definition

Chronic osteomyelitis is a **persistent bone infection** lasting beyond 6 weeks, characterized by **necrotic bone (sequestrum)**, **new bone formation (involucrum)**, and often sinus formation.

Key Pathological Terms

Term	*Definition*
Sequestrum	Dead piece of bone separated from living bone, harboring infection
Involucrum	New bone formed around sequestrum by periosteal reaction
Cloaca	Opening in involucrum through which pus drains
Sinus tract	External opening of infection on the skin

Clinical Features

- Chronic discharging sinus.
- Intermittent swelling, redness.
- Persistent dull bone pain.
- History of prior acute osteomyelitis, open fractures, or surgeries.

Cause of chronicity of infection

1. Presence of unabsorbed and retained sequestra serving as a constant source of infection
2. Unobliterated cavities (dead spaces alive with bacteria)
3. 'Microbiological shift' (change of aerobic cocci to gram negative or anaerobes)
4. Multiple types of bacteria "mixed infection" and anti microbial resistance.

Diagnosis

- *Blood tests*: ESR and CRP elevated chronically.
- *X-ray*: Sequestrum appears as dense devascularized bone; involucrum seen as thickened periosteal new bone.
- *MRI*: Defines soft tissue extent.
- *Sinogram*: If sinus tract present.
- *Bone biopsy*: For definitive microbiological diagnosis.

Management Principles

Step	*Details*
Surgical debridement	Removal of sequestrum and infected tissue (sequestrectomy)
Antibiotic therapy	Culture-directed antibiotics (6–8 weeks)
Stabilization	External fixation if necessary (if bone instability)
Dead space management	Bone grafting, antibiotic-loaded beads, muscle flaps
Reconstruction	If major bone loss—e.g., Ilizarov techniques, vascularized bone grafts

Important Surgical Options

- Sequestrectomy (removal of dead bone).
- Saucerization (widening of cavity for drainage).
- Antibiotic cement beads/spacers.
- Ilizarov external fixator for infected non-union.

Mnemonic for Management: "DASSR"
- *D*ebridement
- *A*ntibiotics
- *S*tabilization
- *S*pace management
- *R*econstruction

Q3. What are the prerequisites of surgery (sequestrectomy and saucerization) for chronic osteomyelitis?

Absolute
- *Radiological*: Well-formed involucrum surrounding the discretely visible sequestrum adequately at least 2/3rd diameter of bone (3 intact walls on two views ensure 3/4th intact walls!).
- *Clinically*: Symptomatic patient with pus discharge or chronic unrelieved disabling pain due to osteomyelitis per se and type A/B host.
- *Ethical*: Salvageable limb and patient willing for prolonged and multiple treatments.

Relative: Stopping antibiotic treatment at least one week prior to surgery (otherwise cultures will be misleading).

Quick Tips for Theory and Viva
- In acute osteomyelitis, **early diagnosis + early IV antibiotics** are key.
- In chronic osteomyelitis, **surgery is essential**—antibiotics alone are not enough!
- Always clearly define **sequestrum and involucrum**—highly scoring if drawn neatly in exam diagrams.

Short answer and Viva Question

Q4. Define musculoskeletal infections. Classify with examples.

Definition

Musculoskeletal infections are **infective conditions affecting bones, joints, muscles, tendons, or surrounding soft tissue** caused by microbial organisms.

Classification
1. *Based on site*:
   - Osteomyelitis
   - Septic arthritis
   - Pyomyositis
   - Tenosynovitis
2. *Based on etiology:*
   - Pyogenic (*Staphylococcus aureus*)
   - Tubercular (*Mycobacterium tuberculosis*)
   - Fungal (e.g., *Candida, Aspergillus*)
3. *Based on duration*:
   - Acute (<2 weeks)
   - Subacute (2–6 weeks)
   - Chronic (>6 weeks)
4. *Based on mode of acquisition*:
   - Hematogenous
   - Direct inoculation
   - Contiguous spread

Q5. Classification of osteomyelitis based on duration, pathology, and etiology.

Duration
- *Acute*: <2 weeks
- *Subacute*: 2–6 weeks
- *Chronic*: >6 weeks

Pathology
- Suppurative (e.g., *Staphylococcus aureus*)
- Non-suppurative (e.g., TB)
- Granulomatous (fungal, TB)

Etiology
- Pyogenic
- Tubercular
- Fungal
- Viral
- Parasitic

Classification of osteomyelitis

A. *Based on the mode of infection*:
  - Hematogenous—via bloodstream (common in children)
  - Contiguous spread—from nearby soft tissue or wound
  - Direct inoculation—trauma, surgery, implants

B. *Based on duration*:
  - Acute (<2 weeks)
  - Subacute (2–6 weeks)
  - Chronic (>6 weeks)

Q6. Cierny–Mader classification (most widely used).

Based on two factors:
1. Anatomic type (bone involvement)
2. Host physiology (patient's immune status)

Anatomic Types

Type	*Description*
I	Medullary osteomyelitis (confined to the medullary canal)
II	Superficial osteomyelitis (involves cortical bone)
III	Localized osteomyelitis (full-thickness bone involvement but stable)
IV	Diffuse osteomyelitis (circumferential bone involvement, instability)

Host Types

Host	*Description*
A	Normal healthy host
B	Systemically or locally compromised host
C	Treatment worse than disease (very poor host; treatment may be avoided)

Example

Patient could be classified as **type III, Host B** osteomyelitis.

Q7. What is the common site of osteomyelitis and why?

(Grant Government Medical College 2014)

Metaphysis

- Hair pin bend arrangement of arterioles
- Relatively less phagocytosis (↓ reticuloendothelial system activity)
- Sluggish flow
- Tortuous blood vessels and skimming of bacteria
- Dead (apoptotic) and degenerating cartilage cells from physeal plate serving as medium for bacterial growth
- Microfractures and local hematoma common in young active children

Q8. What are the causes for diaphyseal osteomyelitis?

- Long standing osteomyelitis in children (grows out to diaphysis)
- Post-traumatic osteomyelitis
- Implant related osteomyelitis
- Tubercular osteomyelitis
- Drug abusers (heroin addicts—pseudomonas)
- Immunocompromised (fungal)
- Salmonella osteomyelitis (often bilateral and may be symmetrical).

Q9. Routes of infection spread in musculoskeletal infections.

(Christian Medical College Vellore 2014)

1. *Hematogenous spread*:
    - Common in children
    - From distant foci like skin or respiratory tract
    - E.g., Acute hematogenous osteomyelitis
2. *Direct inoculation*:
    - Post-trauma or surgery
    - Implant-associated infections
    - E.g., Infection after ORIF
3. *Contiguous spread*:
    - From adjacent soft tissue infections or ulcers
    - Common in diabetics
    - E.g., Diabetic foot osteomyelitis

Q10. Pathophysiology of musculoskeletal infections.

1. **Bacterial colonization** of tissue
2. Activation of **innate immune response**
3. Influx of **neutrophils** → **pus formation**
4. **Inflammatory cytokines** → tissue destruction
5. **Increased intramedullary pressure** → ischemia → necrosis
6. Formation of **sequestrum**, especially in osteomyelitis
7. *Chronic phase*: Biofilm formation, sinus tract, immune evasion

Q11. Biofilms in orthopedic infections (short note).

Definition

Biofilm is a **structured bacterial colony** embedded in self-produced matrix (EPS) that adheres to surfaces like implants.

Characteristics

- Highly **antibiotic-resistant**
- Shields bacteria from **immune clearance**
- Requires **implant removal** for eradication of infection
- Delays healing and causes **chronicity**

Examples

- Prosthetic joint infections
- Infected intramedullary nails or plates

Q12. Role of imaging in diagnosing musculoskeletal infections.

(Jammu University 2013)

- *X-ray*: Detects **periosteal elevation, osteolysis, sequestrum** (late findings)
- *Ultrasound:* Useful in detecting **effusions, abscesses**
- *MRI:*
  - **Most sensitive** modality
  - Shows **bone marrow edema**, **soft tissue involvement**, sinus tracts
- *CT*:
  - Useful for **bone detail**, sequestrum visualization
  - Assists in **guided biopsy**
- *Nuclear imaging*: Bone scan (Tc-99m), PET-CT for **early detection** and **infection mapping**

Q13. Role of laboratory investigations.

Blood Tests

- *CBC*: Leukocytosis
- *ESR, CRP*: Elevated in acute/chronic infection
- *Procalcitonin*: Specific for bacterial infections

Microbiological Tests

- Blood cultures (hematogenous cases)
- Aspirate culture and sensitivity
- Gram stain, AFB stain, fungal cultures

Histopathology

Helps in **tubercular or fungal** cases.

Q14. Role of CRP and procalcitonin.

(Kashmir University)

C-reactive Protein (CRP)

- Acute-phase protein
- **Rapid rise and fall** with infection/inflammation
- Useful for **monitoring treatment response**

Procalcitonin

- More **specific to bacterial infections**
- Rises **faster than CRP** (within 6–12 hours)
- Not elevated in **viral or autoimmune inflammation**

Q15. Pathophysiology of acute osteomyelitis.

1. Bacterial entry via bloodstream or direct trauma
2. Neutrophil influx → pus formation in medullary cavity

3. Increased intramedullary pressure → vascular compromise
4. Ischemia and bone necrosis → formation of sequestrum
5. Reactive new bone formation (involucrum) may follow if not treated early

In Children

- Infection starts in the **metaphysis** due to the rich, slow-flowing blood supply and end-artery configuration

Q16. Etiological factors for acute osteomyelitis.

(Rajendra Institute of Medical Sciences 2016)

1. *Microbial*:
    - *Staphylococcus aureus* (most common)
    - MRSA, *Streptococcus* species, Gram-negative bacilli
    - *Salmonella* in sickle cell disease
    - *Mycobacterium tuberculosis* in endemic areas
2. *Host factors*:
    - Immunocompromised states
    - Diabetes, malnutrition
    - Recent trauma or surgery
    - IV drug use

Q17. Clinical features, diagnosis, and management.

Clinical Features

- Acute onset of **localized bone pain**, **fever**, swelling
- Limitation of movement
- *In children*: **Refusal to bear weight**, pseudoparalysis

Diagnosis

- *Blood tests*: ↑ ESR, CRP, WBC count
- **Blood culture**
- *Imaging*: MRI is most sensitive
- **Bone biopsy/aspiration** for culture and sensitivity

Management

- Empirical IV antibiotics → culture-based antibiotics
- **Surgical drainage** if abscess or no improvement
- Limb support (splint/cast)
- Monitor CRP for response

Q18. Radiological features of acute osteomyelitis.

(AIIMS Bhubaneswar 2014)

X-ray (after 10–14 days)

- Soft tissue swelling
- Periosteal reaction
- Lucent areas indicating lysis

MRI (most sensitive)

- Early **bone marrow edema**
- Soft tissue involvement
- Abscess or sequestrum detection

Ultrasound
Useful in detecting **subperiosteal abscess** in children

Bone Scan/PET-CT
Sensitive but less specific; useful in multifocal cases

Q19. Differential diagnosis of acute osteomyelitis.

Condition	*Differentiating feature*
Septic arthritis	Joint tenderness, effusion, rapid destruction
Ewing sarcoma	Systemic symptoms, diaphyseal involvement
Osteoid osteoma	Night pain, nidus on CT
Cellulitis	No bony tenderness, normal imaging early
Bone infarction	Sickle cell disease, lacks inflammatory markers

Q20. Acute hematogenous osteomyelitis (short note).

(Baba Farid University of Health Sciences 2013)

- Common in **children**
- Affects **metaphysis** of long bones (femur, tibia)
- *Route*: **Hematogenous spread** from minor infections (URTI, skin)
- Presents with **fever, localized pain, pseudoparalysis**
- Treated with **early antibiotics**, sometimes surgical drainage
- *Staphylococcus aureus* is the most common pathogen

Q21. Complications of acute osteomyelitis.

Early
- Septicemia
- Septic arthritis (especially in infants)
- Subperiosteal abscess

Late
- Chronic osteomyelitis
- Growth disturbances (physeal damage)
- Pathological fractures
- Joint stiffness
- Deformity or limb length discrepancy

Q22. Principles of antibiotic therapy in acute osteomyelitis.

Initial Therapy
- **Empirical IV antibiotics** targeting *Staphylococcus aureus, Streptococcus*, and Gram-negatives
- Choice guided by **local sensitivity patterns** and patient factors

Duration
- Typically **4–6 weeks**
- **IV → oral switch** after clinical response (fever, CRP decline)

Monitoring
- Serial **CRP/ESR**, clinical improvement
- Modify based on **culture and sensitivity**

Q23. Role of surgical management in acute osteomyelitis.

(All India Institute of Medical Sciences New Delhi 2013)

Indications
- Failure of medical treatment
- Presence of **abscess**, sequestrum, or sinus
- Diagnostic uncertainty
- **Compartment syndrome**

Procedures
- **Aspiration or incision & drainage**
- **Cortical window** for decompression
- Removal of **necrotic bone or sequestrum** if present
- Drain placement and lavage

Q24. Define chronic osteomyelitis. Classify it.

Definition

Chronic osteomyelitis is a **long-standing infection of bone**, typically lasting >6 weeks, characterized by **necrotic bone (sequestrum), sinus tracts**, and persistent inflammation.

Classification

A. *Based on source:*
   - Hematogenous
   - Post-traumatic/post-surgical
   - Contiguous spread

B. *Based on duration:*
   - Chronic >6 weeks
   - *Subacute*: 2–6 weeks

C. *Cierny-Mader classification:*
   - *Anatomic type (1–4)*:
     - 1: Medullary
     - 2: Superficial
     - 3: Localized
     - 4: Diffuse
   - *Host type (A/B/C)*:
     - A: Healthy
     - B: Compromised
     - C: Surgery not justified due to risks

Q25. Pathophysiology of chronic osteomyelitis.

(Atal Medical and Research University 2012)

1. Persistence of infection after acute phase
2. Sequestrum formation (dead bone harboring bacteria)
3. Involucrum formation (reactive new bone)
4. Development of sinus tracts
5. Biofilm formation on necrotic bone or implants
6. Chronic inflammatory response → bone sclerosis, poor vascularity

Q26. Risk factors for chronic osteomyelitis.

- **Previous acute osteomyelitis**
- Open fractures

- **Surgical implants** (internal fixation, prosthesis)
- Diabetes mellitus
- Immunosuppression
- Peripheral vascular disease
- **Inadequate treatment** of acute infection

Q27. Clinical presentation of chronic osteomyelitis.

(Grant Medical College Mumbai 2009)

- **Chronic discharging sinus**
- Pain and swelling
- Non-healing wound or ulcer
- Sinus fixed to bone or healed puckered scar
- Exposed necrotic bone
- Soft tissue contractures
- **Local tenderness**, limb deformity
- *Occasionally*: Fever, malaise
- History of trauma or surgery

Q28. Radiological features of chronic osteomyelitis.

- *X-ray*:
  - *Sequestrum*: **Dense, necrotic bone fragment**
  - *Involucrum*: **New bone formation around sequestrum**
  - *Cloaca*: **Opening in involucrum** for sinus drainage
  - Sclerosis, periosteal thickening
- *MRI*: Best for soft tissue, sinus tracts, marrow involvement
- *CT scan*: Defines **bone architecture, cloacae, and sequestrum**
- *Bone scan/PET-CT*: Detects **active infection**, especially in multifocal disease

Q29. Treatment options for chronic osteomyelitis.

(Dr DY Patil Vidyapeeth Pune 2011)

Non-surgical
- **Long-term antibiotics** based on culture (4–6 weeks or more)
- Best for **low-grade or inoperable cases**

Surgical
- Debridement of necrotic tissue and sequestrum
- Sinus tract excision
- Dead space management (antibiotic beads, muscle flap)
- Stabilization if bone defect present
- Reconstruction using bone grafts or vascularized flaps

Q30. Surgical principles in chronic osteomyelitis management.

1. Adequate debridement of infected and necrotic tissue
2. Sequestrectomy and curettage
3. Identify and excise sinus tracts
4. *Dead space management*:
   - Antibiotic beads (PMMA)

- Vascularized muscle flap
- Bone transport (ilizarov)

5. *Reconstruction*:
   - Bone grafting
   - Free flaps for coverage
   - External or internal stabilization

Q31. Role of antibiotics in chronic osteomyelitis.

Principles

- **Culture-guided therapy** is essential
- Antibiotics alone are **insufficient** without debridement
- Usually given for **4–6 weeks** post-surgery

Delivery Methods

- **IV or oral** antibiotics
- *Local delivery*: PMMA antibiotic beads, biodegradable carriers
- Monitor using **CRP/ESR** for treatment response

Q32. Short notes on sequestrum and involucrum.

(Goa Medical College Bambolim Goa 2012)

Sequestrum

- A fragment of **necrotic bone** separated from viable bone
- Radiodense, may harbor bacteria
- Requires **surgical removal**

Types of Sequestrum

- *Sequestrum*: Dead bone fragment in osteomyelitis.
  - *Ring sequestrum*: Circumferential, in amputation stump infections.
  - *Button sequestrum*: Small round (seen in eosinophilic granuloma).
  - *Floating sequestrum*: In sinus or cavity.
  - *Coralliform sequestrum*: Perthes
  - *Coke like sequestrum*: Tuberculosis
  - *Feathery sequestrum*: Syphilis
  - *Sand like sequestrum*: Tubercular osteomyelitis in metaphysis
  - *Black*: Amputation stump and long exposure of necrotic bone to air while also attached to parent bone (formation of ferrous sulphide), fungal infection
  - *Green*: Pseudomonal osteomyelitis
- *Involucrum*: Reactive new bone around sequestrum.
- *Cloaca*: Opening in involucrum for pus drainage.

Involucrum

- **Reactive new bone** formed around the sequestrum
- May have **cloacae (openings)** for sinus drainage
- Seen on **X-ray/CT** in chronic osteomyelitis
- Only if three walls of involucrum are seen fully on two perpendicular views should sequestrectomy be undertaken otherwise a pathological fracture will result and it will get converted into infected nonunion.

Q33. Complications of chronic osteomyelitis.

- **Sinus tract formation**
- **Pathological fractures**
- Skeletal **deformity or limb shortening**

- Septic arthritis
- Septicemia
- Soft tissue contractures
- Squamous cell carcinoma in long-standing sinus
- **Amyloidosis** (rare)
- Chronic pain, disability
- Recurrence despite treatment

Q34. Define subacute osteomyelitis. Classify it.

(AIIMS Jodhpur Rajasthan 2011)

Definition

Subacute osteomyelitis is a **low-grade bone infection** that presents between **2 to 6 weeks** after onset. It is **less severe than acute osteomyelitis**, often with **milder symptoms** and a **localized abscess or lytic lesion**.

Clinical Features

- Mild to moderate localized pain
- Low-grade or absent fever
- Minimal systemic symptoms
- Often missed in early stages

Classification

1. *Based on radiological appearance*:
    - *Brodie's abscess*: Localized, intracortical or metaphyseal abscess
    - Metaphyseal lucency with sclerotic rim
    - Subperiosteal lesion
    - Diaphyseal type
    - Epiphyseal type (rare)
2. *Based on anatomic location*:
    - Metaphysis (most common)
    - Diaphysis
    - Epiphysis
    - Vertebrae (rare)

Q35. What is brodie's abscess? Discuss its diagnosis and management.

Definition

Brodie's abscess is a **localized form of subacute osteomyelitis**, characterized by a **walled-off abscess cavity** within the **metaphysis** of long bones.

Common Sites

- Tibia (proximal metaphysis)
- Femur, radius, or calcaneus

Diagnosis

Clinical:

- Chronic dull pain
- No or low-grade fever
- Often in children/adolescents

Radiological

- *X-ray*: Oval/round lytic lesion with **sclerotic margin** in metaphysis
- *MRI*: Confirms abscess, rim enhancement
- *CT*: Defines bony margins and sinus if present

Labs
- Mildly raised or normal ESR/CRP
- Blood cultures usually negative

Management
1. *Conservative (early or small lesions)*: Empirical antibiotics → guided by biopsy/culture
2. *Surgical (larger or symptomatic abscess)*:
   - **Curettage** and **debridement**
   - **Antibiotic bead placement** if needed
   - Post-operative IV antibiotics for 2–4 weeks

Q36. Differential diagnosis of subacute osteomyelitis (short note).

Condition	*Differentiating features*
Bone tumor (e.g., Ewing's sarcoma)	Systemic symptoms, periosteal reaction, diaphyseal location
Osteoid osteoma	No fever, night pain relieved by NSAIDs, nidus seen on CT
Chronic osteomyelitis	Sinus tract, sequestrum, involucrum on imaging
Langerhans cell histiocytosis	Solitary lytic lesion, eosinophilic granuloma
Tubercular osteomyelitis	Constitutional symptoms, caseation, positive GeneXpert

Osteomyelitis after Open Fracture
- *Definition*: Infection of bone secondary to contamination during open fracture.
- *Etiology*: Polymicrobial; common organisms include *Staphylococcus aureus, Pseudomonas.*
- *Management*:
  - Early aggressive debridement.
  - IV antibiotics.
  - Fracture stabilization (external or internal fixation).
  - Sometimes staged reconstruction (Masquelet technique).

Q37. Pyogenic vertebral osteomyelitis.

(Jammu University 2010)

Definition
Bacterial infection of vertebral bodies and intervertebral discs.

Etiology
Hematogenous spread; *Staphylococcus aureus* is most common.

Clinical Features
Back pain, fever, localized tenderness.

Diagnosis
MRI (most sensitive), blood cultures.

Treatment
- IV antibiotics (6–12 weeks).
- Immobilization.
- Surgical decompression if neurological deficit or abscess.

Q38. Chronic recurrent multifocal osteomyelitis (CRMO).

Definition
Non-infectious autoinflammatory bone disorder.

Features

Recurrent episodes of bone pain, swelling, multiple sites.

Diagnosis

Clinical + MRI; cultures negative.

Treatment

- NSAIDs first-line.
- Immunomodulators (e.g., TNF inhibitors) in refractory cases.

Q39. *Salmonella* osteomyelitis.

Common in

Sickle cell disease

Site

Diaphysis of long bones

Diagnosis

Blood cultures, MRI, bone biopsy

Treatment

IV ceftriaxone or fluoroquinolones for 4–6 weeks ± surgical debridement

Summary Flowcharts: Acute Osteomyelitis, Chronic Osteomyelitis

Acute Osteomyelitis: Early Diagnosis and Treatment

Acute osteomyelitis is a bacterial infection of bone, most commonly hematogenous in children and postoperative in adults. Timely diagnosis and antibiotics can prevent chronicity and surgical intervention.

FLOWCHART: Management of acute osteomyelitis.

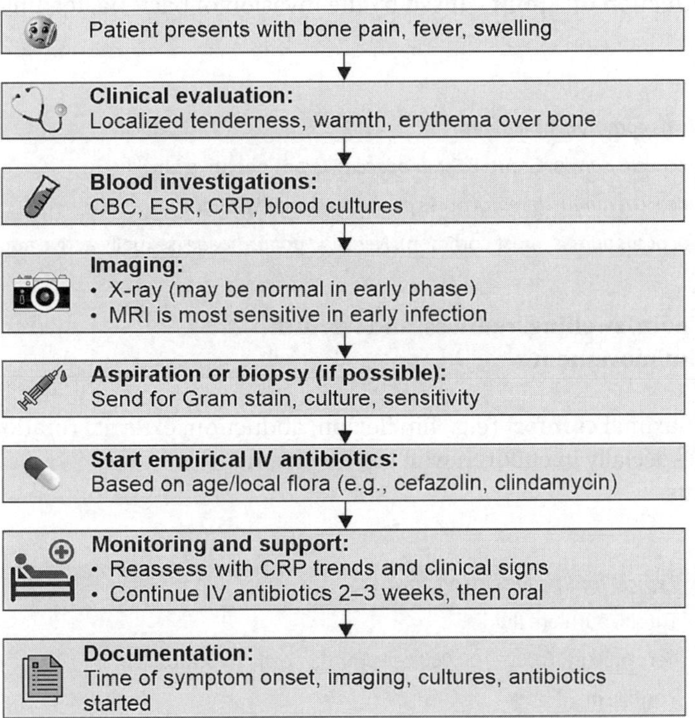

Key Points

- MRI is the best early diagnostic tool for osteomyelitis.
- Blood cultures and local aspiration help guide antibiotic therapy.

- Empirical antibiotics must cover *Staphylococcus aureus* and Streptococci.
- Monitor CRP for response and consider surgical drainage if no improvement.

Chronic Osteomyelitis

Progression from untreated or inadequately treated acute osteomyelitis → Chronic osteomyelitis

↓

Persistent infection + Dead bone (sequestrum)

↓

Sinus tract formation

Clinical features:
- Chronic pain
- Sinus tract discharge
- Bone deformity

Key Mnemonics:
- *Acute*: "Red hot bone" (pain, fever, swelling)
- *Chronic*: "Dead bone and drainage" (sequestrum and sinus)

Septic Arthritis

Q40. Describe septic arthritis with reference to clinical diagnosis, joint aspiration findings, and management.

(Asked in PGI Chandigarh 2022, AIIMS Delhi 2021)

Definition

Septic arthritis is an **acute infection of a joint** caused by the invasion of bacteria, leading to **rapid joint destruction** if not treated urgently.

Common Pathogens

Age Group	***Organisms commonly Involved***
Neonates	*Staphylococcus aureus,* Group B *Streptococcus*, Gram-negative bacilli
Children	*Staphylococcus aureus, Streptococcus pyogenes, Kingella kingae*
Adults	*Staphylococcus aureus* (most common), *Neisseria gonorrhoeae* (sexually active adults)

Clinical Diagnosis
- Acute onset **severe joint pain**, **swelling**, **redness**, and **warmth**.
- Marked **restriction of joint movement.**
- **Fever**, chills, malaise
- Joint held in position of maximal **comfort** (e.g., hip flexion, abduction, external rotation).
- Inability to bear weight (especially in children with hip involvement).
- **Pseudoparalysis** in infants.

Joint Aspiration Findings

Parameter	***Typical finding in septic arthritis***
Appearance	Turbid, purulent fluid
WBC count	Very high (>50,000–100,000 cells/mm^3; mostly neutrophils)
Gram stain	Positive in 50–75%
Culture	Definitive diagnosis
Glucose	Low compared to serum
Protein	Elevated

Management

Stage	*Action*
Immediate	Joint aspiration for diagnosis
Antibiotic therapy	Empirical IV antibiotics (targeting *Staphylococcus aureus*) immediately after cultures
Surgical intervention	Arthrotomy + lavage (especially for hip, shoulder) if severe infection or delayed diagnosis
Joint immobilization	Initial phase (short term)
Physiotherapy	To prevent stiffness post infection control

Empirical Antibiotic Choices
- IV cefazolin or clindamycin (children).
- Vancomycin if MRSA suspected.
- Later tailored based on culture results.

Important Point
Early treatment within **first 24–48 hours** prevents irreversible cartilage destruction!

Q41. Write a note on kocher's criteria for differentiating septic arthritis from transient synovitis.

(Asked in MUHS Maharashtra 2022)

Background
- Designed primarily for differentiating **septic arthritis** from **transient synovitis** in **pediatric hips**.
- Helpful in **early clinical decision-making** before full laboratory results are available.

Kocher's Four Criteria

Criterion	*Significance*
Non-weight bearing on affected side	Strong predictor
ESR > 40 mm/h	Indicates inflammation
Fever > 38.5°C (101.3°F)	Suggests systemic infection
WBC count > 12,000 cells/mm^3	Leukocytosis

Interpretation of Kocher's Criteria

Number of criteria positive	*Probability of septic arthritis*
1/4	~3%
2/4	~40%
3/4	~93%
4/4	~99%

Mnemonic for Kocher's Criteria: "FEWS"
- *F*ever,
- *E*SR raised,
- *W*BC raised,
- *S*tanding not possible (non-weight bearing).

Clinical Tip
- If ≥2 criteria positive → Strong suspicion → Proceed with aspiration and IV antibiotics.
- Always correlate with joint aspiration and imaging findings (e.g., ultrasound showing hip effusion).

Quick Tips for Theory and Viva
- Always emphasize that **joint aspiration** is both diagnostic and therapeutic.
- State clearly that **hip septic arthritis is a true orthopedic emergency**—needs immediate surgical drainage if suspected.

Short answer and viva questions about septic arthritis

Q42. Define septic arthritis. Classify it.

Definition

Septic arthritis is an **acute infection of the joint** caused by pyogenic organisms, leading to **joint inflammation, cartilage destruction**, and potential loss of function.

Classification

A. *Based on source*:
- Hematogenous spread (most common)
- Direct inoculation (e.g. post-surgery, trauma)
- Contiguous spread (e.g. from adjacent osteomyelitis)

B. *Based on organism*:
- *Pyogenic*: *Staphylococcus aureus, Streptococcus,* Gram-negatives
- Tubercular
- Fungal or viral

C. *Based on duration*:
- *Acute*: <2 weeks
- *Subacute*: 2–6 weeks
- *Chronic*: >6 weeks (e.g., TB)

Q43. Etiopathogenesis of septic arthritis.

Etiology
- **Bacteria** (e.g., *Staphylococcus aureus*, MRSA, *Streptococcus, Haemophilus influenzae*)
- *Mycobacterium tuberculosis* in chronic cases

Pathogenesis
1. *Bacterial entry into joint via*:
   - Hematogenous spread
   - Direct inoculation
   - Spread from adjacent tissues
2. Bacteria **adhere to synovium**
3. **Inflammatory response** → cytokine release (IL-1, TNF-α)
4. *Rapid cartilage degradation via*:
   - Enzymes from neutrophils
   - Pressure effects from effusion
5. Can lead to **joint destruction** in 48–72 hours if untreated

Q44. Clinical features and diagnosis.

(Madras Medical College Chennai Tamil Nadu 2010)

Clinical Features
- Sudden onset of **painful, swollen joint**
- **Fever, malaise**
- Joint is **warm, tender, erythematous**
- **Decreased ROM** (guarding due to pain)
- *Most commonly affected*: **Knee, hip, shoulder**

Diagnosis
- **CBC, ESR, CRP**—raised
- **Blood cultures** (positive in 50%)
- *Joint aspiration*: Purulent fluid, ↑ WBC count (>50,000/mm³), ↓ glucose
- Gram stain and culture
- *Imaging*: X-ray, MRI, Ultrasound

Q45. Radiological findings of septic arthritis.

- *X-ray (late signs)*:
    - Joint space **narrowing**
    - Periarticular **osteopenia**
    - **Bone erosions** at articular margins
- *Ultrasound*:
    - Detects **joint effusion**
    - Useful in **hip joint** (especially in children)
- *MRI*: Early detection of **synovial inflammation**, **effusion**, **bone edema**
- *CT*: Helps in **guiding aspiration**, defining joint anatomy

Q46. Differential diagnosis of septic arthritis.

Condition	*Differentiating features*
Reactive arthritis	Recent infection, sterile joint fluid
Gout/Pseudogout	Crystals in fluid, often monoarticular
Rheumatoid arthritis	Symmetrical, multiple joints, RF/anti-CCP positive
Hemarthrosis (bleeding disorders)	No infection signs, history of trauma or hemophilia
Tubercular arthritis	Chronic, insidious onset, caseous tissue

Q47. Synovial fluid analysis in septic arthritis (short note).

[Christian Medical College (CMC) Vellore Tamil Nadu 2008]

Gross Appearance
Turbid or purulent, yellowish

Microscopy
- WBC count > 50,000/mm^3 (mostly neutrophils)
- *Gram stain*: It may show organisms
- *Crystals*: To rule out gout/pseudogout

Culture
- Essential for identifying causative organism
- **Positive in 60–80%**

Glucose
Low (<50 mg/dL) compared to serum glucose

Q48. Principles of management of septic arthritis.

1. *Antibiotics*:
    - Empirical IV antibiotics → switched to targeted therapy after culture
    - Duration: **3–4 weeks IV**, followed by **oral antibiotics**
2. *Joint drainage*: Aspiration, arthroscopic lavage, or open arthrotomy, depending on the joint and response
3. *Immobilization*: Initial rest, followed by **early mobilization** to prevent stiffness
4. *Supportive care*: Analgesia, nutritional support

Q49. Role of arthroscopic lavage.

Indications
- Large joint involvement (e.g., **knee**, shoulder)
- Persistent or **recurrent effusion**
- To **avoid open arthrotomy**

Advantages

- Minimally invasive
- Allows **irrigation + debridement**
- Shorter hospital stay
- Faster recovery and **early mobilization**

Limitations

Not suitable for **deep-seated abscess**, extensive destruction

Q50. Complications of septic arthritis.

(Assam Medical College Dibrugarh 2007)

- Joint destruction and deformity
- Ankylosis (especially in TB arthritis)
- Osteomyelitis (spread to adjacent bone)
- Septicemia
- Growth disturbances (in children, especially hip)
- Chronic arthritis or **recurrent infection**

Q51. Indications for surgical intervention.

- Failure of aspiration/lavage
- Large purulent collections
- Severe joint destruction
- Inaccessible joints (e.g., hip in children)
- Septic arthritis with osteomyelitis

Flowchart Septic Arthritis

Septic arthritis is a medical emergency where bacteria invade a joint, causing inflammation and rapid cartilage destruction. Prompt aspiration and empirical antibiotic initiation are critical to preserve joint function.

FLOWCHART: Management of suspected septic arthritis.

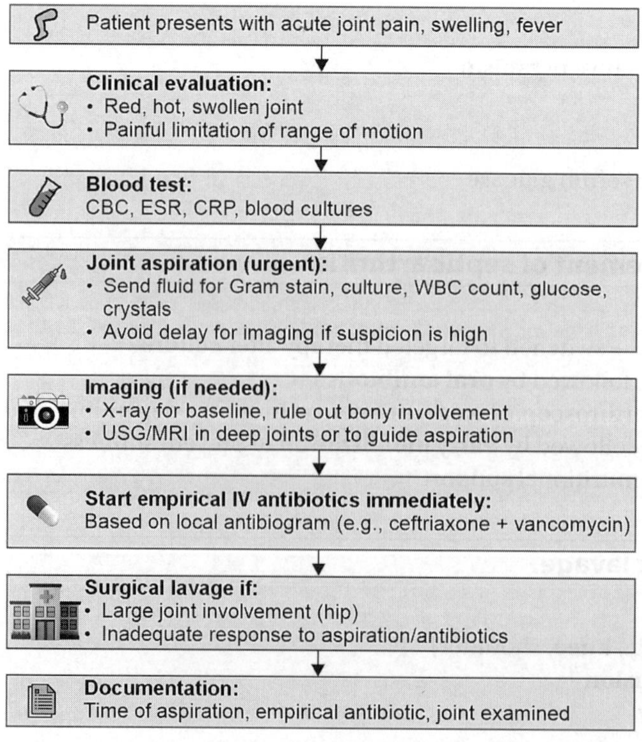

Key Points

- Do not delay joint aspiration in suspected septic arthritis.
- Empirical antibiotics should be started after aspiration.
- Large joints like the hip may need surgical drainage.
- Always send synovial fluid for cell count, culture, and crystals.

Prosthetic Joint Infections (PJI)

Q52. Describe prosthetic joint infections, including the risk factors, diagnosis, and management.

(Asked in JIPMER Puducherry 2022, PGI Chandigarh 2022)

Definition

Prosthetic Joint Infection (PJI) refers to **infection involving a joint prosthesis** and surrounding tissues, leading to implant failure if untreated.

Classification Based on Time of Onset

Type	*Time frame*	*Common organisms*
Early	<3 months	*Staphylococcus aureus*, Gram-negative bacilli
Delayed	3–24 months	Coagulase-negative Staphylococci, *Cutibacterium acnes*
Late	>24 months	Hematogenous spread (e.g., from urinary tract infection)

Risk Factors for PJI

Patient factors	*Surgical factors*
Diabetes mellitus	Poor surgical asepsis
Rheumatoid arthritis	Prolonged operative time
Obesity	Perioperative contamination
Immunosuppression	Revision surgery
Previous joint infection	Multiple surgeries

Diagnosis of PJI

Clinical Features:

- Painful joint (most consistent feature).
- Redness, warmth, swelling.
- Fever may be absent (especially in low-grade infections).

Investigations

Test	*Finding*
ESR and CRP	Elevated
Synovial fluid aspiration	High leukocyte count (>50,000/mm^3), neutrophil predominance
Synovial fluid culture	Positive bacterial growth
Synovial biomarkers	Alpha-defensin test (emerging, highly specific)
Blood cultures	Especially if hematogenous spread suspected
Imaging	X-rays (late), bone scans, PET scans for early detection

Musculoskeletal Infection Society (MSIS) Criteria

- Two positive cultures, or
- Sinus tract communicating with prosthesis, or
- Combination of minor criteria (raised ESR/CRP, elevated synovial WBC, etc.)

Q53. Describe DAIR, one-stage, and two-stage revision for infected prosthetic joints.

(Asked in MUHS Maharashtra 2023, AIIMS Delhi 2022)

Debridement, Antibiotics, and Implant Retention (DAIR)

- *Indication*: Early infection (<3–4 weeks after surgery) or acute hematogenous infections.
- *Procedure*:
  - Open debridement of infected tissue.
  - Exchange modular components (e.g., polyethylene liner in TKR).
  - Retain well-fixed prosthetic components.
  - Start culture-specific IV antibiotics.

One-stage Revision Arthroplasty

- *Indication*:
  - Good soft tissue condition.
  - Known sensitive organism.
  - Patient fit for single-stage major surgery.
- *Procedure*:
  - Remove infected prosthesis.
  - Radical debridement.
  - Immediate re-implantation of new prosthesis.
  - Antibiotics according to cultures.

Advantages

- Single surgery.
- Shorter hospital stay.
- Early rehabilitation.

Disadvantage

Slightly higher risk of reinfection compared to two-stage.

Two-stage Revision Arthroplasty (Gold Standard for Chronic Infection)

- *Indication*:
  - Chronic PJI (>4 weeks).
  - Unknown organism.
  - Poor soft tissues.
- *Procedure*:
  - *Stage 1*:
    - Explant prosthesis.
    - Thorough debridement.
    - Place antibiotic-loaded cement spacer.
    - IV antibiotics (6 weeks).
  - *Stage 2*: Reimplant new prosthesis after confirming infection clearance.

Advantage

Highest success rates (up to 90–95% infection eradication).

Disadvantages

- Two major surgeries.
- Increased morbidity.
- Longer rehabilitation.

Summary Table

Strategy	*Suitable for*	*Main points*
DAIR	Early infections (<3 weeks)	Retain implant + antibiotics
One-stage revision	Select chronic infections	Debridement + immediate reimplant
Two-stage revision	Chronic infections	Remove implant, antibiotics, delayed reimplant

Q54. Define prosthetic joint infections (PJI). Classify them.

Definition

Prosthetic joint infections (PJI) refers to **infection involving a joint prosthesis and surrounding tissue**, typically caused by bacteria adhering to the implant surface, forming a **biofilm**.

Classification

A. *Based on Timing (Zimmerli Classification)*

Type	*Timing*	*Common organisms*
Early	<3 months post-operative	*Staphylococcus aureus*, Gram-negatives
Delayed	3–24 months	Coagulase-negative Staphylococcus
Late	>24 months	Hematogenous spread pathogens

B. *Based on mode*:

- Perioperative (direct inoculation)
- Hematogenous spread
- Contiguous spread (e.g., skin ulcers)

Q55. Risk factors for prosthetic joint infections.

Patient Factors

- Diabetes mellitus
- Rheumatoid arthritis
- Immunosuppression
- Obesity, malnutrition
- Prior joint infection
- Smoking

Surgical Factors

- Poor surgical technique
- Long operating time
- Repeated surgeries/revisions
- Break in asepsis
- Use of drains

Prosthesis-related

- Cementless implants (early phase)
- Surface roughness favoring bacterial adhesion

Q56. Pathophysiology of prosthetic joint infections.

(Himachal Pradesh University Shimla 2013)

1. **Bacterial colonization** of prosthetic surface
2. *Formation of biofilm*:
    - Protects bacteria from antibiotics and immune response
    - Leads to **chronic low-grade infection**
3. **Local tissue damage** due to inflammatory mediators
4. Potential for **loosening**, **sinus formation**, and **implant failure**

Common Organisms

- *Staphylococcus aureus* (including MRSA)
- *Staphylococcus epidermidis*
- Gram-negative bacilli
- Polymicrobial in late-stage infections

Q57. Diagnostic criteria for PJI (short note).

Based on 2018 MSIS (Musculoskeletal Infection Society) Criteria

- *Major criteria (either one confirms PJI):*
    - **Sinus tract** communicating with the prosthesis
    - **Two or more positive cultures** with the same organism
- *Minor criteria (≥3 of 5 suggest PJI):*
    - Elevated **CRP/ESR**
    - Elevated **synovial WBC** or **PMN%**
    - Elevated **synovial alpha-defensin**
    - Positive **intraoperative purulence**
    - Single positive culture

Q58. Principles of management of PJI.

(Kashmir University 2011)

1. *Antibiotic therapy*:
    - Empirical → **culture-guided**
    - IV for 4–6 weeks, sometimes oral follow-up
2. *Surgical options*:
    - DAIR (Debridement, Antibiotics, Implant Retention)—for early infections
    - One-stage exchange—n select chronic cases
    - Two-stage revision—gold standard for chronic PJI
    - Resection arthroplasty (e.g., Girdlestone)—in non-reconstructable cases
    - Amputation—last resort
3. *Supportive measures*:
    - Optimize nutrition, comorbidities
    - Close follow-up with inflammatory markers

Q59. Role of two-stage revision arthroplasty in PJI.

Indications

- **Chronic PJI**, late infections
- **Failed one-stage revision**
- Highly virulent organisms

Procedure

1. *First stage*:
    - Remove infected prosthesis
    - **Thorough debridement**
    - Place **antibiotic-loaded cement spacer**
2. *Interim period*:
    - 6–8 weeks of systemic antibiotics
    - Monitor CRP/ESR
3. *Second stage*: Once infection markers normalize → re-implantation with new prosthesis

Advantages

- High infection eradication rate (~90%)
- Tailored antibiotic therapy

Q60. Antibiotic-loaded cement spacers in PJI (short note).

Definition

Temporary **PMMA cement constructs** containing antibiotics used during first-stage revision to maintain joint space and deliver local antibiotics.

Types
- *Static spacers*: Immobilize joint
- *Articulating spacers*: Allow limited movement

Antibiotics Used
- Gentamicin, vancomycin, tobramycin
- Heat-stable antibiotics compatible with cement

Advantages
- High local antibiotic levels
- Maintains limb length and alignment
- Facilitates reimplantation

Flowchart: Prosthetic Joint Infection (PJI)
- **Etiology**
  - *Early infection (<3 months)*: *Staphylococcus aureus*, Gram-negative bacilli
  - *Delayed infection (3–24 months)*: Coagulase-negative Staphylococci
  - *Late infection (>24 months)*: Hematogenous spread

Pathogenesis

Bacterial adherence to prosthesis

Biofilm formation

Protection from immune system and antibiotics

Persistent infection

Clinical Features
- Pain (most common)
- Swelling
- Warmth and erythema
- Sinus tract formation (late)
- Fever (may be absent in chronic infection)

Diagnosis
- *Blood tests*: ↑ ESR, ↑ CRP
- *Joint aspiration*: Synovial fluid WBC count, Gram stain, culture
- *Imaging*:
  - *X-ray*: loosening, periosteal reaction
  - Nuclear scans (WBC-tagged scan, FDG-PET)
- Intraoperative multiple tissue cultures

Management
- *Acute (<3–4 weeks)*: Debridement, antibiotics, implant retention (DAIR)
- *Chronic infection*:
  - *Two-stage revision arthroplasty*:
    1. Prosthesis removal + debridement + antibiotic spacer
    2. Reimplantation after infection control
- Long-term suppressive antibiotics in selected cases

Key Points
- Biofilm formation is the major barrier to treatment.
- Two-stage revision is gold standard for chronic PJI.
- ESR and CRP are sensitive screening tests.

Quick Tips for Theory and Viva

- Always **classify PJI based on timing** (early, delayed, late).
- Mention **ESR + CRP + Synovial Fluid Analysis** as initial diagnostic steps.
- Know **DAIR** is for early cases; **two-stage revision is gold standard** for chronic cases.

Mnemonic for PJI Management Options: "D-O-T"

- **D**AIR → Early
- **O**ne-stage → Selected
- **T**wo-stage → Chronic

Q61. Define pyomyositis. Classify it.

[King George's Medical University (KGMU) Lucknow Uttar Pradesh 2013]

Definition

Pyomyositis is a **bacterial infection of skeletal muscle**, leading to **intramuscular abscess formation**, often in the **absence of trauma**.

Common Pathogen

- *Staphylococcus aureus* (most common)
- *Others*: *Streptococcus*, Gram-negative bacilli

Classification (Clinical Stages)

Stage	*Features*
1. Invasive	Low-grade fever, localized muscle pain, no abscess
2. Suppurative	Abscess formation, fever, muscle tenderness
3. Septicemic	Systemic toxicity, multiple abscesses, sepsis

Q62. Clinical features and management of pyomyositis.

Clinical Features

- Fever, malaise
- **Localized pain and swelling**
- Tender, firm muscle mass
- **Limited joint movement** (due to adjacent muscle involvement)
- Commonly affects **quadriceps, glutei, iliopsoas**

Investigations

- *CBC*: ↑ WBC
- *ESR/CRP*: Elevated
- *Ultrasound or MRI*: To confirm abscess
- **Aspiration or culture** for organism identification

Management

- *Stage 1*: IV antibiotics (e.g., anti-staph)
- *Stage 2/3*:
  - **Surgical drainage** of abscess
  - Continue antibiotics for 2–4 weeks
  - Supportive care and physiotherapy

Q63. Necrotizing soft tissue infections (NSTI)—short note.

Definition

Necrotizing soft tissue infections (NSTI) are rapidly progressive, **life-threatening infections of fascia, subcutaneous tissue**, and sometimes muscle, characterized by **tissue necrosis and systemic toxicity**.

Types

- *Type I*: Polymicrobial (most common)
- *Type II*: Monomicrobial (*Streptococcus pyogenes*)
- *Type III*: Gas gangrene (*Clostridium*)
- *Type IV*: Fungal (rare)

Clinical Clues

- **Pain out of proportion** to clinical findings
- Erythema, swelling, blisters
- Skin discoloration, **crepitus**, foul-smelling discharge
- Rapid progression to sepsis

Investigations

- **LRINEC score** (CRP, WBC, Hb, sodium, creatinine)
- *CT/MRI*: Fascial edema, gas

Management

1. **Urgent surgical debridement** (life-saving)
2. Broad-spectrum **IV antibiotics** (e.g., piperacillin-tazobactam + clindamycin)
3. **Hemodynamic stabilization**
4. **ICU care** if sepsis is present
5. **Serial debridement** is often needed
6. **NPWT** and later reconstruction (grafts/flaps)

Q64. Principles of surgical debridement in soft tissue infections.

(Himachal Pradesh University Shimla 2016)

Objectives

- Remove all **necrotic, infected, and non-viable tissue**
- Reduce **bacterial load**
- Improve local vascularity
- Prevent further spread of infection

Principles

- **Timely and aggressive** debridement
- Extend beyond visibly infected zones if needed
- Preserve as much **vital tissue** as possible
- Repeat debridement (serial) until clean wound base
- Use **sharp dissection**, avoid blind tunneling

Post-debridement

- Irrigation
- NPWT application
- Antibiotic therapy adjustment
- Plan for reconstruction (skin grafts/flaps)

Q65. Role of negative pressure wound therapy (NPWT).

Definition

Negative pressure wound therapy (NPWT) (VAC therapy) uses **controlled sub-atmospheric pressure** over a sealed wound via a foam dressing connected to a vacuum device.

Mechanism

- Removes **exudate and infection**
- Reduces **edema**

- Improves **blood flow**
- Stimulates **granulation tissue formation**
- **Enhances epithelial migration**
- **Reduces bacterial colonization**
- **Applies negative pressure to uniformly raw wound (wound contraction)**

Indications
- Post-debridement in **soft tissue infections**
- **Open wounds**, flap/graft beds
- Infected surgical wounds
- Delayed primary closure cases

Benefits
- Faster wound healing
- Decreased dressing frequency
- Lower bacterial load
- Bridges time to definitive reconstruction
- Provision of closed, moist wound healing environment
- Control of odor and exudate
- Reduction in complexity and number of surgical procedure

Q66. Role of new-generation antibiotics in musculoskeletal infections.

Examples
- *Linezolid*: Effective against MRSA, VRE
- *Daptomycin*: Bactericidal against resistant Gram-positive cocci
- *Tigecycline*: Broad spectrum including multidrug-resistant organisms
- *Ceftaroline*: β-lactam active against MRSA
- *Delafloxacin*: New fluoroquinolone with Gram+/– activity

Uses
- Prosthetic joint infections
- Osteomyelitis resistant to standard antibiotics
- Infections in immunocompromised patients

Q67. Diabetic foot infections—short note.

(AIIMS Delhi)

Pathogenesis
Neuropathy + ischemia + impaired immunity

Common Organisms
Staphylococcus aureus, Escherichia coli, anaerobes

Classification
Mild, moderate, severe (based on IDSA guidelines)

Another Classification
Wagner, University of Texas

PES Anatomic Staging for Diabetic Foot Osteomyelitis
(Useful specifically for diabetic foot infections)

Based on
- *P*: Perfusion (vascular status)
- *E*: Extent (area and depth of infection)
- *S*: Sepsis (systemic signs of infection)

Management
- **Glycemic control**
- **Wound debridement**
- Culture-based **antibiotics**
- **Off-loading** (orthotics, total contact cast)
- Revascularization if ischemic
- Amputation if non-salvageable

Q68. Role of immunocompromised states in MSK infections.

Conditions
- HIV/AIDS
- Diabetes mellitus
- Cancer/chemotherapy
- Long-term steroid use
- Organ transplant recipients

Effects
- Impaired **neutrophil and macrophage function**
- Increased susceptibility to **opportunistic infections**
- Delayed diagnosis due to **atypical presentations**
- Higher risk of **chronic and disseminated infections**

Q69. Challenges in managing MSK infections in HIV-positive patients.

Key Issues
- Atypical pathogens (e.g., *Mycobacterium avium*, fungi)
- **Delayed healing** and poor response to standard antibiotics
- Drug interactions with **HAART**
- Higher incidence of **septic arthritis, TB, osteomyelitis**
- Surgical wound complications

Q70. Role of hyperbaric oxygen therapy (HBOT).

[King George's Medical University (KGMU) Lucknow Uttar Pradesh 2016]

Principle
Delivers **100% oxygen at increased atmospheric pressure**, improving tissue oxygenation.

Benefits
- Enhances **neutrophil killing**
- Inhibits **anaerobic organisms**
- Promotes **angiogenesis and wound healing**
- Aids in **refractory osteomyelitis, diabetic foot ulcers**

Indications
- Chronic osteomyelitis
- Refractory diabetic foot infections
- Necrotizing fasciitis (adjunctive)

Q71. Role of antibiotic stewardship in Orthopedics.

Goals
- Prevent **overuse and misuse** of antibiotics
- Reduce **antibiotic resistance**

- Promote **culture-based therapy**
- Optimize **dose, duration, and route**

Key Components

- **Multidisciplinary approach** (ID physician, ortho, pharmacist)
- **Documentation** of the indication and plan
- De-escalation once the culture results are available
- Avoid prolonged broad-spectrum use

Q72. Gas gangrene.

- **Also called clostridial myonecrosis**
- *Organism*: *Clostridium perfringens (most common), Clostridium novyi, Clostridium septicum*
- *Pathophysiology*: *C. perfringens* alpha toxin causes muscle necrosis and vessel thrombosis which leads to hemolysis and shock.
- *Gas produced by fermentation of glucose*: Main component is nitrogen
- *Signs*: Sudden pain, crepitus, foul-smelling discharge, blebs and hemorrhagic bullae, "dishwater pus" discharge, altered mental status
- *Triad*:
  - Progressive pain out of proportion to injury
  - Tachycardia not explained by fever
  - Feeling of impending doom
- *Rx*: Urgent surgical debridement, IV penicillin and clindamycin, hyperbaric oxygen, supportive care

Q73. Septic shock.

(Kashmir University 2015)

- *Definition*: Sepsis with hypotension despite fluid resuscitation
- *Rx*: IV fluids, vasopressors (norepinephrine), broad-spectrum antibiotics, ICU care

Q74. Synergistic gangrene (Fournier's gangrene).

- **Polymicrobial necrotizing fasciitis**
- *Sites*: Perineum, limbs
- *Rx*: Broad-spectrum antibiotics + urgent debridement

Q75. Ulcer/Neuritis in leprosy.

- *Cause*: Peripheral nerve involvement → sensory loss
- *Management*: MDT therapy, protective footwear, wound care

Q76. Cellulitis.

(Assam Medical College Dibrugarh 2017)

- *Organism*: *Streptococcus pyogenes, Staphylococcus aureus*
- *Signs*: Warmth, erythema, swelling
- *Rx*: Elevation, IV antibiotics, rest

Q77. Urinary tract infection (UTI)—relevance in ortho.

- **Pre-operative screening** in arthroplasty/spine cases
- *Management*: Urine culture-specific antibiotics, delay elective surgery until treated

Q78. Complications of chronic discharging sinus.

- Squamous cell carcinoma (Marjolin ulcer)
- Osteomyelitis
- Pathological fracture
- Fibrosis
- Secondary infection

Q79. Debridement in orthopedics.

(Assam Medical College Dibrugarh 2012)

- *Types*: Sharp, mechanical, enzymatic, autolytic
- *Indications*: Infected wound, necrotic tissue, osteomyelitis
- *Principles*:
  - Remove all necrotic bone/tissue
  - Preserve vital structures
  - Irrigate thoroughly
  - Send cultures
- *Follow-up*: Antibiotics + secondary closure/grafting

Q80. Leprosy (Musculoskeletal Involvement).

- *Agent*: *Mycobacterium leprae*.
- *Orthopedic manifestations*:
  - Neuropathic joints.
  - Absorption of digits ("pencilling" of bones).
  - Non-healing ulcers.
- *Treatment*: Multidrug therapy (dapsone, rifampicin, clofazimine).

Q81. Maduramycosis (madura foot).

Definition

Chronic granulomatous infection of foot.

Causative agents

Actinomycetes (bacteria) or eumycetes (fungi).

Clinical Features

Swelling, discharging sinuses, granules. Exudates are granular

Diagnosis

- Direct microscopy, biopsy, culture of granules, leucocytosis/neutrophilia, DNA sequencing of conserved genes (HSP65)
- *Radiography*: Cortical thinning; multiple lytic lesions or cavities may be large and few in number with well defined margins (eumycetoma) or small and numerus with ill defined margins (actinomycetoma); osteoporosis

Treatment

- Due to slow, relatively pain free progression of disease, mycetoma is often at advanced stage when diagnosed
- Prolonged antibiotics (actinomycetoma) or antifungals (eumycetoma).
- Surgical debridement often required.
- Amputation in severe cases

Tip

For each infection, remember the key:

- Etiology
- Clinical features
- Diagnosis
- Treatment

Q82. Pyogenic Discitis.

[Rajendra Institute of Medical Sciences (RIMS) Ranchi Jharkhand 2017]

Definition

Infection of the intervertebral disc, usually hematogenous.

Common Organism

Staphylococcus aureus (most common).

Clinical Features

- Severe localized back pain.
- Fever, malaise (variable).
- Restricted spinal movements.
- Neurological deficit rare.

Diagnosis

- ↑ ESR, ↑ CRP.
- *MRI*: Disc space narrowing, end plate changes.
- Blood culture positive in ~50–70%.
- CT-guided disc biopsy if needed.

Treatment

- IV antibiotics 4–6 weeks → oral antibiotics (total 6–12 weeks).
- Spinal rest and immobilization.
- Surgery if abscess, instability, or no response to antibiotics.

Prognosis

- Good with early treatment.
- Delay → risk of abscess, chronic infection.

Q83. Gonococcal arthritis.

- *Agent*: *Neisseria gonorrhoeae.*
- *Features*:
  - Acute septic arthritis in young sexually active adults.
  - Migratory polyarthritis, tenosynovitis, skin lesions.
- *Joints*: Knee, wrist, ankle.
- *Diagnosis*: Synovial fluid gram stain/culture, NAAT.
- *Treatment*: IV ceftriaxone ± joint aspiration.

Q84. Syphilitic bone disease.

- *Causative agent*: *Treponema pallidum.*
- *Congenital*:
  - Clutton's joints (painless bilateral knee hydrarthrosis).
  - Saber shin (anterior bowing of tibia).

- *Acquired*:
    - Gummatous osteitis.
    - Charcot joint (neuropathic arthropathy).
- *Diagnosis*: VDRL, FTA-ABS.
- *Treatment*: Penicillin.

Q85. Musculoskeletal infections by fungi—short note.

(West Bengal University of Health Sciences Kolkata 2011)

Common Fungi

Candida, Aspergillus, Cryptococcus, Histoplasma

Predisposing Factors

- Immunocompromised states
- Indwelling catheters
- Post-surgical patients

Sites

- Vertebrae (fungal spondylodiscitis)
- Joints (fungal arthritis)

Diagnosis

Fungal culture, **KOH mount, histopathology, serology**

Treatment

- Long-term **antifungal therapy** (e.g., amphotericin B, azoles)
- Surgical debridement if necessary

Q86. Lyme disease—short note.

Cause

Borrelia burgdorferi transmitted by **Ixodes tick**

Stages

1. *Early localized*: Erythema migrans
2. *Early disseminated*: Migratory joint pain
3. *Late stage*: **Chronic arthritis**, especially knee

Diagnosis

ELISA, Western blot, PCR

Treatment

- **Doxycycline** or **amoxicillin** (early)
- **Ceftriaxone** for neuro/MSK involvement

Q87. Leprosy (Hansen's disease)—musculoskeletal manifestations.

[Jawaharlal Institute of Postgraduate Medical Education and Research (JIPMER) Puducherry 2010]

- *Agent*: *Mycobacterium leprae.*
- *Skeletal involvement*:
    - Neuropathic joints (Charcot's arthropathy).
    - Bone resorption (pencilling of digits).
    - Osteomyelitis of small bones.
- *Peripheral neuropathy*: Ulnar, common peroneal, posterior tibial nerves.
- *Diagnosis*: Skin smear, biopsy.
- *Treatment*: Multidrug therapy (rifampicin, dapsone, clofazimine).

Q88. Caffey's disease (infantile cortical hyperostosis).

- *Definition*: Rare, self-limiting inflammatory bone disorder of infants.
- *Age*: <6 months; usually presents in the first few weeks.
- *Etiology*: Unknown; possible genetic predisposition (COL1A1 mutation).
- *Clinical features*:
  - Painful swelling (commonly mandible, clavicle, ulna).
  - Irritability, fever, pseudoparalysis.
- *Radiology*: Subperiosteal new bone formation, cortical thickening.
- *Treatment*: Supportive—NSAIDs, resolves spontaneously.

Q89. Recent advances in diagnosing and managing MSK infections.

(Amrita Institute of Medical Sciences Kochi Kerala 2008)

Diagnosis
- PCR and GeneXpert for rapid TB diagnosis
- Next-generation sequencing (NGS) for unknown pathogens
- PET-CT for chronic or multifocal infections

Management
- Antimicrobial-loaded implants
- Silver/iodine coatings to prevent colonization
- Biodegradable antibiotic beads
- One-stage revision arthroplasty in select PJI cases

Q90. Role of molecular diagnostics in MSK infections.

Techniques
1. *Polymerase chain reaction (PCR)*: Detects microbial DNA
2. *GeneXpert*: Rapid TB identification
3. *Next-generation sequencing (NGS)*: Identifies rare or fastidious organisms
4. *Multiplex PCR panels*: Detect multiple pathogens

Advantages
- **High sensitivity**
- Works with **low sample volumes**
- Identifies **non-culturable organisms**
- *Follow-up*: Antibiotics + secondary closure/grafting

Q91. Cytokines and inflammatory markers in MSK infections.

Key Cytokines
- *IL-1, IL-6, TNF-α*: Mediate inflammation, fever, bone destruction
- *IFN-γ*: Enhances macrophage activation

Markers
- *CRP*: Rises quickly, useful for monitoring
- *ESR*: Elevated in chronic infections
- *Procalcitonin*: Specific for bacterial infections
- *Alpha-defensin*: Marker for PJI

Clinical Role

Aid in **diagnosis**, **monitoring treatment**, and **assessing severity**

Q92. Role of biofilm formation in implant-associated infections.

[Kasturba Medical College (KMC) Manipal Karnataka 2013]

What is a Biofilm?

A structured bacterial community enclosed in **self-produced extracellular polymeric substance (EPS)**.

Formation Steps

1. Adhesion to implant surface
2. Colonization and EPS production
3. Maturation into multi-layered structure
4. Detachment and spread to new sites

Clinical Implications

- Highly **resistant to antibiotics** and immune clearance
- Source of **chronic and recurrent infections**
- Requires **implant removal** for eradication

Antibiofilm agents

- Rifampicin has been widely used to prevent biofilms
- *Shot term*: Lactoferrin, xylitol, gallium, farnesol,deferoxamine, EDTA, Dispersin B, Fatty acid gel, nitric oxide
- *Long term*: Quorum sensing inhibitor (RNA III inhibitory peptide, Furanones, autoinducer)

Q93. Role of neutrophils in orthopedic infections (short note).

Functions

- First-line immune cells in **acute bone infections**
- *Kill pathogens via*:
  - Phagocytosis
  - Degranulation
  - Reactive oxygen species (ROS)
  - Formation of **neutrophil extracellular traps (NETs)**

In Osteomyelitis

- Contribute to **pus formation**
- Can exacerbate tissue damage if excessive
- Chronic infections often show **neutrophil dysfunction**

Q94. Molecular basis of chronic osteomyelitis.

(Grant Medical College Mumbai 2017)

Key Mechanisms

1. **Persistent infection** within **biofilm** on necrotic bone or implants
2. **Sequestrum** acts as bacterial reservoir
3. **Downregulation of immune responses** (low antigen presentation, T-cell inhibition)
4. Bacteria enter **stationary phase**, limiting antibiotic efficacy
5. *Upregulation of pro-inflammatory cytokines*: IL-1, IL-6, TNF-α
6. Poor vascularization limits drug delivery

Result

- Chronic inflammation
- Delayed healing
- Sinus formation

Q95. Mechanisms of antibiotic resistance in musculoskeletal infections.

Bacterial Strategies

1. Enzymatic inactivation (e.g., β-lactamases)
2. Target modification (e.g., altered PBPs in MRSA)
3. Efflux pumps expel antibiotics
4. Biofilm formation limits penetration
5. Persistence and dormancy in hostile environments

Clinical Implication

- Requires combination therapy, higher doses, or newer agents
- Reinforces importance of **antibiotic stewardship**

Others Long Questions

Q96. Management of infected non-union of long bones + induced membrane technique.

[Assam Medical College (affiliated to Srimanta Sankaradeva University of Health Sciences) 2020]

Principles of Managing Infected Non-union

1. *Eradication of infection*:
    - Debridement (multiple if needed)
    - Culture-specific antibiotics (6–12 weeks)
2. *Stabilization*:
    - External fixation (Ilizarov preferred)
    - Avoid internal fixation in active infection unless absolutely needed
3. *Dead space management*:
    - Use of antibiotic beads/spacers
    - Induced membrane technique (Masquelet)
4. *Biological augmentation*:
    - Bone grafting
    - Bone transport if needed (Ilizarov)
5. *Soft tissue cover*: Flaps/grafts if soft tissue is compromised

Induced Membrane Technique (Masquelet Technique)

- *Stage 1*:
    - Thorough debridement
    - Insertion of **PMMA cement spacer** (antibiotic-loaded)
    - Spacer induces **vascularized membrane**
    - Wait 4–6 weeks
- *Stage 2*:
    - Remove spacer, preserve membrane
    - Fill cavity with **autologous cancellous bone graft**
    - Membrane aids graft vascularization and infection control

Advantages

- Simple, reproducible
- Useful in large bone defects
- Promotes biologic healing in infected environment

Q97. Acute hematogenous osteomyelitis—pathogenesis + age differences.

Pathogenesis

- Blood-borne spread from remote infection (e.g., throat, skin)

- Bacteria lodge in metaphyseal vessels (slow flow → bacterial adherence)
- Inflammatory response → pus formation
- Increased intraosseous pressure → cortical destruction → sequestrum

Differences by Age

Age group	*Features*
Infants (<1 year)	Vessels cross physis → epiphysis and joint involved early
Children (1–16)	Metaphyseal focus, physis blocks joint spread
Adults	No physis → direct extension into joint

Classification

Early (<3 weeks), delayed, late (>3 months)

Management Principles

1. *Diagnosis*: Clinical signs, CRP/ESR, imaging, aspiration
2. *Surgical management*:
   - *Debridement, antibiotics, implant retention (DAIR)*: Early infections
   - *One-stage exchange*: Low-virulence organisms, good soft tissue
   - *Two-stage exchange*: Gold standard for chronic infection
   - *Removal without reimplantation*: In high-risk patients
3. *Antibiotics*:
   - Empiric → culture-specific
   - Prolonged (6–12 weeks)
4. *Supportive care*: Nutrition, comorbid control, wound care

Short Notes (SN)

Q98. Cervical lymphadenopathy.

(Kashmir University 2010)

- *Causes*: TB, lymphoma, metastatic disease
- *Workup*: FNAC, biopsy, USG
- *Ortho link*: TB spine often presents with cervical nodes

Q99. Nosocomial infections in orthopedics–organisms and prevention.

- *Common organisms*: MRSA, CoNS, *Pseudomonas, Klebsiella, Acinetobacter*
- *Prevention*: Sterile technique, antibiotic prophylaxis, surgical prep, hand hygiene

Q100. Hospital-acquired infection.

- Infections >48 hours after hospital admission
- Includes **SSI, UTI, pneumonia, bloodstream infections**
- Monitored using CDC definitions

Q101. Pyogenic psoas abscess.

(AIIMS Bhubaneswar 2013)

- *Primary*: Hematogenous (rare)
- *Secondary*: TB spine, Crohn's, appendicitis
- *Signs*: Fever, back pain, psoas sign
- *Management*: Imaging + drainage + antibiotics

Q102. Ring sequestrum.

- *Definition*: Circular dead bone surrounded by involucrum
- Common in chronic osteomyelitis or TB spine
- Seen on imaging, often requires debridement

Q103. Garre's sclerosing osteomyelitis.

(Kasturba Medical College Manipal 2018)

- Chronic low-grade osteomyelitis with **dense periosteal reaction**
- Symmetrical thickening of bone and irregularity but with conspicuous absence of abscess and sequestra (Brodie's has abscess but no sequestra)
- **Mandible** commonly affected
- Seen in children
- Treatment is conservative or surgical if symptomatic

Q104. Implant infection.

- **Biofilm formation** on implant surfaces
- Hard to eradicate without removing implant
- Treated with DAIR or revision arthroplasty

Q105. Antimicrobial resistance.

- *Causes*: Overuse, misuse of antibiotics
- *Organisms*: MRSA, VRE, CRE
- *Consequences*: Limited treatment options, higher morbidity
- Urgent need for antibiotic stewardship

Q106. Surgical site infection (SSI) and WHO guidelines.

(Amrita Institute of Medical Sciences 2016)

- *Definition*: Infection within 30 days post-surgery or 90 days with implant
- *WHO prevention*:
    - Pre-operative bath
    - Antibiotics 60 mins before incision
    - Alcohol-based antiseptic
    - Normothermia
    - Glycemic control
    - Limited hair removal

Q107. Vacuum assisted closure (VAC). Discuss contraindications and complications of VAC.

- Negative pressure wound therapy
- Promotes granulation, reduces edema, controls exudate
- Used in chronic wounds, infected wounds, open fractures

Contraindications of VAC

1. Exposed blood vessels (no protective fascia)
2. Untreated osteomyelitis
3. Unexplored fistula
4. Malignant wounds

5. Necrotic tissue with eschar
6. Active bleeding or patient on anticoagulant therapy
7. Untreated malnutrition
8. Non compliant patients

Complications of VAC

1. Pain while removing adhesive tape
2. Retained sponge may lead to infection
3. Dehydration in children due to suction of fluid from wound
4. Maceration of skin
5. Hematoma in surrounding tissue
6. Wound dehiscence in immunocompromised patients

Q108. Radiological features of osteomyelitis and role of MRI.

- *X-ray (late findings)*: Periosteal reaction, osteolytic lesions, sequestrum, involucrum.
- *MRI (modality of choice)*:
  - Detects early marrow edema.
  - High sensitivity for soft tissue extension and abscess.
- *CT*: Useful for detecting sequestra and cortical involvement.
- *Bone scan*: High sensitivity but low specificity.

MRI > **CT** > **X-ray** in early diagnosis.

Q109. Role of antibiotics and indications for surgery in osteomyelitis.

[Assam Medical College (affiliated to Srimanta Sankaradeva University of Health Sciences) 2021]

- **Empirical antibiotics** started after cultures.
- Tailored to causative organism (e.g., *Staphylococcus aureus*).
- *Duration*: IV for 2–6 weeks, followed by oral.
- *Surgery indicated for*:
  - Sequestrum
  - Chronic infection
  - Failure of medical therapy
  - Abscess formation

Q110. Principles of surgical debridement in chronic osteomyelitis.

- Adequate exposure and removal of all necrotic tissue.
- Sequestrectomy and saucerization.
- Culture from debrided tissue.
- Use of local antibiotic spacers.
- Second-stage bone reconstruction (e.g., Masquelet).

Q111. Septic arthritis versus reactive arthritis.

Feature	*Septic arthritis*	*Reactive arthritis*
Cause	Direct infection (bacteria)	Post-infectious immune response
Synovial fluid	Purulent, +ve cultures	Sterile, WBCs ↑
Treatment	Antibiotics + drainage	NSAIDs, DMARDs
Prognosis	Rapid joint destruction possible	Usually self-limiting

Q112. Antibiotic choices in septic arthritis.

(Jammu University 2014)

- *Staphylococcus aureus*: Cefazolin, Vancomycin (if MRSA)
- *Gram-negatives*: Ceftriaxone, Ciprofloxacin
- *Gonococcal*: Ceftriaxone
- *Tubercular*: ATT (RIPE)
- Based on culture/sensitivity and adjusted accordingly.

Q113. Masquelet technique.

- *Two-stage procedure for segmental bone defects*:
  - *Stage 1*: Debridement + PMMA spacer (induces bio-membrane)
  - *Stage 2*: After 6–8 weeks, spacer removed, cavity filled with autograft.
- Encourages vascularization and osteogenesis.

Q114. Local antibiotic delivery in MSK infections.

- **Antibiotic-impregnated PMMA beads/spacers**
- High local concentration, low systemic toxicity.
- Used post-debridement.
- *Common drugs*: Gentamicin, Vancomycin.

Q115. Suppressive antibiotic therapy.

(Sri Ramachandra Institute of Higher Education and Research 2014)

- *Long-term, low-dose antibiotics used*:
  - In elderly/unfit patients
  - Where complete surgical debridement isn't feasible
- *Goal*: Prevent progression, not curative.

Q116. Risk factors for surgical site infection (SSI).

- *Patient factors*: Diabetes, malnutrition, smoking, immunosuppression
- *Surgical factors*: Prolonged duration, poor asepsis, contaminated implants
- *Hospital factors*: Overcrowding, antibiotic misuse

Q117. Surgical site infection (SSI)—definition.

An infection occurring within 30 days of surgery (or within 90 days if implant is placed), involving the incision, deep tissue, or organ space.

Q118. WHO guidelines for prevention of surgical site infections (2016 update).

Preoperative Measures

- Preoperative bathing with soap
- Hair removal only when necessary (clipper, not razor)
- Administer prophylactic antibiotics within 60 minutes before incision
- Screen/treat MRSA in high-risk patients

Intraoperative Measures
- Maintain normothermia
- Maintain blood glucose <180 mg/dL
- Avoid using surgical drains unless indicated
- Antiseptic wound irrigation (e.g., aqueous povidone-iodine)

Postoperative Measures
- Wound dressing for 48 hours
- Sterile technique for dressing changes
- No topical antimicrobial application unless indicated

Q119. Risk factors for surgical site infections.

(Seth Gordhandas Sunderdas Medical College and KEM Hospital 2009)

Patient-related
- Diabetes
- Malnutrition
- Immunosuppression
- Obesity
- Smoking
- Pre-existing infections

Surgery-related
- Prolonged duration
- Blood loss
- Implant use
- Emergency surgery
- Poor aseptic technique

Hospital-related
- Contaminated environment
- Inadequate sterilization
- Overuse of antibiotics

Q120. Postoperative fever—causes.

Follows the "5 W's"
1. *Wind (day 1-2)*: Atelectasis or pneumonia
2. *Water (day 3–5)*: UTI
3. *Wound (day 5–7)*: Surgical site infection
4. *Walking (day 5+)*: DVT/PE
5. *Wonder drugs*: Drug fever

In Orthopedics, also consider
- Septic arthritis
- Osteomyelitis
- Implant-related infection

Q121. Suppurative tenosynovitis.

- *Definition*: Pus in a tendon sheath, commonly in fingers (flexor tendons)
- *Etiology*: Usually due to penetrating injury or spread from local infection (*Staphylococcus aureus* most common)

- *Kanavel's signs (diagnostic)*:
    1. Finger held in flexion
    2. Fusiform swelling
    3. Tenderness along tendon sheath
    4. Pain on passive extension
- *Treatment*:
    1. Urgent surgical drainage
    2. Broad-spectrum antibiotics

Q122. Sequelae of Osteomyelitis in Children

(AIIMS Jodhpur 2019)

- Chronic osteomyelitis
- *Growth disturbances*: Physeal damage → limb length discrepancy or angular deformity
- Pathological fracture
- Joint stiffness or ankylosis
- Sinus tract formation
- Sequestrum/involucrum formation
- Amyloidosis (rare, late)
- Recurrence due to incomplete treatment

Q123. Tom smith arthritis (infantile septic hip).

- Septic arthritis of hip
- Seen in infants
- Head of femur is completely destroyed by the pyogenic process
- *Pathophysiology*: Transphyseal vessels are present in early infancy before the formation of growth plate. This may account for the frequency of septic arthritis of the hip in neonate
- In children, about a third of long bone osteomyelitis is associated with septic arthritis of the adjacent joint

C/F

- Onset is acute with rapid abscess formation
- Can be mistaken for a superficial infection
- Can present later with complaints of limp without any pain
- *O/e*: Affected limb is shorter and hip movements are increased in all directions
- Telescopy test- positive

X-ray

Complete absence of head and neck of femur

Treatment

- Acute Surgical emergency
- Open drainage of hip is the most effective method treatment
- *Sequelae*: AVN femoral head, limb shortening, joint dislocation

Q124. *Mycobacterium tuberculosis* in musculoskeletal infections.

- *Common forms:*
    - Pott's spine
    - Tubercular arthritis
    - Tubercular osteomyelitis
    - Cold abscess

- *Diagnosis*:
    - CB-NAAT/GeneXpert
    - Histopathology (caseating granuloma)
    - AFB staining and culture (Lowenstein–Jensen)
    - ESR, CRP, imaging (X-ray, MRI)
- *Treatment*:
    - ATT (2 months HRZE + 10 months HR)
    - Surgery in case of abscess, deformity, instability

Quick Mindmap: Infections in Orthopedics

- *Infections in orthopedics*:
    - *Acute osteomyelitis*:
        - MRI early detection
        - IV antibiotics + drainage
    - *Chronic osteomyelitis*:
        - Sequestrum, involucrum
        - Surgical debridement
    - *Septic arthritis*:
        - Kocher's criteria
        - Urgent arthrotomy
    - *Tuberculosis of bones and joints*:
        - Spine (Pott's)
        - Hip, knee TB
    - Prosthetic joint infections
    - DAIR, one-stage, two-stage revisions.

3.1 Musculoskeletal Tuberculosis

Qazi Manaan Masood, Rohit Rambani

Q1. Describe the pathology, clinical features, and management of spinal tuberculosis.

(Universities: MUHS – 2022, RGUHS – 2021, DNB – multiple years)

Pathology
- *Causative agent*: *Mycobacterium tuberculosis* (usually *M. tuberculosis* hominis)
- *Spread*: Hematogenous (from lungs or lymph nodes)
- *Site*: Commonly affects **lower thoracic and lumbar vertebrae**
- *Pathogenesis*:
  - Involvement starts in **vertebral body (paradiscal)**, often bilateral
  - Leads to **caseation, necrosis**, vertebral collapse
  - Formation of **cold abscesses** (paravertebral, psoas)
  - Late stage → kyphotic deformity or gibbus

Clinical Features
- *Constitutional symptoms*: Fever, weight loss, malaise, night sweats
- *Back pain*: Dull, localized, worsening at night
- *Spinal deformity*: Kyphosis or gibbus
- *Neurological signs*: Pott's paraplegia (due to cord compression)
- *Cold abscesses*: Psoas abscess (visible in groin or iliac fossa)
- **Restriction of spinal movements**

Investigations
- *Blood tests*: ↑ ESR, CRP
- *Mantoux test*: May be positive
- *X-ray spine*:
  - Disc space narrowing
  - Lytic lesions, vertebral collapse
  - Paravertebral shadow
- *MRI spine*: Gold standard for early detection & cord involvement
- *CT-guided biopsy*: For histopathology and culture
- *CBNAAT/GeneXpert*: Detects MTB and rifampicin resistance

Management

Medical (mainstay):
- *Anti-tubercular therapy (ATT)*: 12-month regimen (2HRZE + 10HR)
- Monitor clinical and radiological improvement

Surgical indications:
- Neurological deficit (Pott's paraplegia)
- Severe kyphosis
- Spinal instability
- Large cold abscesses
- Failure of medical treatment

Surgical Options
- Anterior decompression and fusion
- Posterior decompression and stabilization
- Combined approaches in severe deformity

Supportive

- Spinal orthosis (TLSO)
- Nutritional support
- Neurological rehabilitation if needed

Q2. Classify skeletal tuberculosis. Describe the clinical presentation and management of tuberculosis of the hip joint.

(Universities: RGUHS – 2020, TNMGRMU – 2019, DNB – 2021)

Classification of Skeletal TB

1. *Axial skeleton*:
    - Spine (50%): Pott's disease
    - Sacroiliac joint
2. *Appendicular skeleton*:
    - Hip
    - Knee
    - Shoulder
    - Elbow
3. *Others*:
    - Tuberculous osteomyelitis
    - Dactylitis (spina ventosa in children)

TB Hip - Clinical Presentation

- **Insidious onset hip pain**
- **Limping** and muscle wasting (gluteal, thigh)
- Morning stiffness
- **Restricted hip movement**
- *Deformities*: Flexion, adduction, internal rotation
- *Cold abscess*: In groin or upper thigh
- **Trendelenburg gait**

Stages of Hip TB (Shanmugasundaram Classification)

- *Stage 1 - Synovitis*: Mild effusion, painful limitation of motion
- *Stage 2 - Early arthritis*: Cartilage erosion, joint space narrowing
- *Stage 3 - Advanced arthritis*: Bone destruction, subluxation
- *Stage 4 - Healed with deformity*: Ankylosis, fibrous or bony union

Investigations

- *Blood*: ↑ ESR, CRP
- *X-ray pelvis and hip*: Early–osteopenia; Late–joint destruction
- *MRI*: Early cartilage and synovial involvement
- *USG*: Detect effusion, abscess
- *Aspiration/Biopsy*: CBNAAT, AFB staining, culture

Management

Medical:

- **ATT** for 12 months (as per national guidelines)
- Non-weight bearing until inflammation subsides

Surgical

- Aspiration and drainage (if abscess)
- Synovectomy (Stage 2/3)
- Corrective osteotomy or excision arthroplasty (Stage 4 with deformity)
- Total hip replacement (in healed TB with deformity)

Physiotherapy

- Gentle mobilization
- Prevent contractures

Q3. Describe the pathology, clinical features, investigations, and treatment of Pott's paraplegia.

(Universities: AIIMS – 2023, RGUHS – 2022, DNB – 2020)

Definition

Pott's paraplegia refers to **spinal cord or nerve root compression** due to **tuberculous spondylitis**, resulting in **motor/sensory deficits.**

Types

Timing	*Type*
Early onset	During active disease (granulation, abscess, instability)
Late onset	After healing (bony deformity, fibrosis, scar tethering)

Pathogenesis:

- *Mechanical compression by*:
  - Cold abscess
  - Granulation tissue
  - Sequestrum
  - Vertebral collapse
- **Ischemia** of cord (vascular thrombosis)
- **Cord edema or myelitis** from inflammatory response

Clinical Features

- **Back pain** and spinal tenderness
- **Motor weakness** (spastic or flaccid paraplegia)
- Sensory deficit
- **Bladder/bowel dysfunction**
- Spasticity or flaccidity depending on level/severity

Investigations

- *X-ray spine*: Vertebral collapse, kyphosis
- *MRI spine*: Cord compression, soft tissue, abscess
- *ESR, CRP*: Elevated
- *CBNAAT/Biopsy*: To confirm TB and rule out other causes

Management

Medical:

- **ATT for minimum 12 months**
- Indicated in **mild or early-onset paraplegia**

Surgical Indications

- Progressive neurological deficit
- Lack of response to ATT in 3–4 weeks
- Severe kyphosis/instability
- Large abscesses

Surgical Options

- **Anterior decompression** ± bone grafting
- **Posterior decompression with instrumentation**
- Combined anterior-posterior in severe deformity

Prognosis

- Early-onset has better recovery
- Late-onset due to fibrosis has **poorer prognosis**

Rehabilitation
- Bracing (TLSO), physiotherapy, occupational therapy
- Prevention of pressure sores and contractures

Q4. Tuberculosis of the knee joint—discuss pathology, clinical features, diagnostic methods, and management.

(Universities: MUHS – 2021, DNB – 2019)

Pathology
- **Primary infection** spreads via **hematogenous route** from lungs or lymph nodes
- TB of the knee joint usually begins as **synovitis** → spreads to articular cartilage and subchondral bone
- Formation of **granulation tissue**, **caseation necrosis**, **joint effusion**, and **pannus formation**
- If untreated → joint destruction, fibrosis, and **ankylosis (fibrous or bony)**

Clinical Features
- **Chronic knee pain** with swelling
- **Gradual onset** over weeks/months
- Stiffness and **restricted range of motion**
- **Muscle wasting**, especially quadriceps
- **Cold effusion** (non-tender, fluctuant)
- **Flexion deformity** in advanced stages
- Possible **sinus formation or cold abscess** in neglected cases
- *Constitutional signs*: Low-grade fever, night sweats, weight loss

Diagnostic Methods

Modality	*Use*
X-ray knee	Early: Periarticular osteopenia, effusion; Late: joint space narrowing, erosions
MRI	Sensitive for early detection of synovitis, marrow edema
Synovial fluid aspiration	Cell count, AFB stain, CBNAAT (GeneXpert)
Synovial biopsy	Gold standard for diagnosis—shows epithelioid granulomas, caseation
ESR/CRP	Elevated
Mantoux test	May be positive but non-specific
Culture (Lowenstein–Jensen or BACTEC)	Confirms diagnosis

Management

Medical:
- *ATT for 12 months*: 2 months intensive phase (HRZE), 10 months continuation phase (HR)
- Non-weight-bearing during acute phase
- NSAIDs for pain relief

Surgical Indications
- Failure of conservative treatment
- Abscess drainage
- Synovectomy (especially Stage 2)
- Debridement and joint preservation
- Arthrodesis or total knee arthroplasty (in late-stage, healed TB with ankylosis/deformity)

Rehabilitation
- Physiotherapy to restore ROM
- Splinting during active inflammation
- Long-term follow-up to monitor for recurrence

Q5. Outline diagnostic algorithm and management plan for suspected osteoarticular tuberculosis.

(Universities: PGIMER pattern, DNB – 2022)

Stepwise Diagnostic Algorithm

1. *Clinical suspicion*:
   - Insidious onset monoarticular joint pain
   - Swelling, stiffness, discharging sinus
   - History of TB contact or past TB
2. *Basic investigations*:
   - *Blood*: ESR, CRP (usually raised)
   - *X-ray of joint/bone*: Early—osteopenia; Late—joint space loss, erosions
   - Mantoux test and chest X-ray
3. *Advanced imaging*:
   - *MRI*: Detects early synovitis, marrow edema, soft tissue abscess
   - *CT scan*: Bony involvement, sequestra, surgical planning
4. *Microbiological and histological confirmation*:

Test	*Purpose*
Synovial fluid/tissue biopsy	Histology (granulomas with caseation)
AFB smear and culture	Identifies TB bacilli
CBNAAT (GeneXpert)	Detects MTB and rifampicin resistance
Line probe assay (LPA)	Drug resistance profile (MDR-TB)
PCR-based tests	Rapid detection of TB DNA

Management Plan

1. *Medical management (cornerstone)*:
   - *ATT (DOTS or daily)*: 12-month duration
   - 2HRZE + 10HR (standard regimen)
   - Extended treatment for resistant or non-responding cases
2. *Surgical indications*:
   - Diagnostic (open/synovial biopsy)
   - Drainage of cold abscess
   - Debridement or synovectomy (persistent disease)
   - Arthrodesis for unstable joints
   - Arthroplasty for healed joint with severe damage
3. *Rehabilitation*:
   - Joint mobilization during healing
   - Muscle strengthening
   - Non-weight-bearing → partial → full weight-bearing as healing progresses

Summary Chart—Management Approach:

Step	*What to do*
Initial evaluation	ESR, CRP, X-ray, MRI
Confirm diagnosis	Biopsy, CBNAAT, AFB stain
Start ATT	Standard regimen 12 months
Monitor response	Clinical, lab, radiological
Surgery (if needed)	Based on abscess, instability, or deformity
Rehabilitation	Early mobilization and strength training

Q6. Write a note on the imaging features of spinal tuberculosis.

(Universities: RGUHS – 2023, DNB – 2021)

1. *X-ray findings*:
    - *Paradiscal involvement (most common)*: Early narrowing of disc space
    - Loss of vertebral height (anterior collapse → kyphosis/gibbus)
    - Lytic lesions in vertebral body
    - Paravertebral soft tissue shadow (suggesting cold abscess)
    - Subluxation or dislocation (in late cases)
    - Can appear normal in **early disease**
2. *MRI findings (gold standard)*:
    - Early detection of marrow edema
    - Shows soft tissue involvement and cold abscess
    - Detects epidural extension and spinal cord compression
    - Identifies granulation tissue, sequestra, and pus pockets
    - Helps differentiate **tubercular versus pyogenic lesions**
3. *CT scan*:
    - Provides better bone detail (sequestrum, cortical breach)
    - Detects calcified abscesses
    - Useful in **surgical planning and biopsy guidance**

Summary
- **MRI** is most sensitive and preferred in early stages
- **X-ray and CT** complement by showing late bony changes and helping in surgical planning

Q7. Pott's spine versus pyogenic spondylitis—differentiate.

(Universities: DNB – 2020, MUHS – 2021)

Feature	*Pott's spine (TB)*	*Pyogenic spondylitis*
Onset	Insidious, slow progression	Acute, rapid onset
Age	Young adults	Elderly or immunocompromised
Pain	Mild to moderate, chronic	Severe, acute
Disc involvement	Initially preserved, later involved	Early disc space destruction
Vertebral body	Anterior involvement, wedge collapse	Generalized vertebral involvement
Paravertebral abscess	Large, cold abscess, minimal signs	Smaller, hot abscess, tender
Systemic signs	Constitutional symptoms (fever, weight loss)	High fever, chills
Neurological deficit	Common (Pott's paraplegia)	Less common
Imaging (MRI)	T2 hyperintensity with abscesses and skip lesions	Rapid destruction, disc first
Response to treatment	Good with ATT	Good with antibiotics

Q8. Role of MRI in diagnosis and management of musculoskeletal TB.

Universities: DNB – 2022, AIIMS – 2021

Diagnostic Roles of MRI

1. *Early diagnosis*:
    - Detects **marrow edema** and soft tissue involvement before X-ray
    - Useful in **disc space and early vertebral body changes**
2. *Cold abscess identification*:
    - Well-defined **T2 hyperintense lesions**
    - Shows **extent of abscess**, including psoas and paravertebral

3. *Neural element compression*:
   - Identifies cord compression in Pott's paraplegia
   - Differentiates **abscess versus granulation versus fibrosis**
4. *Multifocal/spinal skip lesions*: Whole-spine MRI can pick up **non-contiguous lesions**

Role in Management
- Guides **surgical planning** (decompression, abscess drainage)
- Monitoring of **treatment response** (e.g., reduction in abscess size)
- Differentiates **active vs healed lesions**

Q9. Discuss antitubercular therapy (ATT) in osteoarticular TB.

(Universities: RGUHS – 2022, DNB – 2021)

Principles of ATT in Bone and Joint TB
1. *Prolonged duration*:
   - *Minimum 12 months (WHO guidelines)*:
     - *2 months of intensive phase*: HRZE
     - *10 months continuation phase*: HR
   - Some guidelines accept 9-month regimens in selected cases
2. *Drugs used*:
   - *H*: Isoniazid
   - *R*: Rifampicin
   - *Z*: Pyrazinamide
   - *E*: Ethambutol
3. *Route*: Oral (IV in selected resistant or GI intolerant cases)
4. *DOTS versus daily regimen*:
   - *Directly observed treatment short-course (DOTS)*: Public health protocol
   - *Daily regimen*: Commonly used in hospitals and institutions for precision
5. *Compliance monitoring*:
   - Regular liver function tests, adherence checks
   - **MDR-TB testing** if no response in 4–6 weeks

   Role of ATT
   - Primary treatment in all cases
   - Helps resolve infection, abscess, and prevents deformity
   - Must be **combined with surgery** in selected patients (abscess, deformity, or non-responders)
6. *Complications of spinal tuberculosis*:
   - *Universities*: MUHS – 2019, TNMGRMU – 2020, DNB – 2019.
   - *Points*: Kyphosis, Pott's paraplegia, deformity progression, late-onset paraplegia.

Q10. Gibbus deformity.

(Asked in: DNB – 2019)

Definition
Gibbus is a **sharp angular kyphotic deformity** of the spine resulting from **anterior wedging or collapse of one or more vertebrae**, most commonly due to **tuberculosis**.

Features
- Commonly seen in **thoracolumbar region**
- Formed by **collapse of anterior vertebral bodies**
- Often associated with **Pott's spine (spinal TB)**

- May result in **Pott's paraplegia** due to spinal cord compression
- **Rigid** and **non-correctable**

Other Causes (less common)
- Congenital kyphosis
- Vertebral hemangioma
- Metastasis or trauma (rare)

Q11. Cold abscess.

(TNMGRMU – 2021)

Definition
A **cold abscess** is a **chronic, fluctuant, non-tender swelling** resulting from **tuberculous liquefaction of caseous tissue**, without classical signs of inflammation.

Features
- **No redness, heat, or severe pain**
- *Contents*: Pus with liquefied necrotic material
- *Common locations*:
  - Psoas abscess (lumbar TB) → presents in groin
  - Paravertebral abscess (thoracic TB)
  - Axillary or supraclavicular (in cervical TB)

Pathway
- Tracks along **fascial planes** (gravity dependent)
- May **point at distant sites** (thigh, iliac fossa)

Management:
- **ATT is primary treatment**
- May require **aspiration or drainage** if large or symptomatic

Q12. Stages of tubercular arthritis.

(DNB – 2020)

Shanmugasundaram Classification (4 Stages)
1. *Stage I—Synovitis*:
   - Joint effusion, hyperemia, synovial hypertrophy
   - Normal X-ray or mild soft tissue swelling
2. *Stage II—Early arthritis*:
   - Cartilage erosion, marginal erosions
   - Early joint space narrowing
3. *Stage III—Advanced arthritis*:
   - Severe bone destruction
   - Subluxation/dislocation
   - Extensive joint space loss
4. *Stage IV—Healing/Ankylosis*:
   - Fibrous or bony ankylosis
   - Joint becomes stiff, deformed, and fused

Clinical Use
- Guides **treatment planning** (conservative vs. surgical)
- Influences **functional outcome**

Q13. Sinus formation in osteoarticular TB.

(MUHS – 2020)

Description

Sinus formation occurs when **cold abscess breaks through skin**, resulting in a **chronic discharging tract**.

Features

- Common in neglected or poorly treated TB
- Discharge is typically **serous or seropurulent**
- Common in **spine, hip, or long bones**
- May lead to **secondary bacterial infection**

Complications

- Persistent sinus → risk of scarring, deformity
- Squamous cell carcinoma transformation (Marjolin's ulcer)—rare
- Osteomyelitis or sequestrum formation

Management

- **Complete course of ATT**
- Sinus excision or **surgical debridement** if chronic or infected
- Proper wound care

Q14. Differential diagnosis of tubercular osteomyelitis.

(DNB – 2021)

Key Differentials

Condition	***Key differentiating features***
Brodie's abscess	Localized chronic pyogenic infection, well-circumscribed on X-ray
Fungal osteomyelitis	Rare, immunocompromised hosts, similar chronic features
Chronic pyogenic osteomyelitis	Sinus with foul-smelling discharge, sequestrum formation
Bone tumors (e.g., Ewing's sarcoma)	Pain + swelling + fever; Onion-skin appearance on X-ray
Langerhans cell histiocytosis	Lytic lesion with soft tissue mass, often in children
Metastasis or lymphoma	Older age, multiple lytic lesions, systemic symptoms

Role of Biopsy

- **Definitive diagnosis** requires **histopathology and microbiology**
- **CBNAAT** or **AFB culture** to confirm TB and drug sensitivity

Bonus: Frequently Clubbed/Integrated Topics

Q15. HIV and musculoskeletal TB – focus on atypical presentations and management differences

Atypical Presentations in HIV

- **Multifocal skeletal TB** (uncommon in immunocompetent)
- *Less common sites*: **shoulder, sternum, ribs, small bones**
- **Minimal or absent constitutional symptoms**
- **Rapid progression** and **poor granulation response**
- **Cold abscesses may be larger**, but systemic signs muted

Diagnostic Considerations

- **Low CD4 count** may result in false-negative Mantoux
- **GeneXpert/CBNAAT** preferred for rapid diagnosis and drug resistance
- **Imaging (MRI)** essential for early lesion detection

Treatment Differences

- **Standard ATT for 12 months**
- **Start ART within 2–8 weeks** of initiating ATT
- Monitor for **IRIS (immune reconstitution inflammatory syndrome)**
- **Drug interactions** between rifampicin and ART (efavirenz preferred)

Summary

HIV alters the presentation and progression of skeletal TB, requiring **heightened suspicion, earlier biopsy, and coordinated ART + ATT initiation.**

Q16. TB of small bones (e.g., foot or hand)—often missed, but increasingly asked.

Sites Involved

- *Foot*: Calcaneus, talus, navicular
- *Hand*: Metacarpals, phalanges → leads to **spina ventosa** in children

Clinical Features

- Chronic pain and swelling
- **Sinus or discharging tract** may be present
- **Minimal systemic symptoms**
- Often **misdiagnosed as osteomyelitis, tumor, or gout**

Radiology

- **Lytic lesions with sclerotic rim**
- Cystic expansion in phalanges in children
- *MRI*: Bone marrow edema, soft tissue abscess

Diagnosis

- **Biopsy + GeneXpert/CBNAAT** is essential
- X-ray may not differentiate TB from other lytic lesions

Treatment

- **ATT for 12 months**
- Surgical curettage only if diagnostic uncertainty or non-response

Summary

TB in small bones is rare and easily missed; **biopsy and imaging** are key to avoid delay in treatment.

Q17. DOTS strategy in skeletal TB—relevance in orthopedic context.

DOTS: Directly observed treatment, short-course

- WHO strategy for TB control
- Delivered via **RNTCP/NTEP in India**

Standard Regimen for Skeletal TB

- *2 months (intensive phase)*: H + R + Z + E
- *10 months (continuation phase)*: H + R
- *Total*: **12 months** recommended for musculoskeletal TB

Advantages of DOTS in Ortho TB

- **Improves compliance** in long-duration treatments
- Reduces risk of **drug resistance**
- **Monitored dosing** through treatment supporters
- Available free under **national programs**

Orthopedic Considerations

- Not all surgical patients are enrolled in DOTS → **integration needed**
- **Daily regimen** preferred in some centers (based on severity, MDR risk)

Summary

DOTS ensures **compliance and monitoring**, especially crucial in **long-course skeletal TB treatment.**

Q18. Role of biopsy and GeneXpert in diagnosis—high-yield due to newer diagnostic trends.

Biopsy

- **Gold standard** for confirming osteoarticular TB
- Provides **histology** (granulomas, caseation)
- Performed under **CT/MRI or USG guidance**

GeneXpert (CBNAAT)

- Rapid molecular test detecting ***Mycobacterium tuberculosis***
- Detects **rifampicin resistance** (MDR-TB screening)
- Gives results in <**2 hours**
- Can be done on **tissue, pus, aspirate**

Advantages

- More sensitive than AFB staining
- Confirms diagnosis even in **paucibacillary skeletal TB**
- Helps in **early targeted therapy**
- WHO-endorsed and **included in NTEP**

Summary

GeneXpert and biopsy are now the **cornerstones of diagnosis** in skeletal TB, offering **early, accurate, and resistance-aware diagnosis**.

Q19. Discuss the diagnosis and management of tuberculosis of the sacroiliac joint.

(DNB – 2022, RGUHS – 2021)

Overview

- **Sacroiliac TB** accounts for **1–5%** of osteoarticular TB
- Often **misdiagnosed** due to its deep location and vague symptoms

Clinical Features

- **Low backache** or buttock pain (unilateral)
- Pain aggravated by walking, prolonged sitting
- **Limping gait**, difficulty turning in bed
- Local tenderness over sacroiliac region
- *Occasionally*: **Cold abscess in gluteal or iliac fossa**
- Constitutional symptoms (weight loss, evening fever)

Physical Examination

- Positive **FABER test (Patrick's test)**
- Tenderness on **sacroiliac compression**
- Limited terminal range of motion at hip

Investigations

Modality	*Findings*
X-ray pelvis (AP view)	Late signs—joint space narrowing, sclerosis, erosion
MRI pelvis	Early detection—marrow edema, joint effusion, abscess
CT scan	Cortical breach, lytic lesions in ilium/sacrum
USG abdomen	Detects psoas or iliac abscess
CBNAAT/Biopsy	From aspirated pus or synovial tissue

Management

Medical:

- **ATT (HRZE for 2 months + HR for 10 months)**
- *Total duration*: 12 months
- Regular follow-up with ESR and imaging

Surgical Indications

- Large cold abscess not responding to meds
- Severe pain or disability
- Diagnostic uncertainty

Procedures

- CT-guided aspiration
- Open debridement (rare)
- Arthrodesis if joint instability persists

Summary

Sacroiliac TB should be suspected in **atypical low back pain**, diagnosed via **MRI and GeneXpert**, and treated with **prolonged ATT ± aspiration**.

Q20. Enumerate differential diagnoses of spinal TB and describe how to differentiate it from malignancy.

(DNB – 2023)

Differential Diagnoses of Spinal TB

- Pyogenic spondylodiscitis
- Metastatic spine disease
- Multiple myeloma
- Lymphoma of spine
- Brucella spondylitis
- Fungal spondylitis
- Vertebral hemangioma or aneurysmal bone cyst

Differentiating Spinal TB from Malignancy

Feature	*Tuberculous spondylitis*	*Spinal malignancy*
Onset	Insidious, slow	Rapid or subacute
Pain	Constant, dull, night pain	Severe, unrelenting, nocturnal
Systemic symptoms	Fever, night sweats, weight loss	Weight loss, fatigue
Neurological deficit	Common in late stages	May be early if cord compression
Vertebral involvement	Anterior part, multiple contiguous vertebrae	Often non-contiguous, posterior elements may be involved
Disc space	Initially preserved, then narrowed	Often spared in early malignancy
Abscess	Cold abscess with calcification	Rare

Continued

Continued

Feature	Tuberculous spondylitis	Spinal malignancy
MRI findings	T2 hyperintensity, paravertebral abscess	Irregular vertebral destruction, no abscess
Biopsy	Granulomas, caseation, AFB	Atypical cells, tumor-specific histology

Summary

Spinal TB can **mimic malignancy**, but **MRI pattern, abscess, and biopsy findings** are key to differentiation.

Q21. Discuss kyphotic deformity in spinal TB—prevention and surgical correction.

(AIIMS pattern – 2021, DNB – 2022)

Pathogenesis

- Vertebral body destruction (especially anterior part)
- Collapse leads to **angular kyphosis** or **gibbus**
- Common at **thoracolumbar junction**
- May lead to **late-onset paraplegia**

Predictors of Severe Kyphosis

- Age <10 years at onset
- More than **2 vertebrae** involved
- **Thoracolumbar or cervical spine** affected
- Delay in treatment initiation
- **Anterior and middle column** collapse

Prevention

- **Early ATT initiation**
- Spinal support with **bracing (TLSO)**
- **Close radiographic follow-up**
- Surgery in high-risk cases (prophylactic decompression/stabilization)

Surgical Correction (Indications)

- **Progressive kyphosis**
- Deformity >50–60°
- **Neurological deficit due to deformity**
- Instability or pain
- Cosmetic or functional impairment

Surgical Techniques

1. *Anterior approach*:
   - Corpectomy + bone grafting (structural support)
   - Suitable for **single-level disease with minimal kyphosis**
2. *Posterior approach*:
   - **Pedicle screw instrumentation**
   - Posterior column osteotomy (e.g., Smith-Petersen or pedicle subtraction)
3. *Combined approach*:
   - For **severe or multi-level deformity**
   - Anterior decompression + posterior stabilization

Timing of Surgery

- Ideally done during **healing phase**
- **Early surgery** in high-risk patients to prevent kyphosis
- **Delayed correction** in healed disease with deformity

Summary

Kyphosis in TB is **preventable** with early treatment and brace support. Severe deformities need **surgical correction using anterior, posterior, or combined approaches**.

Q22. Outline the role of surgery in the treatment of spinal tuberculosis.

(Frequently Asked: DNB – 2020, MUHS – 2019)

Surgery in Spinal TB: Not First-line, but Vital in Select Cases

Indications for Surgery (Mnemonic: NIDEF):

Indication	Details
N: Neurological deficit	Pott's paraplegia (progressive or non-responsive to ATT)
I: Instability	Spinal collapse, risk of worsening deformity
D: Deformity (kyphosis >60°)	Progressive kyphosis, cosmetic or functional issues
E: Epidural abscess	Cord compression due to pus/granulation
F: Failed medical therapy	No improvement after 6–8 weeks of ATT

Surgical Options

- Anterior decompression + bone grafting
- Posterior stabilization (pedicle screws)
- Combined anterior + posterior approach
- Kyphosis correction with osteotomy if needed

Post-operative

- Continue ATT
- Bracing + physiotherapy

Q23. Tuberculosis of the shoulder joint—clinical presentation.

(RGUHS – 2020)

Types of Shoulder TB

- *Caries sicca*: Dry form (commonest)
- *Caries exudata*: Cold abscess, rare
- *Subdeltoid bursitis*: Isolated bursal TB

Clinical Presentation

- **Chronic pain**, swelling over deltoid
- **Global restriction of movement**
- **Muscle wasting** (deltoid, supraspinatus)
- No warmth or redness (cold joint)
- Often mimics **frozen shoulder or rotator cuff tear**
- *Late stages*: fibrous ankylosis

Investigations

- *X-ray*: Joint space narrowing, lytic humeral head
- *MRI*: Early detection of synovitis, marrow changes
- *CBNAAT, biopsy*: Essential for confirmation

Management

- **ATT for 12 months**
- Joint rest in acute phase
- **Physiotherapy** in later stage
- *Surgery if*:
  - Debridement needed
  - Frozen or ankylosed shoulder → arthrolysis or arthroplasty

Conclusion

Shoulder TB often presents as **"caries sicca"** with gradual stiffness and pain—requires **early suspicion, ATT, and supportive therapy**.

Q24. Role of histopathology in diagnosis of osteoarticular TB.

(TNMGRMU – 2022)

Importance
- Helps confirm **granulomatous infection**
- Key when **smear/culture is negative**
- Especially useful in **extrapulmonary TB (bones/joints)**

Histopathological Features
- **Epithelioid granulomas**
- **Langhans giant cells** (multiple peripheral nuclei)
- **Caseous necrosis** in center
- Chronic **lymphoplasmacytic infiltrate**

Sample Collection
- **CT/MRI-guided biopsy** (vertebrae, joint)
- **Open biopsy** if deeper access needed
- Synovial tissue, bone, or cold abscess wall

Conclusion
Histopathology remains **a definitive diagnostic tool**, especially when combined with **CBNAAT or culture**, in **skeletal TB**.

Q25. Immune reconstitution inflammatory syndrome (IRIS) in TB spine.

[DNB – 2023 (newer pattern)]

Definition
IRIS is a **paradoxical worsening of TB symptoms** after starting **antiretroviral therapy (ART)** in HIV patients due to immune recovery.

Pathophysiology
- **Rapid restoration of T-cell immunity** after ART → intense inflammatory response
- Exaggerated reaction to **latent or partially treated TB antigens**

When It Occurs?
- Within **2–12 weeks** of starting ART
- Especially in patients with **low baseline CD4 counts (<50 cells/mm^3)**

Clinical Features in TB Spine
- New or worsening back pain
- Onset of **neurological deficit**
- Increase in **cold abscess size** or appearance of new lesions
- Fever, inflammation despite ongoing ATT

Management
- **Continue ATT and ART**
- Use **NSAIDs** for symptom control
- **Corticosteroids** (e.g., prednisolone) if severe IRIS
- Surgical decompression if new **neurological compression**

Conclusion
IRIS is an **inflammatory flare** post-ART, not drug failure. Recognizing it in TB spine is critical to **avoid misdiagnosis and ensure timely intervention.**

Q26. Langhans giant cell.

(DNB – 2019)

Definition

Langhans giant cells are **multinucleated macrophages** found in **granulomatous inflammation**, especially **uberculosis**.

Histological Features

- Nuclei arranged **peripherally in a horseshoe or ring shape**
- Derived from **epithelioid macrophages**
- Surrounded by **epithelioid cells and lymphocytes**
- Seen along with **caseous necrosis** in TB

Diagnostic Value

- Strongly suggests **chronic granulomatous infection**
- *Also seen in*: TB, sarcoidosis, leprosy, Crohn's disease

Summary

Langhans giant cells are a **hallmark of TB granulomas** and help confirm **histopathological diagnosis** of osteoarticular TB.

Q27. Caries spine.

(MUHS – 2020)

Definition

Caries spine is a historical term for **tuberculous spondylodiscitis**, usually affecting the **thoracic and lumbar spine**.

Pathology

- *Granulomatous infection leads to*:
  - Destruction of vertebral bodies
  - Disc space narrowing
  - Formation of **cold abscess**
  - **Gibbus deformity** in severe cases

Clinical Features

- Chronic back pain
- Paravertebral swelling
- Spinal deformity (kyphosis/gibbus)
- Neurological signs (Pott's paraplegia)

Investigations

- X-ray, MRI
- CBNAAT, biopsy for confirmation

Summary

Caries spine: **TB of spine**, most commonly in **thoracolumbar region**, with potential for **abscess, deformity, and paraplegia**.

Q28. Differential diagnosis of monoarticular arthritis in adults.

(In DNB/PGIMER pattern exams)

Common Causes

Etiology	***Examples***
Infectious	Tuberculosis, septic arthritis
Crystal arthropathy	Gout, pseudogout

Continued

Continued

Etiology	*Examples*
Trauma-related	Hemarthrosis, osteochondral injury
Degenerative	Osteoarthritis (if secondary)
Autoimmune	Early RA (occasionally monoarticular)
Tumors	Pigmented villonodular synovitis (PVNS)

Clinical Differentiation Points
- *TB*: Insidious, cold joint, effusion, no erythema
- *Septic arthritis*: Acute, hot, swollen, tender
- *Gout*: Acute, red, very painful (MTP joint)
- *OA*: Crepitus, limited ROM, older adults

Summary
Always consider **TB in chronic monoarthritis**, especially if **effusion + minimal pain + systemic symptoms** are present.

Q29. Streptomycin in TB—mechanism and orthopedic relevance.

Mechanism of Action
- An **aminoglycoside antibiotic**
- Inhibits **protein synthesis** by binding to the **30S ribosomal subunit** of *Mycobacterium tuberculosis*
- **Bactericidal** against extracellular bacilli

Usage in TB
- Part of the **older first-line ATT regimen**
- Now rarely used due to **toxicity and resistance**
- Used in **MDR-TB cases** as part of second-line therapy

Orthopedic Relevance
- Historically used for **local injection into cold abscesses**
- Was part of regimens for **bone and joint TB before rifampicin era**
- Now mainly of **historical importance or in MDR-TB protocols**

Summary
Streptomycin is an **injectable aminoglycoside** with historic importance in **bone TB treatment**, still used selectively in **drug-resistant cases**.

Q30. Ziehl-Neelsen staining—principle and role in TB diagnosis.

(Basic science question: Occasionally appears in DNB or university papers)

Principle
- Based on **acid-fastness** of *Mycobacterium tuberculosis* due to **mycolic acid** in cell wall
- Once stained with **carbol fuchsin**, they resist **decolorization with acid-alcohol**

Procedure (Simplified Steps)
- Heat-fixed smear flooded with **carbol fuchsin**
- Heated gently (enhances penetration)
- Decolorized with **acid-alcohol**
- Counterstained with **methylene blue**

Result
- **Acid-fast bacilli (AFB)** appear **red**
- Background tissue/cells stain **blue**

Role in Diagnosis

- Detects **TB in pus, sputum, tissue smears**
- Used in **cold abscess, sinus discharge, biopsy samples**
- **Rapid and inexpensive**, but **low sensitivity** in skeletal TB

Summary

Ziehl-Neelsen staining is a **foundational diagnostic tool** in TB, especially useful for **AFB detection in accessible lesions**, though **limited in bone TB.**

Probable Emerging Questions (Based on Guidelines/Updates)

Q31. Discuss the Revised National Tuberculosis Control Program (RNTCP) approach to osteoarticular TB.

New guideline-oriented regimen now called as NTEP (National Tuberculosis Elimination Program).

Core Strategies for Osteoarticular TB

1. *Daily regimen (vs. DOTS earlier)*:
   - All TB patients (including extrapulmonary) are now treated with **daily fixed-dose combinations (FDCs)**
   - Weight-based categorization (Adults: 4 weight bands)
2. *ATT for osteoarticular TB*:
   - *2 months intensive phase*: HRZE
   - *10 months continuation phase*: HR
   - *Total*: **12 months minimum**, longer if indicated
3. *Monitoring and reporting*:
   - Nikshay portal mandatory for case notification and follow-up
   - **Follow-up imaging** advised for bone TB (MRI/X-ray)
4. *Role of DOTS plus/Programmatic management of drug-resistant TB (PMDT)*:
   - *All samples from osteoarticular TB (tissue, pus) are sent for*:
     - CBNAAT/GeneXpert
     - Line probe assay (LPA)
     - Culture (MGIT)
5. *Surgical integration*:
   - *Coordination with orthopedic units for*:
     - Diagnostic biopsy
     - Abscess drainage
     - Stabilization procedures (if required)

Summary

The RNTCP (now **NTEP**) integrates **daily FDCs, drug resistance testing, and digital monitoring** into the care of osteoarticular TB, aiming for **early diagnosis, effective treatment, and relapse prevention**.

Q32. Drug-resistant TB in bones and joints—diagnosis and management.

(DNB – 2022, emerging trend)

Types of drug resistance

Type	*Definition*
MDR-TB	Resistant to isoniazid (H) and rifampicin (R)
XDR-TB	MDR + resistance to fluoroquinolones and injectable 2nd-line drugs

Diagnosis

Test	*Utility*
CBNAAT (GeneXpert)	Rapidly detects MTB + Rifampicin resistance
Line probe assay (LPA)	Detects resistance to H, R, and second-line drugs
Culture and DST (MGIT)	Confirms resistance and guides therapy

Clinical Suspicion
- No improvement after 6–8 weeks of ATT
- Persistent sinus, cold abscess
- Known TB contact with **drug-resistant history**
- Immunocompromised host (e.g., HIV)

Management
MDR-TB:
- Treated with **longer MDR regimen (18–20 months)** or **shorter MDR regimen (9–11 months)** as per NTEP
- Regimen includes **Bedaquiline, Linezolid, Levofloxacin, Clofazimine**, etc.

XDR-TB:
Needs **individualized regimen** with newer drugs (delamanid, pretomanid)

Role of Surgery
- For **diagnosis (biopsy)**
- Drainage of **non-resolving abscesses**
- **Stabilization** if collapse or deformity present

Summary
Drug-resistant TB in bone is on the rise. Diagnosis is based on **GeneXpert, LPA, and culture**, and treatment includes **longer, toxic regimens**, requiring **multidisciplinary management**.

Q33. Classification of spinal TB based on location and extent.

(Asked in: AIIMS style – 2023, possibly NEET SS)

Rajasekaran Classification (Location + Extent)

1. *Based on location within vertebra*:

Type	*Description*
1	Paradiscal involvement
2	Central vertebral body
3	Anterior subligamentous spread
4	Posterior element involvement (rare)

2. *Based on number of vertebrae involved*:
   - Single vertebra
   - Contiguous multilevel involvement
   - Skip lesions (non-contiguous)
3. *Based on stability and deformity risk*:

Stage	*Findings*
A	Stable spine, no kyphosis
B	Potential instability or mild deformity
C	Gross kyphosis, instability, risk of paraplegia

Use in Surgical Planning
- Helps decide approach (anterior/posterior/combined)
- Predicts need for early stabilization (e.g., in types 2–4)
- Useful for **prognostication** of deformity risk

Summary

Rajasekaran classification offers a **comprehensive anatomic and risk-based framework** for spinal TB, essential for **decision-making in surgical management**.

Revision Table (Comparative Format)

TB Spine versus Pyogenic Spondylitis

Feature	*TB spine*	*Pyogenic*
Onset	Insidious	Acute
Fever	Mild	High-grade
Disc involvement	Late	Early
Abscess	Cold abscess (large)	Pus-filled, warm
Vertebral collapse	Common	May occur late
Response to antibiotics	Slow (ATT)	Quick (IV antibiotics)

Flashcard Summary (For Memorization)

Flashcard 1

Q: Most common site for musculoskeletal TB?
A: Spine (50%)—especially thoracic region.

Flashcard 2

Q: First-line anti-TB drugs?
A: H—isoniazid, R—rifampicin, Z—pyrazinamide, E—ethambutol.

Flashcard 3

Q: Indications for surgery in spinal TB?
A: Neurological deficit, severe deformity, instability, failed medical treatment.

Advanced and Less Common Theory Questions—Long/Short Essays

Q34. Pathological basis of deformity in spinal TB and its prevention.

Focus

Mechanics of vertebral collapse, anterior wedge, factors influencing deformity

Pathogenesis

- TB affects the **anterior vertebral body (paradiscal)** → destruction → **collapse**
- Leads to **anterior wedge-shaped vertebrae**
- Progressive collapse causes **angular kyphosis or gibbus**

Deformity Influencers

- **Number of vertebrae** involved
- *Age*: Worse in children <10 years
- *Level*: Thoracolumbar junction is most deforming
- **Delay in diagnosis and treatment**
- **Extent of bone destruction**

Rajasekaran's Prediction of Kyphosis Angle

- **Final kyphosis angle = Initial angle + 30° (on average)**
- Predicts worsening based on early imaging

Prevention

- **Early ATT initiation**
- **Bracing (TLSO)** during active disease

- *Surgical stabilization if*:
  - 2 vertebrae involved
  - Progressive kyphosis
  - Unstable spine
  - Young age (<10 years)

Summary
Kyphotic deformity in spinal TB is due to **anterior column collapse**, and early diagnosis, bracing, and surgical planning can **prevent severe deformity**.

Q35. Describe various surgical approaches in spinal TB with indications.

(TNMGRMU-2019)

Anterior, posterior, combined—pros and cons

Indications for Surgery
- Neurological deficit
- Spinal instability
- Severe/progressive deformity
- Failure of ATT
- Abscess or sequestrum

Approaches

Approach	*Indications*	*Pros*	*Cons*
Anterior	Isolated anterior disease, abscess, cord compression	Direct decompression, access to pathology	Technically demanding (thoracotomy)
Posterior	Kyphosis correction, multilevel disease	Familiar approach, easier stabilization	Limited access to anterior abscess
Combined	Severe deformity, multilevel, panvertebral involvement	Maximum decompression + stability	Longer surgery, more blood loss
Minimally invasive	Emerging, less morbidity	Cosmetically better, early recovery	Limited visualization, experience needed

Summary
Surgical approach in spinal TB depends on **location, extent, and goal (decompression vs. correction)** — often tailored patient-wise.

Q36. Role of biopsy in musculoskeletal TB—technique, types, and interpretation.

FNAC versus open biopsy, MDR screening focus

Purpose
- **Confirm diagnosis** in atypical/extra-pulmonary TB
- **Detect drug resistance** via GeneXpert/LPA
- Rule out mimics (tumor, pyogenic infection)

Types

Type	*Method*	*Use*
FNAC	Needle aspiration from lesion	Limited sample; less accurate in bone TB
Core needle biopsy	CT/USG-guided Tru-cut biopsy	Preferred in spine, joints
Open biopsy	Surgically obtained tissue (e.g., synovium)	Gold standard, especially in MDR cases

Interpretation
- *Histopathology*: **Granulomas, caseation, Langhans cells**
- *CBNAAT (GeneXpert)*: MTB + rifampicin resistance

- *Culture + DST*: Final confirmation and drug sensitivity
- *LPA*: Gene-based resistance profiling

Summary

Biopsy is crucial in **diagnosing and customizing TB treatment**, especially in **MDR cases and atypical presentations**.

Q37. MDR/XDR tuberculosis—implications in orthopedic TB.

Treatment regimens, new drugs like bedaquiline

Definitions
- *MDR-TB*: Resistant to INH + Rifampicin
- *XDR-TB*: MDR + resistance to fluoroquinolone + 2nd-line injectables

Diagnosis
- CBNAAT/GeneXpert
- Line probe assay (LPA)
- Culture with drug sensitivity testing (DST)

Treatment Principles
- Managed under **NTEP PMDT protocols**
- *Longer MDR regimen*: ~18–20 months
- *Shorter MDR regimen*: ~9–11 months (selected patients)

Key Drugs Used

Group	*Examples*
Group A (core)	Bedaquiline, linezolid, levofloxacin
Group B (add-on)	Clofazimine, cycloserine
Group C (other)	Ethambutol, delamanid

Orthopedic Considerations:
- ATT must be **strictly adhered to**
- Surgical debridement/stabilization for **cold abscess, deformity**
- Regular **MRI follow-up**
- Higher relapse risk

Summary

MDR/XDR TB requires **genetic diagnosis, prolonged toxic regimens**, and close orthopedic-surgical coordination.

Q38. Immunopathogenesis of osteoarticular TB.

(AIIMS 2016)

Granuloma, immune evasion, HIV link

Steps in Pathogenesis
- **Hematogenous spread** of MTB to bone/synovium
- Activation of **macrophages** → granuloma formation
- Influx of **CD4+ T cells** → IFN-γ release → further macrophage activation
- **Langhans giant cells**, **epithelioid cells** form
- **Caseation necrosis** in center due to persistent infection

Immune Evasion by MTB
- Inhibits phagosome-lysosome fusion
- Survives intracellularly
- Suppresses T-cell mediated killing

HIV Co-infection

- ↓ CD4 count → defective granuloma formation
- ↑ Risk of dissemination
- Poorer response to ATT
- Higher chance of **IRIS**

Summary

Osteoarticular TB involves **cell-mediated immunity**, granuloma formation, and **immune subversion by MTB**, especially pronounced in **HIV patients**.

Q39. Describe Phemister's triad and its significance.

Seen in tubercular arthritis

Phemister's Triad: **Classic X-ray findings in TB arthritis**

- Juxta-articular osteoporosis
- Peripheral (marginal) erosions
- Gradual joint space narrowing

Significance

- Highly suggestive of **chronic tubercular arthritis**
- Seen in **hip, knee, shoulder TB**
- Helps distinguish from:
    - OA (central cartilage loss)
    - RA (uniform loss + symmetric)
    - Pyogenic arthritis (rapid destruction)

Summary

Phemister's triad is a **diagnostic hallmark on radiographs** in TB joints, indicating **slow, progressive, granulomatous arthritis**.

Q40. Cervical spine TB—peculiarities in diagnosis and treatment.

Odontoid, respiratory risks and dislocation

Unique Features

- Rare (2–5% of spinal TB)
- Involves **atlantoaxial joint, odontoid process**
- Can cause **retropharyngeal abscess** → airway compromise
- High risk of **atlantoaxial dislocation**

Clinical Signs

- Neck pain and stiffness
- **Dysphagia or hoarseness** (due to abscess)
- Neurological signs if cord compression
- **Torticollis or dropped head posture**

Diagnosis

- *MRI*: Soft tissue and cord compression
- *X-ray*: C1–C2 instability
- *CT*: Bone destruction
- Biopsy for confirmation

Treatment

- ATT for 12–18 months
- Halo vest immobilization if instability
- *Surgery*:
  - **Anterior decompression + posterior fusion** if dislocation or abscess
  - C1–C2 fusion in unstable cases

Summary

Cervical TB is **dangerous due to proximity to airway and brainstem**—requires **early MRI, biopsy, and cautious stabilization.**

Additional Short Notes

Q41. DOTS versus daily regimen in skeletal TB.

(Banaras Hindu University – Institute of Medical Sciences 2011)

Recent changes under NTEP (National TB Elimination Program)

Feature	*DOTS (earlier)*	*Daily regimen (current, NTEP)*
Dosing	Intermittent (3 days/week)	Daily fixed-dose combination (FDC)
Supervision	Directly observed treatment (health worker)	Can be self-administered (with follow-up)
Drug formulation	Loose pills	Fixed-dose combination (FDC)
Coverage	Mostly pulmonary TB	Now includes extrapulmonary TB (e.g., bone)
Rationale for shift	Better compliance, reduced resistance	Improves outcomes in MSK TB

Summary

NTEP has shifted to a **daily FDC regimen** even for **skeletal TB**, ensuring better **compliance and outcome monitoring**.

Q42. Caries Sicca.

Dry form of TB arthritis of the shoulder

Features

- Most common form of **TB shoulder**
- *Presents with*:
  - Chronic pain and stiffness
  - Wasting of shoulder muscles
  - No joint effusion or abscess ("dry" type)
  - Global restriction of movement

X-ray

- Juxta-articular osteopenia
- Marginal erosions
- Decreased joint space (in late stages)

Management

- ATT for 12 months
- Gentle mobilization
- Surgery (arthrolysis or debridement) only if fibrous ankylosis occurs

Summary

Caries sicca is a **dry, fibrotic form of TB arthritis**, commonly involving the **shoulder**, with pain, stiffness, and muscle wasting.

Q43. TB tenosynovitis.

Involves tendon sheaths—especially wrist and ankle

Pathology
- TB infects the **synovial lining of tendon sheaths**
- Most commonly affects **flexor tendons of hand or foot**
- Can present as a **slow-growing swelling** along tendon

Clinical Features
- Painless, soft, **fluctuant or rubbery swelling**
- Restriction of tendon movement
- "Rice bodies" (degenerated fibrin masses) may be found inside sheath

Diagnosis
- *MRI*: Shows synovial thickening, fluid
- *Biopsy/Aspiration*: GeneXpert, histopathology

Treatment
- ATT 12 months
- Surgical excision if compressive or non-responsive

Summary
TB tenosynovitis presents as a **painless swelling of tendon sheaths**, especially in **hands and wrists**, and requires biopsy + ATT.

Q44. TB dactylitis.

(Bihar University)

Seen in children—affects short bones of hands/feet

Features
- TB infection of **metacarpals, phalanges, metatarsals**
- Most common in **children under 5 years**
- Presents with **fusiform swelling** of a finger or toe

Radiology
- **Expansile lytic lesion**
- Cortical thinning
- Often described as **spina ventosa** appearance

Diagnosis
- X-ray + MRI
- Biopsy or aspiration + GeneXpert

Treatment
- ATT 12 months
- Rarely needs surgery unless abscess or deformity present

Summary
TB dactylitis causes **cystic expansion of short bones** in children, typically showing the **spina ventosa** sign.

Q45. Spina Ventosa.

Cystic expansion of short tubular bones—pediatric TB

Definition
Radiological term for **ballooned or expanded** appearance of phalanges/metacarpals in TB dactylitis.

Features
- Seen in **children <5 years**
- Involves **short tubular bones** of hand/foot
- Appears as a **cystic, blown-out bone with thinned cortex**

Clinical Significance
- Suggests **chronic granulomatous infection**
- Helps differentiate from pyogenic osteomyelitis

Summary
Spina ventosa—**pediatric TB of short bones** will lead to cystic expansion due to **endosteal granulation and cortical thinning**.

Q46. Use of GeneXpert and line probe assay in MSK TB.

Rapid diagnosis, detects rifampicin resistance

GeneXpert (CBNAAT)
- Detects *Mycobacterium tuberculosis* **DNA**
- Gives result in **<2 hours**
- Detects **rifampicin resistance** (proxy for MDR-TB)
- *Sample*: Pus, tissue, synovium, abscess fluid

Line Probe Assay (LPA)
- Detects resistance to **isoniazid and rifampicin**
- Can also detect resistance to **2nd-line drugs**
- Requires more tissue/sample
- Result in **24–48 hours**

Advantages
- Faster than culture
- Useful in **early diagnosis**, especially in extrapulmonary TB
- Guides **early change in regimen** in MDR cases

Summary
GeneXpert and LPA are critical in **early detection and resistance profiling** of MSK TB, helping initiate the **correct ATT protocol**.

Q47. Role of physiotherapy in osteoarticular TB.

(Sri Ramachandra Institute of Higher Education and Research 2017)

Prevents deformity, maintains ROM

Importance
- Prevents **joint stiffness** and **muscle wasting**
- Maintains **range of motion** during recovery
- Helps correct **posture and spinal alignment**
- Aids **functional recovery** after surgery or immobilization

Phases of Rehabilitation

Phase	*Goal*
Acute (on ATT)	Pain relief, joint rest
Subacute	Begin passive ROM exercises
Recovery	Active mobilization + strengthening
Post-operative (if any)	Gait training, bracing, neuro rehabilitation

Summary
Physiotherapy plays a vital role in **preserving function, preventing deformities**, and **speeding recovery** in TB of bones and joints.

Q48. Paradoxical Reaction in TB.

Worsening despite treatment, common in immunocompromised

Definition
Clinical or radiological worsening of TB lesions **despite adequate ATT**, often seen in **HIV patients or with ART initiation**.

Mechanism
- Restoration of immunity causes **exaggerated inflammatory response** to existing MTB antigens
- A type of **immune reconstitution inflammatory syndrome (IRIS)**

Clinical Features
- New or expanding abscess
- Worsening of spinal lesion or paraplegia
- Fever, constitutional symptoms return

Management
- Continue **ATT and ART**
- Add **NSAIDs or corticosteroids**
- Rarely, surgery needed for decompression

Summary
Paradoxical reaction: **Apparent worsening due to immune recovery**, not drug failure; treat supportively while **continuing ATT**.

Possible Integrated or Cross-Subject Questions

Q49. Tubercular osteomyelitis versus Pyogenic osteomyelitis—compare and contrast.

(Seth Gordhandas Sunderdas Medical College and KEM Hospital 2014)

Feature	***Tubercular osteomyelitis***	***Pyogenic osteomyelitis***
Onset	Insidious, chronic	Acute or subacute
Causative organism	*Mycobacterium tuberculosis*	*Staphylococcus aureus* (most common)
Pain	Dull, mild to moderate	Severe, localized
Systemic features	Mild fever, weight loss, night sweats	High-grade fever, chills
Discharge	Serous or thin, may form sinus	Purulent, foul-smelling
Imaging (X-ray/MRI)	Lytic lesions, sequestra, periosteal thickening	Early marrow edema, periosteal reaction
Cold abscess	Common	Rare
Biopsy/Aspirate	Granulomas, caseation, AFB	PMNs, bacteria on Gram stain
Treatment	ATT for 12 months	IV antibiotics followed by oral; surgical drainage

Summary
TB osteomyelitis presents **slowly**, with **milder symptoms**, often requiring **biopsy for confirmation**, unlike pyogenic, which is **acute and obvious**.

Q50. Impact of diabetes and HIV on musculoskeletal TB.

In Diabetes

- **Impaired immunity** → delayed healing and increased infection risk
- *Poor glycemic control may*:
  - Promote **sinus formation**
  - Cause **non-responsiveness to ATT**
  - Lead to **superadded pyogenic infections**
- Higher risk of **MDR-TB**

In HIV

- Reduced **CD4+ T-cell count** → defective granuloma formation
- TB may present as **multifocal, disseminated, or atypical**
- **Rapid progression** to bone/joint damage
- Increased risk of **IRIS** after starting ART
- Requires **early biopsy + GeneXpert** for diagnosis
- Close **co-management with ART team**

Summary

Diabetes and HIV both **alter presentation**, **delay healing**, and **increase complications** in TB, requiring **tailored monitoring and therapy**.

Q51. Case-based scenario: A 40-year-old presents with chronic back pain and progressive lower limb weakness.

(Common in NEET SS/DNB new pattern)

Likely Diagnosis

→ Spinal tuberculosis with Pott's paraplegia

Clinical Clues

- Chronic backache
- Night sweats, low-grade fever
- Gibbus or tenderness on spine
- Spasticity, hyperreflexia in lower limbs
- Weakness + sensory deficits ± bladder involvement

Investigation Flowchart

- *CBC, ESR, CRP*: Supportive
- *X-ray spine*: Check for wedge collapse, kyphosis
- *MRI spine*: Soft tissue abscess, cord compression
- CBNAAT (GeneXpert) from cold abscess aspirate
- *Biopsy (CT-guided)*: Histology + culture

Management

- Start **ATT (2HRZE + 10HR)** immediately
- *Neurological deficit present*: Surgical decompression
- **Spinal stabilization** if kyphosis or instability
- *Post-operative*: physiotherapy + nutritional support

Summary

The scenario suggests **Pott's spine with paraplegia**, requiring urgent **MRI**, **biopsy**, **ATT**, and often **surgical decompression**.

Q52. National TB elimination program 2025—orthopedic relevance.

Key NTEP Goals
- **Eliminate TB in India by 2025** (5 years ahead of global target)
- Includes **extrapulmonary TB** (e.g., musculoskeletal)

Orthopedic Relevance
- **Mandatory notification** of osteoarticular TB on **Nikshay portal**
- Use of **daily ATT** via **FDCs** (fixed-dose combinations)
- *Emphasis on*:
  - **Early diagnosis** via CBNAAT/LPA
  - **Biopsy confirmation** before long-term ATT
- Integration of **MDR-TB management protocols (PMDT)**
- Support for **rehabilitation and deformity correction surgeries**

Summary
Orthopedists play a crucial role in **early identification, notification, biopsy-based confirmation**, and **rehabilitative care** under NTEP 2025.

Q53. Role of TB notification and contact tracing in orthopedic practice.

(Goa Medical College 2013)

Notification
- All TB cases (including **bone and joint TB**) are **notifiable** by law
- Must be reported via the **Nikshay portal**
- Ensures patients receive **free diagnostics, drugs, and follow-up**

Why Orthopedists Must Notify?
- Musculoskeletal TB is often diagnosed **late or mismanaged**
- Prevents **loss to follow-up** and **drug resistance**
- Helps central database **track outcomes and resistance trends**

Contact Tracing
- Identify **household and close contacts**
- Screen for **symptoms and latent TB**
- Useful especially in **pediatric cases or MDR-TB**

Summary
Orthopedic surgeons have a **public health responsibility** to notify TB cases, aiding in **surveillance, contact tracing, and national elimination goals**.

Rare and Advanced MSK TB Theory Questions

Q54. Tuberculosis of the foot—clinical presentation, diagnosis, and management.

Rare but increasingly seen; navicular and calcaneum most involved

Clinical Presentation
- **Chronic midfoot or heel pain**, especially on weight-bearing
- **Swelling, limping, or sinus** (in advanced cases)
- Often missed/misdiagnosed as **plantar fasciitis, calcaneal bursitis, stress fracture**

Common Sites
- **Calcaneum** (most common)

- **Navicular, cuboid, metatarsals**
- May present as **isolated bone TB** or **joint TB (subtalar, tarsometatarsal)**

Investigations
- *X-ray*: Osteolytic lesion, cystic changes, cortical thinning
- *MRI*: Marrow edema, abscess formation
- *CBNAAT/GeneXpert*: On aspirated pus or tissue
- *Biopsy*: Granulomas, caseation

Management
- **ATT for 12 months**
- Immobilization (POP or boot) in painful phase
- *Surgery*:
  - Curettage ± bone grafting (rare)
  - Debridement in sinuses or deformities

Summary
TB of the foot requires **high suspicion**, especially in **midfoot/heel pain with lytic lesions**, and responds well to **early ATT**.

Q55. Tuberculosis of the elbow joint—diagnostic challenges and differential diagnosis.

(Jammu University)

Mimics RA or JIA, especially in children

Clinical Presentation
- Gradual onset **pain and stiffness**
- **Effusion** in early stages
- **Flexion deformity** in late stage
- Muscle wasting, especially triceps and brachialis
- Often **painless range restriction**

Diagnostic Challenges
- *Often misdiagnosed as*:
  - Juvenile idiopathic arthritis
  - Rheumatoid arthritis
  - Trauma or bursitis
- Minimal systemic signs

Investigations
- *X-ray*:
  - *Early*: Soft tissue shadow, osteopenia
  - *Late*: Joint space narrowing, erosions
- *MRI*: Synovitis, pannus, early bone changes
- *Biopsy + CBNAAT*: For definitive diagnosis

Management
- **ATT 12 months**
- Splinting in early painful phase
- Active physiotherapy in recovery
- *Surgery if*:
  - Synovectomy (persistent synovitis)
  - Arthrolysis (fibrous ankylosis)

Summary
TB elbow is often **subtle and mimics autoimmune arthritis**, requiring **early imaging and biopsy** for diagnosis.

Q56. Tubercular osteomyelitis of long bones—clinical features and radiological differentiation from tumors.

Mimics Ewing's sarcoma, chronic osteomyelitis, Brodie's abscess

Clinical Features
- **Local pain and swelling** (diaphysis or metaphysis)
- **Sinus or discharging wound** (if advanced)
- Mild fever or systemic signs
- Frequently confused with **bone tumors**

Common Sites
- Femur, tibia, humerus, radius
- Diaphyseal involvement common

Radiological Differentiation

Condition	X-ray/MRI features
TB osteomyelitis	Lytic lesion, sequestrum, cortical erosion
Ewing's sarcoma	Onion-skin periosteal reaction, soft tissue mass
Brodie's abscess	Well-defined lytic lesion with sclerotic rim
Chronic pyogenic OM	Involucrum, sequestrum, more aggressive periosteal reaction

Diagnosis:
- *MRI*: Shows abscess, marrow changes
- *Biopsy*: Granulomatous tissue
- *GeneXpert*: For MTB and rifampicin resistance

Management
- ATT 12 months
- Curettage or debridement in chronic/abscess cases

Summary

Tubercular osteomyelitis of long bones **mimics tumors** and needs **biopsy confirmation** to avoid misdiagnosis.

Q57. Tuberculosis of the hand and wrist—types, presentation, and treatment.

[Postgraduate Institute of Medical Education and Research (PGIMER) Chandigarh 2011]

Includes: TB tenosynovitis, dactylitis, synovitis

Types
- *TB tenosynovitis*: Most common
- *TB synovitis*: Affects radiocarpal or intercarpal joints
- *TB dactylitis*: Seen in children (spina ventosa)

Presentation
- **Wrist pain + swelling**, flexor or extensor tendon involvement
- Local warmth is usually absent
- May present as **carpal tunnel syndrome (rare)**
- Multiple **rice bodies** in tendon sheath (on surgery)

Diagnosis
- *MRI*: Synovial thickening, tendon sheath fluid
- Biopsy from synovium or sheath
- GeneXpert/AFB staining

Management
- ATT 12 months
- *Surgical excision of sheath if*:
  - Compression neuropathy
  - Failure to resolve
  - Large abscess or rice bodies

Summary
Hand and wrist TB often affects **tendon sheaths or joints**, causing **painless swelling**, and needs **early diagnosis to preserve function**.

Integrated Clinical Case Style Questions

Q58. A 35-year-old male presents with low back pain and cold abscess tracking into the thigh. Discuss diagnosis and management.

Expectation
Identify psoas abscess from TB spine

Likely Diagnosis
Tuberculous spondylitis with psoas abscess

Clinical Features
- Chronic low back pain
- Limp or flexion deformity at hip
- **Palpable swelling in groin or medial thigh**
- *Abscess may point in*:
  - Inguinal region
  - Upper thigh
  - Iliac fossa

Investigations
- *MRI spine + pelvis - reveals*:
  - Vertebral body destruction
  - Cold abscess tracking along psoas
- *X-ray lumbar spine*: may show vertebral collapse, kyphosis
- *USG abdomen/pelvis*: for collection
- *Aspiration of abscess—send for*:
  - CBNAAT (GeneXpert)
  - AFB stain and culture
- *Blood tests*: ESR, CRP, CBC

Management
- **Start ATT (2HRZE + 10HR)** immediately
- *CT-guided aspiration of psoas abscess if*:
  - Large or causing pain
  - Suspected secondary infection
- *Surgery indicated if*:
  - Neurological signs present
  - Spinal instability or deformity
  - Persistent abscess despite ATT

Summary

Cold abscess in thigh is often due to **tracking of pus from spinal TB via psoas muscle**, and needs **imaging, drainage, and ATT**.

Q59. A 50-year-old patient on ATT develops worsening kyphosis and neurological signs. How will you manage?

(Himachal Pradesh University Shimla 2011)

Highlights paradoxical reaction or late-onset paraplegia

Likely Differential Diagnoses

- *Paradoxical reaction (IRIS)*: Inflammatory flare after immune reconstitution
- *Late-onset Pott's paraplegia*: From progressive kyphosis, fibrosis, or granulation tissue

Evaluation Steps

- *Repeat MRI spine—to assess*:
  - Cord compression (granulation, fibrosis, abscess)
  - Deformity progression
- **Review compliance with ATT**
- *ESR/CRP*: Rule out superinfection
- Rule out MDR-TB via GeneXpert or culture

Management Plan

If paradoxical reaction:

- Continue ATT
- Add **NSAIDs or short-course steroids**
- Monitor for stabilization

If progressive kyphosis with deficit (late-onset paraplegia):

- Surgical decompression + stabilization
- *Usually via*:
  - Anterior corpectomy
  - Posterior instrumentation
  - Kyphosis correction osteotomy if needed

Post-operative

- Continue ATT
- Physiotherapy for neural recovery
- Nutritional and orthotic support

Summary

Worsening signs on ATT warrant **urgent imaging** to differentiate **paradoxical reaction versus true progression**, and may require **surgical correction**.

Q60. Discuss the principles of rehabilitation following surgical treatment of spinal TB.

Focus on physiotherapy, orthotic support, nutritional support

Goals of Rehabilitation

- Prevent **post-operative deformities and contractures**
- Restore **mobility and independence**
- Enhance **neurological recovery**
- Maintain **spinal alignment and function**

Key Components

1. *Physiotherapy*:
    - *Phase-wise mobilization*: Passive → assisted → active
    - Gait training
    - Trunk stability, abdominal and paraspinal strengthening
    - Neuro-rehabilitation in paraplegia cases
2. *Orthotic support*:
    - **TLSO or lumbosacral orthosis** post-surgery
    - Maintains spinal alignment during healing
    - Typically worn for **3–6 months**, depending on fusion and stability
3. *Nutritional support*:
    - **High-protein, high-calorie diet**
    - Supplement **vitamins A, D, B-complex**
    - Essential for **wound healing and immunity**
4. *Social and occupational rehabilitation*:
    - Gradual return to **daily activities**
    - **Workplace adjustments** for manual laborers
    - Counseling for chronic disease coping

Summary

Rehabilitation after spinal TB surgery is **multi-disciplinary**, aiming for **structural healing, neural recovery**, and **functional reintegration**.

Modern Management and Public Health Integration

Q61. Discuss the orthopedic implications of India's goal to eliminate TB by 2025.

[Dr Ram Manohar Lohia Institute of Medical Sciences (RMLIMS) Lucknow 2017]

Involves early diagnosis, surveillance, adherence, and DOTS

National Target

India, under **NTEP**, aims to **eliminate TB by 2025**, ahead of the global 2030 target.

Orthopedic Implications

1. *Early diagnosis*:
    - High suspicion in **chronic monoarthritis, cold abscesses, spinal deformities**
    - Use of **MRI, CBNAAT, and biopsy** for confirmation
    - Avoid mislabeling as trauma, tumor, or RA
2. *Prompt notification*:
    - Report every case of MSK TB on **Nikshay** portal
    - Enables **tracking, free drug access, and patient support**
3. *Ensuring treatment adherence*:
    - Monitor **compliance to daily ATT**
    - Educate patients on need for **long-duration therapy (12 months)**
    - Use **DOTS supervisors or family monitors**
4. *Rehabilitation and follow-up*:
    - Long-term follow-up to detect **recurrence or deformity**
    - Document **treatment outcomes and complications**

Summary

Orthopedic surgeons are vital in achieving TB elimination through **early detection**, **structured therapy**, and **public health coordination**.

Q62. Role of multidisciplinary team (MDT) in managing osteoarticular TB.

Integration of orthopedics, ID, radiology, microbiology, public health

MDT is critical due to:
- Complex presentations
- Need for **integrated diagnostics and long-term care**

Core MDT Members and Roles

Discipline	*Role*
Orthopedics	Diagnosis, biopsy, surgical debridement, stabilization
Radiology	MRI/X-ray interpretation, USG/CT-guided aspiration
Microbiology	AFB stain, culture, CBNAAT, line probe assay
Infectious disease	Drug regimens (especially MDR/XDR TB), ATT adjustments
Public health/NTEP	DOTS, patient tracking, nutrition support, contact tracing
Physiotherapy	Rehabilitation planning, mobility recovery
Social worker	Adherence, socio-economic aid, stigma reduction

Summary
An MDT ensures **accurate diagnosis, comprehensive treatment, and rehabilitation**, reducing **morbidity, relapse, and disability** in MSK TB.

Q63. Role of AI and digital tools in TB diagnosis in orthopedic practice.

Recent push in PGIMER, AIIMS, NTEP for TB digitization

Key Applications of AI and Digital Health

1. *AI in imaging*:
    - *AI-based software for X-ray and MRI interpretation*:
        - Detecting **vertebral collapse, disc loss, abscesses**
        - AIIMS & PGIMER trials on **automated spine TB detection**
2. *Digital microscopy and AFB detection*:
    - Image recognition for **automated ZN stain interpretation**
    - Faster and more sensitive smear reading
3. *Nikshay portal integration*:
    - Web-based national TB notification platform
    - Links **orthopedic units, labs, drug supply, and follow-up tracking**
    - Monitors adherence and outcomes
4. Predictive algorithms:
    - *AI used to forecast*:
        - MDR risk
        - Poor compliance probability
        - Risk of relapse or paradoxical reaction

Future Directions
- **Mobile-based tools** for remote TB triage
- Integration with **radiology PACS** for real-time alerts
- **e-Nikshay AI dashboards** for hospital MDTs

Summary
AI and digital platforms are enhancing **early detection, decision-making, and public health tracking** of TB—even in **orthopedic practice**.

Pharmacological and Resistance-based Questions

Q64. Discuss the mechanism of action, side effects, and monitoring of ATT drugs relevant to orthopedic TB

(Assam Medical College Dibrugarh 2013)

Includes INH, RIF, Ethambutol, Pyrazinamide, Streptomycin

Drug	Mechanism of action	Major side effects	Monitoring
Isoniazid (INH)	Inhibits mycolic acid synthesis → disrupts cell wall	Hepatitis, peripheral neuropathy (↓ B6), rash	LFTs, pyridoxine (B6) supplementation
Rifampicin (RIF)	Inhibits DNA-dependent RNA polymerase	Hepatitis, orange urine, drug interactions	LFTs, watch for ART/rifampin interactions
Pyrazinamide (PZA)	Disrupts membrane energetics, intracellular action	Hepatotoxicity, hyperuricemia, arthralgia	LFTs, uric acid (if joint pain)
Ethambutol (EMB)	Inhibits arabinosyl transferase → cell wall damage	Optic neuritis, red-green color blindness	Visual acuity, color vision monthly
Streptomycin (STM)	Aminoglycoside → inhibits 30S ribosome	Ototoxicity, nephrotoxicity	Audiometry, renal function tests

Summary

Understanding **mechanism, organ toxicity, and monitoring** is key to managing MSK TB patients on ATT, especially **elderly or comorbid cases**.

Q65. How do you modify ATT in hepatic dysfunction?

Common in case-based OSCE/spotters

ATT and Hepatotoxicity

- **INH, rifampicin, and pyrazinamide** are all **potentially hepatotoxic**
- In **pre-existing or ATT-induced liver injury**, ATT must be **adjusted to avoid further hepatic damage**

Strategies

Mild hepatic dysfunction (LFTs <3× ULN, no symptoms):

- **Continue standard ATT** with **close monitoring**
- Add **pyridoxine** for INH support

Moderate-severe hepatic dysfunction (LFTs >3–5× ULN or symptomatic):

Modified ATT regimen	Includes
Non-hepatotoxic (safe) options	Ethambutol + Streptomycin + Levofloxacin
If some hepatotoxicity acceptable	Ethambutol + Rifampicin + Levofloxacin

General Measures

- Stop ATT temporarily if ALT/AST > 5× ULN or jaundice present
- Reintroduce drugs **one at a time** (Rifampicin → INH → PZA, if tolerated)
- Consider **specialist consultation** for TB-HIV or cirrhosis

Summary

ATT in liver dysfunction should be **customized**, prioritizing **non-hepatotoxic agents** and **frequent LFT monitoring**.

Q66. Discuss the role of second-line drugs in drug-resistant musculoskeletal TB

[Christian Medical College (CMC) Vellore Tamil Nadu 2017]

Include bedaquiline, linezolid, fluoroquinolones

Indications

- **MDR-TB (resistance to INH + RIF)**
- **XDR-TB** or treatment failure after standard ATT
- As per **NTEP PMDT** guidelines

Key Second-line Drugs

Drug	Mechanism	Side Effects
Bedaquiline	Inhibits ATP synthase (bactericidal)	QT prolongation, hepatotoxicity
Linezolid	Inhibits 50S ribosome, prevents translation	Myelosuppression, optic neuropathy
Levofloxacin/Moxifloxacin	Fluoroquinolones → DNA gyrase inhibition	Tendinopathy, QT prolongation
Clofazimine	Binds DNA, bactericidal	Skin discoloration, GI upset
Cycloserine	Cell wall inhibitor	Psychiatric symptoms, seizures
Delamanid	Blocks mycolic acid synthesis	QT prolongation

Administration:

- Usually **6–7 drugs** in MDR regimen (intensive phase: 6–9 months)
- *Duration*: **18–20 months** total
- Requires **DOTS Plus centers** and specialist input

Summary

Second-line agents are lifesaving in **MDR/XDR musculoskeletal TB**, but need **monitoring for toxicity** and **adherence support**.

Miscellaneous High-level Questions

Q67. Describe the types and management of kyphotic deformity in TB spine.

Include Rajasekaran's classification and surgical correction strategies

Types of Kyphotic Deformity (Rajasekaran Classification)

Type	Features
I	Healed lesion, no instability or progression
II	Progressive kyphosis with risk of paraplegia
III	Healed lesion but instability/deformity persists
IV	Gross kyphosis with late-onset paraplegia

Predictors of Severe Kyphosis

- Age <10 years
- Involvement of >2 vertebrae
- Thoracolumbar location
- Delay in ATT initiation
- Involvement of anterior/middle columns

Management

Non-surgical:

- **Brace (TLSO)** during active phase
- Close radiological monitoring

Surgical indications:

- Kyphosis > 50–60°
- Progressive deformity
- Neurological signs
- Cosmetic/functional impairment

Surgical Strategies

Approach	*Goal*
Anterior decompression	Remove collapsed body, relieve cord
Posterior instrumentation	Stabilize spine, correct deformity
Osteotomy (e.g., pedicle subtraction)	For severe, rigid kyphosis
Combined anterior + posterior	For multilevel deformity

Summary

Rajasekaran's system helps **grade deformity severity** and plan **timely surgical correction** to prevent paraplegia or functional disability.

Q68. Post-tubercular sequelae in joints—diagnosis and management.

(Narayana Medical College Nellore Andhra Pradesh 2017)

Includes fibrous ankylosis, deformities, growth disturbances

Common Sequelae

Type	*Example*
Fibrous ankylosis	Hip/knee stiffness with loss of ROM
Bony ankylosis	Fusion in end-stage joint TB
Growth disturbance	Epiphyseal TB—limb length discrepancy
Joint deformity	Varus/valgus at knee or foot
Secondary OA	Due to cartilage damage

Diagnosis

- History of **past TB**
- *X-ray*: Joint narrowing, sclerosis, malalignment
- Functional assessment (ROM, limb length)

Management

Conservative:

- Physiotherapy
- Orthosis/bracing for stability
- Shoe raise or gait aid

Surgical:

- Arthrolysis for fibrous ankylosis
- Corrective osteotomy for deformity
- Total joint replacement (THR/TKR) in painful stiff joints
- Epiphysiodesis or lengthening procedures in children

Summary

Post-TB joint sequelae cause **chronic disability** and may require **rehabilitation or reconstructive surgery** based on deformity and joint function.

Q69. Compare TB arthritis with rheumatoid arthritis—clinical and radiological features.

Common differential diagnosis for monoarthritis

Feature	*TB arthritis*	*Rheumatoid arthritis (RA)*
Onset	Insidious, chronic	Insidious, symmetrical
Joint involvement	Monoarticular, weight-bearing joints	Polyarticular, small joints (MCP/PIP)

Continued

Continued

Feature	***TB arthritis***	***Rheumatoid arthritis (RA)***
Constitutional signs	Fever, weight loss common	Fatigue, malaise
Joint exam	Effusion, cold joint, limited ROM	Warm, swollen, painful joints
Radiological	*Phemister triad*: Osteoporosis, erosions, space narrowing	Uniform narrowing, periarticular erosion
Lab	ESR ↑, CBNAAT+, AFB/Biopsy+	RF/Anti-CCP+, CRP↑

Summary

TB arthritis is typically **monoarticular, slow, and cold**, while RA is **inflammatory, symmetric, and seropositive**—biopsy helps confirm TB.

Q70. Describe the complications of skeletal TB and their management.

[Kasturba Medical College (KMC) Manipal Karnataka 2014]

Includes pathological fractures, sinuses, ulcers, infections

Common Complications

Complication	***Site***	***Management***
Pathological fracture	Long bones, vertebrae	ATT + stabilization (cast or internal fixation)
Cold abscess	Spine, psoas, iliac	ATT ± image-guided aspiration or drainage
Sinus formation	Over joints or bone	Prolonged ATT, curettage if persistent
Discharging ulcer	Skin overlying lesion	Dressing + debridement + ATT
Superadded infection	Especially with sinuses	Antibiotics + debridement + culture guidance
Late-onset paraplegia	Kyphotic spine TB	Decompression surgery + ATT

General Principles

- Continue **full-course ATT**
- Address **nutritional deficits and immunity**
- Rule out **MDR-TB** if poor healing
- Use **surgical intervention selectively** for non-healing lesions

Summary

Skeletal TB can lead to **severe local and systemic complications**, which require **prolonged therapy, surgical care, and close follow-up**.

Recent Pattern-based and Image-based Questions (Spotters/OSCE)

Q71. Identify and describe the radiograph of Pott's spine with gibbus deformity.

Classic image-based spotter in PG/viva

Radiographic Features

- *Vertebral body destruction*: Typically anterior
- *Loss of disc space*: Seen in paradiscal TB
- *Wedge-shaped collapse* of involved vertebrae
- *Angular kyphosis ("gibbus")*: Sharp posterior angulation
- *May see paravertebral shadow*: Due to cold abscess
- Healed cases show **fusion and deformity**

Common Levels

- Thoracic > Thoracolumbar > Lumbar

Additional Clues

- Gibbus usually forms when **≥2 adjacent vertebrae collapse**
- In severe cases → **late-onset paraplegia** risk

Summary

X-ray of Pott's spine with gibbus deformity shows **anterior vertebral collapse**, **disc space loss**, and **sharp angular kyphosis**, diagnostic of **spinal TB**.

Q72. Cold abscess tracking to the groin—likely source? Investigation?

(Frequently asked in OSCE and image-based NEET SS)

Diagnosis

Cold abscess from spinal TB tracking via psoas muscle

Likely Source

- **Lumbar spine TB (L2–L4)**
- Pus follows **psoas sheath** → appears in **inguinal region**, **upper medial thigh**, or **iliac fossa**

Key Features

- **Painless**, fluctuant swelling
- No redness or warmth
- May be **bilateral** in some cases

Investigations

- *MRI spine + pelvis*: To locate vertebral lesion and abscess tract
- *Ultrasound*: Fluid collection
- *Aspiration—send for*:
    - CBNAAT (GeneXpert)
    - AFB stain
    - Histopathology

Summary

Groin cold abscess often originates from **lumbar spinal TB**, tracking through **psoas**, best evaluated with **MRI and guided aspiration**.

Q73. Identify Ziehl-Neelsen stain image—describe relevance in TB diagnosis.

Common image in practicals or OSCEs

What You See

- **Bright red, rod-shaped bacilli** on a **blue background**
- Seen in sputum, pus, or biopsy smear

Principle of ZN Stain

- Acid-fastness due to **mycolic acid** in MTB cell wall
- Stained with **carbol fuchsin**, decolorized with **acid-alcohol**, counterstained with **methylene blue**

Use in Orthopedic TB

- Performed on **aspirated pus**, sinus discharge, biopsy
- **Low sensitivity** in bone TB (~30–40%)
- Still important for **rapid diagnosis** and **legal documentation**

Alternatives

- **CBNAAT (GeneXpert)** now preferred for sensitivity + rifampicin resistance
- Culture (MGIT) or **histology** for confirmation

Summary
Ziehl-Neelsen stain is a **classical test** to demonstrate **AFB in TB**, useful in **osteomyelitis, abscesses**, and TB sinus evaluation, though now largely supported by **molecular methods**.

Ultra-Rare, Fringe, and Emerging Theory Questions on Musculoskeletal TB

Q74. Tubercular involvement of the costovertebral or sternoclavicular joints – clinical relevance and management

Rare sites; often misdiagnosed as tumor or pyogenic arthritis

Clinical Relevance
- Rare (<1% of skeletal TB)
- Presents with **painful swelling near sternum or posterior thorax**
- *Can mimic*:
  - Tumor (e.g., chondrosarcoma)
  - Septic arthritis
  - Fungal osteomyelitis
- Seen more in **HIV-positive or immunosuppressed patients**

Clinical Features
- Dull ache, local swelling
- Restricted shoulder/chest movement (in SCJ involvement)
- Occasionally draining sinus

Investigations
- *MRI/CT chest wall*: Defines soft tissue and bony changes
- *Biopsy/Aspiration*: Mandatory for diagnosis
  - CBNAAT, AFB stain, histology
- *X-ray*: May show erosion, joint space widening

Management
- **ATT for 12 months**
- *Surgery if*:
  - Large abscess
  - Suspected malignancy
  - Instability or failure to respond

Summary
TB of costovertebral or sternoclavicular joints presents **atypically**, often mimicking tumors, and requires **early imaging + biopsy + ATT**.

Q75. Tuberculous bursitis—common sites, presentation, and treatment.

[Assam Medical College (affiliated to Srimanta Sankaradeva University of Health Sciences) 2018]

For example, Trochanteric or olecranon TB bursitis

Common Sites

Bursa	*Location*
Trochanteric	Over greater trochanter
Olecranon	Posterior elbow
Prepatellar	Over patella
Subdeltoid	Below deltoid (shoulder)

Clinical Presentation

- Chronic **painless swelling** over bursa
- May form **cold abscess or sinus**
- **No redness or warmth**
- Often **misdiagnosed as bursitis of other origin or neoplasm**

Diagnosis

- *USG/MRI*: Shows thickened bursal wall, fluid
- *Aspiration or excision biopsy*: Send for GeneXpert, AFB, histopathology

Management

- **ATT for 12 months**
- *Surgical bursectomy if*:
  - Cold abscess
  - Persistent symptoms
  - Diagnostic doubt (tumor mimic)

Summary

TB bursitis often affects **trochanteric or olecranon bursae**, presenting as **chronic fluctuant swellings**, requiring **biopsy and ATT.**

Q76. Spinal TB in children—growth-related complications and treatment challenges.

Angular deformity, kyphosis, growth plate disruption

Why It's Special?

- Children's spine is **more flexible**, but vertebral growth plates are **vulnerable**
- Early collapse → **gibbus deformity**
- Higher risk of **neurological involvement**

Growth-related Complications

- Vertebral wedging or collapse
- Angular kyphosis (Rajasekaran type II or IV)
- Late-onset paraplegia
- Compensatory hyperlordosis

Challenges in Management

- Risk of **progression even after healing**
- Need for **frequent radiologic monitoring**
- *Surgical decisions complicated by*:
  - Growth potential
  - Implant size
  - Deformity correction goals

Management Principles

- **Early ATT (12–18 months)**
- **Bracing (TLSO)** for prevention of deformity
- *Surgery if*:
  - Kyphosis > 50–60°
  - Neurological deficit
  - Spinal instability

Summary

Spinal TB in children demands **close monitoring for growth-related deformities**, with a low threshold for **surgical stabilization and correction.**

Q77. Tuberculosis of the pubic symphysis—diagnosis and management.

(Rajasthan University of Health Sciences Jaipur 2017)

Very rare; seen in postpartum or immunosuppressed patients

Clinical Features

- Pain in **lower pelvis or pubic area**
- Difficulty in **walking, standing up**
- Local tenderness over **pubic symphysis**
- *May mimic*:
  - Osteitis pubis
  - Pelvic fracture
  - Septic arthritis or tumor

Epidemiology

- Rare site of skeletal TB
- *More common in*:
  - Postpartum females
  - HIV-positive patients
  - Post-surgical or catheterized patients

Investigations

- *MRI pelvis*: Shows erosion, abscess
- *X-ray*: May show joint widening, rarefaction
- *CT-guided aspiration or open biopsy—definitive*: CBNAAT, AFB, histology

Management

- ATT for 12 months
- Rest and pelvic support
- Surgical drainage if abscess present or biopsy needed

Summary

Pubic symphysis TB is a **rare but important mimic** of pelvic pain syndromes and requires **imaging, biopsy, and ATT**, especially in **postpartum or immunocompromised patients**.

Advanced Surgical Questions

Q78. Three-column concept in spinal TB surgery—relevance in approach selection.

Denis' theory used to assess spinal stability in TB.

Denis' Three-column Theory

Column	Structures
Anterior column	Anterior longitudinal ligament (ALL), anterior half of vertebral body and disc
Middle column	Posterior half of vertebral body, posterior longitudinal ligament (PLL)
Posterior column	Pedicles, laminae, spinous process, ligamentum flavum, interspinous ligaments

Relevance in Spinal TB

- **Paradiscal TB** begins in anterior/middle columns
- **Instability** occurs when **≥2 columns** are destroyed
- *Guides whether to*:
  - Decompress anteriorly

- Stabilize posteriorly
- Use **360° fusion (combined approach)** in panvertebral disease

Clinical Use

- If **only anterior column** involved → ATT + brace
- If **anterior + middle** → may require anterior decompression
- If **posterior column + kyphosis** → posterior stabilization needed

Summary

Three-column model helps **classify spinal TB severity**, predict **instability**, and choose **surgical approach** appropriately.

Q79. Anterior instrumentation versus posterior stabilization in spinal TB—current evidence.

[All India Institute of Medical Sciences (AIIMS) Jodhpur Rajasthan 2018]

Posterior-only approach increasingly preferred

Traditional Approach

- *Anterior decompression and grafting were standard for*:
  - Cord compression
  - Vertebral body destruction
  - Abscess drainage

Drawbacks of Anterior Instrumentation

- Technically demanding (thoracotomy, retroperitoneal)
- Poor fixation in osteoporotic TB bone
- *Risks*: Vascular injury, poor kyphosis correction

Posterior Stabilization—Current Evidence

Advantages	*Studies supporting*
One-stage decompression + fixation	Rajasekaran et al., Jain AK, global reviews
Better correction of kyphosis	Singh et al. (2020), Global Spine Journal
Shorter operative time, less morbidity	PGIMER, AIIMS studies, NEET-SS clinical consensus

Current Recommendation

- *Posterior-only stabilization is now*:
  - Preferred for most thoracolumbar TB
  - Effective in **kyphosis correction + decompression**
  - Often combined with **transpedicular decompression**

Summary

Posterior-only stabilization is now evidence-backed as **safe, effective, and versatile** in spinal TB, replacing anterior constructs in many cases.

Q80. Minimally invasive surgical options in spinal TB—discuss indications and outcomes.

(King George's Medical University 2016)

Thoracoscopic decompression, percutaneous fixation

Why Minimally Invasive?

- TB patients are often **malnourished/immunocompromised**
- *MIS reduces*:
  - Blood loss
  - Wound infection
  - Hospital stay

Minimally Invasive Options

Technique	Indication
Thoracoscopic anterior decompression	Mid-thoracic TB with cord compression
Percutaneous pedicle screw fixation	Lumbar/thoracolumbar TB without severe deformity
Mini-open retroperitoneal approach	L2–L5 vertebral body disease (abscess, wedge collapse)
Endoscopic biopsy + drainage	Diagnostic or for isolated cold abscesses

Outcomes (per Recent Studies)
- Similar kyphosis correction to open surgery
- Lower morbidity and better cosmesis
- Requires specialized expertise and instrumentation
- AIIMS, PGIMER, and global meta-analyses endorse MIS for early-stage TB spine

Summary
Minimally invasive spine TB surgery offers **safe, cosmetically better options** with outcomes similar to open surgery, especially in **early, localized disease**.

Complications and Special Situations

Q81. Surgical management of healed TB with severe kyphotic deformity.

(Banaras Hindu University – Institute of Medical Sciences 2018)

Include pedicle subtraction osteotomy, vertebral column resection (VCR), halo-pelvic traction.

Context
- Deformity often persists despite healing
- *May cause*:
  - Late-onset paraplegia
  - Functional limitation
  - Cosmetic concern

Surgical Options Based on Severity

Deformity	Surgical approach
< 40° kyphosis	Posterior instrumentation with compression
40°–60° kyphosis	Pedicle subtraction osteotomy (PSO)—wedge removal from posterior elements
> 60° kyphosis, rigid	Vertebral column resection (VCR)—complete removal of one or more vertebral bodies
Fixed or massive deformity	Halo-pelvic traction—gradual deformity correction before surgery

Adjunct Measures
- **Neuro-monitoring** during deformity correction
- Post-operative **orthosis (TLSO)** for 3–6 months
- Continue **ATT** if any suspicion of reactivation

Summary
Healed TB with severe kyphosis requires complex correction like **PSO or VCR**, often staged with **traction and multidisciplinary planning**.

Q82. TB arthritis with co-existing rheumatoid arthritis—how does management change?

Dual pathology: Immunosuppression and diagnostic masking.

Challenges
- RA can **mask TB arthritis** (monoarthritis in a polyarticular setting)

- **Immunosuppressive drugs** (e.g., methotrexate, steroids) may **reactivate latent TB**
- TB can be **mistaken for RA flare**

Diagnosis Approach
- Consider TB in **RA patient with monoarthritis**, non-responsive joint
- **Synovial biopsy + CBNAAT** is crucial
- **Avoid steroids or DMARDs** until infection ruled out

Treatment Modifications

Condition	*Management strategy*
Active TB + active RA	Start ATT first, delay immunosuppressants by 4–6 weeks
Quiescent TB, active RA	Resume DMARDs cautiously under supervision
Joint damage from both	Consider arthroplasty after TB is healed

Summary
RA with TB arthritis requires **careful diagnostic separation, prioritizing TB treatment**, and **delayed reintroduction of immunosuppressants.**

Q83. Management of pathological fracture through tubercular focus.

(Baba Farid University of Health Sciences 2019)

Pathological fracture in tubercolosis is rare, complex – requires internal fixation + prolonged ATT.

Definition
Fracture occurring through a bone weakened by **active TB infection.**

Common Sites
- Femur, tibia, humerus, spine
- May occur **spontaneously or after minimal trauma**

Management Plan
1. *Confirm diagnosis*:
   - MRI + biopsy from fracture site
   - CBNAAT, culture, histology
2. *Start ATT immediately*:
   - HRZE for at least 12–18 months
   - Nutritional and systemic support
3. *Surgical stabilization*:

Approach	*Indication*
Internal fixation (IM nail or plate)	For long bone fractures—provides early mobilization
External fixator	If there's a draining sinus or infection
Spinal instrumentation	If through collapsed vertebra

   - Use **antibiotic-loaded cement** if infected
   - Combine with **debridement** if needed
4. *Post-operative monitoring*:
   - Watch for **non-union, implant loosening**
   - Continue **long-term ATT**, especially in MDR suspicion

Summary
TB-related pathological fractures need **early ATT + stable fixation**, ideally after **biopsy confirmation**, with **careful surgical planning.**

Multidisciplinary/Research-based Questions

Q84. Discuss clinical scoring systems used in assessing severity and prognosis in spinal TB.

For example, Modified Frankel grading, Rajasekaran's kyphosis angle prediction

A. Modified Frankel Grading (Neurological Severity):

Grade	Neurological status
A	Complete motor and sensory loss
B	Sensory preserved, no motor function
C	Motor present but non-functional
D	Motor useful but not normal
E	Normal motor and sensory function

Used pre- and post-operatively to assess cord compression severity and recovery.

B. Rajasekaran's Kyphosis Prediction Formula (Spinal Deformity Risk)

Final kyphosis angle (°) = 5 + (30 × number of vertebral bodies lost)

- Predicts deformity risk in children and adults
- Used for planning **surgical correction timing**

C. Other Scores

- **ASIA Impairment Scale** – similar to Frankel, for international use
- **Spinal Instability Score (Tuli's criteria)** – includes pain, neurodeficit, mobility, radiology

Summary

Scoring systems like **Modified Frankel and Rajasekaran's angle** help stratify **neurological severity and deformity risk**, guiding **surgical urgency and prognosis**.

Q85. Write briefly on recent advances in diagnosis of MSK TB.

(AIIMS Bhubaneswar 2018)

Include PET-CT, nucleic acid amplification tests, MGIT culture.

A. Nucleic Acid Amplification Tests (NAATs)

Tool	Use
CBNAAT (GeneXpert)	Detects MTB + rifampicin resistance in 2 hours
Line probe assay (LPA)	Detects INH + RIF resistance via DNA hybridization

Used on pus, synovial fluid, biopsy tissue: Rapid, sensitive for early TB and **MDR-TB**

B. Mycobacterial Growth Indicator Tube (MGIT) Culture

- Liquid culture system (faster than LJ medium)
- **Gold standard for drug sensitivity**
- Time to positivity: 10–14 days

C. FDG-PET CT (Positron Emission Tomography)

- Detects **metabolically active TB lesions**
- *Useful in*:
  - Multifocal TB
  - Post-therapy response assessment
  - TB vs tumor differential

D. Others

- *Interferon gamma release assays (IGRA)*: Limited role in bone TB
- PCR-based diagnostic panels (e.g., Truenat MTB)

Summary
Advances like **CBNAAT, LPA, PET-CT, and MGIT** enable **rapid, reliable detection** of musculoskeletal TB and **drug resistance profiling**.

Q86. Genetic predisposition and immunogenetics in extrapulmonary TB—future prospects.

(Rajendra Institute of Medical Sciences 2017)

HLA associations, TLR polymorphisms, PGI/AIIMS research focus.

Why It Matters?
- Not all exposed individuals develop TB
- **Host genetic factors** influence **susceptibility and extrapulmonary TB (EPTB)** development

A. HLA Associations
- Certain **HLA-DR and HLA-DQ alleles** linked to increased risk
- **HLA-DRB1*15**—associated with **extrapulmonary and skeletal TB** (observed in PGIMER studies)

B. Toll-Like Receptor (TLR) Polymorphisms

Receptor	*Polymorphism*	*Effect*
TLR2, TLR4	Single-nucleotide polymorphisms (SNPs)	Alter innate immune response to MTB
TLR8	X-linked polymorphisms	Explored in male-predominant spinal TB

C. Cytokine Gene Variants
- **TNF-α, IFN-γ, IL-12** pathway mutations → impaired granuloma formation
- Contribute to **chronicity or dissemination**

D. Current Research
- **AIIMS and PGIMER Chandigarh** conducting GWAS and targeted sequencing
- *Aim*: Predict **high-risk individuals**, personalize **vaccine/therapy response**

Summary
Understanding **genetic predisposition** via **HLA typing and TLR polymorphisms** is a future avenue for **precision TB care**, particularly in **extrapulmonary presentations**.

AIIMS/DNB—Style Integrated Questions

Q87. Case: A patient with long-standing HIV presents with foot pain, discharging sinus, and night sweats. What is your differential? How will you confirm and manage?

Focus: Immunocompromised host with extrapulmonary TB features.

Differential Diagnosis

Condition	*Key Clues*
Tuberculous osteomyelitis	Night sweats, sinus, chronicity, HIV risk
Chronic pyogenic osteomyelitis	Foul discharge, fever, bone destruction
Fungal osteomyelitis	Immunosuppressed, non-resolving infection
Atypical mycobacteria	Disseminated in AIDS, non-tuberculous species
Neoplastic lesion (rare)	Persistent sinus, lytic lesion mimicking tumor

Clinical Evaluation
- *Local*: Swelling, tenderness, sinus, reduced ROM
- *Systemic*: Fever, weight loss, HIV ART history
- Examine for **other TB foci (lungs, spine, nodes)**

Investigations

- *X-ray/CT foot*: Osteolysis, sequestra
- *MRI foot*: Abscess, marrow edema
- *Pus/biopsy from sinus*:
  - CBNAAT (GeneXpert MTB/RIF)
  - AFB stain and culture (MGIT)
  - Fungal culture (in HIV+)
- ESR/CRP, CBC
- *HIV profile*: CD4 count, viral load

Management

- **Start ATT** if TB confirmed (even in extrapulmonary site)
- Continue ART – modify if drug interactions (e.g., rifampicin)
- **Debridement** if sequestrum or abscess
- Nutrition, wound care
- Consider **steroids** if IRIS suspected post-ART start

Summary

This HIV-positive patient likely has **tubercular osteomyelitis of foot**, and management includes **biopsy-confirmed diagnosis, ATT, surgical debridement, and ART coordination**.

Q88. Compare pyogenic spondylodiscitis, brucella spondylitis, and TB spine—write a diagnostic algorithm.

[Assam Medical College (affiliated to Srimanta Sankaradeva University of Health Sciences) 2019]

Important comparison in endemic regions and PG theory exams.

Clinical Comparison Table

Feature	*TB spine*	*Pyogenic*	*Brucella*
Onset	Insidious	Acute/subacute	Subacute
Fever	Low-grade, evening rise	High-grade, with chills	Undulant or absent
Pain	Severe, localized back pain	Acute back pain	Milder pain, sacroiliac often involved
Neurological signs	Common (due to kyphosis/abscess)	Less common	Rare
Cold abscess	Common	Rare	Absent
Vertebral involvement	Anterior, multiple bodies	Single vertebra, rapid destruction	Single-disc involvement
Lab	ESR↑, AFB+, GeneXpert+	Neutrophilia, positive blood culture	SAT/Rose Bengal test+, blood culture+

Imaging Clues

- *TB*: Paradiscal, anterior vertebral body, gibbus
- *Pyogenic*: Endplate destruction, vertebral collapse, disc height loss
- *Brucella*: Disc-space narrowing, SI joint involvement, no collapse

Diagnostic Algorithm

- **Clinical presentation + endemic area**
- *Blood tests*:
  - CBC, ESR, CRP
  - SAT/Rose Bengal (Brucella)
  - Blood culture (Brucella, pyogenic)

- *MRI spine*: Look for disc space, abscess, vertebral involvement
- *Biopsy/Aspirate*:
  - CBNAAT for TB
  - Bacterial/fungal culture
  - Histopathology

Treatment Outline

Condition	*Treatment*
TB	ATT (12 months), surgery if needed
Pyogenic	IV antibiotics (6–8 weeks), then oral, debridement
Brucella	Doxycycline + Rifampin for ≥6–12 weeks

Summary

This algorithm distinguishes **TB, brucella, and pyogenic spondylitis** based on **clinical, imaging, serologic, and biopsy data**, guiding targeted therapy.

CHAPTER 4

Musculoskeletal Tumors

Ashish Gulia, Aman Koul, Vipin Sharma

Q1. Describe the clinical approach to diagnosing soft tissue tumors.

(Kashmir University)

History
- Duration, growth rate, pain
- Trauma, systemic signs, previous malignancy

Examination
- Size, location, depth (superficial vs. deep fascia)
- Consistency, mobility, pulsatility
- Neurovascular involvement

Imaging
- Ultrasound for superficial lesion
- MRI—investigation of choice (defines extent, depth, vascularity)
- CT scan for calcification and bony involvement
- PET-CT for metastasis in malignant lesions

Definitive Diagnosis
- **Core needle biopsy or incisional biopsy**
- Followed by histopathology and immunohistochemistry

Q2. Discuss the role of biopsy in orthopedic tumors.

Purpose
- Confirm diagnosis
- Grade and stage the tumor
- Guide treatment planning

Types
- *FNAC*: Screening; limited use
- *Core needle biopsy (Tru-cut)*: Most common, image-guided
- *Incisional biopsy*: For large, accessible tumors
- *Excisional biopsy*: Only for small, superficial benign lesions

Guiding Principles
- **Biopsy tract must be within planned excision zone**
- Avoid contamination of other compartments

- Performed after imaging (MRI)
- Prefer image-guided biopsy for deep lesions
- Done by **orthopedic oncologist/surgical team**

Q3. Radiological approach to bone tumors.

- *Plain radiograph (first-line)*: Site, zone, margin, matrix (e.g., osteoid, chondroid, lytic/blastic)
- *CT scan*: Better cortical detail, periosteal reaction, mineralization
- *MRI*: Soft tissue involvement, marrow changes, neurovascular encasement
- *Bone scan*: Detect multifocality or metastasis
- *PET-CT*: Useful for staging and assessing response to therapy

Q4. Role of dynamic contrast-enhanced MRI in soft tissue tumors.

Principles
- Repeated imaging post-contrast
- Evaluates tumor vascularity and perfusion kinetics

Applications
- Differentiate benign versus malignant tumors
- Tumor grading
- Assess response to neoadjuvant chemotherapy

Benign Bone Tumors

Q5. Classify various benign bone tumors with examples.

(Asked in PGI Chandigarh 2021, AIIMS Delhi 2022)

Classification of Benign Bone Tumors

Category	*Examples*
Bone-forming tumors	Osteoid osteoma, osteoblastoma
Cartilage-forming tumors	Osteochondroma, enchondroma, chondroblastoma
Fibrous tissue tumors	Fibrous cortical defect, non-ossifying fibroma
Vascular tumors	Hemangioma
Others	Giant cell tumor (GCT), aneurysmal bone cyst (ABC), simple bone cyst

Key Tip
- *Bone-forming*: Osteoid.
- *Cartilage-forming*: Chondroid.

Simple Mnemonic: "Big Cute Friends Often Help Grow."
(Bone, Cartilage, Fibrous, Others, Hemangioma, GCT)

Q6. Define musculoskeletal tumors. Classify based on histology and behavior?

Definition

Musculoskeletal tumors are **abnormal proliferations of mesenchymal origin**, affecting **bone, cartilage, muscle, fat, or connective tissue**.

Classification

A. Based on Histologic Origin

Tissue	*Examples*
Bone	Osteosarcoma, osteoid osteoma
Cartilage	Chondrosarcoma, enchondroma
Fibrous tissue	Fibrosarcoma, desmoid
Fat	Lipoma, liposarcoma
Muscle	Rhabdomyosarcoma, leiomyoma
Vascular	Hemangioma, angiosarcoma

B. Based on Biological Behavior

- *Benign*: For example, osteochondroma, chondroblastoma
- *Locally aggressive*: For example, giant cell tumor
- *Malignant*: For example, osteosarcoma, ewing's sarcoma

Q7. WHO classification of bone tumors (2020 revision).

Categories

- *Bone-forming tumors*:
  - *Benign*: Osteoid osteoma
  - *Malignant*: Osteosarcoma
- *Cartilage-forming tumors*:
  - *Benign*: Enchondroma, osteochondroma
  - *Malignant*: Chondrosarcoma
- *Fibrous tumors*: Desmoid, fibrosarcoma
- *Vascular tumors*: Hemangioma, angiosarcoma
- *Other tumors*: Ewing's sarcoma, adamantinoma
- Undifferentiated/Unclassified tumors

Q8. Differences between benign and malignant bone tumors.

Feature	*Benign*	*Malignant*
Growth rate	Slow	Rapid
Local invasion	None/minimal	Present
Metastasis	Absent	Present (lungs, bone)
Symptoms	Often asymptomatic	Pain, swelling, systemic features
Radiology	Well-defined, sclerotic margins	Ill-defined, cortical breach

Q9. Describe osteoid osteoma with reference to clinical features, radiology, and management.

(Asked in MUHS Maharashtra 2022, RGUHS Karnataka 2022)

Definition

Osteoid osteoma is a **small, benign, osteogenic tumor** characterized by a **nidus (<2 cm)** surrounded by **reactive sclerosis**.

Clinical Features

- Night pain **relieved dramatically by NSAIDs** (especially aspirin).
- Common in young males (10–30 years).

- Most common site: **proximal femur**, tibia, posterior elements of spine.
- Limp or stiffness if near joints.
- Pain worse at night, unrelated to activity.

Radiology
- *X-ray*: Small, radiolucent nidus with surrounding reactive sclerosis.
- *CT scan*: Best to localize the nidus clearly.
- *MRI*: Shows bone marrow and soft tissue edema but may obscure nidus.

Management

Method	*Details*
Medical treatment	NSAIDs for symptom control (small lesions)
Minimally invasive	CT-guided radiofrequency ablation (RFA) (gold standard now)
Surgical excision	Reserved for inaccessible lesions or failed RFA

Important Tip
- CT is investigation of choice.
- RFA is the preferred treatment today.

Q10. Osteoid osteoma versus osteoblastoma—differences.

Feature	*Osteoid osteoma*	*Osteoblastoma*
Size	<1.5 cm (nidus)	>2 cm
Pain	Severe, night pain, NSAID-relieved	Mild, dull, less NSAID-responsive
Location	Diaphysis of long bones	Spine (posterior elements), flat bones
Radiology	Sclerotic rim, lucent nidus	Expansile lesion, less sclerosis
Treatment	RFA or excision	Surgical curettage or excision
Malignant potential	None	Rare (may mimic aggressive lesions)

Q11. Write a note on enchondroma with reference to diagnosis and differential diagnosis.

(Asked in JIPMER Puducherry 2022)

Definition

Enchondroma is a **benign cartilage tumour** arising within the **medullary cavity** of bone.

Common Sites
- Small bones of hand and feet (phalanges, metacarpals).
- Proximal humerus, femur.

Clinical Features
- Usually **asymptomatic**, found incidentally.
- Pathological fracture may be first presentation.
- Rarely causes swelling or deformity.

Radiology

Imaging	*Findings*
X-ray	Well-circumscribed lytic lesion with "rings and arcs" (chondroid matrix calcification)
MRI	Homogenous low to intermediate T1 and high T2 signal

Differential Diagnosis

Condition	Key differences
Low-grade chondrosarcoma	Painful lesion, cortical breach, soft tissue extension
Bone infarct	More sclerotic, serpiginous borders
Fibrous dysplasia	Ground-glass appearance on X-ray

Management

- Observation if asymptomatic.
- Curettage and bone grafting if fracture risk or symptomatic.

Important Tip

Pain in an enchondroma suggests possibility of **malignant transformation** (very rare)!

Q12. Osteochondroma—clinical presentation and complications?

Definition

Most common benign bone tumor, composed of **cartilage-capped bony projection** that arises from **metaphysis** and is continuous with the **cortex and medulla** of the host bone.

Clinical Presentation

- Painless, slow-growing **bony swelling**
- Common in **distal femur, proximal tibia, humerus**
- May present with **mechanical symptoms**, deformity, or neurovascular compression

Complications

- Mechanical irritation (bursa formation, impingement)
- Nerve compression (e.g., peroneal nerve)
- Fracture at stalk
- Growth deformities in children
- *Rarely*: Malignant transformation to chondrosarcoma (~1%)

Q13. Multiple hereditary exostoses (MHE)—genetics and complications.

(PMCH Patna 2019)

Definition

Autosomal dominant disorder characterized by **multiple osteochondromas**, typically involving **metaphyseal regions** of long bones.

Genetics

- Mutation in ***EXT1* or *EXT2* genes**
- Affects **heparan sulphate biosynthesis** → abnormal cartilage proliferation

Clinical Features

- Multiple **bony swellings**
- **Limb deformities** (e.g., genu valgum, limb length discrepancy)
- **Short stature**
- Family history often positive

Complications

- Skeletal deformities
- Neurovascular compression
- Malignant transformation (up to 5%)
- Joint movement restriction

Q14. Describe in detail giant cell tumour (GCT) of bone, its pathology, clinical features, and the treatment.

(Asked in AIIMS Delhi 2022, PGI Chandigarh 2022)

Definition

Giant cell tumour (GCT) is a **locally aggressive benign tumor** composed of **stromal mononuclear cells** and **multinucleated giant cells**.

Pathology

- Abundant multinucleated giant cells uniformly distributed among stromal cells.
- Stromal cells are **neoplastic**.

Common Sites

- **Epiphysis of long bones**.
- *Around knee*: Distal femur, proximal tibia most common.

Clinical Features

- Pain and swelling around joint.
- Limitation of joint motion.
- Pathological fracture may occur.
- Usually affects young adults (20–40 years).

Radiology

Imaging	*Findings*
X-ray	Eccentric, expansile lytic lesion involving epiphysis, "soap-bubble" appearance
MRI	Soft tissue involvement, marrow edema

Management

Stage/Severity	*Treatment*
Localized	Extended curettage + adjuvant (phenol, cryotherapy) + bone graft/cement
Recurrent	Repeat curettage or wide excision
Unresectable/Metastatic	Denosumab (RANKL inhibitor therapy)
Very aggressive cases	Wide excision ± reconstruction (endoprosthesis)

Important Points

- **Denosumab** is a targeted therapy for GCT (inhibits RANKL pathway).
- Pulmonary metastases can occur even though tumor is histologically benign.

Q15. Campanacci classification of GCT.

Grade	*Radiological appearance*	*Management implication*
I	Well-defined margins with intact cortex	Curettage and grafting
II	Well-defined margins with cortical thinning/expansion	Extended curettage, cement
III	Ill-defined margins with cortical breach/soft tissue extension	Wide excision ± reconstruction

Q16. Recurrence and malignant transformation in GCT.

Recurrence

- Occurs in up to **20–30%** of cases after curettage
- Higher with inadequate margins, aggressive lesions
- Local recurrence presents with pain/swelling
- Monitored with periodic **MRI/X-ray**

Malignant Transformation

- Rare (<2%)
- May occur **de novo** or secondary to **radiotherapy**
- Transforms into **high-grade sarcoma (e.g., osteosarcoma)**
- Requires **wide excision and chemotherapy**

Q17. Role of denosumab in GCT.

(GMERS Medical College Rajasthan University of Health Sciences 2018)

Mechanism

RANKL inhibitor: Suppresses osteoclast activity and giant cells

Indications

- Unresectable tumors
- High-risk anatomical sites (spine, pelvis)
- Neoadjuvant to reduce tumor size before surgery

Benefits

- Reduces **tumor volume** and vascularity
- Facilitates **joint preservation**

Limitations

- Requires prolonged use
- Risk of **rebound recurrence** after stopping
- May obscure histology due to tumor ossification

Quick Tips for Theory and Viva

- Always start bone tumor answers with **classification**.
- In osteoid osteoma, **night pain relieved by NSAIDs** is a **buzzword**!
- In enchondroma, **"rings and arcs" calcification** is key X-ray feature.
- For GCT, **epiphyseal location + soap-bubble lytic lesion** must be mentioned early.

Q18. Giant cell tumor (GCT) variants.

- *Classical GCT*: Epiphyseal-metaphyseal lesion, soap-bubble appearance
- *Variants*:
  - Aneurysmal bone cyst changes
  - Malignant GCT (sarcomatous transformation)
  - Secondary ABC

Malignant Bone Tumors

Q19. Classify different malignant bone tumors.

(Asked in PGI Chandigarh 2021, RGUHS Karnataka 2022)

Classification of Malignant Bone Tumors

Category	*Examples*
Primary malignant tumors	Osteosarcoma, Ewing's sarcoma, chondrosarcoma, fibrosarcoma
Hematopoietic tumors	Multiple myeloma, primary bone lymphoma
Secondary (metastatic)	Carcinoma metastases (breast, lung, prostate, kidney, thyroid)

Important Points

- *Osteosarcoma*: Most common primary malignant bone tumor in young adults.
- *Metastasis*: Most common overall malignancy in bone in adults.

Mnemonic for Primary Malignant Tumors: "Every Odd Cancer Forms Fear."
(Ewing, osteosarcoma, chondrosarcoma, fibrosarcoma)

Q20. Basic principles of diagnosing bone tumors.

(BJ Medical College Ahmedabad 2014)

1. *History and clinical exam*: Age, duration, pain, swelling, trauma history
2. *Imaging*: X-ray → MRI → CT → PET/bone scan
3. *Labs*:
   - CBC, ESR, CRP
   - ALP, LDH, calcium (in some tumors)
4. *Biopsy*:
   - Essential for definitive diagnosis
   - Must be planned with oncologic surgery

Q21. Radiological approach to MSK Tumors.

- *X-ray (first-line)*:
  - Site, size, margins
  - Cortical breach, periosteal reaction, matrix mineralization
- *MRI*: Best for soft tissue extent, marrow involvement, skip lesions
- *CT*: Bony detail, mineralization, cortical thinning
- *PET-CT/Bone scan*: Staging, metastasis, skip lesions

Q22. Role of CT, MRI, and PET in bone tumors.

[Government Medical College (GMC) Srinagar 2013]

Modality	*Role*
CT scan	Bony architecture, cortical integrity, chest staging
MRI	Extent, marrow invasion, neurovascular relation
PET scan	Whole-body staging, response to therapy, recurrence detection

Q23. Importance of bone scan.

- Uses **technetium-99m MDP**
- Detects **osteoblastic activity**
- *Useful in*:
  - **Metastasis screening**
  - Multifocal lesions
  - Local recurrence
  - Cold spot in **multiple myeloma**

Q24. Bone biopsy in tumors—short answer?

Definition

Procedure to obtain tissue from a bone lesion to confirm diagnosis (benign vs. malignant) and plan treatment.

Types
- *Core needle biopsy*: Image-guided, preferred for deep lesions.
- *Open biopsy*: For superficial or inconclusive lesions.
- *FNAC*: Limited role; poor for grading.

Principles
- Planned **with definitive surgeon**.
- Use **longitudinal incision**, avoid vital structures.
- Biopsy tract must be **resectable** during tumor surgery.
- **Post-imaging** biopsy only.
- Avoid contaminating compartments or causing hematoma.

Indications
- Suspected primary/malignant bone tumor
- Metastasis to bone
- Unclear radiological diagnosis

Complications
- Tumor seeding
- Hematoma
- Infection
- Inadequate sample

Orthopedic Importance
A properly planned biopsy preserves limb salvage. A wrongly done biopsy may necessitate amputation.

Q25. Enneking's surgical staging system.

(IMS and SUM Hospital 2012)

Stage	*Grade*	*Local Extent*	*Metastasis*
IA	Low	Intracompartmental	No
IB	Low	Extracompartmental	No
IIA	High	Intracompartmental	No
IIB	High	Extracompartmental	No
III	Any	Any	Yes

Use
Guides surgical margins: Wide, marginal, radical, etc.

Q26. TNM staging in bone tumors.

Component	*Description*
T	Tumor size (T1 <8 cm, T2 >8 cm)
N	Node involvement (N0/N1)
M	Metastasis (M0/M1)
G	Grade (G1: low, G2: high)

Used for **prognosis and treatment planning** in malignant tumors.

Q27. Chemotherapy and radiotherapy in MSK tumors.

Chemotherapy
- *Indications*: Osteosarcoma, Ewing's sarcoma

- Neoadjuvant + adjuvant
- *Drugs*: Doxorubicin, cisplatin, ifosfamide

Radiotherapy

- Ewing's sarcoma, chordoma, multiple myeloma
- Palliative in bone metastasis
- Used when **surgical resection not feasible**

Q28. Genetic and molecular markers.

(Bihar University of Health Sciences 2012)

Tumor	*Genetic marker*
Ewing's sarcoma	t(11;22)(q24;q12): EWSR1-FLI1
Synovial sarcoma	t(X;18)(p11;q11): SS18-SSX
Chondrosarcoma	IDH1/IDH2 mutations
Osteosarcoma	p53, *Rb* gene mutations
Giant cell tumor	H3F3A mutation
Myxoid liposarcoma	FUS-DDIT3 fusion

Q29. Oncological margins in MSK tumors?

Margin type	*Description*
Intralesional	Through tumor → not oncologically safe
Marginal	Through pseudo capsule → risk of recurrence
Wide	Through normal tissue around tumor → preferred
Radical	Entire compartment excised → for high-grade tumors

Principles

Margins depend on **tumor grade**, location, and **soft tissue involvement**.

Q30. Describe pathology, radiology, and management of osteosarcoma.

(Asked in AIIMS Delhi 2022, MUHS Maharashtra 2023)

Definition

Osteosarcoma is a **high-grade malignant tumor** of bone in which **neoplastic cells produce osteoid (immature bone)**.

Pathology

- Originates from primitive bone-forming mesenchymal cells.
- Histology shows malignant osteoblasts producing osteoid matrix.
- *Variants*: Conventional, telangiectatic, small-cell, surface osteosarcomas.

Common Sites

- Metaphysis of long bones.
- Around the knee (distal femur > proximal tibia).

Radiology

Imaging	*Findings*
X-ray	Mixed lytic and sclerotic lesion; Codman's triangle; sunburst appearance
MRI	Defines intraosseous and soft tissue extent
CT chest	Mandatory for lung metastases screening
Bone scan	To detect skip lesions or metastases

Important Radiological Signs

- *Codman's triangle*: Periosteal elevation.
- *Sunburst appearance*: Radiating spicules of new bone.

Management

Step	*Details*
Biopsy	Confirm diagnosis (core needle biopsy preferred)
Neoadjuvant chemotherapy	MAP regimen (methotrexate, adriamycin, cisplatin)
Surgical resection	Wide excision with limb salvage surgery (preferred) or amputation if necessary
Adjuvant chemotherapy	Postoperative chemotherapy
Monitoring	CT chest for lung metastasis follow-up

Key Concept

Limb salvage > **Amputation** whenever feasible today.

Prognosis

5-year survival ~60–70% with modern multimodal therapy.

Q31. Define osteosarcoma. Classify its types.

Definition

Osteosarcoma is a **high-grade malignant bone tumor** characterized by the **direct production of osteoid (immature bone) by malignant cells**.

Classification

A. *Based on location*:

- *Central (intramedullary)*: Conventional, telangiectatic
- *Surface (juxtacortical)*: Parosteal, periosteal, high-grade surface

B. *Based on histology*

Type	*Features*
Conventional	Most common (~90%), high-grade
Telangiectatic	Blood-filled spaces, mimics ABC
Parosteal	Low-grade, arises on bone surface
Periosteal	Cartilage-producing, intermediate grade
Small-cell variant	Mimics Ewing's sarcoma

Q32. Role of neoadjuvant chemotherapy in osteosarcoma.

(RIMS 2015)

Benefits

- Shrinks tumor preoperatively
- Kills micro metastases early
- Facilitates **limb-salvage surgery**
- Helps assess **histological response** (good: >90% necrosis)

Regimen

MAP protocol: Methotrexate + Adriamycin (doxorubicin) + Cisplatin

Q33. Differences—conventional, telangiectatic and parosteal osteosarcoma.

Feature	*Conventional*	*Telangiectatic*	*Parosteal*
Grade	High-grade	High-grade	Low-grade
Site	Metaphysis, central	Metaphysis, central	Bone surface (posterior distal femur)
Appearance	Mixed lytic-sclerotic	Cystic, fluid-filled	Dense ossified mass
Imaging	Sunburst, Codman	Fluid levels on MRI	Dense, lobulated surface mass
Treatment	Chemotherapy + Surgery	Chemotherapy + Surgery	Wide excision ± Chemotherapy

Q34. Differential diagnosis of osteosarcoma.

(Rajasthan University of Health Sciences 2012)

Condition	*Differentiating clues*
Ewing's sarcoma	Diaphyseal, onion-skin periosteal reaction
Osteomyelitis	Fever, raised inflammatory markers
ABC	Fluid levels on MRI, no osteoid production
Chondrosarcoma	Older age group, cartilage matrix
Bone metastasis	Elderly, known primary, multiple lesions

Q35. Poor prognostic factors in osteosarcoma.

- **Poor histological response** to chemotherapy (<90% necrosis)
- **Metastasis at presentation** (especially lung)
- Tumor size >8 cm
- **Axial or pelvic location**
- Elevated **ALP, LDH**
- **Skip lesions**

Q36. Principles of limb-salvage surgery in osteosarcoma.

Goals
- Achieve **oncologically safe margins**
- Preserve **limb function**
- Avoid local recurrence

Key Principles
- **Wide resection** of tumor with healthy margins
- *Reconstruction*:
  - **Modular tumor prosthesis**
  - **Biological (allograft/autograft)**
  - **Rotationplasty** (in selected cases)
- Requires pre-operative planning with **MRI + biopsy correlation**
- **Post-operative chemotherapy** continues based on necrosis grade

Q37. What are the clinical features, imaging, and treatment of Ewing's sarcoma?

(Asked in PGI Chandigarh 2022, JIPMER Puducherry 2022)

Definition

Ewing's sarcoma is a **highly malignant small round blue cell tumor** of bone and soft tissue, common in children and adolescents.

Clinical Features

- Pain and swelling over affected area.
- Fever, weight loss, fatigue (can mimic infection).
- Common in diaphysis of long bones, pelvis, ribs.

Imaging

Imaging	*Findings*
X-ray	"Onion-skin" (lamellated) periosteal reaction; permeative bone destruction
MRI	Defines extent of marrow involvement and soft tissue mass
CT chest	For lung metastasis detection

Management

Step	*Details*
Biopsy	Confirms diagnosis (CD99 positivity on IHC)
Neoadjuvant chemotherapy	VAC (vincristine, adriamycin, cyclophosphamide) regimen ± Ifosfamide, Etoposide
Local control	Surgery (wide excision) or radiotherapy
Adjuvant chemotherapy	Postoperative continuation

Important Point

Ewing's sarcoma is **highly radiosensitive**, but surgery is preferred if feasible.

Prognosis

5-year survival ~60% if localized at diagnosis.

Q38. Role of chemotherapy and radiotherapy in Ewing's sarcoma.

Chemotherapy

- Mainstay of treatment
- *Protocol*: VDC/IE
  - Vincristine, doxorubicin, cyclophosphamide
  - Ifosfamide, etoposide

Radiotherapy

- *Indications*:
  - Unresectable tumors
  - Post-operative margin positivity
  - Palliative for pain relief
- *Dose*: 45–55 Gy

Q39. Ewing's sarcoma versus osteosarcoma—differences.

Feature	*Ewing's sarcoma*	*Osteosarcoma*
Age	5–25 years	10–25 years
Location	Diaphysis	Metaphysis
Radiology	Onion-skin periosteal reaction	Sunburst, Codman triangle
Histology	Small round blue cells	Malignant osteoid production
Genetic Marker	EWSR1-FLI1 (t11;22)	p53, Rb, no specific translocation
Treatment	Chemotherapy + surgery/RT	Neoadjuvant chemotherapy + surgery
Radiosensitivity	High	Low

Q40. Chondrosarcoma—diagnosis and treatment options.

(Asked in MUHS Maharashtra 2022)

Definition

Chondrosarcoma is a **malignant cartilage-forming tumor** of bone, typically occurring in middle-aged to elderly adults.

Common Sites

Pelvis, femur, proximal humerus, ribs.

Clinical Features

- Deep, dull aching pain (progressive).
- Swelling or palpable mass (large lesions).

Diagnosis

Test	*Findings*
X-ray	Lytic lesion with cortical destruction; "rings and arcs" calcification
MRI	Defines marrow and soft tissue involvement
Biopsy	Confirms diagnosis—atypical chondrocytes in lacunae

Treatment

- **Wide surgical excision** is the **treatment of choice.**
- Chemotherapy and radiotherapy are generally ineffective.
- High-grade chondrosarcomas require more aggressive surgery.
- Pelvic tumors may require complex reconstructions after resection.

Important Point

Unlike osteosarcoma and Ewing's, **chondrosarcoma is chemotherapy and radio-resistant—surgery is mandatory**.

Prognosis

- Depends on the grade.
- *Low-grade tumors*: ~90% survival.
- *High-grade tumors*: Poorer outcomes.

Q41. Clinical features, radiology, and management of chondrosarcoma?

Clinical Features

- *Age*: 40–70 years
- **Dull, progressive pain** and swelling
- Common in **pelvis, femur, humerus, scapula**
- May arise **de novo** or from **osteochondroma/enchondroma**

Radiological Features

- *X-ray*:
  - Lytic lesion with **ring-and-arc calcifications**
  - Endosteal scalloping, cortical thinning
- *CT*: Better for mineralization
- *MRI*: Marrow and soft tissue extent

Management

- **Surgical excision with wide margins**
- Chondrosarcoma is **chemoresistant and radioresistant**
- High-grade or unresectable tumors may need **palliative radiotherapy**

Q42. Differences—conventional, dedifferentiated, and mesenchymal chondrosarcoma.

Feature	Conventional	Dedifferentiated	Mesenchymal
Age	>40 years	>50 years	10–30 years
Grade	Low to high	High-grade	High-grade
Growth	Slow	Rapid	Aggressive
Histology	Hyaline cartilage	Cartilage + high-grade spindle cells	Small round blue cells
Treatment	Surgery only	Surgery + chemotherapy	Surgery + chemotherapy/radiotherapy
Prognosis	Fair	Poor	Intermediate

Quick Tips for Theory and Viva

- Always classify malignant bone tumors into **primary, hematopoietic, metastatic**.
- Know **osteosarcoma—osteoid production**; **Ewing's—onion skinning**; **chondrosarcoma—rings and arcs calcification**.
- Quote **neoadjuvant chemotherapy** → **surgery** → **adjuvant chemotherapy** for osteosarcoma and Ewing's.
- Stress **surgery only** for chondrosarcoma (radioresistant as they are radioresistent).

Metastatic Bone Disease

Q43. What are the common primary tumors causing bone metastasis?

(Asked in PGI Chandigarh 2022, AIIMS Delhi 2021)

Definition

Bone metastasis occurs when **cancer cells from a primary site** spread hematogenously to bones.

Most Common Primary Tumors Causing Bone Metastasis

Primary tumor	Notes
Breast carcinoma	Most common in females
Prostate carcinoma	Most common in males (often blastic lesions)
Lung carcinoma	Common source of lytic lesions
Thyroid carcinoma	Tends to produce lytic, expansile metastases
Kidney (renal cell carcinoma)	Tends to cause highly vascular lytic lesions
Others	GI malignancies, melanoma

Key Patterns

- **Blastic (sclerotic) lesions** → Prostate, breast (partially).
- **Lytic lesions** → Lung, kidney, thyroid, GI cancers.
- **Mixed lytic-blastic** → Breast cancer.

Mnemonic: "BLT with Kosher Pickle"

- *Breast*
- *Lung*
- *Thyroid*
- *Kidney*
- *Prostate*

Q44. Describe management principles of metastatic bone disease.

(Asked in MUHS Maharashtra 2022, RGUHS Karnataka 2023)

Pathophysiology of metastatic bone disease

- **Hematogenous spread** of malignancy to bone (mostly axial skeleton)

- Tumor cells activate **osteoclasts** → bone resorption
- *Common primaries*: Breast, prostate, lung, kidney, thyroid

Clinical Features
- Bone pain, fractures, spinal cord compression
- Hypercalcemia symptoms

Principles of Management

Goal	*Strategy*
Pain relief	Radiotherapy, analgesics
Stabilization of impending/pathological fractures	Surgical fixation
Local tumor control	Radiotherapy, surgery
Control systemic disease	Chemotherapy, hormonal therapy, targeted therapy
Maintain quality of life	Palliative multidisciplinary care

Surgical Indications
- Impending fracture (Mirel's score >8).
- Established pathological fracture.
- Unstable or painful lesions.
- Neurological deficit (in case of spinal metastasis).

Surgical Options
- *Intramedullary nailing* (long bone metastases).
- *Cement augmentation* (e.g., PMMA cementoplasty).
- *Endoprosthetic replacement* (e.g., proximal femur).
- *Spinal decompression and stabilization.*

Radiotherapy

External beam radiation therapy (EBRT) for pain control and local tumor control.

Medical Management
- **Bisphosphonates** (zoledronic acid) or **denosumab** to reduce skeletal-related events.
- Systemic therapy based on primary tumor.

Key Point

Aim is **palliation, pain control, stabilization**, not cure in most cases.

Q45. Describe Mirel's scoring system for impending pathological fractures.

(Asked in JIPMER Puducherry 2022)

Purpose

Mirel's score helps predict the risk of pathological fracture in a bone metastasis.

Components of Mirel's Score

Parameter	*Score = 1*	*Score = 2*	*Score = 3*
Site	Upper limb	Lower limb	Peritrochanteric region
Pain	Mild	Moderate	Functional pain (severe, at rest)
Lesion type	Blastic	Mixed	Lytic
Size	<1/3 diameter	1/3–2/3 diameter	>2/3 diameter

Interpretation

Total score	*Risk of fracture*	*Recommendation*
≤7	Low risk	Conservative treatment
8	Moderate risk	Consider prophylactic fixation
≥9	High risk	Prophylactic surgical stabilization recommended

Mnemonic for Mirel's Components: "SPLiT"
- *S*ite
- *P*ain
- *L*esion type
- *T*hickness (size)

Important Tip
A score ≥8–9 indicates **prophylactic fixation** to prevent catastrophic fracture and improve quality of life.

Q46. Management principles—pathological fractures due to tumors.

Principles
- *Identify underlying pathology*: Biopsy before fixation
- Assess fracture stability
- *For metastasis*:
  - If survival >6 months → **internal fixation + cementing**
  - Shorter life expectancy → **palliative care**

Fixation Techniques
- Intramedullary nails for long bones
- Cement augmentation
- Spinal decompression and instrumentation in cord compression

Post-operative care
- Early mobilization
- Adjunct **radiotherapy** for local control

Quick Tips for Theory and Viva
- Always mention **breast** > **prostate** > **lung** as top causes of bone metastasis.
- Stress that **bone metastases are managed palliatively**, not curatively.
- Quote **Mirel's score** confidently when discussing risk assessment.
- Emphasize that **stabilization + radiotherapy** are core strategies for painful bone metastasis.

Q47. Describe various principles of limb salvage surgery (LSS).

Principles of limb salvage surgery (LSS)
Limb salvage surgery is a surgical approach aimed at removing bone or soft tissue tumors while preserving the limb's function, stability, and appearance. It is commonly used in the treatment of **malignant bone tumors**, such as **osteosarcoma** and **Ewing sarcoma**.

Core Principles of LSS
1. *Oncologic safety*:
   - **Wide surgical margins** are essential to ensure complete tumor removal.
   - *Must follow Enneking's principles*: Excision must be **wide or radical**, based on the tumor's location and extent.
   - Avoid tumor spill during surgery.
2. *Limb function preservation*:
   - Maintain adequate **joint mobility, stability, and weight-bearing ability**.
   - Prioritize function over cosmesis.
   - Functional reconstruction should aim for a limb that is **pain-free and usable**.
3. *Reconstruction*: After tumor removal, reconstruct the limb using—
   - **Endoprosthesis** (modular or custom-made implants)
   - **Biological reconstruction** (autograft, allograft, or rotationplasty)
   - **Allograft-prosthetic composites**
   - **Vascularized fibular grafts** in some cases.

4. *Multidisciplinary approach*:
   - *Surgery must be coordinated with*:
     - **Medical oncology** (for chemotherapy)
     - **Radiology** (MRI/CT for planning)
     - **Pathology** (margin assessment)
     - **Rehabilitation team** (post-operative function)
5. *Patient selection*:
   - Adequate response to **neoadjuvant therapy** (e.g., chemotherapy).
   - Tumor should be **resectable** with negative margins.
   - No major neurovascular involvement that can not be reconstructed.
6. *Infection and complication control*:
   - Ensure **meticulous surgical technique**.
   - Use of **antibiotic prophylaxis**, proper soft tissue coverage (e.g., muscle flaps).
   - Monitor for **prosthetic loosening, fracture, or infection**.
7. *Cosmesis and psychological outcome*:
   - Consider **body image, self-esteem, and quality of life**.
   - *In pediatric patients*: Account for **growth potential** and **limb-length discrepancy**.

Q48. What are the indications and contraindications for limb salvage surgery?

(Asked in PGI Chandigarh 2021, AIIMS Delhi 2022)

Definition

Limb salvage surgery (LSS) is a surgical procedure where a **limb with a malignant or aggressive benign tumor** is **preserved**, removing only the tumor while ensuring **adequate oncological margins**, instead of amputation.

Indications for LSS

Indication	*Examples*
Resectable bone/soft tissue sarcomas	Osteosarcoma, Ewing's sarcoma
Good neurovascular status	Major nerves and vessels not involved or reconstructable
Responsive to neoadjuvant therapy	Tumor shrinkage improving resectability
Patient acceptance and compliance	Willingness for rigorous follow-up

Contraindications for LSS

Contraindication	*Notes*
Extensive neurovascular involvement	Major artery and nerve encasement
Poor soft tissue coverage	Cannot achieve good closure post-resection
Inadequate margins possible	High risk of local recurrence
Uncontrolled infection	Risk of postoperative complications
Poor general health	Inability to tolerate complex surgery
Pathological fracture with contamination	Risk of seeding tumor cells

Important Tip

- **Wide resection margin** must be achievable to ensure oncologic safety.
- LSS should **not compromise survival** compared to amputation.

Q49. Describe the steps and oncological principles of limb salvage surgery.

(Asked in MUHS Maharashtra 2023, JIPMER Puducherry 2022)

Oncological Principles of LSS

- *Preoperative staging*:
  - MRI of local site (extent of tumor).

- CT Chest for metastasis.
- Bone scan or PET-CT (to detect skip lesions).
- *Planning of resection*:
  - Wide excision with a cuff of healthy tissue.
  - Identification of neurovascular structures.
  - Margins based on Enneking's surgical staging.
- *En bloc tumor resection*: Tumor removed in one piece without violating capsule.
- *Reconstruction*:
  - Bone defect filled by:
    - Modular megaprosthesis
    - Allograft reconstruction
    - Vascularized bone grafts
    - Arthrodesis (in select cases)
- *Soft tissue coverage*:
  - Muscle flaps, free flaps if needed.
  - Adequate coverage critical to prevent infection.
- *Adjuvant therapy*: Chemotherapy and/or radiotherapy based on histology and margins.

Q50. Surgical margins (Enneking classification).

Margin type	*Definition*
Intralesional	Through tumor (poor oncological outcome)
Marginal	Through reactive zone (higher recurrence risk)
Wide	Through healthy tissue (goal in LSS)
Radical	Entire compartment removal

Q51. Describe the role of modular prostheses and mega prosthesis in LSS.

(Asked in RGUHS Karnataka 2022)

Definition

Modular prostheses and **megaprostheses** are large segmental joint replacement devices used to reconstruct bone and joint defects after tumor resection.

Advantages of Modular/Megaprostheses

Advantage	*Explanation*
Immediate mechanical stability	Early weight bearing possible
Customizable	Modular segments can match defect size
Shorter surgical time	Compared to custom-made prostheses
Better function	Compared to arthrodesis

Common Sites for Megaprosthesis Use

- Proximal femur (after osteosarcoma resection).
- Distal femur (most common for knee tumors).
- Proximal humerus
- Total femur (extensive tumors).

Complications of Megaprosthesis

- Infection
- Aseptic loosening
- Mechanical failure (fracture of prosthesis)
- Soft tissue failure leading to instability (especially around shoulder and knee).

Important Tip
Infection remains the **biggest challenge** after limb salvage with prosthesis.

Q52. Tumor prosthesis—definition, indications, advantages, and limitations.

Definition
A **custom or modular metal prosthesis** used to replace resected bone and joint structures following tumor excision.

Indications
- **Limb salvage** after wide excision
- Failed biological reconstructions
- Non-reconstructable fractures with tumor

Advantages
- **Immediate weight bearing**
- Shorter surgical time
- Predictable function

Limitations
- Cost
- **Mechanical failure** over time
- **Infection risk**

Quick Tips for Theory and Viva
- Start your answer with a clear definition of LSS and **oncological safety**.
- Always emphasize **wide margins** and **proper reconstruction**.
- Quote **modular prosthesis = flexibility + early mobilization**.
- Know that **megaprosthesis** use has revolutionized outcomes post-tumor resection.

Q53. Amputation versus limb salvage surgery—very brief answer.

Definition
- *Amputation*: Complete removal of the limb to achieve oncological clearance.
- *Limb salvage surgery (LSS)*: Tumor excision with adequate margins while preserving and reconstructing the limb.

Indications

Amputation	*Limb salvage*
Major neurovascular involvement	Tumor resectable with safe margins
Extensive soft tissue loss	Good response to chemotherapy
Fungating/infected tumors	Adequate reconstruction possible
Failed limb salvage	Patient fit and cooperative

Advantages

Amputation	*Limb salvage*
Simple, quicker surgery	Preserves limb function and appearance
Lower recurrence risk	Better psychological acceptance

Disadvantages

Amputation	*Limb salvage*
Psychological trauma	Technically demanding
Need for prosthesis	Higher complication risk

Key Points

- *Oncological safety is paramount*: Clear margins are non-negotiable.
- *Preference*: Limb salvage if feasible without compromising cure.

Quick Mindmap: Tumors in Orthopedics

- *Tumors in orthopedics*:
  - *Benign bone tumors*:
    - Osteoid osteoma
    - Enchondroma
    - Giant cell tumor (GCT)
  - *Malignant bone tumors*:
    - Osteosarcoma
    - Ewing's sarcoma

Q54. Tumor-induced osteomalacia.

(Goa Medical College 2011)

Definition

Rare paraneoplastic syndrome due to **phosphaturic mesenchymal tumors**, causing **hypophosphatemic osteomalacia.**

Pathophysiology

- Tumor secretes **FGF23** → inhibits phosphate reabsorption
- ↓ 1,25$(OH)_2$ vitamin D
- ↓ Bone mineralization

Features

Bone pain, muscle weakness, fragility fractures.

Diagnosis

- ↑ FGF23, ↓ phosphate, ↓ vitamin D
- *Localization*: PET-DOTATATE, MRI

Treatment

- **Tumor excision** is curative
- Until then, phosphate and calcitriol supplements

Q55. Malignant transformation of osteochondroma.

Incidence

- 1% in solitary osteochondroma
- 5–25% in MHE

Indicators of Malignant Change

- Increased size after skeletal maturity
- Pain at rest or night pain
- Thick cartilage cap >2 cm on MRI
- Soft tissue mass or lysis at base

Most Common Malignancy

Secondary chondrosarcoma

Management

- **Wide local excision** of suspicious lesion
- **Histopathological confirmation**

Q56. Ollier's disease and Maffucci's syndrome.

Ollier's Disease

- **Non-hereditary**, multiple enchondromas (enchondromatosis)
- *Presents in childhood with*:
    - Limb length discrepancy
    - Pathological fractures
    - Deformities (e.g., genu valgum)
    - Commonly affects **unilateral limb**

Complication

Risk of **malignant transformation to chondrosarcoma (~25–30%)**

Q57. Maffucci's syndrome.

(Goa Medical College 2011)

- **Ollier's disease + soft tissue hemangiomas**
- *Associated with*:
    - Phleboliths in soft tissues
    - Increased risk of **visceral malignancies** (pancreas, brain)

Q58. Fibrous dysplasia—description and types.

Definition

Benign, developmental fibro-osseous disorder where **normal bone is replaced by fibrous tissue and immature woven bone.**

Etiology

Caused by **activating mutation in *GNAS* gene** → ↑ cAMP

Types

Type	*Features*
Monostotic	Involves a single bone (~70–80% cases)
Polyostotic	Multiple bones; often unilateral; deformities common

Common Sites

- Femur, tibia, ribs, skull, jaw
- **"Shepherd's crook deformity"** in proximal femur

Q59. McCune–Albright syndrome—clinical significance.

Triad

- Polyostotic fibrous dysplasia
- **Café-au-lait spots**
- *Endocrinopathy*: Most commonly **precocious puberty** in girls

Cause

Postzygotic mutation in ***GNAS* gene** → mosaicism.

Other Endocrine Manifestations

- Hyperthyroidism
- Cushing's syndrome
- Growth hormone excess

Clinical Significance
- Early diagnosis critical
- Requires **multidisciplinary management**
- Risk of **fractures and deformities**

Q60. Aneurysmal bone cyst (ABC)—clinical features and management.

(Grant Government Medical College 2009)

Definition
Benign, **expansile, blood-filled cystic lesion**, often in **metaphysis of long bones or posterior elements of spine.**

Etiology
Can be **primary (*USP6* gene rearrangement)** or **secondary to other tumors (e.g., GCT)**

Clinical Features
- **Pain, swelling, and rapid growth**
- May cause **neurological symptoms** if spinal
- Common in <20 years

Radiology
- *X-ray*: Eccentric, expansile lytic lesion with **"blow-out" or soap-bubble** appearance
- *MRI*: **Fluid-fluid levels** (characteristic)

Management
- Curettage and bone grafting
- Selective arterial embolization
- Sclerotherapy (e.g., polidocanol)
- *Rarely*: En bloc resection

Q61. ABC versus SBC—differences.

Feature	*Aneurysmal bone cyst (ABC)*	*Simple bone cyst (SBC)*
Age	<20 years	<20 years
Location	Metaphysis (long bones, spine)	Proximal humerus/femur
Radiology	Expansile, fluid-fluid levels	Central, well-defined, "fallen fragment sign"
Symptoms	Pain, swelling	Often asymptomatic; pathological fracture
Management	Curettage, embolization, sclerotherapy	Observation, steroid injection, curettage

Q62. Sclerotherapy in simple bone cysts.

Definition
Minimally invasive method where sclerosant is injected into the cyst to promote healing.

Common Agents
Polidocanol, Ethibloc, doxycycline, or alcohol.

Procedure
- Percutaneous aspiration of fluid → sclerosant injection under image guidance
- Often repeated every 6–8 weeks

Indications
- SBCs at high fracture risk
- Recurrent or large cysts

Advantages

- **Non-surgical**, outpatient procedure
- Faster return to activity
- Avoids complications of open surgery

Q63. Define chondrosarcoma. Classify its types based on histology.

(Kasturba Medical College Manipal 2008)

Definition

Chondrosarcoma is a **malignant tumor of cartilage-producing cells**, usually arising in **adults >40 years**, with **no osteoid formation**.

Classification (Histological Types)

Type	*Features*
Conventional	Most common (85%), slow-growing
Dedifferentiated	High-grade, aggressive, poor prognosis
Mesenchymal	Rare, affects young, resembles Ewing's
Clear cell	Epiphyseal, low-grade
Myxoid	Contains abundant myxoid matrix

Q64. Chordoma—definition, features, locations, and management.

Definition

Chordoma is a **rare malignant tumor** derived from **notochordal remnants**, producing **physaliphorous cells**.

Clinical Features

- **Slow-growing, locally aggressive**
- Presents with **pain, neurologic deficits** due to location
- Most common in **sacrococcygeal region**, **clivus**, and **mobile spine**

Common Locations

- *Sacrum* (50%)
- *Clivus* (35%)
- *Thoracolumbar spine* (15%)

Management

- **Wide surgical excision** is the mainstay
- **Carbon-ion radiotherapy or proton beam therapy** adjunctively
- Recurrence is common; **long-term follow-up required**

Q65. Differential diagnosis of chordoma.

Condition	*Differentiating features*
Chondrosarcoma	Ring-and-arc calcifications, no physaliphorous cells
Metastasis	Known primary, multifocal, lacks vacuolated cells
Giant cell tumor (GCT)	Younger age, purely lytic lesion, epiphyseal
Plasmacytoma	Age >50, punched-out lesion, positive for CD138
Notochordal rest	Benign, small, asymptomatic, discovered incidentally

Q66. Fibrosarcoma of bone—features and management.

(Jawaharlal Institute of Postgraduate Medical Education and Research 2012)

Definition

Primary malignant tumor composed of **fibroblasts producing collagen**, without osteoid or cartilage.

Clinical Features

- *Age*: 30–60 years
- **Pain and swelling**
- *Sites*: femur, tibia, pelvis
- Pathologic fractures may occur

Radiological Features

- Lytic lesion with ill-defined margins
- No matrix mineralization
- Cortical destruction and soft tissue extension

Management

- **Wide surgical resection**
- May be followed by **radiotherapy or chemotherapy**, especially in high-grade lesions

Q67. Differences between fibrosarcoma and malignant fibrous histiocytoma (MFH).

Feature	*Fibrosarcoma*	*Malignant fibrous histiocytoma (MFH)*
Origin	Fibroblasts	Pleomorphic spindle cells + histiocyte-like cells
Histology	Herringbone pattern	Storiform-pleomorphic pattern
Age	30–60 years	>40 years
Sites	Femur, tibia	Pelvis, femur, retroperitoneum
Prognosis	Guarded	Poor (high recurrence/metastasis)
Treatment	Surgery ± radiotherapy	Wide excision ± adjuvant therapy

Miscellaneous Musculoskeletal Tumors

Q68. Adamantinoma—pathology, clinical features, and treatment.

(Kashmir University)

Pathology

- Rare **low-grade malignant tumor** of epithelial origin
- Thought to arise from **remnants of embryonic epithelium**
- *Histology*: **Biphasic** pattern—epithelial cells in fibrous stroma

Clinical Features

- *Age*: 10–40 years
- *Common site*: **Tibia (anterior cortex)**
- **Slow-growing swelling**, often painless
- May cause deformity or pathologic fracture

Treatment

- **Wide surgical excision** or segmental resection
- Amputation if extensive
- **Chemotherapy and radiotherapy are not effective**

Q69. Hemangioma of bone—clinical features, radiology, and management.

Definition

Benign vascular tumor of bone; often an **incidental finding.**

Clinical Features

- Usually **asymptomatic**
- May present with **pain or pathological fracture**
- *Common sites*: **Vertebrae (body), skull**

Radiology

- *X-ray*: Corduroy or honeycomb appearance
- *CT*: Polka-dot sign (vertebral hemangioma)
- *MRI*: High T2 signal

Management

- Observation in asymptomatic cases
- **Vertebroplasty**, embolization, or excision if symptomatic

Soft Tissue Tumors

Q70. Describe classification, diagnosis, and management principles of soft tissue sarcomas.

(Asked in AIIMS Delhi 2022, PGI Chandigarh 2021)

Definition

Soft tissue sarcomas are a **heterogeneous group of malignant tumors** arising from **mesenchymal tissues** such as muscle, fat, fibrous tissue, blood vessels, and peripheral nerves.

Classification of Soft Tissue Sarcomas

Tissue of origin	*Examples*
Adipose tissue	Liposarcoma
Fibrous tissue	Fibrosarcoma, dermatofibrosarcoma protuberans (DFSP)
Muscle tissue	Rhabdomyosarcoma (skeletal), leiomyosarcoma (smooth)
Vascular tissue	Angiosarcoma
Peripheral nerve sheath	Malignant peripheral nerve sheath tumor (MPNST)
Synovial tissue	Synovial sarcoma

Diagnosis

Clinical Features

- Painless enlarging mass (most common).
- Late onset of pain or neurovascular symptoms (compression).
- Deep-seated mass >5 cm is suspicious for malignancy.

Investigations

Modality	*Findings*
MRI	Best for local staging—defines size, extent, relationship to neurovascular structures
Biopsy	Core needle biopsy preferred for diagnosis
CT chest	Mandatory to rule out lung metastases (most common site)
PET-CT	For metastatic work-up in some cases

Histopathology

Helps determine **grade**, **type**, and **margins**.

Management Principles

Step	Details
Wide surgical excision	Gold standard; negative margins essential
Radiotherapy	Adjuvant or neoadjuvant to improve local control
Chemotherapy	Role in high-grade sarcomas (e.g., rhabdomyosarcoma, synovial sarcoma)
Limb salvage preferred	Amputation reserved for unresectable tumors

Important Point

- *Wide margins*: Tumor + cuff of normal tissue excised.
- *R0 resection*: Negative margins (goal of surgery).

Q71. Liposarcoma—features and management.

(Asked in MUHS Maharashtra 2023)

Definition

Liposarcoma is a **malignant tumor of adipocytic origin**, most commonly affecting adults aged 40–60 years.

Types of Liposarcoma

Type	Features
Well-differentiated	Slow-growing, low metastatic potential
Myxoid	Most common type; intermediate grade
Round cell	High-grade, aggressive variant
Pleomorphic	Highly aggressive
Dedifferentiated	Transformation from well-differentiated to high-grade

Clinical Features

- Deep, slow-growing mass (often painless initially).
- *Common sites*: Thigh, retroperitoneum.

Diagnosis

- MRI shows fatty mass with thickened septa (in well-differentiated types).
- Core biopsy confirms histological type.

Management

Treatment	Details
Surgery	Wide excision with clear margins
Radiotherapy	Adjuvant radiotherapy for high-grade tumors
Chemotherapy	Limited role except in high-grade or metastatic disease

Prognosis

- Depends on histologic subtype.
- *Well-differentiated*: Good prognosis.
- *Pleomorphic and dedifferentiated*: Poor prognosis.

Q72. Synovial sarcoma—clinical features and radiological findings.

(Asked in JIPMER Puducherry 2022)

Definition

Synovial sarcoma is a **high-grade soft tissue sarcoma**, often arising near joints, but not from synovium itself.

Clinical Features

- Slowly growing deep soft tissue mass near large joints (especially knee, ankle).
- Pain in around 50% of cases.
- Often occurs in young adults (15–40 years).

Radiological Findings

Imaging	*Findings*
X-ray	May show soft tissue mass ± calcifications
MRI	Heterogeneous "triple signal intensity" pattern on T2-weighted images (hypo-, iso-, hyperintense areas)
CT chest	For lung metastasis screening

Key Radiologic Sign

"Triple sign" on MRI: Areas of solid tumor, hemorrhage, and necrosis.

Diagnosis

- *Core needle biopsy*:
    - *Histology*: Biphasic pattern (spindle cells + epithelial-like cells) or monophasic.
- *Immunohistochemistry*: Positive for cytokeratin, EMA.

Management

Treatment	*Details*
Surgery	Wide excision with negative margins
Radiotherapy	Adjuvant radiotherapy common
Chemotherapy	Ifosfamide and doxorubicin-based regimens used for high-risk cases

Prognosis

5-year survival ~50–60% depending on size, grade, and metastasis.

Quick Tips for Theory and Viva

- Soft tissue sarcoma management is **wide excision first, radiotherapy often adjunct**.
- Liposarcoma is usually **slow-growing** unless pleomorphic type.
- In Synovial Sarcoma, **young adults + near joints + MRI triple sign** should trigger suspicion.

Mnemonic for Soft Tissue Sarcoma Management: "See Real Care"

- *S*urgery (wide excision)
- *R*adiotherapy (adjuvant)
- *C*hemotherapy (selected cases)

Q73. Classification based on histology and behavior.

A. Based on Histology

Type	*Examples*
Adipocytic	Lipoma, liposarcoma
Fibrous	Fibroma, fibrosarcoma
Muscle	Rhabdomyosarcoma, leiomyoma
Vascular	Hemangioma, angiosarcoma
Nerve sheath	Schwannoma, MPNST

B. Based on Behavior

- *Benign*: Lipoma, fibroma
- *Intermediate*: Desmoid tumor
- *Malignant*: Liposarcoma, synovial sarcoma

Q74. Lipoma versus liposarcoma—differences.

Feature	*Lipoma*	*Liposarcoma*
Nature	Benign	Malignant
Age group	Any, often middle-aged	Adults >40
Location	Superficial (subcutaneous)	Deep-seated (retroperitoneal, thigh)
Consistency	Soft, mobile	Firm, nodular
Imaging (MRI)	Homogeneous fat signal	Heterogeneous, non-fatty components
Treatment	Excision if symptomatic	Wide excision ± chemotherapy

Q75. Wide local excision in soft tissue sarcomas.

Definition

Surgical removal of tumor with a **margin of 1–2 cm** of healthy tissue

Importance

- Ensures **oncological control**
- Reduces local recurrence
- Preserves limb function versus radical procedures

Requirements

- Pre-operative **MRI planning**
- Intra-operative margin assessment
- Followed by **adjuvant radiotherapy** if margins close/positive

Q76. Radiotherapy principles in soft tissue sarcoma.

Indications

- High-grade sarcomas
- Positive/close surgical margins
- Inoperable tumors

Types

- **External beam radiotherapy (EBRT)**
- *Pre-operative*: Shrinks tumor, allows smaller surgical margins
- *Post-operative*: Targets residual microscopic disease

Dose

50–66 Gy over 5–6 weeks

Side Effects

Fibrosis, joint stiffness, wound complications (especially pre-operative RT)

Q77. Rhabdomyosarcoma versus leiomyosarcoma—differences.

(Madras Medical College 2012)

Feature	*Rhabdomyosarcoma*	*Leiomyosarcoma*
Origin	Skeletal muscle	Smooth muscle
Age	Children, adolescents	Adults >40
Common sites	Head/neck, genitourinary, limbs	Retroperitoneum, uterus, extremities
Histology	Small round blue cells	Spindle-shaped cells

Continued

Continued

Feature	Rhabdomyosarcoma	Leiomyosarcoma
Treatment	Surgery + chemotherapy + radiotherapy	Surgery ± chemotherapy/radiotherapy
Prognosis	Variable (depends on subtype)	Poor if high-grade

Q78. Common tumor-like conditions mimicking musculoskeletal tumors.

Tumor-like lesions are **non-neoplastic conditions** that radiologically or clinically resemble bone tumors but lack neoplastic histology.

Common Tumor-like Lesions

Condition	Key features
Fibrous dysplasia	Ground-glass appearance; painless swelling
Bone cysts	Lytic, metaphyseal (SBC, ABC); seen in children/adolescents
Osteomyelitis	Mimics Ewing's/osteosarcoma in early stages
Eosinophilic granuloma	Lytic lesion, children, skull/spine/long bones
Stress fractures	Sclerotic or periosteal reaction; mimics malignancy
Infarct	Central serpiginous calcification; resembles enchondroma
Paget's disease	Bone enlargement, cortical thickening, sclerosis

Q79. Differential diagnosis of lytic bone lesions in young adults.

Category	Conditions	Typical clues
Benign tumors	Unicameral bone cyst, ABC, enchondroma	Well-defined margins, central
Aggressive tumors	Osteosarcoma, Ewing's sarcoma, GCT	Ill-defined margins, periosteal reaction
Infective	Subacute osteomyelitis, Brodie's abscess	Local pain, systemic signs
Metabolic	Hyperparathyroidism (brown tumor)	Subperiosteal resorption, multiple sites
Others	Fibrous dysplasia, Langerhans cell histiocytosis	Diaphyseal, vertebral involvement

Q80. Differential diagnosis of sclerotic bone lesions.

(Christian Medical College Vellore 2014)

Cause category	Conditions	Distinguishing features
Benign tumors	Osteoma, osteoid osteoma	Small nidus, night pain relieved by NSAIDs
Malignant tumors	Osteoblastic metastasis (e.g., prostate, breast)	Multiple lesions, axial skeleton
Bone-forming tumors	Osteosarcoma	Sunburst appearance, metaphyseal lesion
Infective	Chronic osteomyelitis, TB	Sequestrum/involucrum on imaging
Metabolic	Osteopetrosis	Diffuse sclerosis, bone marrow failure
Paget's disease	Cotton wool appearance, thickened cortex	

Q81. Distinguishing infective, metabolic and neoplastic bone lesions—principles.

Feature	Infective	Metabolic	Neoplastic
Onset	Acute/Subacute	Chronic	Variable
Pain	Localized, throbbing	Diffuse, mild	Progressive, constant
Systemic signs	Often present (fever, CRP↑)	Usually absent	May occur in malignancy
Radiology	Lytic, periosteal reaction	Diffuse changes (osteopenia, sclerosis)	Lytic/sclerotic, soft tissue mass
Labs	↑WBC, ↑ESR, ↑CRP	Deranged Ca^{2+}, phosphate, PTH	ALP, LDH ↑ in aggressive tumors
Histopathology	Inflammatory cells, necrosis	Increased bone turnover	Tumor cells, mitotic activity

Q82. Changes in bone tumors.

[Assam Medical College (affiliated to Srimanta Sankaradeva University of Health Sciences) 2019]

Types of Changes

Change type	Features and examples
Reactive bone changes	Periosteal reactions (onion-skin, sunburst)
Cystic degeneration	Seen in GCT, aneurysmal bone cysts
Calcification	Popcorn calcification in chondrosarcoma
Necrosis	Common in high-grade malignancies
Fibrous transformation	*Fibrous dysplasia*: Ground-glass matrix
Pathologic fractures	In lytic lesions (e.g., metastasis, GCT)

Radiological Clues

- *Codman's triangle*: Aggressive periosteal elevation
- Sclerosis in osteoblastic tumors (osteosarcoma)
- Lytic in osteolytic tumors (GCT, metastases)

Q83. Osteochondroma—key points.

Definition

Benign cartilage-capped bony outgrowth from the metaphysis, often near the knee.

Etiology

- Abnormal growth plate development
- *Genetic link*: EXT1/EXT2 mutations in hereditary multiple exostoses (HME)

Radiology

- Bony projection in continuity with the cortex and medullary canal
- Sessile or pedunculated appearance

Histology

- Mature trabecular bone core
- Cartilaginous cap (usually <1.5 cm in adults)

Clinical Features

- Painless swelling
- May cause nerve, vessel compression or deformity

Treatment

- Observation if asymptomatic
- Excision if painful, growing, or suspected malignant transformation

Complication

Rare malignant transformation to chondrosarcoma (~1% in solitary; 5–25% in HME)

Q84. Immunohistochemistry (IHC).

IHC is used to identify tumor lineage and subtype via antigen markers:

- *CD99*: Strongly positive in Ewing's sarcoma (membranous pattern)
- *S100*: Seen in chondroid tumors, neural tumors, and melanoma
- *Cytokeratin*: Positive in metastatic carcinomas; confirms epithelial origin

Q85. Common locations of bone tumors.

- *Osteosarcoma*: Commonly affects metaphysis (distal femur, proximal tibia, humerus)

- *Ewing's sarcoma*: Diaphyseal region, often pelvis or femur
- *Chondroblastoma*: Epiphyseal lesions in skeletally immature patients (proximal humerus, femur)

Q86. Age distribution.

- *<20 years*: Osteosarcoma, Ewing's sarcoma (high-grade, aggressive)
- *20–40 years*: Giant cell tumor (epiphyseal, benign but locally aggressive)
- *>40 years*: Chondrosarcoma, multiple myeloma, bone metastasis (commonly from breast/prostate/lung)

Q87. Lichtenstein's classification.

Classifies bone tumors by tissue type:

- *Osteoid-forming*: Osteoid osteoma, osteoblastoma, osteosarcoma
- *Chondroid*: Enchondroma, chondroblastoma, chondrosarcoma
- *Fibrous*: Fibrous dysplasia, fibrosarcoma
- *Cystic*: UBC, ABC
- *Vascular*: Hemangioma, hemangioendothelioma
- *Miscellaneous*: Adamantinoma, chordoma

Q88. Pattern of bone destruction.

- *Geographic*: Well-marginated lytic lesions, often benign or low-grade tumors
- *Moth-eaten*: Multiple small lytic areas, typical of aggressive malignancy
- *Permeative*: Poorly defined, infiltrative destruction; seen in Ewing's, lymphoma

Q89. Periosteal reactions.

- *Solid*: Benign or slow-growing (e.g., osteoid osteoma)
- *Laminated (onion-skin)*: Seen in Ewing's sarcoma
- *Sunburst*: Seen in osteosarcoma due to aggressive periosteal reaction
- *Codman triangle*: Lifted periosteum due to rapid lesion growth

Q90. Langerhans cell histiocytosis.

- Rare disorder of dendritic cells
- *Eosinophilic granuloma*: Solitary bone lesion
- *Vertebra plana*: Collapse of vertebral body
- *Other variants*:
  - *Hand-Schüller-Christian*: Triad of skull lesions, diabetes insipidus, exophthalmos
  - *Letterer-Siwe*: Aggressive multisystem disease in infants

Q91. Pseudotumors

- Non-neoplastic lesions mimicking tumors on imaging
- *Includes*:
  - Bone cysts (UBC, ABC)
  - Osteomyelitis
  - Fibrous dysplasia
  - Brown tumors (seen in hyperparathyroidism)
  - Important to differentiate radiologically and histologically to avoid overtreatment

Q92. Multiple myeloma.

(Grant Government Medical College 2011)

Definition

Multiple myeloma (MM) is a malignant neoplasm of **monoclonal plasma cells** that proliferate within the bone marrow, producing abnormal immunoglobulins and leading to extensive **skeletal destruction**, **anemia**, **renal dysfunction**, and **immunodeficiency**.

Etiology and Risk Factors
- Age > 50 years (median age ~70 years)
- Male predominance
- African descent (higher prevalence)
- Ionizing radiation exposure
- Chronic antigenic stimulation
- Genetic predisposition (monoclonal gammopathy of undetermined significance—MGUS - as a precursor)

Pathophysiology
- Monoclonal plasma cells proliferate in bone marrow → osteolysis via **RANKL overexpression**
- Produce **M-protein** (monoclonal immunoglobulin or light chains)
- Inhibit osteoblast activity → lytic lesions
- Light chain deposition → **renal tubular damage**
- Immunosuppression due to decreased normal immunoglobulins

Clinical Features (Mnemonic: CRAB)

Symptom	*Mechanism*
C: HyperCalcemia	Bone resorption due to osteolytic lesions
R: Renal insufficiency	Light chain cast nephropathy, hypercalcemia
A: Anemia	Bone marrow suppression
B: Bone pain	Due to lytic lesions, especially in spine, ribs, skull

Other Features
- Recurrent infections
- Pathological fractures (vertebrae, ribs, femur)
- Neurological deficits (cord compression, plasmacytoma)
- Hyperviscosity syndrome (in IgA myeloma)

Skeletal Manifestations
- Punched-out lytic lesions on skull X-rays ("raindrop skull")
- Vertebral compression fractures
- Diffuse osteopenia
- Pathological fractures in long bones
- Spinal cord compression (due to plasmacytoma or fracture)

Investigations
1. *Laboratory tests:*
    - *CBC*: Normocytic normochromic anemia
    - *ESR*: Markedly elevated
    - *Serum protein electrophoresis (SPEP)*: **M-protein spike**
    - *Serum free light chain assay*: κ/λ ratio abnormal
    - *Serum calcium*: Elevated
    - *Renal function*: Elevated creatinine, urea
2. *Urine studies*: Urine Bence Jones protein (light chains)
3. *Bone marrow biopsy*: 10% monoclonal plasma cells confirm diagnosis

4. *Radiology*:
    - *Skeletal survey*: Multiple lytic lesions, vertebral compression
    - *MRI spine*: Detects early marrow changes, cord compression
    - *PET-CT*: For staging and follow-up

Diagnostic Criteria (IMWG: International Myeloma Working Group)

Diagnosis confirmed if:
- Clonal bone marrow plasma cells ≥10% **or** biopsy-proven plasmacytoma, and
- One or more myeloma-defining events (CRAB criteria or biomarkers like >60% plasma cells, FLC ratio >100)

Differential Diagnosis
- Metastatic bone disease
- Osteoporosis
- Lymphoma
- MGUS (precancerous)
- Solitary plasmacytoma

Management
1. *Supportive management*:
    - *Bisphosphonates (zoledronate or pamidronate)*: ↓ bone resorption
    - *Pain control*: NSAIDs, opioids, radiotherapy
    - Treatment of hypercalcemia and renal failure
    - Blood transfusions, hydration, diuretics
    - Vertebroplasty/kyphoplasty for spinal fractures
2. *Definitive therapy*:
    - For transplant-eligible patients (<65 years, good performance status):
        - *Induction chemotherapy*: For example, Bortezomib + Lenalidomide + Dexamethasone (VRD)
        - **Autologous stem cell transplant (ASCT)**
    - *Non-transplant candidates*:
        - Chemotherapy or immunomodulators ± steroids
        - Proteasome inhibitors (bortezomib)
        - Monoclonal antibodies (daratumumab)

Orthopedic Role
- **Biopsy** of suspected lesions (usually after SPEP and marrow studies)
- Management of pathological fractures:
    - **Prophylactic fixation** of impending fractures (Mirels' score)
    - **Internal fixation or arthroplasty** for fractures
- **Spinal decompression and stabilization** in cord compression
- Coordination with hematologist for systemic therapy

Prognosis
- *Median survival*: 5–7 years (with current therapy)
- *Prognostic markers*: β2 microglobulin, albumin levels, cytogenetics [del17p, t(4;14)]

Recent Advances
- **CAR-T cell therapy** for relapsed/refractory cases
- *Monoclonal antibodies*: Daratumumab, elotuzumab
- *Proteasome inhibitors*: Carfilzomib, ixazomib
- *Immunomodulators*: Pomalidomide, lenalidomide

Key Points for Exam
- Always mention the **CRAB** criteria
- Emphasize **M-protein**, Bence Jones protein, and marrow findings
- *Orthopedic focus*: **Diagnosis**, **fracture care**, **biopsy**, and **multidisciplinary management**

Q93. Plasmacytoma—short theory answer.

(Maharashtra University of Health Sciences 2012)

Definition

Plasmacytoma is a **localized monoclonal plasma cell tumor**, presenting without systemic features of multiple myeloma.

Types

1. *Solitary bone plasmacytoma (SBP)*:
    - Arises in bones (vertebrae, ribs, pelvis).
    - Appears as a single lytic lesion.
    - May progress to multiple myeloma.
2. *Extramedullary plasmacytoma (EMP)*:
    - Occurs in soft tissues, especially the upper respiratory tract (nasopharynx, sinuses).
    - Less likely to become systemic.

Clinical Features

- Localized bone pain, swelling, or fracture (SBP).
- Nasal obstruction or mass (EMP).
- No CRAB features (hypercalcemia, renal failure, anemia, bone lesions elsewhere).

Investigations

- *X-ray/MRI*: Single lytic lesion.
- *Biopsy*: Monoclonal plasma cells.
- *Bone marrow*: <10% plasma cells.
- *Serum protein electrophoresis*: May show low M-protein.
- Whole-body imaging to rule out systemic disease.

Treatment

- *Radiotherapy (mainstay)*: 40–50 Gy over 4–5 weeks.
- *Surgery*: Rarely indicated, except for spinal instability or cord compression.
- Surveillance for progression to multiple myeloma.

Prognosis

- EMP has better prognosis.
- SBP progresses to multiple myeloma in 50–70% over 10 years.

Q94. Fibrous lesions of bone.

- *Examples*: Fibrous dysplasia (FD), non-ossifying fibroma (NOF).
- *Features*: Ground-glass appearance (FD); usually metaphyseal.
- *Treatment*:
    - Observation if asymptomatic.
    - Curettage and bone grafting if symptomatic or risk of fracture.

Q95. Chondroblastoma.

- **Benign epiphyseal tumor** in adolescents.
- *Sites*: Proximal humerus, distal femur.
- *Treatment*:
    - Intralesional curettage and bone grafting.
    - Extended curettage (with adjuvant like phenol or cryotherapy) if aggressive.

Q96. Chondromyxoid fibroma (CMF).

- **Rare benign metaphyseal tumor** (proximal tibia common).

- *Treatment*:
  - Extended curettage ± bone grafting.
  - Rarely wide excision for recurrences.

Q97. Diaphyseal aclasis (hereditary multiple exostosis).

(Seth Gordhandas Sunderdas Medical College and KEM Hospital 2012)

- **Autosomal dominant disorder** with multiple osteochondromas.
- *Treatment*:
  - Observation if asymptomatic.
  - Excision if pain, deformity, or suspected malignant change.

Q98. Primitive neuroectodermal tumor (PNET).

- **Highly malignant small round cell tumor**, part of Ewing's family.
- *Treatment*:
  - Neoadjuvant chemotherapy → Surgery/radiotherapy → Adjuvant chemotherapy.
  - Multimodal therapy essential.

Q99. Round cell tumors of bone.

- *Examples*: Ewing's sarcoma, PNET, lymphoma of bone.
- *Treatment*:
  - Combination chemotherapy, local control by surgery/radiotherapy.
  - Based on specific diagnosis.

Q100. Cystic lesions of bone.

- *Unicameral bone cyst (UBC)*:
  - Aspiration and steroid injection.
  - Curettage and bone grafting if large or pathological fracture.
- *Aneurysmal bone cyst (ABC)*:
  - Extended curettage with adjuvant (phenol, cryotherapy).
  - Bone grafting.

Q101. Schwannoma.

- Benign peripheral nerve sheath tumor.
- *Treatment*: Complete surgical excision preserving the nerve.

Q102. Pyknodysostosis.

- Genetic osteosclerotic disorder (cathepsin K mutation).
- *Treatment*:
  - No specific cure.
  - Fracture prevention and management.
  - Dental care, orthopedic correction of deformities.

Q103. Synovial chondromatosis.

- Benign cartilaginous nodules in joints.

- *Treatment*:
  - Synovectomy with removal of loose bodies.
  - Arthroscopic or open surgery.

Q104. Musculoskeletal manifestations of neurofibromatosis (NF1).

(Kasturba Medical College Manipal 2012)

- *Skeletal manifestations*: Scoliosis, pseudoarthrosis (especially tibia), bone dysplasia.
- *Treatment*:
  - Bracing for scoliosis if mild.
  - Surgical correction for severe scoliosis or pseudoarthrosis.
  - Observation or surgery based on deformity severity.

Q105. Gamma camera (nuclear medicine imaging).

- *Use*: Detection of bone metastasis, infection, prosthesis loosening.
- *Treatment relevance*: Guides treatment planning (e.g., identifies sites needing biopsy or fixation).

Q106. Differential diagnosis (D/Ds) of cystic lesions in the upper end of the tibia.

Common Causes
- Simple bone cyst (unicameral)
- Aneurysmal bone cyst (ABC)
- Fibrous dysplasia
- Giant cell tumor (epiphyseometaphyseal in adults)
- Chondromyxoid fibroma
- Non-ossifying fibroma
- Infective cyst (Brodie's abscess)

Evaluation
- Age, symptoms, radiographic features
- MRI for internal structure
- Biopsy if suspicious

Q107. Pigmented villonodular synovitis (PVNS).

(Jawaharlal Institute of Postgraduate Medical Education and Research 2012)

Clinical Picture
- Young adult with **chronic monoarthritis** (usually knee)
- Swelling, mild pain, joint stiffness
- Joint effusion, palpable mass

Pathology
- Synovial proliferation with **hemosiderin deposition**
- **Benign but locally aggressive**

Differential Diagnosis
- Synovial chondromatosis
- TB arthritis
- RA
- Hemophilic arthropathy

Management
- *MRI*: Shows low signal due to hemosiderin

- **Arthroscopic or open synovectomy**
- **Radiotherapy** for recurrence or diffuse cases

Q108. Epiphyseal multiloculated lesion in 30-year-old female (likely GCT).

Differential Diagnosis
- **Giant cell tumor (GCT)**—most likely
- **Chondroblastoma** (younger age group)
- Clear cell chondrosarcoma
- Infection (e.g., Brodie's abscess)
- PVNS with bone involvement

Features Favoring GCT
- *Age*: 20–40 years
- *Location*: Epiphyseometaphyseal
- *Imaging*: **Lytic, expansile, narrow transition zone**

Management
- **Curettage + Bone grafting or PMMA cement**
- Extended curettage with burr/phenol
- **Wide excision** if recurrent/aggressive
- **Denosumab** for unresectable cases or recurrence
- Regular follow-up for lung metastasis

Q109. Giant cell variants.

- GCT of bone (benign)
- Giant cell-rich osteosarcoma
- Brown tumor (hyperparathyroidism)
- Aneurysmal bone cyst
- Chondroblastoma

Q110. Chondromyxoid fibroma (CMF).

- Rare benign tumor, metaphyseal location
- *Age*: Adolescents/young adults
- *Radiology*: **Eccentric, lytic lesion**, sclerotic margin
- *Histology*: Chondroid + myxoid matrix
- *Treatment*: **Curettage and grafting**

Q111. Shepherd's crook deformity.

- **Coxa vara** deformity with bowed femoral neck
- Seen in **polyostotic fibrous dysplasia**, also McCune-Albright syndrome
- *Correction*: Osteotomy

Q112. Eosinophilic granuloma.

- Localized form of **Langerhans cell histiocytosis**
- Solitary lytic lesion in bone (skull, spine, femur)
- May cause vertebra plana
- *Treatment*: Curettage, sometimes resolves spontaneously

Q113. Chemotherapy for osteosarcoma.

- **Neoadjuvant chemotherapy** before surgery
- *Drugs*: **MAP protocol**—methotrexate, adriamycin (doxorubicin), cisplatin
- Improves limb salvage and survival
- Response to chemotherapy guides prognosis

Q114. Surface osteosarcomas.

- *Types*:
  - Parosteal (low-grade, best prognosis)
  - Periosteal (intermediate grade)
  - High-grade surface osteosarcoma
- All arise from bone surface, not medulla
- *Management*: **Wide excision**, chemotherapy based on grade

Q115. Fine needle aspiration cytology (FNAC).

- Minimally invasive diagnostic tool
- *Often used in*:
  - **Soft tissue tumors**
  - **Secondary bone lesions**
  - Lymph nodes
- May be limited in primary bone tumors (biopsy preferred)

Q116. Tumor markers.

- *Osteosarcoma*: ALP, LDH (prognostic)
- *Ewing's sarcoma*: CD99 (MIC2), FLI1
- *Multiple myeloma*: M-protein
- *Choriocarcinoma (metastasis)*: β-HCG
- **PSA** for prostate metastasis to bone

1. Nerve Sheath Tumors

Benign

- *Schwannoma (neurilemmoma)*: Encapsulated, eccentric, positive for **S-100**.
- *Neurofibroma*: Non-encapsulated, central, seen in **NF1**, also S-100 positive.

Malignant

- *Malignant peripheral nerve sheath tumor (MPNST)*: Aggressive, high recurrence; associated with NF1.
- *Markers*: S-100 (focal), SOX10, EMA.

2. Kahler's Disease (Multiple Myeloma)

- Plasma cell malignancy involving bone marrow.
- *Clinical*: Bone pain, anemia, renal failure, hypercalcemia.
- *X-ray*: "Punched-out" lytic lesions (especially skull, spine).
- *Diagnosis*: M-protein (SPEP), Bence Jones proteins, marrow plasmacytosis (>10%).
- *Treatment*: Chemotherapy (bortezomib, lenalidomide), bisphosphonates.

3. Osteoid-forming Tumors

Tumor type	*Benign*	*Malignant*
Osteoid-forming	Osteoid osteoma, osteoblastoma	Osteosarcoma (classical type)

- *Osteoid osteoma*: Night pain, relieved by NSAIDs, nidus <1.5 cm.
- *Osteosarcoma*: Commonest primary malignant bone tumor (excluding MM). Sunburst pattern, Codman's triangle.

4. Location and Age Distribution of Bone Tumors

Tumor	*Common location*	*Age group*
Osteosarcoma	Metaphysis of long bones	Adolescents
Ewing's sarcoma	Diaphysis	5–25 years
Giant cell tumor	Epiphysis	20–40 years
Chondrosarcoma	Pelvis, proximal femur	>40 years
Osteoid osteoma	Cortex of long bones	10–30 years

5. Immunohistochemistry in Bone Tumors

Marker	*Tumor Indicated*
CD99	Ewing's sarcoma
S-100	Chondroid tumors, nerve sheath tumors
Cytokeratin	Carcinomas, chordomas
Vimentin	Mesenchymal tumors
Desmin	Rhabdomyosarcoma
HMB-45	Melanoma

6. Cartilage (Chondroid)-forming Tumors

Benign	*Malignant*
Enchondroma	Chondrosarcoma
Osteochondroma	Dedifferentiated CS
Chondroblastoma	Clear cell CS

- *Enchondroma*: Small bones of hand; asymptomatic.
- *Chondrosarcoma*: Painful, slow-growing, resistant to chemotherapy/radiation.

7. Cystic Lesions (Benign vs. Malignant)

Benign	*Malignant (Mimic cystic)*
Unicameral bone cyst (UBC)	Telangiectatic osteosarcoma
Aneurysmal bone cyst (ABC)	Giant cell-rich osteosarcoma
Fibrous dysplasia	Malignant transformation (rare)
Non-ossifying fibroma	–

8. Round Cell Tumors/Sarcomas

- *Common tumors*:
    - **Ewing's sarcoma** (CD99+)
    - **Lymphoma of bone** (CD45+)
    - Mesenchymal chondrosarcoma
    - Neuroblastoma metastasis
    - Small cell osteosarcoma

- *Histology*: Small round blue cells with scant cytoplasm.
- *Diagnosis*: IHC + Cytogenetics [e.g., t(11;22) for Ewing's].

9. Vascular Tumors of Bone

Benign	*Malignant*
Hemangioma (vertebra)	Angiosarcoma
Lymphangioma	Epithelioid hemangioendothelioma (EHE)

- *Hemangioma*: Corduroy or polka-dot vertebral pattern.
- *EHE*: Low-grade malignancy; biopsy + IHC (CD31, ERG+).

Quick Recap Table (Short Note Mnemonics)

SN topic	*Key points*
GCT variants	ABC, brown tumor, chondroblastoma, osteosarcoma (giant cell rich)
CMF	Rare, metaphyseal, curettage
Shepherd's crook	Coxa vara in fibrous dysplasia
Eosinophilic granuloma	Vertebra plana, skull lesion
Chemotherapy in osteosarcoma	MAP protocol
Surface osteosarcomas	Parosteal, periosteal, high-grade surface
Multiple myeloma	CRAB + raindrop skull + M-protein
FNAC	Screening tool, less reliable in primary bone tumors
Megaprosthesis	Limb salvage after tumor resection
Tumor markers	ALP, LDH, CD99, M-protein

FLOWCHART: Showing summary/approach to treatment of musculoskeletal tumour.

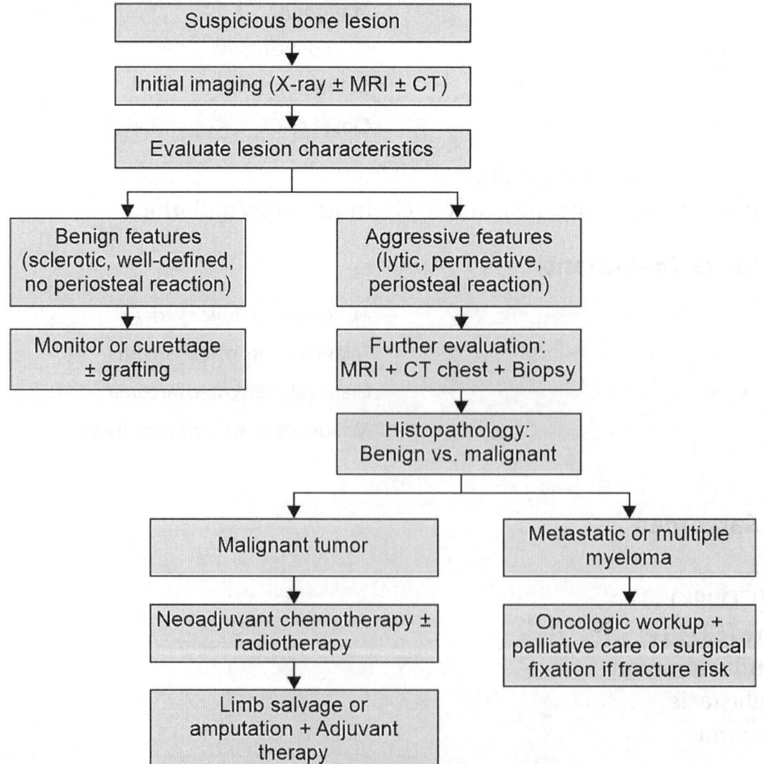

CHAPTER 5

Metabolic Bone Diseases and Endocrine Disorders

Bhat Jameel Mohd Jabbar, Sparsh Dagoria, Rifaaqat Ghani

Q1. Definition and classification of metabolic bone disease?

Definition

Metabolic bone diseases are disorders of bone strength due to abnormalities in minerals (Ca, $P0_4$), vitamin D, bone mass or turnover.

Classification
- Osteoporosis
- Osteomalacia
- Rickets
- Paget's disease
- Hyperparathyroidism-related bone disease
- Renal osteodystrophy
- Inherited disorders (e.g., osteogenesis imperfecta)

Q2. What is the role of calcium, phosphorus and vitamin D in bone health?

(BJ Medical College Ahmedabad 2012)

- *Calcium*: Essential for bone mineralization; regulated by PTH and vitamin D.
- *Phosphorus*: Critical in hydroxyapatite formation; balance with calcium is vital.

Role of Vitamin D in Bone Health
- *Functions*:
  - ↑ Calcium and phosphate absorption
  - Mineralization of bone
- *Deficiency leads to*:
  - Rickets in children
  - Osteomalacia in adults
  - Ultimately contributes to osteoporosis

Calcium in Bone Metabolism
- *Bone structure*: About 99% of the body's calcium is stored in bones and teeth, where it forms hydroxyapatite crystals $[Ca_{10}(PO_4)_6(OH)_2]$ that give bones strength and rigidity.
- *Mineral reservoir*: Bones act as a reservoir to maintain stable calcium levels in the blood, which is vital for muscle contraction, nerve transmission, and blood clotting.
- *Regulation*: Parathyroid hormone (PTH) increases blood calcium by stimulating bone resorption (breakdown of bone tissue). Calcitonin helps reduce blood calcium levels by inhibiting bone resorption.

Phosphorus in Bone Metabolism
- *Structural role*: About 85% of body phosphorus is in bones, where it combines with calcium to form hydroxyapatite.
- *Energy and cell function*: Phosphorus is involved in energy production (as ATP) and is a component of DNA, RNA, and cell membranes.
- *Bone remodeling*: Balanced phosphorus levels are essential for healthy bone remodelling. Excess phosphorus, especially with low calcium, can lead to bone loss.

Balance and Interaction
- The calcium-to-phosphorus ratio is crucial: imbalances can impair bone health.
- Chronic kidney disease, malnutrition, or hormonal imbalances can disrupt calcium-phosphorus metabolism, leading to conditions like osteomalacia or osteoporosis.

Q3. What is the role of parathyroid hormone (PTH) in bone metabolism?

Source: Chief cells of parathyroid gland
- *Stimulated by*: Low serum calcium
- *Acts on*:
  - *Bone*: Stimulates osteoclasts (via RANKL pathway) → ↑ Ca^{2+} release
  - *Kidney*:
    - ↑ Calcium reabsorption
    - ↓ Phosphate reabsorption
    - ↑ Activation of vitamin D (1-alpha hydroxylase)
  - *Gut (indirectly)*: Via activated vitamin D → ↑ Ca^{2+} absorption

Net effect: ↑ Serum Ca^{2+}, ↓ Serum phosphate

Pathology
- Hyperparathyroidism → osteitis fibrosa cystica, subperiosteal resorption
- Pseudohypoparathyroidism → resistance to PTH action
- **Chronic high PTH** → bone resorption
- **Intermittent PTH** (e.g., teriparatide) → anabolic effect

Q4. What is the role of fibroblast growth factor 23 (FGF-23), aging and alkaline phosphatase in bone metabolism?

(WBUHS 2012)

FGF-23
- Secreted by osteocytes.
- Lowers phosphate levels by:
  - Decreasing renal phosphate reabsorption
  - Inhibiting 1,25-dihydroxyvitamin D synthesis
- Elevated in tumor-induced osteomalacia, X-linked hypophosphatemia

Aging and Bone Metabolism
- Decreased osteoblast activity
- Increased osteoclast activity → net bone loss
- Reduced estrogen/testosterone → loss of antiresorptive effect
- *Results*: Osteopenia, osteoporosis, increased fracture risk

Alkaline Phosphatase (ALP)
- Produced by osteoblasts; marker of bone formation.
- *Elevated in*:
  - Bone growth (children)
  - Osteomalacia
  - Paget's disease
  - Healing fractures

Q5. Describe the role of various hormones in the development of bone.

Hormone	*Role in bone*
Parathyroid hormone (PTH)	Increases bone resorption indirectly, enhances Ca^{2+} reabsorption
Vitamin D (calcitriol)	Enhances Ca^{2+} and phosphate absorption from gut
Calcitonin	Inhibits osteoclast activity
Estrogen	Inhibits bone resorption, promotes osteoblast survival
GH and IGF-1	Stimulates bone growth and proliferation
Thyroid hormones	Stimulates bone turnover

Q6. Write a note on bone homeostasis and remodeling.

Bone Remodelling

- *Cyclical process involving*:
  - Osteoclasts—bone resorption
  - Osteoblasts—bone formation

Phases

- Activation—pre-osteoclast recruitment
- Resorption—osteoclast-mediated
- Reversal—apoptosis of osteoclasts, osteoblast recruitment
- Formation—osteoid deposition and mineralization

Homeostasis

- Balance between resorption and formation maintains bone mass
- Regulated by mechanical loading, hormones, cytokines

Q7. Discuss the assessment of metabolic bone disorders.

[Assam Medical College (Affiliated to Srimanta Sankaradeva University of Health Sciences) 2021]

Role of Dual-energy X-ray Absorptiometry (DEXA)

- Gold standard for assessing bone mineral density (BMD)
- Measures spine, hip, and forearm.
- Used for diagnosis, screening, and treatment monitoring.
- *Reported as*:
  - *T-score*: Comparison with young adult mean (used for diagnosis)
  - *Z-score*: Comparison with age-matched mean (used in children)

WHO Criteria (Based on T-score)

- *Normal*: > –1
- *Osteopenia*: –1 to –2.5
- *Osteoporosis*: < –2.5
- *Severe osteoporosis*: < –2.5 + fragility fracture

Role of Biochemical Tests

Test	*Significance*
Serum calcium	↓ in osteomalacia, ↑ in hyperparathyroidism
Serum phosphate	↓ in rickets, ↑ in CKD
Alkaline phosphatase	↑ in high bone turnover (Paget's, osteomalacia)
PTH	Elevated in primary/secondary hyperparathyroidism
25(OH) vitamin D	↓ in rickets/osteomalacia
Bone turnover markers	CTX (resorption), P1NP (formation)

Revision Flowchart

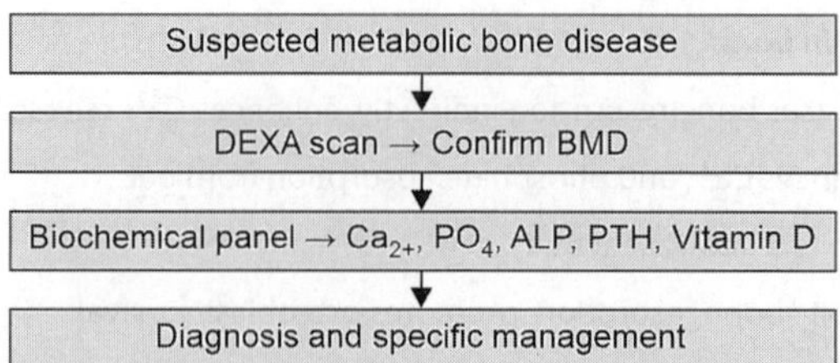

Q8. Define osteoporosis. Describe risk factors, diagnosis and management.

(Asked in: AIIMS Delhi 2022, PGI Chandigarh 2021, MUHS 2022)

Definition

Osteoporosis is a systemic skeletal disorder characterized by decreased bone mass and deterioration of bone microarchitecture, leading to increased fracture risk.

Classification

- *Primary type 1*: Postmenopausal
- *Primary type 2*: Senile (age-related)
- *Secondary*: Due to medications (e.g., glucocorticoids), diseases (e.g., hyperparathyroidism)

Risk Factors

- Postmenopausal status (estrogen deficiency)
- Age >65
- Steroid use
- Smoking, alcoholism
- Rheumatoid arthritis
- Low BMI
- Family history

Pathophysiology of Osteoporosis

- Imbalance between **bone resorption and formation**.
- Increased osteoclast activity > osteoblast function.
- Estrogen deficiency, aging, immobility, and corticosteroids are major contributors.

Diagnosis

- DEXA scan = Gold standard; T-score $\leq -2.5 \rightarrow$ osteoporosis
- FRAX score (WHO tool) estimates 10-year fracture risk
- **Rule out** secondary causes (thyroid, calcium, vitamin D, renal profile)

Management

Factors: Age, sex, BMI, smoking, alcohol, steroids, previous fracture, rheumatoid arthritis.

These factors are used to guide treatment decisions, especially in osteopenia.

- *Non-pharmacological*:
  - Weight-bearing exercises
  - Calcium (1,000–1,500 mg/day), vitamin D3 (800 IU/day)
  - Fall prevention
- *Pharmacological*:
  - *Antiresorptive*: Bisphosphonates (alendronate), denosumab
  - *Anabolic*: Teriparatide (recombinant PTH)
  - *SERM*: Raloxifene for postmenopausal women
- *Follow-up*: Repeat DEXA every 1–2 years

Q9. Discuss pharmacological management of osteoporosis.

1. *Bisphosphonates*:
   - *MOA*: Inhibit osteoclast-mediated bone resorption.
   - *Indications*: **First-line** therapy for postmenopausal, steroid-induced, or senile osteoporosis.
   - *Commonly used*: Alendronate, risedronate, zoledronic acid.
     - **Alendronate**
   - *Class*: Amino-bisphosphonate
   - *Mechanism*: Inhibits osteoclast-mediated bone resorption
   - *Dose*: 70 mg once weekly (oral)
   - *Precautions*: Take on empty stomach with water; remain upright for 30–60 minutes
   - *Side effects*: Esophagitis, osteonecrosis of jaw, atypical femoral fractures
2. *Denosumab*:
   - *Type*: Monoclonal antibody (anti-RANKL)
   - *Mechanism*: Inhibits osteoclast formation and activity
   - *Dose*: 60 mg subcutaneously every 6 months
   - *Indications*: Postmenopausal osteoporosis, bone metastases
   - *Side effects*: Hypocalcemia, infections, rebound bone loss on discontinuation
3. *Teriparatide*:
   - *Type*: Recombinant human PTH (1–34)
   - *Mechanism*: Intermittent administration → ↑ osteoblastic activity
   - *Dose*: 20 mcg SC daily (maximum 2 years)
   - *Indications*:
     - Severe osteoporosis (T-score < –3 or fracture + T-score < –2.5)
     - Failed prior therapy
   - *Contraindications*: Paget's disease, prior radiation therapy, malignancy
4. *SERMs:*
   - *Selective estrogen receptor modulators*: For example, Raloxifene.
   - Mimic estrogen in bones but antagonize it in breast/uterus.
   - Useful for **postmenopausal osteoporosis** with added benefit of breast cancer risk reduction.

Q10. Discuss complications of long-term bisphosphonates.

- Atypical femoral fractures
- Osteonecrosis of the jaw (ONJ)
- Esophagitis (oral forms)
- Drug holiday may be considered after 3–5 years in low-risk patients.

Q11. What is Singh's index for osteoporosis?

(IMS and SUM Hospital 2013)

Definition

Radiographic method to assess trabecular patterns in the proximal femur.

Grades

- *Grade VI*: All trabecular groups are visible and well-defined — normal bone density.
- *Grade V*: Mild reduction in trabecular density; principal tensile and compressive trabeculae are still prominent.
- *Grade IV*: Loss of some trabeculae, especially the secondary tensile group; early signs of osteopenia.
- *Grade III*: Only principal compressive trabeculae are prominent; others are disappearing—moderate osteoporosis.
- *Grade II*: Marked loss of trabeçulae; only a few compressive trabeculae remain—severe osteoporosis.
- *Grade I*: Almost total loss of trabecular pattern—very severe osteoporosis.

Limitations

Subjective, not quantitative. Superseded by DEXA in current practice.

Q12. What is steroid-induced osteoporosis?

- Glucocorticoids inhibit osteoblasts and promote resorption.
- Occurs early (within 6 months of therapy).
- *Prevention*: Calcium, vitamin D, bisphosphonates.
- *Screening*: DEXA if long-term steroids are planned.

Q13. Describe post-menopausal osteoporosis.

- *Etiology*: Estrogen deficiency → ↑ bone resorption.
- *Prevention*:
  - Calcium (1,000–1,200 mg/day) and vitamin D (800 IU/day)
  - Weight-bearing exercise, fall prevention
- *Pharmacologic*:
  - Bisphosphonates (first-line)
  - Denosumab
  - SERMs (e.g., raloxifene)
  - Teriparatide (severe cases)
- *Monitoring*: DEXA every 2 years

Q14. Difference between osteoporosis and osteopenia.

Parameter	*Osteopenia*	*Osteoporosis*
T-score	–1 to –2.5	< –2.5
Bone loss	Mild	Severe
Fracture risk	Increased slightly	High
Treatment	Lifestyle ± medications (calcium and vitamin D supplement)	Requires pharmacologic treatment

Q15. Discuss osteomalacia—causes, features, and management.

(Asked in: AIIMS Delhi 2022, PGI 2021)

Defective mineralization of osteoid in adults, commonly due to vitamin D deficiency.

Pathophysiology
- ↓ Vitamin D → ↓ calcium absorption → hypocalcemia → ↑ PTH → bone resorption
- Impaired mineralization of osteoid matrix → soft bones, pain, fractures.

Causes
- Nutritional vitamin D deficiency
- Malabsorption (celiac, post-gastrectomy)
- CKD (renal rickets)
- Drug-induced (phenytoin, rifampicin)

Clinical Features
- Bone pain and tenderness (especially hips/spine)
- Proximal myopathy
- Waddling gait
- Fragility fractures

Investigations
- ↓ Serum Ca, ↓ PO_4, ↑ ALP, ↑ PTH
- *X-ray*: Looser's zones (pseudofractures), osteopenia
- Biochemical findings in osteomalacia

Parameter	*Change*
Calcium	↓ or normal
Phosphate	↓
Alkaline phosphatase (ALP)	↑
PTH	↑
25(OH) vitamin D	↓

Management

- High-dose vitamin D (cholecalciferol) IM/oral
- Calcium supplementation
- Treat underlying cause

Q16. Describe rickets—types, radiology, and differences.

(Asked in: MUHS 2022, RGUHS 2023)

- *Rickets*: Defective mineralization of growth plate cartilage in children.
- *Types*:
  - Nutritional (vitamin D deficiency)
  - Vitamin D–dependent (type 1 and 2)
  - Hypophosphatemic
  - Renal rickets

1. *Nutritional rickets:*
   - Delayed milestones
   - Genu varum (bow legs), frontal bossing
   - Rachitic rosary (swollen costochondral junctions)
   - Widened wrists
   - Irritability, muscle weakness
2. *Vitamin D–resistant rickets—hypophosphatemic rickets*:
   - X-linked dominant (PHEX gene defect) → renal phosphate wasting
   - Serum phosphate ↓ despite normal calcium/vitamin D
   - *Treatment*:
     - Oral phosphate supplements
     - Calcitriol (active Vit D analogs)
     - Burosumab (anti-FGF23 monoclonal antibody in XLH)
3. *Vitamin D–dependent rickets*:
   - *Type 1*: Deficiency of 1α-hydroxylase → ↓ calcitriol
     - *Treatment*: Calcitriol
   - *Type 2*: End-organ resistance to calcitriol
     - *Treatment*: High-dose calcitriol + calcium

Feature	*Nutritional rickets*	*Renal rickets (CKD)*
Ca, PO_4	↓ Ca, ↓ PO_4	↓ Ca, ↑ PO_4
ALP, PTH	↑ ALP, ↑ PTH	↑ ALP, ↑↑ PTH
Vitamin D	↓	Normal/↓
Radiology	Cupping, fraying	Same + secondary changes
Rx	Vitamin D, Ca	Phosphate binders, Vitamin D analogs

Role of Calcium and Phosphate in Rickets

- Essential for normal bone mineralization
- *Nutritional rickets*: Supplement both if deficient

- *Hypophosphatemic rickets*: Requires high-dose phosphate
- Vitamin D enhances both calcium and phosphate absorption from gut.

Radiological features

Looser's zones (pseudofractures):

- Radiolucent bands perpendicular to bone surface (e.g., ribs, femoral neck)
- Pathognomonic for osteomalacia
- Represent incomplete stress fractures due to poor mineralization.

Treatment

Based on etiology—vitamin D, phosphate, or specific therapy (e.g., calcitriol in type 1).

Q17. Differentiate between rickets and osteomalacia.

Feature	*Rickets (children)*	*Osteomalacia (adults)*
Growth plate	Affected	Not affected
Symptoms	Genu varum, widening wrists, rachitic rosary	Bone pain, waddling gait
Radiology	Cupping, fraying, splaying of metaphyses	Looser's zones, pseudofractures
Cause	Vitamin D deficiency, phosphate disorders	Vitamin D deficiency, renal disease

Q18. Describe renal osteodystrophy and role of FGF-23.

Definition

Bone pathology due to CKD → secondary hyperparathyroidism

Features

- Osteitis fibrosa cystica (↑ PTH)
- Osteomalacia, adynamic bone disease
- **Rugger-jersey spine**

FGF-23

- Secreted by osteocytes
- ↑ in CKD → ↓ phosphate reabsorption and ↓ vitamin D activation

Q19. Discuss the pathology, clinical features, and management of Paget's disease.

(Asked in: PGI 2022, MUHS 2023, AIIMS 2021)

Definition

Localized disorder of abnormal bone remodeling, with increased resorption followed by chaotic bone formation.

Pathology

- Excess osteoclastic activity → disorganized lamellar bone
- "Mosaic pattern" on histology

Common Sites

Skull, pelvis, femur, tibia

Pathophysiology of Paget's Disease

- A chronic bone remodeling disorder.
- *Three phases*:
  1. *Lytic phase*: ↑ osteoclastic activity → bone resorption
  2. *Mixed phase*: Disorganized osteoblast/osteoclast activity
  3. *Sclerotic phase*: Excessive, disorganized bone formation
- *Result*: Structurally weak, deformed bone.

Clinical Features
- Bone pain
- Skull enlargement (increased hat size)
- Hearing loss
- Bowing of legs
- High-output cardiac failure (rare)

Radiological Features
- *Skull*: Cotton wool appearance
- *Spine*: Picture frame vertebrae
- *Long bones*: Bowing, cortical thickening, mixed sclerotic-lytic lesions
- *Pelvis*: Coarsened trabeculae and widened iliopectineal lines

Investigations
- *Role of alkaline phosphatase (ALP)*:
  - **Marker of disease activity**
  - Elevated in active disease
  - *Used to monitor*:
    - Disease progression
    - Treatment response (should decrease post-treatment)
- *X*-ray:
  - Lytic → mixed → sclerotic phases
  - Cotton-wool skull, blade-of-grass lesion
- *Bone scan*: Increased uptake

Complications
- Pathological fractures
- Secondary osteoarthritis (e.g., hip, knee)
- Hearing loss (due to skull involvement)
- High-output cardiac failure (rare)
- *Sarcomatous transformation (1–3%)*:
  - Rare but serious complication (usually osteosarcoma)
  - Suspect in:
    - Sudden ↑ in bone pain
    - Swelling, pathological fracture
    - Rapid ↑ ALP despite bisphosphonates
  - Poor prognosis

Treatment
- Bisphosphonates (zoledronic acid is the drug of choice)
- Analgesics
- Orthopedic correction if deformity or fracture

Role of Bisphosphonates in Treatment
- *First-line*: **IV zoledronate** or **oral alendronate**
- *Mechanism*: Inhibit osteoclasts → reduce bone turnover
- *Effects*: Decrease bone pain, normalize ALP, improve radiographic features

Q20. Describe hyperparathyroidism.

(Asked in: PGI 2022, RGUHS 2022)

Types
- *Primary*: Autonomous PTH secretion (e.g., parathyroid adenoma)
- *Secondary*: Due to chronic hypocalcemia (e.g., CKD)
- *Tertiary*: Autonomous PTH secretion after long-standing secondary hyperparathyroidism (e.g., post-renal transplant)

1. *Primary hyperparathyroidism*:
    - Caused by excessive **PTH** → ↑ osteoclastic activity.
    - *Bone findings*:
        - Osteopenia/Osteoporosis
        - Subperiosteal bone resorption (classic on radial side of middle phalanges)
        - Brown tumors (localized bone lesions)
        - Salt and pepper skull on X-ray
        - Osteitis fibrosa cystica
2. *Secondary hyperparathyroidism*:
    - Stimulated by **chronic hypocalcemia** due to:
        - Chronic kidney disease (CKD) → ↓ vitamin D activation
        - Vitamin D deficiency
        - Malabsorption
    - Prolonged stimulation → parathyroid gland hyperplasia → ↑ PTH secretion
    - *Leads to*:
        - Renal osteodystrophy
        - Bone pain, fragility

Biochemistry
- *Primary*: ↑ Ca, ↓ PO_4, ↑ ALP
- *Secondary*: ↓ Ca, ↑ PO_4, ↑ ALP

Radiological Features
- *Subperiosteal resorption*: Especially radial aspect of fingers
- *Salt and pepper skull*: Granular demineralization
- *Rugger jersey spine*: Dense vertebral endplates (in secondary HPT)
- *Brown tumors*: Expansile lytic lesions

Management
- *Primary*: Parathyroidectomy
- *Secondary*: Phosphate binders, active vitamin D (calcitriol), renal transplant
- *Bone lesions*: Rarely need curettage or fixation.

Q21. What is osteitis fibrosa cystica?

- Severe form of hyperparathyroid bone disease.
- *Histology*: ↑ osteoclastic resorption, marrow fibrosis.
- *Radiology*:
    - **Cystic bone lesions**, cortical thinning
    - Associated with **Brown tumors**

Q22. What are the indications for parathyroidectomy?

- Symptomatic hypercalcemia
- Osteoporosis or fragility fractures
- Age <50 with elevated calcium
- Nephrolithiasis or CKD
- Markedly elevated serum calcium or PTH

Q23. What is Brown's tumor?

- Reactive bone lesions due to high PTH
- Composed of fibrous tissue, osteoclasts, and hemorrhage
- Mimic neoplasms on imaging

- *Common sites*: Pelvis, ribs, mandible, long bones
- **Reversible** post-parathyroidectomy

Q24. Describe renal osteodystrophy.

Definition

A spectrum of bone disorders in **chronic kidney disease (CKD)** due to disturbances in calcium, phosphate, PTH, and vitamin D metabolism.

Classification (Based on Bone Turnover and Mineralization)

- *High turnover*:
  - Secondary hyperparathyroidism
  - Osteitis fibrosa cystica
- *Low turnover*:
  - **Adynamic bone disease**
  - Osteomalacia (due to vitamin D deficiency or aluminum toxicity)
- **Mixed uremic osteodystrophy** (features of both high and low turnover)

Pathophysiology of Renal Osteodystrophy

- *CKD leads to*:
  - ↓ phosphate excretion → hyperphosphatemia
  - ↓ active vitamin D (calcitriol) → hypocalcemia
  - ↑ PTH secretion (secondary hyperparathyroidism)
  - Disturbed bone remodeling, mineralization, and turnover
- Over time, **parathyroid hyperplasia** may lead to tertiary HPT

Q25. What are the skeletal manifestations of CKD-MBD (chronic kidney disease–mineral and bone disorder)?

[Government Medical College (GMC) Srinagar 2012]

- Bone pain and deformities
- Pathological fractures
- Vertebral collapse
- **Subperiosteal bone resorption**
- **Rugger jersey spine**
- Growth retardation in children

Q26. Write a short note on adynamic bone disease.

- **Low bone turnover**, minimal osteoblast/osteoclast activity
- Often due to **over-suppression of PTH** (e.g., excessive vitamin D or calcium)
- *Features*:
  - Fracture risk
  - Vascular calcifications
  - Hyporesponsive bone to PTH
- *Diagnosis*: Bone biopsy (gold standard)

Q27. Discuss the role of phosphate binders.

- Used to reduce **serum phosphate** levels, slowing secondary hyperparathyroidism
- *Types*:
  - Calcium-based (e.g., calcium acetate/carbonate)
  - Non-calcium-based (e.g., sevelamer, lanthanum)
- Avoids phosphate retention and vascular calcification

Q28. What are the orthopedic complications of renal osteodystrophy.

- Pathological fractures (especially vertebrae, femur, ribs)
- Delayed fracture healing
- Bone pain and deformities
- Tendon ruptures (e.g., quadriceps, Achilles)
- Increased risk during orthopedic surgery due to poor bone quality

Q29. Classify osteogenesis imperfecta and describe management principles.

(Asked in: PGI 2021, JIPMER 2022, MUHS 2022)

Definition

Osteogenesis imperfecta (OI) is a genetic disorder characterized by fragile bones that break easily, often with little or no trauma. It is commonly known as "brittle bone disease."

Causes

- Most cases are caused by mutations in the *COL1A1* or *COL1A2* genes, which encode type I collagen, a major structural protein in bone and connective tissue.
- It is usually inherited in an autosomal dominant manner, though some forms are autosomal recessive.

Sillence Classification

Type	*Severity*	*Features*
I	Mild	Blue sclera, hearing loss
II	Perinatal lethal	Fractures at birth
III	Severe	Progressive deformities
IV	Moderate	Normal sclera, fractures

Clinical Features

- Fragile bones, multiple fractures
- Blue sclerae
- Dentinogenesis imperfecta
- Hearing loss
- Short stature

Management

- Bisphosphonates (pamidronate IV)
- Intramedullary rodding (Fassier-Duval rods)
- Bracing, physiotherapy
- Genetic counseling

Q30. Describe the skeletal manifestations of fluorosis.

(Asked in: AIIMS 2022, PGI 2021, MUHS 2023)

Definition

A chronic metabolic bone disease caused by **excessive fluoride intake**, leading to abnormal bone mineralization.

Causes

- Drinking water with high fluoride (>1.5 ppm)
- Industrial exposure (aluminum smelting, phosphate fertilizers)
- Fluoride-containing coal combustion
- Tea overconsumption (tea contains fluoride)

Clinical Features
- Joint stiffness
- Spinal rigidity
- Decreased mobility
- Ossification of ligaments (interosseous membrane, sacrospinous)

Radiology
- Osteosclerosis (especially axial skeleton)
- Ligamentous calcification
- Interosseous membrane ossification
- Diffuse increased bone density, "rugger-jersey spine"
- Bone thickening, especially in pelvis and vertebrae

Differential Diagnosis
- Paget's disease
- Osteopetrosis
- Renal osteodystrophy
- Diffuse idiopathic skeletal hyperostosis (DISH)
- Sclerotic bone metastases (e.g., prostate cancer)

Differentiation based on **history of exposure, lab tests, and bone biopsy if needed**

Management
- *Primarily preventive*:
  - Reduce fluoride intake (defluorinated water)
  - Public health measures in endemic areas
- *Symptomatic treatment*:
  - Analgesics, physiotherapy
  - Surgery for severe deformities or neurological compression (e.g., decompression laminectomy)
  - Rehabilitation for joint stiffness
- Surgery is only for severe deformity

Q31. Describe radiological features of various metabolic disorders.

(Rajasthan University of Health Sciences 2012)

Condition	*Classic radiology*
Osteomalacia	Looser's zones, decreased density
Rickets	Cupping, fraying, widening
Paget's	Cotton-wool skull, mixed lesions
HPT	Subperiosteal resorption, salt and pepper skull
Fluorosis	Dense bones, calcified ligaments
OI	Wormian bones, thin cortices

Q32. Osteopetrosis—definition and genetic classification.

Definition

A group of rare genetic disorders characterized by increased bone density due to defective osteoclast-mediated bone resorption.

Genetic Classification
- *Autosomal recessive (malignant infantile)*: Severe, presents early
- *Autosomal dominant (benign adult)*: Milder, later onset
- *X-linked*: Rare

Pathophysiology

Defect in osteoclast function or differentiation → failure of bone resorption

- Results in dense but brittle bones
- *Skeletal features*: Frequent fractures
- Cranial nerve compression (due to narrowed foramina)
- Osteomyelitis (especially mandible)
- Erlenmeyer flask deformity
- Bone marrow failure (pancytopenia)

Skeletal Manifestations of Osteopetrosis

- "Bone within a bone" appearance
- Radiographic hallmark of **osteopetrosis**
- Seen especially in vertebrae, phalanges, and pelvis
- Represents endochondral bone encased in abnormally dense bone matrix

Q33. Write a short note on bone marrow transplantation in osteopetrosis.

- Curative in severe infantile (malignant) type
- Introduces normal osteoclast precursors → improves hematopoiesis and bone turnover
- Most effective if done early

Q34. Write a short note on hypophosphatasia.

- Rare metabolic disorder caused by **alkaline phosphatase deficiency**
- *Features*:
  - Poor bone mineralization
  - Fractures, rickets-like changes
  - Premature loss of teeth
- *Management*:
  - **Asfotase alfa** (enzyme replacement therapy)
  - Supportive care, fracture management

Q35. Melorheostosis—short note.

- Rare sclerosing bone disorder
- "**Dripping candle wax**" appearance on radiographs
- Affects long bones unilaterally
- *Causes*:
  - Pain
  - Contractures
  - Joint stiffness
- *Treatment*: Symptomatic (physiotherapy, surgery for deformity)

Q36. Pyknodysostosis—short note.

- **Autosomal recessive**, mutation in **cathepsin K** gene (affects osteoclasts)
- *Features*:
  - Short stature
  - Delayed closure of cranial sutures

  - Fragile bones
  - Dental anomalies
  - Osteosclerosis
- Differentiated from osteopetrosis by **acroosteolysis** (resorption of terminal phalanges)

Q37. Camurati–Engelmann disease—short note.

- Rare autosomal dominant disorder
- Characterized by **diaphyseal dysplasia**
- *Features*:
  - Limb pain
  - Muscle weakness
  - Waddling gait
  - Cortical thickening of long bones (especially femur)
- *Diagnosis*: Radiographs, genetic testing
- *Management*: Corticosteroids, physical therapy

Q38. Write a short note on role of aluminium toxicity in bone disease.

(Bihar University of Health Sciences 2012)

- Seen in **patients with chronic kidney disease** on dialysis using aluminum-containing phosphate binders
- *Leads to adynamic bone disease*:
  - Suppression of bone turnover
  - Impaired mineralization
- *Clinical effects*:
  - Bone pain
  - Fractures
  - Muscle weakness
- *Diagnosis*: Bone biopsy, serum aluminium levels

Q39. Describe the impact of osteoporosis on fracture healing.

- *Osteoporosis leads to*:
  - Decreased bone density and strength
  - Increased risk of fragility fractures (especially vertebral, hip, and wrist)
  - Delayed union or non-union due to poor bone stock
  - Fixation failure due to compromised screw hold in osteoporotic bone
- *Management tip*: Use augmented fixation (e.g., locking plates, bone grafts), address the underlying osteoporosis

Q40. Write a note on diabetes mellitus—skeletal implications.

Effects

- Increased fracture risk
- Impaired bone formation (osteoblast dysfunction)
- Charcot arthropathy
- Delayed healing
- Diffuse idiopathic skeletal hyperostosis (DISH)

Q41. Effect of diabetes mellitus on bone healing—short note.

- *Hyperglycemia impairs*:
    - Collagen synthesis
    - Angiogenesis and cell proliferation
    - Osteoblastic activity
- Increased risk of infection, non-union, and implant loosening
- Glycemic control is critical pre- and post-operatively

Q42. Describe the influence of chronic kidney disease (CKD) on fracture healing.

(Seth Gordhandas Sunderdas Medical College and KEM Hospital 2015)

- *CKD causes renal osteodystrophy, affecting bone quality*:
    - Abnormal calcium-phosphate metabolism
    - Vitamin D resistance
    - Secondary hyperparathyroidism
- *Complications*:
    - Fragile bones with poor remodeling capacity
    - Delayed union, pathological fractures
- Treatment includes correcting metabolic imbalances and ensuring proper bone turnover

Q43. Write a note on metabolic bone disease-related periprosthetic fractures.

- *Occurs around implants (e.g., hip/knee arthroplasty) in patients with*: Osteoporosis, osteomalacia, or renal osteodystrophy
- *Pathophysiology*: Weak bone → inadequate support for prosthesis → increased risk of fracture
- *Management*:
    - Stabilize fracture and revise or secure implant
    - Treat underlying metabolic bone disease concurrently
- *Treatment*: Stop aluminum exposure, use chelating agents (e.g., deferoxamine)

Q44. Describe prevention and management of fragility fractures.

Definition

Fractures from low-energy trauma (e.g., fall from standing).

Prevention

- Treat underlying osteoporosis
- *Fall risk reduction*: Balance training, remove home hazards

Management

- Surgical fixation
- Osteoporosis treatment (bisphosphonates, teriparatide, etc.)
- Secondary fracture prevention programs (e.g., FLS → fracture liaison services)

Q45. Describe bony changes in scurvy.

(West Bengal University of Health Sciences 2013)

Etiology

Vitamin C deficiency → defective collagen synthesis

Radiological signs
- White line of Frankel (dense provisional zone)
- Wimberger's ring (scorbutic ring sign)
- Pelkan spurs
- Trummerfeld zone (lucent metaphysis)

Clinical
Painful limbs, pseudoparalysis, gum bleeding

Treatment
Vitamin C supplementation (100–500 mg/day), diet correction

Q46. What is Rugger–Jersey spine?

Definition
Sclerotic bands at vertebral endplates with radiolucent center

Seen in
Secondary hyperparathyroidism (especially renal osteodystrophy)

Mechanism
Disordered bone turnover and mineralization

Q47. Describe hypocalcemia—causes and treatment.

Definition
Serum calcium < 8.5 mg/dL

Causes
- Hypoparathyroidism
- Vitamin D deficiency
- Chronic kidney disease
- Acute pancreatitis
- *Drugs*: Bisphosphonates, calcitonin

Symptoms
Tetany, Chvostek and Trousseau signs, seizures

Treatment
- *Acute*: IV calcium gluconate
- *Chronic*: Oral calcium + Vitamin D (calcitriol in CKD)

Q48. Describe hypercalcemia.

Causes
- Primary hyperparathyroidism
- Malignancy (PTHrP, bone mets)
- Vitamin D intoxication
- Sarcoidosis, thiazides

Skeletal effects
Subperiosteal resorption, osteopenia, fractures

Treatment
- Hydration + loop diuretics
- Bisphosphonates, calcitonin
- Dialysis if severe

Q49. What are the skeletal manifestations of acromegaly?

(Atal Medical and Research University 2012)

Cause

GH excess (pituitary adenoma)

Features

- Enlarged hands/feet, prognathism
- Spade-like terminal phalanges
- Vertebral enlargement → kyphosis
- Arthropathy (cartilage overgrowth)

Q50. Explain the diagnostic approach to metabolic bone diseases.

Examples

Osteoporosis, osteomalacia, rickets, osteoporosis, Paget's, fluorosis

History and Clinical Clues

- Bone pain, fractures, deformities
- Family history
- Dietary deficiency, renal disease, medications

Investigations

Test	*Findings in metabolic bone diseases*
Serum calcium	↓ in osteomalacia, ↑ in hyperparathyroidism
Phosphate	↓ in rickets, ↑ in renal disease
ALP	↑ in osteomalacia, Paget's disease
PTH	↑ in secondary hyperparathyroidism
Vitamin D	↓ in osteomalacia and rickets
X-rays	Looser's zones, codfish vertebrae
DEXA scan	Osteoporosis
Bone biopsy	Rarely done (diagnosis unclear)

Q51. Describe peak bone mass (PBM).

(Grant Medical College Mumbai 2011)

Definition

Peak bone mass (PBM) refers to the maximum bone density and strength an individual achieves, typically between **20–30 years of age**.

Significance

- Acts as a **bone bank** for later life.
- Higher PBM reduces the risk of osteoporosis and fragility fractures in old age.

Factors Affecting PBM

- Genetics (60–80%)
- *Nutrition*: Adequate calcium, vitamin D, protein
- *Physical activity*: Especially weight-bearing exercises
- *Hormonal status*: Estrogen/testosterone levels

- *Lifestyle*: Smoking and alcohol reduce PBM
- *Diseases/Medications*: Chronic illness or corticosteroids ↓ PBM

Q52. Describe Gaucher's disease.

Etiology

Autosomal recessive lysosomal storage disorder due to **β-glucocerebrosidase deficiency**.

Pathology

Accumulation of glucocerebroside in macrophages → "Gaucher cells".

Skeletal manifestations

- Osteopenia, bone pain, Erlenmeyer flask deformity of femur
- AVN of femoral head
- Pathological fractures

Diagnosis

Enzyme assay, bone marrow showing Gaucher cells.

Treatment

Enzyme replacement therapy (imiglucerase), bisphosphonates for bone.

Q53. Discuss Fanconi's syndrome.

Etiology

Proximal renal tubular dysfunction → impaired reabsorption of glucose, phosphate, bicarbonate, amino acids.

Causes

Inherited (Fanconi anemia), acquired (ifosfamide, tenofovir, Wilson's disease).

Orthopedic Impact

- Hypophosphatemic rickets
- Bone deformities and fractures due to osteomalacia

Treatment

Phosphate, vitamin D supplementation, manage underlying cause.

Q54. Write a note on hemophilia.

Types

A (Factor VIII deficiency), B (Factor IX deficiency); X-linked recessive.

Orthopedic Relevance

- *Hemarthrosis*: Especially knee, elbow, ankle
- Chronic arthropathy → joint deformities
- Pseudotumors in bone/soft tissue due to bleeding

Diagnosis

Prolonged aPTT, normal PT; factor assay.

Management

- Factor replacement therapy
- Joint protection, physiotherapy
- Synovectomy or joint replacement in end-stage

Q55. Write a note on sickle cell disease (SCD).

(Narayana Medical College Nellore Andhra Pradesh 2011)

Etiology

Autosomal recessive; HbS polymerization → vaso-occlusion.

Musculoskeletal manifestations

- **Dactylitis** (hand-foot syndrome)
- AVN of femoral/humeral head
- Osteomyelitis (commonly *Salmonella*)
- Growth retardation, bone infarcts

X-ray

"Hair-on-end" skull, bone sclerosis.

Treatment

Hydroxyurea, transfusions, supportive care. Surgery for AVN or osteomyelitis.

Q56. Write a short note on thalassemia.

Etiology

Inherited defect in globin chain synthesis (α or β).

Skeletal manifestations

- Marrow hyperplasia → frontal bossing, "chipmunk facies"
- Osteopenia, vertebral collapse
- Erlenmeyer flask deformity

X-ray

"Hair-on-end" skull, cortical thinning.

Treatment

Regular transfusions, iron chelation, bone marrow transplant.

Q57. Write a note on myositis ossificans progressiva (fibrodysplasia ossificans progressiva).

(Jammu University 2013)

Definition

Rare genetic disorder (ACVR1 mutation) → heterotopic ossification of muscle/connective tissue.

Clinical Features

- Starts in childhood, progressive stiffness
- Ankylosis of joints, restricted chest wall movement
- Hallux valgus (early sign)

X-ray

Heterotopic bone formation in characteristic patterns.

Avoid

Trauma, surgery, intramuscular injections (may worsen ossification).

Management

Supportive; bisphosphonates, corticosteroids (short-term), gene therapy under trial.

CHAPTER 6

Inflammatory Disorders, Crystal Arthropathy, and Degenerative Disorders

Anoop Kumar, Sachin Kudyar, Ankita Khajuria

Q1. Define inflammatory arthritis and classify its types.

Definition

- A group of autoimmune or autoinflammatory disorders characterized by **synovial inflammation**, **morning stiffness**, and **joint destruction** if untreated.

Classification

1. **Autoimmune Inflammatory Arthritis:**
    - Rheumatoid arthritis (RA)
    - Systemic lupus erythematosus (SLE)
    - Psoriatic arthritis (PsA)
    - Juvenile idiopathic arthritis (JIA)
2. **Seronegative Spondyloarthropathies:**
    - Ankylosing spondylitis (AS)
    - Reactive arthritis
    - Enteropathic arthritis
    - Psoriatic arthritis
3. **Crystal-induced Arthritis:**
    - Gout (monosodium urate)
    - Pseudogout (calcium pyrophosphate)

Q2. Differentiate between inflammatory and non-inflammatory arthritis.

Feature	*Inflammatory arthritis*	*Non-inflammatory arthritis (OA)*
Onset	Gradual or acute	Gradual
Morning stiffness	>30 minutes, improves with activity	<30 minutes, worsens with activity
Swelling	Soft tissue swelling	Bony enlargement (osteophyte formation)
Systemic symptoms	Common (fever, fatigue)	Rare
Inflammatory markers	↑ ESR, ↑ CRP	Usually normal
Synovial fluid	Inflammatory (WBC > 2,000/mm^3)	Non-inflammatory (WBC < 2,000/mm^3)

Q3. Pathophysiology of inflammatory arthritis.

- Initiated by **immune dysregulation** → activated **T-cells and B-cells** →
- Release of **pro-inflammatory cytokines** (TNF-α, IL-1, IL-6)
- Synovial membrane becomes **hyperplastic (pannus)**
- Destruction of **cartilage and bone** via **osteoclast activation**
- *Result:* **Joint deformity**, **pain**, **loss of function**

Q4. Role of cytokines in inflammatory arthritis.

- *TNF-α:* Central to inflammation; promotes angiogenesis and pannus formation
- *IL-1:* Stimulates synovial fibroblasts, cartilage degradation
- *IL-6:* Promotes acute phase response, osteoclast differentiation
- *IL-17:* Produced by Th17 cells, enhances neutrophil recruitment and joint damage
- *Targeted therapies:* Anti-TNF (e.g., infliximab), IL-6 inhibitors (e.g., tocilizumab)

Q5. Immunopathogenesis of rheumatoid arthritis (RA).

(Kashmir University 2011)

1. *Genetic predisposition:* HLA-DR4, DR1 association
2. **Trigger (infection, smoking)** → **autoantigen presentation**
3. Activation of **CD4+ T-** and **B-cells**
4. *Production of autoantibodies*:
   - **Rheumatoid factor (RF)**
   - **Anti-citrullinated protein antibodies (ACPA)**
5. **Immune complex formation** → complement activation
6. Synovial inflammation → pannus → joint erosion and deformity

Rheumatoid Arthritis

Q6. Define rheumatoid arthritis and discuss its classification criteria.

Definition

A chronic, systemic autoimmune disease primarily affecting **synovial joints** with **symmetric, erosive polyarthritis** and systemic inflammation.

Classification Criteria – 2010 ACR/EULAR: Total score ≥6/10 indicates definite RA:

Domain	*Points*
Joint involvement	1–5 points (based on number and type of joints)
Serology (RF, ACPA)	0–3 points
Acute phase reactants (ESR, CRP)	0–1 point
Duration of symptoms (>6 weeks)	1 point

Q7. Describe the pathogenesis and management of rheumatoid arthritis. (AIIMS Delhi 2022).

Pathogenesis

- Autoimmune disease targeting synovium
- *Key players:* T-cells, B-cells, cytokines (TNF-α, IL-1)
- Leads to pannus formation, cartilage erosion, bone destruction

Clinical Features
- Morning stiffness > 1 hour
- Symmetrical joint involvement (MCP, PIP, wrist)
- Rheumatoid nodules

Investigations
- RF (+ in ~70%), anti-CCP (more specific)
- ESR/CRP elevated, X-ray shows joint space narrowing, erosions

Management
- NSAIDs, steroids (short-term)
- DMARDs (methotrexate, leflunomide)
- Biologics (TNF inhibitors: Etanercept, infliximab)
- Physical therapy, joint protection

Q8. Clinical features of RA and its extra-articular manifestations.

Articular
- **Symmetric small joint involvement** (MCP, PIP, wrists)
- Morning stiffness >1 hour
- Swan-neck, boutonnière deformities
- Ulnar deviation, Z-thumb

Extra-articular
- *Skin:* Rheumatoid nodules
- *Eyes:* Scleritis, keratoconjunctivitis sicca (part of Sjögren's)
- *Lungs:* Interstitial lung disease, pleuritis
- *Heart:* Pericarditis, increased CV risk
- *Hematologic:* Anemia of chronic disease, Felty's syndrome (RA + neutropenia + splenomegaly)
- *Neurologic:* Peripheral neuropathy, entrapment syndromes

Q9. Radiological and laboratory findings in RA.

Radiology
- *Early:* Soft tissue swelling, juxta-articular osteopenia
- *Late:* Joint space narrowing, erosions, subluxations

Labs
- ↑ ESR, ↑ CRP
- *Rheumatoid factor (RF):* Positive in ~70%
- *Anti-CCP (ACPA):* Highly specific (~95%) for RA
- Normocytic normochromic anemia

Q10. Role of disease-modifying anti-rheumatic drugs (DMARDs).

Purpose
Halt disease progression, reduce joint damage

Types
1. **Conventional synthetic DMARDs:**
    - Methotrexate (first-line)
    - Sulfasalazine
    - Leflunomide
    - Hydroxychloroquine

2. **Biologic DMARDs:**
   - *Anti-TNF*: Infliximab, etanercept
   - *IL-6 inhibitors*: Tocilizumab
   - *B-cell therapy*: Rituximab
   - *T-cell costimulation inhibitor*: Abatacept
3. **Targeted Synthetic DMARDs:** JAK inhibitors (e.g., Tofacitinib)

Regular monitoring of liver function, blood counts, and infections is essential.

Q11. Surgical management options for RA.

Indicated for
- Severe joint damage
- Intractable pain or deformity
- Functional impairment

Procedures
- *Synovectomy:* Early disease with persistent synovitis
- *Joint replacement (arthroplasty):* Hip, knee, MCPs
- *Joint fusion (arthrodesis):* Wrist, ankle, or unstable joints
- *Tendon reconstruction:* For ruptures due to tenosynovitis

Q12. Rheumatoid nodules and their clinical significance.

(Assam Medical College Dibrugarh 2010)

Definition
Firm, non-tender subcutaneous nodules usually over pressure areas (elbow, forearm)

Histology
Central fibrinoid necrosis surrounded by palisading histiocytes

Significance
- Seen in **seropositive RA**
- Associated with more **severe disease**
- May be complicated by ulceration or infection

Q13. Extra-articular manifestations of RA.

(PGI Chandigarh 2023)

- *Pulmonary:* ILD, pleuritis
- *Cardiac:* Pericarditis
- *Eye:* Scleritis, keratoconjunctivitis sicca
- *Skin:* Rheumatoid nodules
- *Hematological:* Anemia of chronic disease, Felty's syndrome

Q14. Define seronegative spondyloarthropathies and classify them.

Definition
- A group of chronic inflammatory rheumatic diseases characterized by:
  - **Negative rheumatoid factor (RF)**
  - **Axial and peripheral arthritis**
  - **Enthesitis** (inflammation at tendon/ligament insertion sites)
  - **Association with HLA-B27**

Classification (PEARS)

- *P*soriatic arthritis
- *E*nteropathic arthritis (IBD-associated)
- *A*nkylosing spondylitis (AS)
- *R*eactive arthritis (ReA)
- *S*pondyloarthritis undifferentiated/juvenile SpA

Ankylosing Spondylitis

Q15. Clinical features and radiology in ankylosing spondylitis.

(JIPMER Puducherry 2021)

Clinical Features

- Young male (15–40 years)
- Chronic **low back pain**, worse in morning, improves with activity
- **Bamboo spine**, reduced spinal mobility (Schober's test ↓)
- **Peripheral arthritis** (hips/shoulders)
- **Enthesitis** (Achilles, plantar fascia)
- *Extra-articular:* Uveitis, aortic regurgitation, apical lung fibrosis

Radiological Findings

- *Sacroiliitis:* Bilateral, symmetric (earliest sign)
- *Syndesmophytes:* Vertical ossifications between vertebrae
- *Bamboo spine:* Late finding on X-ray
- MRI is useful for early sacroiliitis

Management

- NSAIDs, DMARDs, physiotherapy
- Anti-TNF agents in refractory cases

Q16. Discuss the role of HLA-B27 in seronegative arthritis.

- Present in ~90–95% of **AS** patients
- *Associated with:*
  - **Reactive arthritis (~60–80%)**
  - **Psoriatic arthritis with axial involvement**
  - **Enteropathic arthritis**
- Not diagnostic but suggests a strong **genetic predisposition**
- Role in **antigen presentation and molecular mimicry**

Psoriatic Arthritis

Q17. Explain psoriatic arthritis (PsA), its clinical subtypes, and radiological features.

Clinical Subtypes (CASPER criteria)

1. **Asymmetric oligoarthritis**
2. **Symmetric polyarthritis** (RA-like)
3. **Distal interphalangeal (DIP)** involvement
4. **Arthritis mutilans**
5. **Axial/spinal** involvement

Clinical Clues
- Psoriatic skin or nail changes (pitting, onycholysis)
- Dactylitis ("sausage digits")
- Enthesitis

Radiological Findings
- **Pencil-in-cup** deformity
- **Asymmetric** sacroiliitis
- Bone proliferation and erosions without osteoporosis

Q18. Differentiate psoriatic arthritis versus rheumatoid arthritis.

(TNMGR Chennai 2022)

Feature	*Psoriatic arthritis*	*Rheumatoid arthritis*
Symmetry	Often asymmetric	Symmetric
DIP involvement	Common	Rare
RF	Usually negative	Positive (~70%)
Skin lesions	Psoriasis	Absent
Nail pitting	Common	Rare
Subcutaneous nodules	Absent	Present

Reactive Arthritis

Q19. Discuss reactive arthritis and its management.

Definition
Acute arthritis triggered by **GI or GU infections** (e.g., *Chlamydia, Shigella, Salmonella, Campylobacter*)

Classic Triad (Reiter's Syndrome)
- **Arthritis** (asymmetric, lower limbs)
- **Urethritis**
- **Conjunctivitis**

Other Features
Keratoderma blennorrhagicum (skin), circinate balanitis

Management
- *NSAIDs*: First-line
- **Antibiotics** (if ongoing infection)
- **DMARDs** for persistent arthritis
- Steroid pulse therapy/injections for monoarthritis

Enteropathic Arthritis

Q20. Explain enteropathic arthritis and its association with inflammatory bowel disease (IBD).

Associated with
- **Crohn's disease** and **ulcerative colitis**

Patterns

1. *Axial involvement*: Similar to AS (independent of bowel activity)
2. *Peripheral arthritis*:
   - *Type 1*: Acute, pauciarticular, flares with IBD activity
   - *Type 2*: Chronic, polyarticular, independent of bowel disease

Management

- Treat underlying IBD
- NSAIDs cautiously (may worsen IBD)
- Sulfasalazine, TNF-α inhibitors (e.g., infliximab) for severe cases

Gout

Q21. Pathophysiology and management of gout.

(RGUHS Karnataka 2023)

Pathophysiology

- Monosodium urate crystal deposition in joints
- Trigger inflammation via NLRP3 inflammasome → IL-1β

Clinical Features

- Acute monoarthritis (MTP joint - podagra)

Diagnosis

- *Polarized microscopy:* Negatively birefringent needle-shaped crystals
- Serum uric acid (may be normal during acute attack)

Management

- *Acute:* NSAIDs, colchicine, steroids
- *Chronic:* Allopurinol, febuxostat (urate-lowering agents)
- *Lifestyle:* Avoid alcohol, purine-rich food

Q22. Radiological features of chronic gout.

(AIIMS Delhi 2021)

- Punched-out erosions with overhanging edges (Martel's sign)
- Preserved joint space
- Tophi may be visible on X-ray

Q23. Discuss the pathogenesis and clinical features of gout.

Pathogenesis

- Caused by **monosodium urate (MSU) crystal deposition** in joints due to **hyperuricemia**
- *Triggered by:*
  - Overproduction (e.g., myeloproliferative disorders)
  - Underexcretion (renal impairment, diuretics)

Inflammation Mechanism

MSU crystals activate **NLRP3 inflammasome** → IL-1β release → neutrophilic inflammation

Clinical Features

- Acute monoarthritis—**podagra** (1st MTP joint) most common
- Rapid onset, intense pain, redness, swelling
- Often nocturnal
- Recurrent attacks if untreated
- *Chronic:* **Tophi**, joint deformities, uric acid nephropathy

Q24. Explain the diagnostic criteria for gout and pseudogout.

gout (MSU)

- *Synovial fluid:* Needle-shaped, **negatively birefringent** crystals (yellow parallel to compensator)
- Serum uric acid may be high but **not diagnostic alone**
- *Imaging:* "Punched-out erosions with overhanging edges"
- ACR/EULAR classification criteria (based on clinical, lab, imaging)

Pseudogout (CPPD)

- Caused by **calcium pyrophosphate dihydrate (CPPD) crystal** deposition
- Affects larger joints — **knee** is most common
- *Crystals:* **Rhomboid-shaped, positively birefringent** (blue parallel)
- *X-ray:* **Chondrocalcinosis** (cartilage calcification)

Q25. Discuss the role of synovial fluid analysis in crystal-induced arthritis.

Key Diagnostic Modality:

- **Differentiating gout from pseudogout and septic arthritis**
- *Confirmatory test for crystal type:*
  - *MSU*: Needle-shaped, negative birefringence
  - *CPPD*: Rhomboid, positive birefringence

Other Findings

- Elevated WBC count (usually 2,000–50,000/mm^3)
- *Exclude infection:* Gram stain and culture essential
- Helps guide acute management decisions

Q26. Describe tophaceous gout and its complications.

Tophaceous Gout

- *Chronic phase of gout with tophi formation*:
  - Firm nodular deposits of **MSU crystals**
  - *Sites*: Ears, olecranon bursa, fingers, Achilles tendon

Complications

- Joint deformity and **destruction**
- Skin ulceration and secondary infection
- *Renal complications:* Urate nephropathy, nephrolithiasis
- Functional disability

Management

- Urate-lowering therapy (allopurinol, febuxostat)
- Lifestyle modifications
- Surgical excision in severe/deforming cases

Pseudogout

Q27. Clinical features and treatment of pseudogout.

(PGI Chandigarh 2022)

Pathophysiology
Deposition of calcium pyrophosphate dihydrate (CPPD) crystals

Sites
Knee, wrist, shoulder

Diagnosis
Polarized microscopy: Positively birefringent rhomboid-shaped crystals

Treatment
- *Acute:* NSAIDs, colchicine
- *Recurrent:* Low-dose colchicine prophylaxis

Q28. Gout versus pseudogout comparison.

(MUHS Maharashtra 2023)

Feature	*Gout*	*Pseudogout*
Crystal type	Monosodium urate	Calcium pyrophosphate
Shape	Needle-shaped	Rhomboid-shaped
Birefringence	Negative	Positive
Common joint	1st MTP	Knee

Q28(A). Describe purine metabolism.

Purines (adenine, guanine) are nitrogenous bases involved in DNA/RNA synthesis. Their metabolism includes:

Synthesis
- *De novo pathway:* Starting from ribose-5-phosphate → IMP (inosine monophosphate) → AMP/GMP
- *Salvage pathway:* Hypoxanthine and guanine are recycled via **HGPRT** enzyme

Catabolism
- Purines are degraded to hypoxanthine → xanthine → **uric acid**
- *Enzyme:* **Xanthine oxidase** catalyzes both steps

Clinical Relevance
- **Humans lack uricase** (which converts uric acid to allantoin), so uric acid builds up
- Overproduction or under-excretion → **hyperuricemia** → **gout**

Q28(B). Write a short note on uricosuric agents.

These drugs increase uric acid excretion by **inhibiting renal tubular reabsorption.**

Drug	*Mechanism*	*Uses*	*Contraindications*
Probenecid	Inhibits URAT1 transporter in renal tubules	Chronic gout (under-excretors)	Renal stones, CrCl <50 mL/min
Sulfinpyrazone	Similar to probenecid	Less commonly used	GI irritation, blood dyscrasias
Lesinurad (newer)	Inhibits URAT1 and OAT4	Adjunct with xanthine oxidase inhibitors	Only approved in combination therapy

Note: Adequate hydration is essential to prevent uric acid nephrolithiasis.

Q28(C). Write a short note on drugs for gout and gouty arthritis.

A. For Acute Gout (Pain and Inflammation):

Drug	*Mechanism*	*Notes*
NSAIDs	Inhibit COX → ↓ prostaglandins	First-line (e.g., indomethacin, naproxen)
Colchicine	Inhibits microtubules → ↓ neutrophil chemotaxis	GI toxicity common (diarrhea)
Steroids	Anti-inflammatory	Used in renal failure or contraindicated NSAIDs

B. For Chronic Gout (Hyperuricemia Control):

1. **Uricostatic (Inhibit Uric Acid Production)**

Drug	*Mechanism*	*Use*
Allopurinol	Xanthine oxidase inhibitor (non-selective)	First-line in chronic gout
Febuxostat	Selective xanthine oxidase inhibitor	Safer in mild renal disease

Start after acute attack is resolved. Co-prescribe NSAID/colchicine to prevent flare.

2. **Uricolytic (Convert Uric Acid to Allantoin)**

Drug	*Mechanism*	*Use*
Rasburicase	Recombinant uricase	Tumor lysis syndrome, severe gout
Pegloticase	Pegylated uricase	Refractory chronic gout (IV only)

Treatment Approach Summary

Condition	*Treatment*
Acute gout	NSAIDs or colchicine or steroids
Chronic gout	Allopurinol or febuxostat + lifestyle modification
Under uric acid excreter patients	Add uricosuric (e.g., probenecid)
Over-producers or renal disease	Xanthine oxidase inhibitors (not uricosurics)
Severe/refractory gout	Pegloticase or rasburicase

Key Points for Viva

- **Don't start allopurinol during an acute attack**
- **HGPRT deficiency → Lesch–Nyhan syndrome (↑ uric acid)**
- **Monitor uric acid levels and renal function regularly**
- *Dietary advice:* Avoid red meat, alcohol, shellfish, fructose

Miscellaneous Inflammatory Arthritides

Q29. Discuss juvenile idiopathic arthritis (JIA) and its subtypes.

Definition

Chronic arthritis in children <16 years of age, lasting >6 weeks, of unknown cause.

Subtypes (ILAR Classification)

1. *Oligoarticular JIA*: ≤4 joints in first 6 months (most common)
   - Early onset, ANA positive, risk of **uveitis**
2. *Polyarticular JIA (RF-negative/positive)*: ≥5 joints
   - RF+ resembles adult RA; RF– has better prognosis
3. *Systemic JIA (Still's disease)*: Arthritis + fever, rash, hepatosplenomegaly
   - **IL-1 and IL-6 mediated**; high ferritin
4. *Enthesitis-related arthritis (ERA)*: Boys >8 years, HLA-B27+, SI joint involvement

5. *Psoriatic JIA*: Arthritis + psoriasis, dactylitis, nail pitting
6. *Undifferentiated*: Doesn't fit above criteria

Q30. Explain systemic lupus erythematosus (SLE) arthritis and its differentiation from RA.

SLE Arthritis Features
- Non-erosive, symmetrical polyarthritis (often hands, wrists)
- *Jaccoud's arthropathy:* Reducible deformities (due to ligament laxity)
- *Associated with other systemic features:* Malar rash, nephritis, serositis

Key Differences from RA

Feature	*SLE arthritis*	*Rheumatoid arthritis*
Joint damage	Non-erosive	Erosive, destructive
Deformities	Reducible (Jaccoud's)	Fixed (due to joint destruction)
Systemic features	Multisystem (skin, renal, CNS)	Primarily articular + nodules
Autoantibodies	ANA, anti-dsDNA, anti-Sm	RF, anti-CCP
Gender predilection	Female (9:1)	Female (3:1)

Q31. Discuss palindromic rheumatism and its clinical significance.

Definition
- Recurrent episodes of **acute, self-limited mono/polyarthritis** lasting hours to days
- Joints return to normal between attacks

Clinical Features
- Sudden joint pain, swelling, erythema
- No joint damage between episodes
- Often a **prodrome to RA** (30–50% evolve into RA)

Investigations
- RF or anti-CCP may be positive
- *Imaging:* Normal during asymptomatic phases

Management
- NSAIDs during attacks
- Hydroxychloroquine or methotrexate for frequent/recurrent episodes
- Monitor for transition to RA

Osteoarthritis

Q32. Pathogenesis and management of knee OA.

(JIPMER Puducherry 2023)

Definition

A degenerative joint disease characterized by progressive **loss of articular cartilage**, subchondral bone changes, and osteophyte formation.

Pathogenesis
1. **Mechanical stress + biochemical changes** → chondrocyte dysfunction
2. **Matrix degradation** (↓ aggrecan, collagen II)

3. **Synovial inflammation** (low-grade)
4. **Bone remodeling** → osteophytes, subchondral sclerosis
5. **Joint space narrowing + cartilage erosion**

Risk Factors
Age, obesity, joint trauma, malalignment, genetics

Management
- *Non-pharmacological:* Weight loss, physiotherapy
- *Pharmacological:* NSAIDs, intra-articular steroids, hyaluronic acid
- *Surgical:* HTO, TKR

Q33. Describe the radiological features of osteoarthritis.

X-ray (Weight-bearing AP/Lateral View)
- **Joint space narrowing** (asymmetric)
- **Osteophyte formation** (marginal)
- **Subchondral sclerosis**
- **Subchondral cysts**
- Malalignment (varus/valgus deformities in knee OA)

Mnemonic: "LOSS"
- *L*oss of joint space
- *O*steophytes
- *S*ubchondral sclerosis
- *S*ubchondral cysts

Q34. Describe various differentiating features of osteoarthritis versus inflammatory arthritis.

Feature	*Osteoarthritis*	*Inflammatory arthritis*
Joint space	Asymmetric narrowing	Symmetric narrowing
Osteophytes	Present	Rare
Erosions	Absent	Present (marginal)
Subchondral sclerosis	Common	Less prominent
Soft tissue swelling	Mild	Prominent
Joints involved	Weight-bearing (hip, knee)	Small joints, wrists (RA)

Q35. Describe various radiological grading of osteoarthritis—Kellgren and Lawrence (K&L) classification.

This is the **most widely used radiographic grading system** for osteoarthritis (OA), particularly for the **knee and hip joints.**

Kellgren and Lawrence Grading (1957)

Grade	*Radiological findings*	*Interpretation*
0	No radiographic features of OA	Normal
1	Doubtful joint space narrowing, possible osteophytic lipping	Suspected early OA
2	Definite osteophytes, possible joint space narrowing	Mild OA

Continued

Continued

Grade	*Radiological findings*	*Interpretation*
3	Moderate osteophytes, definite joint space narrowing, some sclerosis, possible deformity	Moderate OA
4	Large osteophytes, marked joint space narrowing, severe sclerosis, definite bony deformity	Severe OA

Common Sites Evaluated Radiologically

- *Knee:* Medial/lateral tibiofemoral, patellofemoral compartments
- *Hip:* Superolateral joint space, osteophytes, subchondral sclerosis
- *Spine:* Disc space narrowing, osteophytes, sclerosis of vertebral endplates

Key Radiological Features of OA

- Joint space narrowing (asymmetric)
- Subchondral sclerosis
- Osteophyte formation
- Subchondral cysts
- Joint deformity (late stage)

Q36. Discuss the role of viscosupplementation in osteoarthritis.

Viscosupplementation like intra-articular hyaluronic acid (HA)

Mechanism

- Supplements synovial fluid viscosity
- Reduces pain, improves lubrication and shock absorption

Indications

- **Mild-to-moderate OA**, especially **knee OA**
- Poor response to NSAIDs or contraindications to surgery

Efficacy

- Modest pain relief (~6 months)
- Controversial benefit, more effective in younger patients with early OA

Contraindications

Infection, allergy to HA or avian proteins

Q37. Total hip replacement in OA.

(TNMGR Chennai 2022)

Indications

Severe OA with pain, disability not relieved by conservative treatment

Outcomes

Pain relief, functional restoration, improved quality of life

Complications

DVT, dislocation, loosening, infection

Q38. Radiographic features of OA.

(RGUHS Karnataka 2022)

- Narrowed joint space (especially medial compartment)
- Osteophytes
- Subchondral cysts
- Sclerosis

6.13 Miscellaneous Joint Diseases

Q39. Pigmented villonodular synovitis (PVNS).

Definition

A benign proliferative disorder of the **synovium** leading to **joint swelling**, pain, and **hemosiderin deposition**.

Types

- **Localized** (e.g., tendon sheath nodules)
- **Diffuse** (intra-articular, usually knee or hip)

Diagnosis

- *MRI:* Hypo- to isointense on T1; **"blooming artifact"** on T2 (due to hemosiderin)
- Synovial biopsy confirms diagnosis.

Treatment

- **Arthroscopic or open synovectomy**
- Targeted therapies (e.g., CSF1 inhibitors) in recurrent cases

Q40. Synovial chondromatosis.

Definition

Metaplastic formation of **cartilaginous nodules** in synovium → can ossify.

Radiological Features

- Multiple **calcified intra-articular loose bodies**
- Joint space preservation in early stages
- *X-ray and CT:* "Rice grain" or "popcorn" calcifications

Treatment

Synovectomy + removal of loose bodies

Q41. Hemophilic arthropathy.

Cause

Repeated **hemarthroses** in hemophilia A/B → chronic synovitis and joint destruction

Clinical Features

- Painful, swollen joints (especially **knees, elbows, ankles**)
- Flexion contractures
- Muscle wasting

Management

- **Factor VIII/IX replacement**
- Physical therapy
- Synovectomy (chemical, radiosynovectomy, surgical)
- Joint replacement in severe cases

Q42. Differential diagnosis of monoarthritis versus polyarthritis.

Type	*Common causes*
Monoarthritis	Septic arthritis, gout, trauma, hemarthrosis
Polyarthritis	RA, SLE, PsA, viral arthritis, post-infectious arthritis

Key Investigations
Synovial fluid analysis, blood tests (ESR/CRP, RF, ANA), imaging

Q43. Post-traumatic arthritis.

Definition
Secondary OA due to **previous joint injury** (fracture, ligament tears)

Clinical Features
- Pain, stiffness, swelling
- Deformity or instability

Management
- NSAIDs, physical therapy
- Corrective osteotomy
- Arthroplasty in end-stage cases

Q44. Charcot's joint (neuropathic arthropathy).

Definition
Progressive joint destruction due to **loss of protective sensation**

Causes
Diabetes mellitus (most common), syringomyelia, leprosy, tabes dorsalis

Clinical Features
- Swollen, painless joint
- Deformity ("rocker-bottom" foot in diabetics)
- Instability

Radiology
Joint disorganization, fragmentation, debris, sclerosis

Management
- Off-loading, braces/casts
- Surgical fusion or arthroplasty in selected cases

CHAPTER 7

Regional Orthopedic Pathologies

7.1 Shoulder Disorders

Priti Ranjan Sinha, Khalid Muzzafar, Omeshwar Singh

Q1. Anatomy of the shoulder joint.

The shoulder complex comprises four joints:

1. *Glenohumeral (GH) joint:* A ball-and-socket synovial joint between the humeral head and glenoid fossa.
2. *Acromioclavicular (AC) joint:* Articulation between the acromion and clavicle.
3. *Sternoclavicular (SC) joint:* Junction of the sternum and clavicle.
4. *Scapulothoracic articulation:* Functional joint between the scapula and thoracic wall.

The GH joint is stabilized by the labrum, capsule, ligaments, and rotator cuff muscles.

Q2. Biomechanics of the glenohumeral joint.

The GH joint offers six degrees of freedom, enabling extensive mobility. Stability is maintained through.

- *Static stabilizers:* Labrum, capsule, ligaments, and negative intra-articular pressure.
- *Dynamic stabilizers:* Rotator cuff muscles and scapular stabilizers.

Proper function requires coordinated muscle activity to prevent impingement and maintain joint congruency.

Q3. Static and dynamic stabilizers of the shoulder.

- *Static stabilizers:* Glenoid labrum, joint capsule, glenohumeral ligaments, and negative intra-articular pressure.
- *Dynamic stabilizers:* Rotator cuff muscles (SITS), deltoid, biceps brachii, and scapular muscles.

These structures work synergistically to maintain shoulder stability during movement.

Q4. Blood supply and innervation of the shoulder joint.

- *Blood supply:* Anterior and posterior circumflex humeral arteries (branches of the axillary artery), suprascapular artery, and circumflex scapular artery.
- *Innervation:* Axillary, suprascapular, and lateral pectoral nerves.

Q5. Anatomy and function of the rotator cuff.

The rotator cuff comprises four muscles:

1. *Supraspinatus:* Initiates abduction of the arm.
2. *Infraspinatus:* Responsible for external rotation.
3. *Teres minor:* Assists in external rotation.
4. *Subscapularis:* Facilitates internal rotation.

These muscles stabilize the glenohumeral joint by keeping the humeral head centered in the glenoid fossa during arm movements.

Q6. Scapulohumeral rhythm and clinical relevance.

Scapulohumeral rhythm refers to the coordinated movement between the scapula and humerus during arm elevation. Typically, for every 2° of GH movement, there is 1° of scapulothoracic movement. Disruption can lead to shoulder dysfunction and impingement.

Q7. Biomechanics of throwing injuries in the shoulder.

Overhead throwing involves phases: wind-up, cocking, acceleration, deceleration, and follow-through. The shoulder endures high stresses, particularly during the cocking and deceleration phases, leading to injuries like SLAP lesions, rotator cuff tears, and impingement.

Q8. Coracoacromial arch and its significance.

The coracoacromial arch, formed by the coracoid process, acromion, and coracoacromial ligament, provides a protective vault over the humeral head. It prevents superior dislocation but can contribute to impingement syndromes if the space beneath is reduced.

Q9. Importance of the glenoid labrum in shoulder stability.

The glenoid labrum deepens the glenoid cavity, enhancing joint congruency and stability. It serves as an attachment for ligaments and the biceps tendon. Injuries to the labrum, such as SLAP or Bankart lesions, can compromise shoulder stability.

Q10. Kinematics of shoulder abduction and external rotation.

During abduction:

- The supraspinatus initiates movement.
- The deltoid continues abduction.
- Scapular upward rotation complements GH movement.

External rotation involves the infraspinatus and teres minor muscles. Proper kinematics are essential to prevent impingement and ensure efficient movement.

Q11. Rotator cuff tear—causes, diagnosis, and management.

(Asked in: AIIMS Delhi 2022, PGI Chandigarh 2021)

Definition

- Tear of the **rotator cuff muscles**—mainly **supraspinatus**, but may also involve infraspinatus, subscapularis, and teres minor.
- Leads to **pain and dysfunction** of the shoulder.

Causes

1. *Traumatic*:
   - Fall on an outstretched arm.
   - Shoulder dislocation in elderly.
2. *Degenerative*:
   - Age-related tendon wear and tear.
   - Chronic impingement under the acromion.
   - Hypovascularity ("critical zone" near supraspinatus insertion).
3. *Secondary factors*: Smoking, diabetes, hypercholesterolemia.

Clinical Features

Symptoms:
- Shoulder pain (worse at night, with overhead activities).
- Weakness (especially in abduction and external rotation).
- Limited range of motion.

Tests:
- *Empty can test:* Supraspinatus function.
- *Drop arm test:* Large tears.
- *External rotation lag sign:* Infraspinatus tear.
- *Lift-off test:* Subscapularis tear.

Diagnosis

X-ray: May show high-riding humeral head (cuff tear arthropathy).

Ultrasound: Quick, operator-dependent.

MRI shoulder:
- Investigation of choice.
- Shows tear size, retraction, fatty infiltration of muscles.

Management

Non-surgical:
- Indicated for partial tears, elderly, or low-demand patients.
- NSAIDs, physiotherapy (ROM and strengthening exercises).
- Subacromial steroid injections (carefully used).

Surgical:
- Full-thickness tears, active individuals, or failed conservative management.
- Arthroscopic or open rotator cuff repair (suture anchors).
- Debridement ± subacromial decompression if irreparable.

Post-operative rehabilitation:
- Sling immobilization initially.
- Gradual physiotherapy (passive → active exercises).

Q12. Classification of rotator cuff tears and surgical options.

(Asked in: MUHS Maharashtra 2022, JIPMER Puducherry 2022)

Classification

Based on Size (DeOrio and Cofield Classification):

Size	Description
Small	<1 cm
Medium	1–3 cm
Large	3–5 cm
Massive	>5 cm or involving ≥2 tendons

Based on Location

- Supraspinatus only
- Supra + Infraspinatus
- Pan-cuff tear (supra + infra + subscapularis)

Based on Chronicity

Acute traumatic versus Chronic degenerative.

Surgical Options

Arthroscopic repair:

- Preferred method now.
- Suture anchors and double-row repairs.
- Less morbidity, faster recovery.

Mini-open or open repair: For large/massive tears with poor tissue quality.

Partial repairs: If complete repair not possible (massive, retracted tears).

Tendon transfers: Latissimus dorsi or lower trapezius transfer for irreparable posterosuperior cuff tears.

Reverse shoulder arthroplasty: End-stage rotator cuff arthropathy with pseudoparalysis.

Q13. Pathophysiology of subacromial impingement syndrome.

Subacromial impingement syndrome (SAIS) occurs when the rotator cuff tendons and subacromial bursa are compressed between the humeral head and the acromion during arm elevation. This leads to inflammation, pain, and reduced shoulder function. Contributing factors include anatomical variations (e.g., hooked acromion), overuse, and muscle imbalances.

Q14. Neer classification of impingement syndrome.

Neer's classification outlines the progression of rotator cuff impingement:

- *Stage I:* Edema and hemorrhage (typically in patients <25 years); reversible with conservative treatment.
- *Stage II:* Fibrosis and tendinitis (ages 25–40); may require surgical intervention.
- *Stage III:* Bone spurs and tendon rupture (usually >40 years); often necessitates surgical repair.

Q15. Hawkins–Kennedy and Neer impingement tests.

- *Hawkins-Kennedy test:*
  - The examiner flexes the patient's shoulder and elbow to 90°, then internally rotates the arm.
  - Pain indicates subacromial impingement.
- *Neer test:*
  - With the scapula stabilized, the examiner passively flexes the patient's arm overhead.
  - Pain suggests impingement of the rotator cuff tendons under the acromion.

Q16. Internal impingement syndrome in overhead athletes.

Definition

Internal impingement occurs when the undersurface of the rotator cuff impinges against the posterosuperior glenoid rim during abduction and external rotation, common in overhead athletes.

Etiology

- Repetitive overhead activities leading to microtrauma.
- Glenohumeral internal rotation deficit (GIRD).

Symptoms
- Posterior shoulder pain during throwing motions.
- Decreased performance.

Management
- *Conservative:* Physical therapy focusing on posterior capsule stretching and rotator cuff strengthening.
- *Surgical:* Indicated if conservative measures fail; involves debridement or repair of torn structures.

Q17. Internal impingement of the shoulder.

(Himachal Pradesh University Shimla 2015)

Internal impingement occurs when the **posterior-superior aspect of the rotator cuff (supraspinatus and infraspinatus)** gets pinched between the **greater tuberosity of the humerus and the posterosuperior glenoid rim** during **abduction and external rotation**—particularly in **overhead athletes** (e.g., baseball pitchers, swimmers).

Mechanism
- Repetitive overhead motion → **posterior capsular tightness** and **glenohumeral internal rotation deficit (GIRD)** → posterosuperior contact between rotator cuff and glenoid rim/labrum.
- Associated with **posterior labral tears, partial articular-side rotator cuff tears (PASTA lesions)**.

Clinical Features
- Posterior shoulder pain during throwing
- *Positive posterior impingement test:* Pain in abduction + external rotation
- Often coexists with internal rotation loss (GIRD)

Diagnosis
- MRI shows articular-sided partial cuff tears or posterior labral damage
- Arthroscopy is gold standard

Management
- *Non-operative:* Rest, scapular stabilization, posterior capsule stretching
- *Surgical (if refractory)*: Arthroscopic debridement or cuff/labrum repair

Q18. Indications and techniques of rotator cuff repair surgery.

Indications
- Persistent pain and dysfunction despite conservative treatment.
- Acute full-thickness tears, especially in active individuals.
- Progressive weakness or loss of shoulder function.

Techniques
- *Arthroscopic repair:* Minimally invasive; uses small incisions and a camera to guide repair.
- *Mini-open repair:* Combines arthroscopy with a small open incision for tendon repair.
- *Open repair:* Traditional method involving a larger incision; used for complex or massive tears.

Q19. Role of physiotherapy in rotator cuff injuries.

Physiotherapy is crucial in both non-operative and post-operative management:
- *Pain management:* Modalities such as ice, heat, and electrical stimulation.
- *Restoration of range of motion (ROM):* Stretching and mobilization exercises.
- *Strengthening:* Targeted exercises to improve rotator cuff and scapular muscle strength.
- *Functional training:* Activities to restore daily function and prevent recurrence.

Q20. Massive irreparable rotator cuff tears.

Definition

Tears involving two or more tendons, often >5 cm in size, with significant tendon retraction and muscle atrophy.

Management

- *Conservative:* Physical therapy focusing on deltoid and periscapular muscle strengthening; pain management with NSAIDs or injections.
- *Surgical options:*
  - Partial repair
  - Tendon transfers (e.g., latissimus dorsi transfer)
  - Superior capsular reconstruction
  - Reverse shoulder arthroplasty in cases with pseudoparalysis or cuff tear arthropathy.

Exam Tip

When writing about rotator cuff tears:

- **First mention supraspinatus involvement and night pain**—key clinical clues.
- **MRI is the gold standard** for diagnosis.
- In classification, **always mention size-based grading**—it's commonly asked!
- In surgical options, **clearly distinguish repair versus replacement (reverse prosthesis for cuff tear arthropathy)**.

Shoulder Instability

Q21. Types of shoulder instability.

(Asked in: AIIMS Delhi 2021, RGUHS Karnataka 2022)

Definition

Shoulder instability is defined as inability to maintain the humeral head centered in the glenoid fossa during shoulder motion.

Types of Instability

Based on direction:

Type	*Description*
Anterior instability (most common)	Due to forced abduction, external rotation
Posterior instability	After seizures, electric shocks, trauma
Inferior instability	Rare; sulcus sign positive (e.g., multidirectional instability)

Multidirectional instability

Based on cause:

- Traumatic (TUBS—Traumatic, Unidirectional, Bankart lesion, Surgery needed).
- Atraumatic (AMBRI—Atraumatic, Multidirectional, Bilateral, Rehabilitation, Inferior capsular shift if needed).

Q22. Multidirectional instability (MDI).

Definition

Instability of the shoulder in **more than one direction** (anterior, posterior, and inferior), often due to **capsular laxity**.

Features

- Young, athletic, or hypermobile individuals
- May have sulcus sign, positive apprehension test
- Often bilateral and atraumatic

Management
- *Physiotherapy first-line:* Strengthen dynamic stabilizers (rotator cuff, scapular stabilizers)
- *Surgical (if failed rehabilitation)*:
    - Arthroscopic capsular plication
    - Open inferior capsular shift

Q23. Management of recurrent anterior dislocation.

Non-surgical
First-time dislocation without bone loss → Immobilization in external rotation sling (some evidence).

Surgical (For Recurrent Dislocators)
Procedures:
- *Arthroscopic bankart repair:*
    - For soft tissue Bankart lesions.
    - Suture anchors used to reattach labrum.
- *Latarjet procedure:*
    - For bone loss >20–25% of glenoid.
    - Coracoid transfer to anterior glenoid.
- *Remplissage:* Filling of engaging Hill-Sachs lesions with infraspinatus tendon (to prevent engagement).

Post-operative care:
- Sling *immobilization* 3–4 weeks.
- Gradual rehabilitation with strengthening of dynamic stabilizers (rotator cuff and scapular muscles).

Q24. Bankart and Hill–Sachs lesions—describe and treatment options.

(Asked in: PGI Chandigarh 2022, MUHS Maharashtra 2023)

Bankart Lesion
Definition
Avulsion of the **anteroinferior labrum** from the glenoid rim.
- Leads to loss of stability ("essential lesion" of recurrent anterior dislocation).

Types
- *Soft tissue bankart:* Labral tear only.
- *Bony bankart:* Glenoid rim fracture with labral tear.

Treatment
- Arthroscopic Bankart repair (suture anchors).
- Bony Bankart → May need bone grafting if large fragment.

Q25. Hill–Sachs lesion.

Definition
Compression fracture of the posterolateral humeral head due to impaction against the anterior glenoid rim during dislocation.

Clinical Importance
Larger Hill-Sachs lesions engage with glenoid → recurrent instability.

Treatment Options
- *Small, non-engaging:* No surgery needed.
- *Moderate-sized engaging lesions:*
    - **Remplissage** procedure (posterior capsulotenodesis).

- *Very large lesions:*
    - Humeral head bone grafting.
    - Shoulder replacement (in elderly, non-reconstructable cases).

Exam Tip
When writing about shoulder instability:

- **Always mention TUBS versus AMBRI**, and **anterior instability is the most common.**
- *For Bankart and Hill-Sachs:*
    - **Bankart lesion is labrum injury, Hill-Sachs lesion is humeral head defect.**
    - **Bankart → Repair labrum, Hill-Sachs → Remplissage if engaging.**
- **Latarjet procedure** is a buzzword in cases with significant glenoid bone loss.

Q26. Classification and management of shoulder instability.

Classification

- *By direction:*
    - *Anterior:* Most common; often due to trauma.
    - *Posterior:* Less common; may result from seizures or electric shocks.
    - *Multidirectional:* Involves instability in multiple directions; often atraumatic.
- *By frequency:*
    - *Acute:* First-time dislocation.
    - *Recurrent:* Multiple episodes of dislocation or subluxation.
- *By etiology:*
    - *Traumatic:* Resulting from injury.
    - *Atraumatic:* Due to generalized ligamentous laxity or repetitive microtrauma.

Management

- *Conservative:*
    - Physical therapy focusing on strengthening dynamic stabilizers.
    - Activity modification.
- *Surgical:*
    - Indicated for recurrent dislocations or failed conservative treatment.
    - Procedures include Bankart repair, capsular shift, or Latarjet procedure.

Q27. Discuss the morbid anatomy and management of recurrent shoulder dislocation.

Morbid Anatomy
Recurrent shoulder dislocation most commonly involves **anterior instability**, typically following trauma. Key anatomical lesions:

- *Bankart lesion:* Detachment of the anteroinferior labrum from the glenoid rim.
- *Hill-Sachs lesion:* Compression fracture/posterolateral defect of the humeral head due to impaction against the anterior glenoid.
- *Capsular laxity:* Stretching or tearing of the anterior capsule.
- *Glenoid bone loss:* Erosion of the anteroinferior glenoid rim, contributing to instability.
- *Hagl lesion:* Humeral avulsion of glenohumeral ligament.
- *ALPSA lesion:* Medially displaced, healed Bankart lesion with intact periosteum.

Management
Depends on **age, activity level, type of instability, and associated lesions.**

1. *Non-operative (initial episodes or low-demand patients):*
    - Immobilization followed by physiotherapy focusing on scapular and rotator cuff strengthening.
    - Not preferred in young, active patients due to high recurrence.

2. *Surgical options (recurrent cases or failed conservative management):*
   - **Arthroscopic Bankart Repair** (for soft tissue Bankart lesions with <20% bone loss).
   - *Latarjet procedure (for >20–25% glenoid bone loss)*: Transfer of coracoid with conjoined tendon.
   - *Remplissage:* For engaging Hill-Sachs lesion—fills defect using infraspinatus tendon.
   - *Capsular shift /plication:* For capsular redundancy/laxity.
   - *Bone grafting or Eden-Hybinette:* For large bony defects.

Q28. Describe the pathogenesis of recurrent anterior shoulder dislocation and discuss arthroscopic bankart repair.

[Dr Ram Manohar Lohia Institute of Medical Sciences (RMLIMS) Lucknow 2014]

Pathogenesis of Recurrent Anterior Shoulder Dislocation

- *Mechanism:* Forced abduction, external rotation, and extension → anterior translation of humeral head.
- *First-time dislocation damages stabilizing structures:*
  - *Static stabilizers:* Labrum, glenoid bone, capsule, glenohumeral ligaments.
  - *Dynamic stabilizers:* Rotator cuff, scapular stabilizers.
- Inadequate healing leads to **persistent capsulolabral detachment** (Bankart lesion), resulting in recurrent dislocations.
- *Risk factors:* Young age (<25), male gender, contact sports, hyperlaxity.

Arthroscopic Bankart Repair

Indication: Anterior instability with soft tissue Bankart lesion and glenoid bone loss <15-20%.

Surgical Steps

1. *Positioning*: Beach-chair or lateral decubitus.
2. *Portal placement*: Standard posterior viewing portal + anterior working portals.
3. *Evaluation*: Glenoid bone loss, Hill-Sachs lesion, labral condition.
4. *Preparation*: Debridement of glenoid neck to promote healing.
5. *Anchor placement*: 3–4 suture anchors (bioabsorbable or metal) placed from 3 to 6 o'clock (right shoulder).
6. *Capsulolabral repair*: Sutures tied to reattach labrum and tighten capsule.

Advantages

- Minimally invasive
- Faster recovery
- Lower morbidity

Limitations

- Higher failure in contact athletes or significant bone loss.
- Requires surgical expertise.

Q29. Classify dislocations of glenohumeral joint. Discuss about neglected posterior dislocation of shoulder in a young adult male.

Classification of Glenohumeral Dislocations

1. *By direction*:
   - Anterior (95%)
   - Posterior (2–4%)
   - Inferior (luxatio erecta)
   - Superior (very rare)
2. *By duration*:
   - *Acute:* <3 weeks
   - *Chronic/Neglected:* >3 weeks
3. *By associated lesions*: Bony Bankart, Hill-Sachs, reverse Hill-Sachs, fracture-dislocations

Neglected Posterior Dislocation in Young Adult

Pathophysiology:

- *Often missed on AP X-ray; seen in:*
  - Seizures (epilepsy), electrocution, trauma.
- Leads to **locked posterior dislocation**, reverse Hill-Sachs lesion (anteromedial humeral head defect).

Clinical features:

- Limited external rotation
- Flattened anterior shoulder
- Positive jerk test/posterior drawer test

Imaging:

- **Axillary view**, **CT** to assess bone loss
- **MRI** for soft tissue

Management

Depends on:

- Duration
- Size of reverse Hill-Sachs lesion
- Range of motion

1. *<3 weeks*: Closed reduction may be attempted.
2. *>3 weeks/locked dislocation*:
   - *McLaughlin procedure:* **Subscapularis tendon transfer into reverse Hill-Sachs.**
   - *Modified McLaughlin:* **Lesser tuberosity osteotomy and transfer.**
   - **Allograft reconstruction** or **Hemiarthroplasty** if large defect (>40%).
3. *Arthroplasty*: In elderly or with massive bone loss.

Early diagnosis is key. Delayed treatment leads to stiffness, arthritis.

Q30. Reverse shoulder arthroplasty (RSA).

Definition

Prosthesis design where the ball is placed on the glenoid and the socket on the humerus—"reverse" of anatomy.

Indications

- Cuff tear arthropathy
- Failed conventional arthroplasty
- Complex proximal humerus fractures in elderly
- Tumor reconstructions

Biomechanics

Shifts center of rotation medially and inferiorly → increases deltoid efficiency.

Components

- Glenosphere (glenoid ball)
- Humeral socket

Advantages

- Deltoid acts as main elevator in absence of rotator cuff
- Good pain relief and functional outcome

Complications

- Scapular notching
- Instability
- Infection
- Axillary nerve injury

Q31. Tubs versus AMBRI classification of shoulder instability.

[King George's Medical University (KGMU) Lucknow Uttar Pradesh 2011]

TUBS

- *T*raumatic onset.
- *U*nidirectional instability.
- *B*ankart lesion often present.
- *S*urgery often required.

This classification describes patients with a history of trauma leading to unidirectional instability, typically anterior, often associated with a Bankart lesion. Surgical intervention is commonly needed.

AMBRI

- *A*traumatic onset.
- *M*ultidirectional instability.
- *B*ilateral involvement.
- *R*ehabilitation is the first line of treatment.
- *I*nferior capsular shift surgery if conservative measures fail.

This classification pertains to patients with generalized ligamentous laxity leading to multidirectional instability. Initial management is conservative, focusing on rehabilitation.

Q32. Superior labrum anterior to posterior (SLAP) tears.

Definition

SLAP tears involve injury to the superior part of the glenoid labrum, extending from anterior to posterior, where the biceps tendon anchors.

Etiology

- Repetitive overhead activities (e.g., throwing athletes).
- Trauma (e.g., fall on an outstretched arm).

Symptoms

- Deep shoulder pain.
- Clicking or catching sensations.
- Decreased performance in overhead activities.

Diagnosis

- Clinical tests (e.g., O'Brien's test).
- MRI arthrography for detailed imaging.

Management

- *Conservative:* Physical therapy, NSAIDS.
- *Surgical:* Arthroscopic repair for persistent symptoms.

Q33. Snyder classification of SLAP tears.

The Snyder classification categorizes SLAP lesions into four types:

- *Type I:* Fraying of the superior labrum with intact biceps anchor.
- *Type II:* Detachment of the superior labrum and biceps anchor from the glenoid.
- *Type III:* Bucket-handle tear of the superior labrum with intact biceps anchor.
- *Type IV:* Bucket-handle tear extending into the biceps tendon.

This classification aids in determining the appropriate surgical intervention.

Q34. Clinical tests for diagnosing SLAP lesions.

Common Tests

- *O'Brien's test (active compression test):* Pain or clicking during internal rotation that decreases with external rotation suggests a SLAP lesion.
- *Crank test:* Pain or clicking with axial loading and rotation of the shoulder indicates labral pathology.
- *Biceps load test II:* Pain during resisted elbow flexion in a supinated position suggests a SLAP tear.

These tests help in clinical diagnosis, often supplemented by imaging studies.

Q35. Role of arthroscopy in labral injuries.

Arthroscopy is a minimally invasive surgical technique that allows for:

- *Diagnosis:* Direct visualization of labral tears and assessment of joint stability.
- *Treatment:* Repair of labral tears using suture anchors, debridement of frayed tissue, and addressing associated pathologies.

Advantages

- Smaller incisions leading to reduced postoperative pain.
- Faster recovery times.
- Improved visualization of intra-articular structures.

Arthroscopy has become the standard approach for managing labral injuries due to its efficacy and minimally invasive nature.

Biceps Tendon Pathologies

Q36. Anatomy and biomechanics of the long head of the biceps tendon (LHBT).

(Assam Medical College Dibrugarh 2015)

Anatomy

- *Origin:* Supraglenoid tubercle of the scapula and the superior glenoid labrum.

Course

Traverses the shoulder joint intra-articularly, exits through the bicipital groove of the humerus, and merges with the short head to form the biceps brachii muscle.

Biomechanics

- Acts as a humeral head depressor, aiding in shoulder stability during abduction.
- Contributes to elbow flexion and forearm supination, with the long head being more efficient in supination.
- Functions as an anterior stabilizer of the shoulder, especially during overhead activities.

Q37. Biceps tendinitis and its management.

Definition

Inflammation of the LHBT, often due to overuse or repetitive overhead activities.

Clinical Features

- Anterior shoulder pain exacerbated by lifting or overhead motions.
- Tenderness over the bicipital groove.
- Possible clicking or snapping sensation.

Management

- *Conservative:*
  - Rest and activity modification.
  - Ice application to reduce inflammation.
  - Nonsteroidal anti-inflammatory drugs (NSAIDs).
  - Physical therapy focusing on stretching and strengthening exercises.
  - Corticosteroid injections in refractory cases.
- *Surgical:* Considered if conservative measures fail; options include biceps tenotomy or tenodesis.

Q38. Clinical features and treatment of biceps tendon rupture.

Types

- *Proximal rupture:* Typically involves the LHBT.
- *Distal rupture:* Involves the tendon insertion at the radial tuberosity.

Clinical Features

- Sudden, sharp pain in the upper arm.
- Audible "pop" at the time of injury.
- Visible bulge in the upper arm ("Popeye sign").
- Weakness in elbow flexion and forearm supination.

Management

- *Conservative:*
  - Rest and immobilization with a sling.
  - Ice application and NSAIDs for pain control.
  - Physical therapy to restore function.
- *Surgical:* Indicated for active individuals or those requiring full strength; involves tendon repair or reconstruction.

Q39. Indications and techniques of biceps tenotomy versus tenodesis.

[Institute of Medical Sciences Banaras Hindu University (BHU) Varanasi 2011]

Biceps Tenotomy

- *Procedure:* Simple release of the LHBT from its origin.
- *Indications:*
  - Older, low-demand patients.
  - Persistent pain despite conservative treatment.
- *Advantages:*
  - Shorter surgical time.
  - Faster recovery
- *Disadvantages:*
  - Potential for "Popeye" deformity.
  - Possible cramping or fatigue in the biceps muscle.

Biceps Tenodesis

- *Procedure:* Reattachment of the LHBT to the humerus, maintaining its length-tension relationship.
- *Indications:*
  - Younger, active patients.
  - Cosmetic concerns regarding muscle contour.
- *Advantage:* Preservation of biceps function and appearance.
- *Disadvantages:*
  - Longer recovery period.
  - Potential for surgical complications.

Frozen Shoulder (Adhesive Capsulitis)

Q40. Frozen shoulder—stages, clinical features, and management.

(PGI Chandigarh 2022, MUHS Maharashtra 2022)

Definition

Frozen shoulder (adhesive capsulitis) is a condition of the shoulder characterized by **progressive painful restriction of both active and passive movements** due to **chronic inflammation and fibrosis** of the joint capsule.

Etiology
- Idiopathic (primary frozen shoulder)—commonest.
- *Secondary:*
  - Diabetes mellitus (strongest risk factor).
  - Thyroid disorders.
  - Post-trauma or post-surgery.

Clinical Features

Symptoms:
- Gradual onset of pain (especially night pain).
- Progressive stiffness.
- Difficulty in overhead activities.

Examination findings:
- Restriction of both **active and passive** movements.
- **External rotation** is the earliest and most severely restricted movement.

Stages (Reeves Staging)

Stage	Description	Duration
Stage I: Freezing (painful phase)	Pain dominates; progressive loss of movement	10–36 weeks
Stage II: Frozen (stiff phase)	Pain decreases; stiffness persists	4–12 months
Stage III: Thawing (recovery phase)	Gradual return of motion	12–42 months

Diagnosis
- Clinical diagnosis.
- X-ray to rule out other causes (e.g., arthritis, calcific tendinitis).
- MRI if secondary pathology suspected.

Management

Conservative (Mainstay):
- **NSAIDs** for pain control.
- *Physiotherapy:*
  - Pendulum exercises
  - Passive stretching
  - Active-assisted ROM exercises
- **Intra-articular steroid injections** during freezing phase.

Surgical (For resistant cases)
- **Manipulation under anesthesia (MUA)**.
- **Arthroscopic capsular release** (gold standard if severe).

Key Goal

Pain control + gradual recovery of movement.

Q41. Pathophysiology and treatment options for adhesive capsulitis.

(JIPMER Puducherry 2023)

Pathophysiology

Underlying process: Inflammatory process → capsular fibrosis and thickening → adhesion formation → joint volume reduction.

Histological features:
- Chronic synovitis
- Fibrosis of the rotator interval, coracohumeral ligament, and capsule.

Vascular changes: Neovascularization with fibroblastic proliferation.

Treatment Options

Stage-wise management:

Stage	Treatment Focus
Freezing	Pain control (NSAIDs, steroid injections), gentle ROM
Frozen	Aggressive physiotherapy to improve ROM
Thawing	Continuation of strengthening and stretching exercises

Advanced Options
- Manipulation under anesthesia (MUA) if failure after 3–6 months of therapy.
- Arthroscopic capsular release if MUA contraindicated (e.g., osteoporosis, fragile bones).
- Hydrodilatation (saline steroid injection to distend joint capsule).

Q42. Adhesive capsulitis and its stages.

Stages
1. *Freezing stage (painful phase)*: Gradual onset of shoulder pain with increasing stiffness. Movement becomes limited, especially at night. This stage typically lasts from 6 weeks to 9 months.
2. *Frozen stage (stiffness phase)*: Pain may diminish, but the shoulder remains stiff, making daily activities challenging. This stage can last from 4 to 6 months.
3. *Thawing stage (recovery phase)*: Gradual improvement in shoulder mobility and a decrease in pain. Full or near-full recovery occurs over 6 months to 2 years.

Q43. Write a short note on the role of intra-articular corticosteroid injections in frozen shoulder.

(PGI Chandigarh 2014)

Intra-articular corticosteroid injections are effective in the early stages of adhesive capsulitis:
- *Mechanism:* Reduce synovial inflammation, thereby decreasing pain and improving range of motion.
- *Efficacy:* Significant pain relief and functional improvement observed within 4 to 6 weeks post-injection.
- *Considerations:* Best utilized during the freezing stage for optimal outcomes.

Q44. Explain the role of hydrodilatation in the management of frozen shoulder.

Hydrodilatation, also known as distension arthrography, involves the injection of saline, corticosteroids, and local anesthetics into the glenohumeral joint to stretch the capsule:
- *Purpose:* Break adhesions and improve joint mobility.
- *Procedure:* Performed under imaging guidance to ensure accurate delivery.
- *Outcomes:* Early improvements in disability and range of motion have been reported, with comparable effectiveness to corticosteroid injections in long-term outcomes.

Q45. Discuss the surgical management options for refractory adhesive capsulitis.

Surgical intervention is considered when conservative treatments fail after 4 to 6 months:

- *Manipulation under anesthesia (MUA):* The shoulder is forcibly moved to break adhesions while the patient is under anesthesia.
- *Arthroscopic capsular release:* Minimally invasive surgery to release the contracted capsule and restore mobility.
- *Combined approach:* Some cases may benefit from both MUA and arthroscopic release for optimal results.

These surgical options have shown to decrease the duration of the disease and improve range of motion effectively.

Exam Tip

When writing about frozen shoulder:

- **Start with definition focusing on both active and passive movement restriction.**
- **Stages with names (freezing, frozen, thawing)** must be mentioned.
- **State early restriction of external rotation** clearly.
- For pathophysiology, **mention fibrosis + synovitis + capsular thickening.**

Arthritis and Degenerative Conditions of the Shoulder

Q46. Classify glenohumeral osteoarthritis and discuss its management.

Classification

- *Primary osteoarthritis:* Degenerative changes without a known cause.
- *Secondary osteoarthritis:* Resulting from trauma, inflammatory diseases, or rotator cuff pathology.

Walch Classification of Glenoid Morphology

- *Type A:* Centered humeral head.
  - *A1:* Minor central erosion.
  - *A2:* Major central erosion.
- *Type B:* Posterior subluxation of the humeral head.
  - *B1:* Posterior wear without significant bone loss.
  - *B2:* Posterior wear with significant bone loss.
- *Type C:* Severe retroversion (>25°) of the glenoid, often congenital.

Management

- *Non-surgical:*
  - Physical therapy to maintain range of motion.
  - NSAIDs for pain control.
  - Intra-articular corticosteroid injections.
- *Surgical:*
  - Total shoulder arthroplasty (TSA) for advanced cases with intact rotator cuff.
  - Hemiarthroplasty if the glenoid is unaffected.
  - Reverse total shoulder arthroplasty (RTSA) for cases with rotator cuff deficiency.

Q47. Write a short note on rheumatoid arthritis of the shoulder joint.

[Jawaharlal Institute of Postgraduate Medical Education and Research (JIPMER) Puducherry 2011]

Rheumatoid arthritis (RA) is a systemic autoimmune disease that commonly affects the shoulder joint, leading to synovial inflammation, cartilage destruction, and joint deformity.

Clinical Features

- Bilateral shoulder pain and stiffness.
- Reduced range of motion.
- Crepitus during movement.

Management

- *Medical:*
  - Disease-modifying antirheumatic drugs (DMARDs) to control systemic inflammation.
  - NSAIDs and corticosteroids for symptom relief.
- *Physical therapy:* Exercises to maintain joint mobility and strength.
- *Surgical:* Arthroplasty (TSA or RTSA) in cases of severe joint destruction.

Q48. Discuss the indications for total shoulder arthroplasty.

Indications

- Severe primary or secondary osteoarthritis with significant pain and functional limitation.
- Inflammatory arthritis (e.g., RA) with joint destruction.
- Post-traumatic arthritis with joint incongruity.
- Osteonecrosis of the humeral head.
- Intact rotator cuff muscles to ensure prosthesis stability.

Q49. Compare total shoulder arthroplasty versus hemiarthroplasty.

Feature	*Total shoulder arthroplasty (TSA)*	*Hemiarthroplasty (HA)*
Components replaced	Humeral head and glenoid	Humeral head only
Indications	Glenohumeral OA with glenoid involvement	OA with intact glenoid
Rotator Cuff Status	Intact	Intact
Outcomes	Better pain relief and function	Variable outcomes
Complications	Glenoid loosening	Progressive glenoid erosion

Q50. Explain the role of reverse total shoulder arthroplasty in cuff tear arthropathy.

(Narayana Medical College Nellore Andhra Pradesh 2017)

Reverse total shoulder arthroplasty (RTSA) is designed for patients with rotator cuff tear arthropathy, where conventional TSA is contraindicated due to rotator cuff deficiency.

Mechanism

- Reverses the normal ball-and-socket configuration, placing the ball on the glenoid and the socket on the humerus.
- Allows the deltoid muscle to compensate for the deficient rotator cuff, enabling shoulder elevation and abduction.

Indications

- Massive, irreparable rotator cuff tears with arthritis.
- Failed previous shoulder arthroplasty.
- Complex fractures in elderly patients.

Q51. Shoulder resurfacing arthroplasty—short note.

Conservative alternative to traditional arthroplasty where only **damaged humeral head surface is replaced**.

Indications

- Young patients with focal OA or AVN
- Intact rotator cuff

Advantages

- Bone-preserving
- Easier revision if needed

Limitations
Not ideal for severe deformity or glenoid damage

Q52. Write a short note on the management of post-traumatic arthritis of the shoulder.

Post-traumatic arthritis results from joint injuries leading to cartilage damage and subsequent degenerative changes.

Management
- *Non-surgical:*
  - NSAIDs for pain control.
  - Physical therapy to restore range of motion and strength.
  - Activity modification to reduce joint stress.
- *Surgical:*
  - Arthroscopic debridement in early stages.
  - Hemiarthroplasty or TSA in advanced cases with significant joint destruction.

Arthroscopic Shoulder Surgery

Q53. Indications and advantages of arthroscopic shoulder surgery.

(JIPMER Puducherry 2022, CMC Vellore 2023)

Introduction
- **Arthroscopy** is a minimally invasive surgical technique using a small camera and specialized instruments inserted into the joint via small incisions.
- Shoulder arthroscopy has revolutionized management of many **soft tissue and intra-articular pathologies**.

Indications
Rotator cuff disorders:
- Partial or full-thickness rotator cuff tears.
- Impingement syndrome (subacromial decompression).

Instability:
- Bankart lesion repair (anterior instability).
- Remplissage for Hill-Sachs lesions.

Labral tears: SLAP (Superior Labrum Anterior to Posterior) tear repair.

Other indications:
- Subacromial bursitis
- Adhesive capsulitis (capsular release)
- Synovial disorders (rheumatoid arthritis, PVNS)
- Loose body removal

Advantages
Minimally invasive: Small incisions → less soft tissue damage.

Better visualization: Ability to visualize all compartments of shoulder.

Faster recovery:
- Less postoperative pain.
- Early rehabilitation.

Cosmetic benefit: Minimal scarring.

Simultaneous Diagnosis + Treatment
Ability to assess intra-articular pathology in real-time.

Disadvantages (Briefly)
- Steep learning curve.
- Risk of neurovascular injury (rare).
- Fluid extravasation complications (swelling, respiratory distress if massive).

Q54. Various portals shoulder arthroscopy.

Basic Portals
1. *Posterior portal*:
   - Viewing portal
   - 2 cm inferior and medial to posterolateral acromion
2. *Anterior portal*:
   - Working portal
   - Just lateral to the coracoid, via the rotator interval
3. *Anterolateral portal*: Subacromial space access
4. *Lateral portal*: For rotator cuff repair
5. *Neviaser portal (supraspinatus fossa):* SLAP repairs

Uses
- Diagnostic arthroscopy
- Bankart repair
- Rotator cuff repair
- Debridement and synovectomy

Complications
- Neurovascular injury (especially axillary and musculocutaneous nerves)
- Portal site pain
- Infection (rare)

Q55. Arthroscopic management of rotator cuff tears.

(PGI Chandigarh 2022, MUHS Maharashtra 2023)

Arthroscopic Rotator Cuff Repair

Procedure:
- Suture anchors placed into the greater tuberosity of humerus.
- Sutures passed through torn rotator cuff tendon.
- Knotted securely to reattach tendon.

Techniques:
- Single-row repair (simpler, faster).
- Double-row or transosseous-equivalent repair (more footprint coverage, better healing rates).

Post-operative:
- Sling immobilization initially.
- Gradual passive → active-assisted → active physiotherapy protocol.

Q56. Arthroscopic management of shoulder instability.

Bankart Repair
- Avulsed anterior inferior labrum reattached to glenoid rim using suture anchors.
- Restoration of capsulolabral tension improves shoulder stability.

Remplissage Procedure

- For engaging Hill-Sachs lesions.
- Posterior capsule and infraspinatus tendon fixed into the humeral head defect arthroscopically to prevent engagement.

Latarjet (if needed)

Arthroscopic-assisted coracoid transfer in cases with significant glenoid bone loss (>20%).

Q57. Complications of shoulder arthroscopy.

Complication	*Notes*
Shoulder stiffness	Most common
Infection	Rare due to closed technique
Neurovascular injury	Rare but serious
Fluid extravasation	Can lead to airway compromise if massive

Exam Tip

When writing about shoulder arthroscopy:

- **Always begin by listing indications neatly**.
- For rotator cuff and instability, **mention suture anchor-based repairs**.
- In complications, **highlight stiffness and neurovascular injury** briefly at the end.

Nerve Injuries and Neuropathies Affecting the Shoulder

Q58. Discuss the causes and management of axillary nerve injury.

Causes

- Anterior shoulder dislocation (most common).
- Humeral neck fractures.
- Improper intramuscular injections in the deltoid region.
- Iatrogenic injury during shoulder surgery.
- Compression from improper use of crutches.

Clinical Features

- Weakness of deltoid (loss of abduction beyond 15–30°).
- Flattening of the shoulder contour.
- Loss of sensation over the "regimental badge" area (deltoid patch).

Management

- *Conservative:* Observation and physiotherapy for neuropraxia.
- *Surgical:* Nerve repair or grafting if no recovery after 3–6 months.
- *Rehabilitation:* Deltoid strengthening and shoulder mobility exercises.

Q59. Explain the clinical features of suprascapular nerve entrapment.

Sites of Entrapment

- Suprascapular notch (affects both supraspinatus and infraspinatus).
- Spinoglenoid notch (affects infraspinatus only).

Clinical Features

- Deep, dull pain in the posterior-lateral shoulder.

- Weakness in abduction (supraspinatus) and external rotation (infraspinatus).
- Atrophy of supraspinatus and/or infraspinatus.
- No sensory loss (nerve is mostly motor).

Diagnosis
- EMG and nerve conduction studies.
- MRI to rule out ganglion cysts compressing the nerve.

Management
- Activity modification, physiotherapy.
- Surgical decompression if conservative treatment fails.

Q60. Write a short note on quadrilateral space syndrome.

Definition
Compression of the axillary nerve and posterior circumflex humeral artery in the quadrilateral space.

Borders of the Quadrilateral Space
- *Superior:* Teres minor
- *Inferior:* Teres major
- *Medial:* Long head of triceps
- *Lateral:* Surgical neck of humerus

Clinical Features
- Vague shoulder pain, often posterior.
- Weakness of deltoid and teres minor.
- Paresthesia over deltoid patch.
- Worsens with overhead activity.

Diagnosis
- MRI, MR neurography
- EMG shows axillary nerve dysfunction.

Treatment
- Rest, physiotherapy
- Surgical decompression for refractory cases.

Q61. Discuss Parsonage-Turner syndrome (brachial neuritis) and its management.

Definition
Acute idiopathic brachial plexopathy, often triggered by viral illness, vaccination, or surgery.

Pathophysiology
Likely immune-mediated inflammation of the brachial plexus.

Clinical Features
- Sudden, severe shoulder/arm pain.
- Followed by patchy motor weakness and muscle atrophy.
- Most commonly affects suprascapular, long thoracic, and axillary nerves.

Diagnosis
- Clinical suspicion.
- EMG and nerve conduction studies.
- MRI may show denervation changes in shoulder girdle muscles.

Management

- Pain control (NSAIDs, corticosteroids in acute phase).
- Physiotherapy to maintain ROM and muscle strength.
- Most recover in 6–18 months, though some have residual weakness.

Q62. Explain the role of electrodiagnostic studies in shoulder neuropathies.

Electrodiagnostic Studies Include

- Nerve conduction velocity (NCV)
- Electromyography (EMG)

Applications

- *Localization of nerve injury:* Distinguishes between root, plexus, or peripheral nerve injury.
- *Severity and prognosis:* Differentiates between neuropraxia, axonotmesis, and neurotmesis.
- *Diagnosis of specific conditions:*
  - Axillary nerve injury
  - Suprascapular nerve entrapment
  - Quadrilateral space syndrome
  - Brachial neuritis

Timing

Most effective 3 weeks post-injury (allows for Wallerian degeneration).

Miscellaneous Shoulder Conditions

Q63. Discuss the etiology and management of scapular winging.

[Kasturba Medical College (KMC) Manipal Karnataka 2016]

Etiology

- *Neurological causes:*
  - Long thoracic nerve injury → serratus anterior palsy (most common).
  - Spinal accessory nerve injury → trapezius dysfunction.
  - Dorsal scapular nerve injury → rhomboid palsy.
- **Muscle weakness/Atrophy**
- *Structural abnormalities:* Scapulothoracic bursitis, trauma.

Clinical Features

- Prominent medial scapular border (especially on pushing against a wall).
- Shoulder fatigue or weakness.
- Limited overhead activity or scapular dyskinesis.

Management

- *Conservative:* Physical therapy (serratus anterior and scapular stabilizer strengthening).
- *Surgical:* Muscle transfer (e.g., pectoralis major transfer), nerve repair in selected cases.

Q64. Write a short note on snapping scapula syndrome.

Definition

Audible or palpable "snapping" or "grinding" during scapulothoracic motion.

Causes

- Scapulothoracic bursitis.
- Bony abnormalities (e.g., osteochondroma, scapular dyskinesis).
- Muscle imbalance or atrophy.

Clinical Features

- Snapping or grinding over the medial scapula.
- Pain with overhead activities.
- Often worsened with repetitive motion (athletes, swimmers).

Management

- NSAIDs, rest, physical therapy.
- Corticosteroid injections for bursitis.
- Surgical resection of bony lesions if refractory.

Q65. Explain the clinical significance and treatment of OS acromiale.

Definition

Failure of fusion of one or more of the four ossification centers of the acromion.

Clinical Significance

- May be asymptomatic.
- Can contribute to shoulder impingement or rotator cuff pathology.
- Pain with overhead activities.

Diagnosis

X-ray, MRI (to differentiate from fractures or other acromial pathology).

Management

- *Conservative:* Activity modification, NSAIDs, physiotherapy.
- *Surgical:* Excision or internal fixation if symptomatic and fails conservative management.

Q66. Discuss the biomechanics and management of swimmer's shoulder.

(Amrita Institute of Medical Sciences Kochi Kerala 2011)

Definition

Overuse injury due to repetitive overhead activity in swimmers.

Biomechanics

- *Repetitive internal rotation + adduction leads to:*
  - Rotator cuff impingement.
  - Glenohumeral instability.
  - Scapular dyskinesis.
  - Labral stress.

Clinical Features

- Anterior shoulder pain.
- Weakness, fatigue, decreased stroke efficiency.

Management

- *Phase 1:* Pain control (rest, NSAIDs, cold packs).
- *Phase 2:* Physiotherapy to correct muscle imbalances, scapular stability.
- *Phase 3:* Return to sport with modified technique.

Q67. Discuss the role of kinetic chain rehabilitation in shoulder pathologies.

Concept

Shoulder function is linked to the entire kinetic chain: Lower limbs, pelvis, trunk, scapula.

Importance

- Weak core or hips → compensation by shoulder.
- Ensures optimal force generation and energy transfer.

Applications

Rehabilitation of rotator cuff, impingement, SLAP lesions, overhead athlete injuries.

Rehabilitation Focus

- Proximal stability (core, trunk).
- Scapular mechanics.
- Postural alignment and neuromuscular control.

Goal

Restore **efficiency** and prevent **recurrence** by integrating full-body mechanics.

Surgical Procedures and Rehabilitation of the Shoulder

Q68. Write a short note on superior capsular reconstruction (SCR) for irreparable rotator cuff tears.

Definition

A procedure to restore shoulder function by reconstructing the superior capsule using a graft when rotator cuff tears are irreparable.

Indications

- Massive, irreparable rotator cuff tears.
- Intact deltoid and functional glenohumeral joint.
- Younger, active patients.

Technique

- Graft (fascia lata or dermal allograft) anchored to glenoid and greater tuberosity.
- Acts as a spacer and prevents superior migration of the humeral head.

Benefits

- Pain relief.
- Improved range of motion and function.
- Delays need for reverse shoulder arthroplasty.

Q69. Explain the role of rehabilitation in post-surgical shoulder conditions.

Phases of Rehabilitation

1. *Immobilization phase (0–6 weeks)*:
   - Sling use
   - Passive range of motion (PROM).
2. *Early mobilization phase (6–12 weeks)*:
   - Gradual increase in active ROM.
   - Scapular stabilization exercises.
3. *Strengthening phase (12+ weeks)*:
   - Isometric → isotonic exercises.
   - Functional training.

Importance

- Prevents stiffness and adhesions.
- Promotes tendon healing.
- Restores strength and motion.
- Customized for procedure (e.g., cuff repair vs. instability surgery).

Q70. Discuss the indications for coracoacromial ligament release.

Indications

- *Part of subacromial decompression for:*
  - Chronic impingement syndrome
  - Subacromial bursitis not responsive to conservative therapy
  - Acromioplasty with severe anterior acromial spur

Concerns

Over-release may compromise anterosuperior stability (especially in cuff-deficient shoulders).

Technique

Arthroscopic or open excision of the coracoacromial ligament.

Q71. Explain the role of platelet-rich plasma (PRP) in shoulder injuries.

(PGI Chandigarh 2011)

What is PRP?

- Autologous concentration of platelets from whole blood.
- *Contains growth factors:* PDGF, TGF-β, VEGF.

Indications in Shoulder

- Partial rotator cuff tears.
- Tendinopathies (e.g., biceps, supraspinatus).
- Post-surgical augmentation.
- Adhesive capsulitis (as intra-articular injection).

Evidence

- Mixed results in literature.
- Most effective for mild to moderate tendinopathy.
- Adjunct to conservative or surgical management.

Q72. Thoracic outlet syndrome (TOS).

Thoracic outlet syndrome refers to a group of conditions caused by **compression of neurovascular structures** (brachial plexus, subclavian artery, or subclavian vein) as they pass through the **thoracic outlet**—the space between the clavicle and the first rib.

Anatomy of the Thoracic Outlet

The thoracic outlet is bordered by:

- *Anteriorly:* Anterior scalene muscle
- *Posteriorly:* Middle scalene muscle
- *Inferiorly:* First rib
- *Superiorly:* Clavicle

Three potential sites of compression:

1. **Interscalene triangle** (bounded by anterior and middle scalene + 1st rib)
2. **Costoclavicular space** (between clavicle and 1st rib)
3. **Subcoracoid/Subpectoralis minor space**

Classification

1. *Neurogenic TOS (nTOS)—more than 90% of cases:*
   - Compression of **brachial plexus** (C5–T1 roots)
2. *Venous TOS (vTOS)*:
   - Compression of **subclavian vein** (effort thrombosis/Paget–Schroetter syndrome)

3. *Arterial TOS (aTOS):*
    - Compression of **subclavian artery** (rare; often due to cervical rib or anomaly)

Etiology/Causes

- *Congenital:*
    - Cervical rib (C7 rib)
    - Fibrous bands or muscular anomalies
- *Acquired:*
    - Trauma (clavicle fracture, whiplash)
    - Repetitive overhead activity (e.g., swimmers, painters)
    - Poor posture or hypertrophied scalene/pectoralis minor muscles

Clinical Features

Neurogenic TOS (most common):

- *Pain, numbness, tingling in ulnar distribution (C8–T1):* Little and ring finger
- Weakness or atrophy of intrinsic hand muscles (e.g., Gilliatt–Sumner hand)
- Symptoms worsen with overhead activity

Venous TOS:

- Arm swelling, heaviness
- Cyanosis, venous distension
- Possible effort thrombosis

Arterial TOS:

- Limb coolness, pallor, decreased pulses
- Claudication or ischemia of the hand
- May have bruit or thrill

Diagnosis

Clinical tests:

- *Adson's test:* Diminished radial pulse with head turned toward affected side and deep breath (compression of subclavian artery)
- *Roos test (EAST test):* Hands elevated and repeatedly open/close for 3 minutes → reproduction of symptoms
- *Wright's test:* Arm abducted + external rotation → pulse loss or symptoms
- *Costoclavicular test:* Exaggerated military posture to elicit symptoms

Imaging:

- *X-ray neck:* To detect cervical rib
- *Doppler US:* For vascular compromise
- *MRI/MRA:* Soft tissue and vascular detail
- *CT angiography/venography:* For arterial or venous TOS
- *EMG/NCS:* Helps rule out other causes of neuropathy

Management

Conservative (first-line in most cases):

- Postural correction and physiotherapy
- Avoid aggravating activities
- NSAIDs for pain relief
- Botox injections (for tight scalene muscles in select cases)

Surgical (indicated when conservative fails or in vascular TOS):

- **First rib resection** (via transaxillary or supraclavicular approach)
- *Scalenectomy:* Removal of anterior/middle scalene
- **Fibrous band or cervical rib excision**
- **Thrombectomy + venoplasty** (for venous TOS with clot)
- **Bypass grafting or patch angioplasty** (for arterial TOS)

Prognosis

- *Neurogenic TOS:* ~60–70% respond to conservative therapy; surgery improves symptoms in >80% if appropriately selected
- *Venous/Arterial TOS:* Early surgical intervention yields good outcomes

Key Points to Remember

- Neurogenic TOS is the most common form.
- Cervical rib and repetitive strain are common causes.
- Always confirm with imaging; be cautious to differentiate from cervical radiculopathy.
- Surgery is reserved for refractory or vascular cases.

Q73. Torticollis (including spasmodic torticollis).

Torticollis is a condition characterized by abnormal, asymmetrical head or neck position due to muscle spasm or structural anomalies.

Types

- *Congenital muscular torticollis (CMT):* Fibrosis and shortening of the **sternocleidomastoid (SCM)** muscle.
- *Spasmodic torticollis (cervical dystonia):*
  - Involuntary, intermittent or sustained contraction of neck muscles.
  - **Neurological disorder**—idiopathic or secondary (e.g., Parkinson's, trauma).
  - *Abnormal head postures:* rotational (torticollis), tilting (laterocollis), flexion (anterocollis), extension (retrocollis).

Management

- *CMT:* Stretching, physiotherapy; surgical SCM release if unresolved after 1 year.
- *Spasmodic:* Botulinum toxin injections (1st-line), anticholinergics, deep brain stimulation (in resistant cases).

Q74. Cleidocranial dysostosis.

Autosomal dominant skeletal dysplasia due to ***RUNX2* gene mutation**.

Key Features

- Hypoplastic/aplastic clavicles → shoulders meet at midline
- Delayed closure of fontanelles
- Dental abnormalities
- Short stature, scoliosis
- Wide pubic symphysis

Diagnosis

Clinical + radiographs (absent clavicle, wormian bones)

Management

- *Orthopedic:* Scoliosis monitoring
- *Dental:* Prosthodontic treatment
- Genetic counseling

Q75. Scapular dyskinesia.

Definition

Abnormal movement or positioning of the scapula during shoulder motion.

Causes

- Muscle imbalance (serratus anterior, trapezius, rhomboids)
- Nerve injury (long thoracic, spinal accessory)
- Labral tears, shoulder impingement

Types
- *Type I:* Inferomedial border prominence
- *Type II:* Medial border prominence
- *Type III:* Superior scapular elevation
- *Type IV:* Symmetric motion (normal)

Management
- *Rehabilitation:* Scapular stabilization, posture correction
- Treat underlying pathology (nerve injury, rotator cuff tear)

Q76. Painful arc syndrome.

Shoulder pain during mid-range abduction (typically 60–120°), painless at start and end of motion.

Causes
- Subacromial impingement (supraspinatus tendon under acromion)
- Rotator cuff tendinopathy
- Subacromial bursitis
- AC joint arthritis (>160° pain)

Management
- NSAIDs, physiotherapy
- Subacromial injection
- Arthroscopic decompression if conservative fails

Q77. Management of bone marrow edema syndrome.

A self-limiting condition characterized by **painful bone marrow edema** without osteonecrosis, often in the hip/knee.

Imaging
MRI: Hypointense on T1, hyperintense on T2/STIR.

Management
- *Conservative:* Protected weight-bearing, NSAIDs
- Bisphosphonates or iloprost (experimental)
- Usually resolves in 3–6 months

Q78. Functional classification of muscles around the shoulder.

(Goa Medical College Bambolim Goa 2014)

Muscle group	*Muscles*	*Function*
Scapular stabilizers	Trapezius, serratus anterior, rhomboids, levator scapulae	Anchor scapula to thorax
Glenohumeral movers	Deltoid, pectoralis major, latissimus dorsi	Gross movement
Rotator cuff (stabilizers)	Supraspinatus, infraspinatus, teres minor, subscapularis (SITS)	Dynamic stability
Flexors	Anterior deltoid, coracobrachialis, biceps (long head)	Forward elevation
Extensors	Posterior deltoid, latissimus dorsi, teres major	Extension
Abductors	Supraspinatus (0–15°), deltoid (15–90°), trapezius/serratus (>90°)	Arm abduction
External rotators	Infraspinatus, teres minor	External rotation
Internal rotators	Subscapularis, pectoralis major, latissimus dorsi	Internal rotation

Q79. Indications and techniques of shoulder arthrodesis.

Indications
- Irreparable brachial plexus injury
- Paralysis (deltoid and rotator cuff dysfunction)
- Recurrent dislocation (non-reconstructable)
- Post-infective arthritis or failed arthroplasty

Prerequisites for Good Results
- Intact elbow and hand function
- Pain-free joint before fusion
- Adequate bone stock

Optimal Position for Fusion
30° abduction, 30° flexion, 30° internal rotation

Techniques
- Open approach
- Internal fixation (plates, screws)
- Bone grafting if needed
- *Common approach:* Deltoid-splitting

Q80. Milwaukee shoulder syndrome.

Destructive shoulder arthropathy due to **calcium hydroxyapatite crystal deposition**, leading to **rotator cuff rupture** and joint destruction.

Clinical Features
- Elderly women
- Recurrent large hemorrhagic effusions
- Limited ROM, subluxation
- Pseudoparalysis

Radiological Features
- Superior migration of humeral head
- Joint space narrowing
- Soft tissue calcification

Differential Diagnosis
- Charcot joint
- Rheumatoid arthritis
- Septic arthritis
- Cuff tear arthropathy (not due to crystal)

Management
- NSAIDs, aspiration
- Physical therapy
- Arthroplasty if joint is severely damaged

Q81. Calcific tendinitis of the shoulder.

Deposition of **calcium hydroxyapatite crystals** in the rotator cuff tendons, usually the **supraspinatus**. It's a **self-limiting** condition with painful episodes.

Phases
1. **Formative phase**—asymptomatic
2. **Resorptive phase**—intense pain due to inflammation and increased vascularity
3. **Post-calcific**—healing

Clinical Features
- Sudden onset of severe shoulder pain, often nocturnal
- Limited ROM
- Middle-aged women commonly affected

Imaging
- *X-ray:* Cloud-like or well-demarcated calcium deposits
- *USG:* Hyperechoic deposit with shadowing
- *MRI:* Edema around deposit

Management
- *Acute phase:* NSAIDs, rest, ice
- Needle aspiration/lavage (barbotage)
- Ultrasound-guided steroid injection
- ESWT (shockwave therapy)
- Arthroscopic removal for chronic or refractory cases

Q82. Burner (stinger) syndrome.

A **transient brachial plexus injury**, commonly seen in **contact sports** (football, wrestling), caused by **traction or compression** of nerve roots (typically C5–C6).

Mechanism
- Shoulder depressed + head tilted to opposite side → traction
- Direct blow to supraclavicular region → compression

Clinical Features
- Sudden **burning, stinging, or electric shock sensation** down the arm
- Unilateral, transient weakness or numbness (typically deltoid, biceps)
- No neck pain (rules out cervical disc disease)

Diagnosis
- Clinical diagnosis
- MRI if symptoms persist >24–48 hours
- EMG/NCS for persistent weakness

Management
- Most resolve within minutes
- Rest, NSAIDs
- Return-to-play only if full strength/sensation restored
- Recurrent episodes may need spine evaluation for cervical stenosis

Q83. Spinoglenoid notch cyst.

A **paralabral cyst** that forms at the **spinoglenoid notch**, often associated with a **posterior labral tear**, and may compress the **suprascapular nerve**.

Anatomy Note
Suprascapular nerve passes through **suprascapular notch** → innervates **supraspinatus**, then through **spinoglenoid notch** → **infraspinatus**

Clinical Features

- **Isolated infraspinatus atrophy and weakness** (external rotation)
- Dull posterior shoulder pain
- No sensory deficits (motor-only nerve)

Diagnosis

- *MRI:* Shows cyst and labral tear
- *EMG:* Denervation of infraspinatus

Management

- *Initial:* Observation if asymptomatic or mild
- **Aspiration** under US guidance (high recurrence)
- *Definitive:* Arthroscopic **labral tear repair + cyst decompression**

Q84. Klippel–Feil syndrome (KFS)—summary.

(King George's Medical University 2011)

Definition

Congenital fusion of **two or more cervical vertebrae** due to segmentation failure during embryogenesis.

Classic Triad

1. Short neck
2. Low posterior hairline
3. Limited neck mobility

Classification (Feil)

- *Type I:* Extensive cervical and upper thoracic fusion
- *Type II:* 1–2 cervical fusions ± hemivertebrae
- *Type III:* Cervical fusion + lower spine anomalies

Associated Anomalies

- **Sprengel deformity** (elevated scapula)
- **Scoliosis**, spina bifida
- **Hearing loss**
- **Cardiac/renal anomalies**
- **Cleft palate**

Diagnosis

- *X-ray:* Fused cervical vertebrae
- *MRI/CT:* For spinal cord or bony details
- *Echo/USG:* To assess associated anomalies

Management

- *Conservative:* Observation, physio, neck protection
- *Surgical:* For instability, myelopathy, or scoliosis

Prognosis

Good if no neurological involvement; monitor for instability and progressive deformities.

Q85. Costo-clavicular syndrome.

Definition

A form of **thoracic outlet syndrome (TOS)** where the **neurovascular bundle (especially subclavian vein/artery)** is compressed between the **clavicle and the first rib** (in the costoclavicular space).

Causes

- Posture (e.g., military shoulder posture)
- Carrying heavy loads
- Clavicle fractures or callus
- Congenital anomalies

Symptoms

- Pain, numbness, or tingling in the arm
- Arm fatigue with overhead activity
- *Vascular signs:* Swelling, cyanosis, loss of pulse with shoulder retraction

Clinical Test

Costoclavicular maneuver (Military brace test): Exaggerated shoulder retraction reduces radial pulse

Management

- Postural correction, physiotherapy
- Surgical decompression (first rib resection or clavicle osteotomy) in severe cases

Q86. Sprengel shoulder.

A **congenital elevation of the scapula** due to failure of its normal descent during embryogenesis.

Key Features

- Unilateral (usually left side)
- Restricted shoulder abduction
- Cosmetic deformity (visible high scapula)
- Associated with **Klippel–Feil syndrome**, scoliosis, or omovertebral bone (fibrous or bony band connecting scapula to cervical spine)

Diagnosis

Clinical + X-ray/CT (shows elevated scapula, omovertebral bone)

Management

- *Mild:* Observation, physiotherapy
- *Moderate to severe (functional or cosmetic impairment):* **Surgical correction (Woodward procedure)**

Q87. Deltopectoral approach.

A standard **anterior surgical approach to the shoulder**, used in **arthroplasty**, **fracture fixation**, and **shoulder reconstruction**.

Anatomical Landmarks

- Interval between **deltoid (lateral)** and **pectoralis major (medial)**
- The **cephalic vein** runs in the groove and is preserved (or retracted laterally)

Structures at Risk

- Cephalic vein
- Musculocutaneous nerve (deep, medially)
- Axillary nerve (inferolateral)

Advantages

- Good exposure to proximal humerus, joint capsule, and subscapularis
- Muscle-sparing

Common Uses
- Shoulder arthroplasty (total/hemi/reverse)
- ORIF of proximal humerus fractures
- Tumor resection

Q88. Scapulohumeral rhythm.

Coordinated movement between the **glenohumeral joint** and **scapulothoracic articulation.**

Ratio
For every **2° of glenohumeral** movement, there's **1° of scapular rotation** (2:1 ratio).

Clinical Relevance
Disruption seen in shoulder impingement, rotator cuff tears, scapular dyskinesia → reduced overhead function and shoulder pain.

Q89. Biomechanics of throwing injuries in the shoulder.

(AIIMS Bhubaneswar 2011)

- *Phases:* Wind-up → Early Cocking → Late Cocking → Acceleration → Deceleration → Follow-through.
- *Common injuries:*
    - SLAP tears (late cocking)
    - Internal impingement
    - Posterior capsular tightness (GIRD)
    - Rotator cuff tendinopathy or tears
- High stress on **posterior capsule, labrum**, and **rotator cuff** in deceleration and follow-through.

Q90. Axillary nerve injury—causes and management.

Causes
- Shoulder dislocation (anterior)
- Proximal humerus fracture
- Iatrogenic (surgery)

Clinical
- Deltoid weakness, loss of shoulder abduction
- Sensory loss over **regimental badge area**

Management
- Observation (neuropraxia), EMG
- Surgical exploration if no recovery in 3–6 months

Q91. Suprascapular nerve entrapment.

Sites
- **Suprascapular notch** (affects supraspinatus + infraspinatus)
- **Spinoglenoid notch** (isolated infraspinatus)

Symptoms
- Dull posterior shoulder pain
- Weakness in external rotation (infraspinatus)

Diagnosis
MRI (muscle atrophy), EMG

Treatment
Physio, nerve release surgery if persistent

Q92. Quadrilateral space syndrome—short note.

(West Bengal University of Health Sciences 2013)

Compression of the **axillary nerve** and **posterior circumflex humeral artery** in the quadrilateral space.

Borders
- Teres minor (top), teres major (bottom), long head of triceps (medial), humerus (lateral)

Symptoms
- Posterolateral shoulder pain
- Deltoid/teres minor weakness
- Worse with overhead activity

Diagnosis
MRI, EMG

Management
Rest, physio, surgical decompression if needed

Q93. Parsonage–Turner syndrome (brachial neuritis).

Idiopathic brachial plexopathy, often post-viral or post-vaccination

Symptoms
- Sudden shoulder/arm pain → weakness/atrophy (usually suprascapular or long thoracic nerve)
- Delayed weakness after pain

Diagnosis
EMG, clinical

Management
- Analgesia, physiotherapy
- Steroids (in early phase)
- Recovery over months

Q94. Swimmer's shoulder—biomechanics and management.

(Kasturba Medical College Manipal 2011)

Biomechanics
- Repetitive overhead motion → **impingement**, **instability**, and **muscle imbalance**
- Common in freestyle and butterfly strokes

Management
- Stroke correction
- Strengthening scapular stabilizers, rotator cuff
- NSAIDs, rest; rarely surgery

Q95. Role of platelet-rich plasma (PRP) in shoulder injuries.

- Autologous plasma enriched with **platelets and growth factors**
- Proposed to enhance **tendon and soft tissue healing**

Uses
- Partial rotator cuff tears
- Tendinopathies
- Subacromial bursitis

Evidence
- Mixed; better for early/mild degenerative tendinopathy
- Not first-line; adjunct to physiotherapy

Q96. Role of imaging in shoulder pathologies.

- *X-ray:* Fractures, arthritis, acromion type, dislocations.
- *Ultrasound:* Dynamic cuff evaluation, bursa, fluid collections.
- *MRI:* Soft tissue (labrum, rotator cuff, cartilage, AVN).
- *CT scan:* Glenoid morphology, bony Bankart, preoperative planning.
- *MR arthrography:* Labral tears (SLAP, Bankart), capsular laxity.
- *Y-view:* For shoulder dislocations (posterior).

Q97. Traumatic posterior dislocation of the shoulder.

(Amrita Institute of Medical Sciences 2013)

Diagnosis
- *Mechanism:* Seizures, electrocution, trauma.
- Arm in internal rotation, limited external rotation.
- *X-rays:* "Light bulb sign", "rim sign", **Y-view** essential.
- **CT scan** to assess reverse Hill-Sachs defect.

Management
- *Acute:* Closed reduction.
- *Chronic:* McLaughlin procedure, reverse remplissage, arthroplasty if severe.

Q98. Humeral head osteonecrosis.

Etiology
Steroid use, alcohol, trauma, sickle cell disease.

Diagnosis
- *X-ray:* Crescent sign.
- *MRI:* Gold standard (early diagnosis).

Treatment
- *Early:* Bisphosphonates, core decompression.
- *Late:* Hemiarthroplasty or total shoulder arthroplasty.

Q99. Post-traumatic shoulder stiffness.

Causes
Adhesions, capsular fibrosis, improper rehabilitation.

Types
Intrinsic (fractures, cuff tear), extrinsic (DM, thyroid).

Management
- Physiotherapy, analgesia.
- MUA, arthroscopic capsular release if persistent.

Q100. Surgical approaches to shoulder joint.

1. *Deltopectoral:* Most common; used in arthroplasty, ORIF.
2. *Deltoid-splitting:* For lateral procedures.
3. *Posterior (modified judet):* For posterior fracture dislocations.
4. *Superior (transacromial):* Rarely used.

Q101. Complications of rotator cuff repair.

- Re-tear or failed healing
- Adhesive capsulitis
- Infection
- Deltoid detachment (open surgery)
- Shoulder stiffness

Q102. Tendon transfer procedures around shoulder.

Indications

Irreparable cuff tears, brachial plexus injury.

Examples

- Latissimus dorsi transfer (for posterosuperior cuff tear).
- Lower trapezius transfer.
- Pec major transfer (subscapularis loss).
- Steindler flexorplasty (for elbow flexion in brachial plexus injury).

SHORT THEORY/VIVA QUESTIONS

Q No.	*Question*	*Answer*
4	Neer test	Impingement test where shoulder is passively flexed with scapula stabilized. Pain = positive.
6	Apprehension test	Arm abducted and externally rotated. Apprehension = anterior instability.
11	Lift-off test	Tests subscapularis. Hand behind back lifted off. Inability = positive.
13	Hawkins–Kennedy test	Forward flexed arm forcibly internally rotated. Pain = subacromial impingement.
15	Types of acromion	Flat (Type I), Curved (II), Hooked (III – associated with impingement).
16	Y-view	Lateral scapular X-ray to detect posterior dislocation or fracture.
18	Sulcus sign	Inferior translation of humeral head = inferior instability.
19	Codman's paradox	Arm abducted and flexed appears externally rotated without actual rotation.
22	Cross-body adduction test	Arm adducted across chest. Pain = AC joint pathology.
25	Drop arm test	Passive abduction to 90°, then ask to lower slowly. Drop = cuff tear.
28	Latarjet indications	(1) Glenoid bone loss >20%, (2) Failed soft-tissue repair.
29	Pseudoparalysis	Inability to actively elevate shoulder despite full passive ROM. Seen in massive cuff tear.
31	GIRD	>20° loss of internal rotation compared to contralateral side. Common in throwers.
32	Complications of RCR	(1) Retear, (2) Adhesive capsulitis.
33	Acromioplasty	Surgical reshaping of acromion to relieve impingement.
34	Buford complex	Congenital absence of anterior superior labrum with thick MGHL. Variant, not pathology.
35	DDx of shoulder pain	Rotator cuff tear, frozen shoulder, impingement, OA, calcific tendinitis.
36	Open bankart repair	Open surgical reattachment of labrum to anterior glenoid for instability.

7.2 Elbow Disorders

Vipin Sharma, Azhar Ud Din, Nitin Choudhary

Basic Anatomy and Biomechanics of the Elbow Joint

Q1. Describe the anatomy of the elbow joint in detail.

- *Type:* Synovial hinge joint.
- *Articulations:*
  - Humeroulnar (trochlea with ulna).
  - Humeroradial (capitulum with radial head).
  - Proximal radioulnar joint (for pronation/supination).
- *Bones involved:* Humerus, ulna, radius.
- *Capsule:* Encloses all three articulations; lax anteriorly/posteriorly.

Q2. Distal humerus functional anatomy.

- *Articular parts:* Trochlea (ulna), capitellum (radius)
- *Carrying angle:* ~13° valgus
- *Columns:* Medial and lateral columns—act as struts
- *Fossa:* Coronoid, olecranon, radial—allow full ROM
- **Ulnar nerve** passes posterior to medial epicondyle
- Important for surgical approach (e.g., triceps-sparing vs. splitting)

Q3. Discuss the biomechanics of the elbow joint.

- *Movements:*
  - **Flexion-extension** (hinge mechanics).
  - **Pronation-supination** (proximal radioulnar joint).
- *Range:*
  - *Flexion:* ~0° to 140–150°.
  - *Supination/Pronation:* ~85° each.
- *Stability:*
  - *Static:* Bony congruity, collateral ligaments.
  - *Dynamic:* Muscles (biceps, triceps, brachialis).

Q4. Write a short note on the carrying angle and its clinical significance.

- *Definition:* Angle between humerus and forearm when extended and supinated.
- *Normal:*
  - *Males:* ~5–10°.
  - *Females:* ~10–15° (wider pelvis).
- *Clinical relevance:*
  - *Cubitus valgus/varus:* Seen in malunions.
  - Important during fracture evaluation and surgical correction.

Q5. Describe the ligaments and stabilizers of the elbow joint and their functions.

(Dr DY Patil Vidyapeeth 2013)

- *Ulnar collateral ligament (UCL):*
  - Anterior, posterior, and transverse bundles.
  - Resists valgus stress.
- *Radial collateral ligament (RCL):*
  - Lateral epicondyle to annular ligament.
  - Resists varus stress.
- *Annular ligament:*
  - Wraps radial head.
  - Allows radial head rotation.
- *Quadrate ligament and oblique cord:* Support proximal radioulnar joint.

Static stabilizers
- *Medial (ulnar) collateral ligament (MCL):* Resists valgus
- *Lateral (radial) collateral ligament (LCL):* Resists varus
- *Annular ligament:* Stabilizes radial head
- **Joint capsule**

Dynamic stabilizers
- Biceps and brachialis (anterior)
- Triceps (posterior)
- Wrist extensors and flexors (medial/lateral dynamic support)

Q6. Explain the vascular supply and innervation of the elbow joint.

- *Arterial supply:*
  - Rich anastomotic network around the elbow.
  - Branches from brachial, radial, and ulnar arteries.
- *Innervation:*
  - *Median nerve:* Anterior capsule.
  - *Radial nerve:* Lateral aspect.
  - *Ulnar nerve:* Medial aspect.
  - *Hilton's Law:* Nerves supplying muscles crossing joint also innervate joint.

Q7. Discuss the biomechanics of elbow flexion and extension.

- *Flexion:*
  - *Muscles:* Biceps brachii, brachialis, brachioradialis.
  - *Normal ROM:* 0°–145°.
- *Extension:*
  - Triceps brachii.
- *Axis of motion:* Passes through trochlea and capitulum.
- *Functional arc:* ~30° to 130° for ADLs.

Q8. Write a short note on the role of the ulnar collateral ligament in elbow stability.

(Maharashtra University of Health Sciences 2019)

- **Main valgus stabilizer**, especially during overhead sports.
- Injured in throwing athletes → "Tommy John injury".

- *Reconstruction:* **Tommy John surgery** (UCL reconstruction with tendon graft).
- Essential in resisting medial overload stress.

Factors Responsible for Post-traumatic Elbow Stiffness and Its Management

Causes

A. *Intrinsic factors (intra-articular)*:
  - Intra-articular adhesions
  - Articular incongruity
  - Cartilage loss
  - Osteophytes
  - Synovitis

B. *Extrinsic factors (extra-articular)*:
  - Capsular contracture (anterior capsule most commonly)
  - Collateral ligament contracture
  - Heterotopic ossification (HO)
  - Muscle shortening (brachialis, triceps)
  - Skin/graft contracture

C. *Neurogenic/Miscellaneous*:
  - Pain inhibition
  - Reflex sympathetic dystrophy

Management

1. *Non-operative*:
   - Indicated for early stiffness (<3 months)
   - Passive stretching and physiotherapy
   - Static/dynamic splints (e.g., Turnbuckle splint)
   - Continuous passive motion (CPM)
2. *Operative*:
   - **Open/Arthroscopic capsular release**
   - Excision of HO
   - Contracture release of ligaments/muscles
   - Interposition arthroplasty (for ankylosis)
   - Total elbow arthroplasty (in elderly with arthritis)

Q9. Discuss the causes and management of elbow stiffness.

Causes

- *Intrinsic:* Joint capsule fibrosis, intra-articular adhesions, osteophytes, articular surface incongruity.
- *Extrinsic:* Muscle/tendon tightness, heterotopic ossification (HO), skin grafts, scars, burns.
- *Neurogenic:* Reflex sympathetic dystrophy, spasticity (e.g., post-stroke or TBI).

Evaluation

- Clinical exam (range of motion, flexion-extension arc).
- *Imaging:* X-ray, CT (osteophytes, HO), MRI (soft tissue contracture).

Management

- *Non-operative:*
  - Physical therapy (stretching, splints—static/dynamic).
  - NSAIDs for inflammation, CPM machines.
- *Operative:*
  - Open or arthroscopic **arthrolysis**.
  - HO excision if mature and symptomatic.

Q10. Explain the indications and techniques of elbow arthrolysis.

Indications
- Stiff elbow with motion arc <100° and functional limitation.
- Failure of ≥6 months of conservative treatment.
- Post-traumatic contractures, intra-articular adhesions, capsular thickening.

Techniques
- *Open arthrolysis:*
  - Anterior/posterior approaches.
  - Capsulectomy, removal of osteophytes or hardware.
- *Arthroscopic arthrolysis:*
  - Minimally invasive.
  - Requires experience; risk to neurovascular structures.

Post-operative Care
- Immediate physiotherapy.
- Possible use of continuous passive motion (CPM).
- NSAIDs or radiotherapy to prevent HO.

Q11. Write a short note on heterotopic ossification around the elbow.

Definition
Abnormal formation of mature lamellar bone in non-osseous tissue (usually around joint capsules, muscles).

Common Causes
- Trauma (e.g. elbow dislocation/fracture).
- Burns, TBI, SCI.
- Surgical interventions (e.g., ORIF).

Symptoms
- Progressive stiffness, pain, palpable mass.
- Decreased ROM, particularly extension.

Diagnosis
X-ray, bone scan (early), CT for maturity assessment.

Management
- NSAIDs (e.g., indomethacin).
- Surgical excision (only after maturity—6–12 months post-trauma).
- Radiation therapy for prevention.

Q12. Discuss the role of radiation therapy in preventing heterotopic ossification.

Mechanism
- Inhibits osteoprogenitor cell proliferation and differentiation.
- Anti-inflammatory effects on early HO formation.

Indications
- High risk of HO recurrence after excision.
- Prophylaxis post-elbow or hip surgery in high-risk patients.

Protocol
- **Single dose (7–8 Gy)** within **72 hours post-operative** (or pre-operative within 24 hours).
- Can be combined with NSAIDs.

Advantages
- Effective prophylaxis.
- Minimally invasive.

Limitations
- Radiation exposure.
- Cost/logistics in some settings.

Elbow Arthritis and Degenerative Conditions

Q13. Discuss the classification and treatment of elbow osteoarthritis.

(Jammu University)

Classification
- *Primary OA:* Rare; idiopathic, typically in manual laborers or athletes.
- *Secondary OA:* Post-traumatic (fracture, dislocation), inflammatory (RA), crystal arthropathy (gout), infection.

Symptoms
Pain, stiffness (especially extension), locking (loose bodies), loss of terminal ROM.

Treatment
- *Conservative:*
  - NSAIDs, activity modification, physical therapy, bracing.
  - Intra-articular corticosteroid injections.
- *Surgical:*
  - **Arthroscopic debridement** (osteophyte removal, capsular release).
  - **Interposition arthroplasty** (young patients with intact bone).
  - *Total elbow arthroplasty (TEA):* Advanced OA with functional limitation.

Q14. Explain the management of rheumatoid arthritis of the elbow.

Pathophysiology
Synovial inflammation → pannus formation → cartilage erosion and joint destruction.

Clinical Features
- Pain, swelling, stiffness, progressive deformity (valgus), instability.
- May be bilateral and symmetrical.

Management
- *Medical:* DMARDs (methotrexate), biologics (TNF inhibitors), NSAIDs.
- *Rehabilitative:* Physiotherapy for ROM and function.
- *Surgical:*
  - *Synovectomy:* Early disease.
  - **Radial head excision** (in select cases).
  - *Total Elbow Arthroplasty (TEA):* Advanced stage, pain, deformity.

Q15. Write a short note on synovial osteochondromatosis of the elbow.

Definition
Benign condition involving synovial metaplasia forming cartilaginous nodules which may ossify and detach as loose bodies.

Clinical Features
- Pain, stiffness, swelling, mechanical symptoms (clicking, locking).
- Gradual onset

Radiology
- *X-rays:* Multiple intra-articular calcified bodies.
- *MRI:* Detects early non-calcified nodules.

Treatment
Synovectomy + removal of loose bodies (arthroscopic or open).

Q16. Discuss the indications and outcomes of total elbow arthroplasty.

(Kasturba Medical College Manipal 2016)

Indications
- Advanced arthritis (RA, post-traumatic, OA).
- Low-demand elderly patients with severe pain and dysfunction.
- Non-reconstructable distal humerus fractures in the elderly.

Contraindications
Active infection, high-demand patients, inadequate bone stock, neuropathic joint.

Outcomes
- Good pain relief and function in selected patients.
- Lifespan ~10–15 years.
- Restrictions on lifting (typically <5 kg).

Contraindications of Total Elbow Replacement (TER)
Absolute contraindications:
- *Active or recent infection (local or systemic):* For example septic arthritis, osteomyelitis
- *Neuropathic (Charcot) joint:* Poor soft tissue envelope and proprioception
- *Inadequate or non-functional extensor mechanism:* Triceps insufficiency
- *Complete paralysis of the limb:* No functional gain expected
- *Severe bone loss not amenable to reconstruction:* No stable implant fixation possible

Relative contraindications:
- *Young, high-demand patients (<60 years):* Due to high risk of implant loosening or early failure
- *Non-compliance or inability to follow post-operative restrictions:* For example uncontrolled seizures, cognitive issues
- *Insufficient soft tissue coverage:* For example previous radiation, multiple surgeries
- *Significant flexion contracture (>90°):* Difficult to correct and poor functional gain
- *Uncontrolled systemic illness:* For example uncontrolled diabetes, cardiac instability

Special consideration:
- *TER is primarily reserved for:*
    - Rheumatoid arthritis with joint destruction
    - Elderly low-demand individuals with complex distal humerus fractures
    - Post-traumatic arthritis unresponsive to other treatments

Complications: Loosening, infection, triceps insufficiency, and periprosthetic fracture.

Q17. Explain the role of elbow arthroscopy in degenerative conditions.

Indications
- Early to moderate OA, loose bodies, impinging osteophytes, capsular contractures.

Advantages
- Minimally invasive, faster recovery, precise debridement.
- Less morbidity compared to open surgery.

Procedures

Debridement, removal of loose bodies, osteophyte excision, and capsular release.

Outcomes

- Improved pain and ROM in carefully selected cases.
- Not indicated in severe OA or instability.

Neuropathies and Nerve Injuries Affecting the Elbow

Q18. Discuss the causes and treatment of cubital tunnel syndrome.

(Amrita Institute of Medical Sciences 2011)

Definition

Compression of the **ulnar nerve** at the elbow, especially in the **cubital tunnel** behind the medial epicondyle.

Causes

- Repetitive elbow flexion/extension
- Direct trauma
- Osteophytes or arthritis at the elbow
- Subluxation of the ulnar nerve
- Ganglion cysts

Clinical Features

- Numbness/tingling in the 4th and 5th fingers
- Weak grip strength
- Wasting of hypothenar and interossei muscles
- Positive Tinel's sign at the elbow
- Clawing of ulnar digits in severe cases

Treatment

- *Conservative:* Activity modification, night splint in extension, NSAIDs
- *Surgical:* Ulnar nerve decompression (in situ or anterior transposition), medial epicondylectomy

Q19. Explain the clinical features and management of radial tunnel syndrome.

Definition

Compression of the **radial nerve** (posterior interosseous branch) in the radial tunnel between the **brachioradialis and ECRB**.

Clinical Features

- Dull, aching pain over the lateral forearm (mimics lateral epicondylitis)
- Tenderness 3–5 cm distal to lateral epicondyle
- Pain with resisted supination or middle finger extension
- No sensory loss (unlike superficial radial nerve injury)

Management

- *Conservative:* NSAIDs, rest, splinting, physical therapy
- *Surgical:* Radial tunnel decompression in refractory cases

Q20. Write a short note on posterior interosseous nerve syndrome.

Definition

A motor neuropathy caused by compression of the **posterior interosseous nerve (PIN)**, a deep branch of the radial nerve.

Causes
- Compression at arcade of Frohse
- Trauma, masses (lipoma), fibrous bands

Clinical Features
- Weakness/paralysis of finger and thumb extensors (EIP, EPL)
- No sensory loss (purely motor branch)
- "Finger drop" or difficulty extending fingers/thumb

Treatment
- Conservative initially
- Surgical decompression if persistent or progressive

Q21. Discuss the management of ulnar nerve entrapment at the elbow.

Sites of Entrapment
- Cubital tunnel (most common)
- Arcade of Struthers
- Between the two heads of FCU

Management
1. *Non-operative (mild/moderate cases):*
   - Activity modification
   - Elbow extension splint at night
   - NSAIDs
   - Nerve gliding exercises
2. *Surgical (severe or refractory):*
   - In situ decompression
   - Anterior transposition (subcutaneous, submuscular, or intramuscular)
   - Medial epicondylectomy

Indications for Surgery
- Failure of conservative treatment
- Motor weakness or muscle atrophy
- Electrodiagnostic evidence of severe compression

Q22. Explain Froment's sign and its significance in ulnar nerve palsy.

(Kashmir University)

Froment's Sign
- A clinical test for **ulnar nerve palsy**.
- Patient attempts to grasp a piece of paper between thumb and index finger.

Positive Test
- **Flexion of the IP joint of the thumb** indicates **weakness of adductor pollicis** (ulnar nerve) and compensation by **flexor pollicis longus** (median nerve).

Significance
- Indicates **ulnar nerve dysfunction**, especially motor involvement.
- Often used in evaluation of **cubital tunnel syndrome** or **Guyon's canal syndrome**.

Q23. Explain the management of Panner's disease.

Definition
Osteochondrosis of the **capitellum** in children aged 5–10 years.

Etiology
Repetitive microtrauma leading to avascular necrosis of the capitellum.

Clinical Features
- Gradual onset of lateral elbow pain
- Stiffness and limited range of motion
- Tenderness over lateral condyle

Radiology
Capitellar flattening, sclerosis, fragmentation on X-ray

Management
- *Conservative:*
  - Rest from sports (especially throwing)
  - NSAIDs
  - Physical therapy for ROM
- Prognosis is excellent; self-limiting condition

Q24. Write a short note on little league elbow.

Definition
Overuse injury of the medial elbow in young athletes, especially **throwing sports**.

Mechanism
Repetitive valgus stress leads to apophysitis or fragmentation of the **medial epicondyle** growth plate.

Clinical Features
- Pain over medial elbow during/after throwing
- Decreased throwing velocity
- Tenderness at medial epicondyle

Radiographs
Widening, fragmentation, or avulsion of the medial epicondylar apophysis.

Treatment
- Rest and cessation of throwing
- Ice, NSAIDs, physical therapy
- Gradual return to sports
- Surgery in severe avulsion or nonunion cases

Miscellaneous Conditions of the Elbow

Q25. Discuss the clinical features and management of olecranon bursitis.

(AIIMS Jodhpur 2014)

Definition
Inflammation of the **olecranon bursa**, located between the olecranon and skin.

Etiology
- Acute trauma or repetitive microtrauma (e.g., prolonged pressure)
- Infection (septic bursitis)
- Gout, RA, or idiopathic

Clinical Features
- Swelling over the olecranon
- Pain may be mild or absent in aseptic cases
- Redness, warmth, and tenderness in septic bursitis

Diagnosis
- Clinical exam
- **Aspiration** if infection suspected → cell count, Gram stain, culture, crystals

Management
- *Aseptic:* Rest, NSAIDs, compression, aspiration
- *Septic:* Antibiotics ± aspiration or incision and drainage
- *Refractory/Recurrent:* Surgical bursectomy

Q26. Explain the diagnosis and treatment of distal biceps tendinopathy.

Definition
Painful degeneration or inflammation of the distal biceps tendon at its insertion on the radial tuberosity.

Etiology
- Overuse injury (e.g., repetitive lifting or pronation/supination)
- Microtears or tendinosis

Clinical Features
- Pain and tenderness in the antecubital fossa
- Pain aggravated by resisted elbow flexion or supination
- No obvious deformity (vs. rupture)

Diagnosis
Clinical + MRI (to assess tendinosis versus partial tear)

Treatment
- Rest, activity modification
- NSAIDs, ice
- Physical therapy (eccentric loading)
- PRP or corticosteroid injections
- Surgery for chronic or refractory cases

Q27. Write a short note on snapping elbow syndrome.

Definition
A condition characterized by a **clicking/snapping sound** during elbow motion, due to mechanical impingement or instability.

Types
1. *Lateral snapping*: Due to annular ligament or radial head issues
2. *Medial snapping*: Ulnar nerve subluxation over the medial epicondyle
3. *Intra-articular snapping*: Loose bodies, synovial plica, or impinging osteophytes

Clinical Features
- Audible/palpable snap during flexion/extension
- ± pain or ulnar nerve symptoms

Diagnosis
Dynamic ultrasound or MRI

Treatment
- Conservative (NSAIDs, activity modification)
- Surgery (e.g., ulnar nerve transposition, osteophyte excision)

Q28. Discuss the pathology and management of pigmented villonodular synovitis (PVNS) of the elbow.

Definition
A rare, benign but locally aggressive **proliferative disorder of the synovium**, characterized by hemosiderin deposition.

Types
- Localized or Diffuse

Pathology
- Synovial hyperplasia with villous and nodular projections
- Hemosiderin pigmentation
- May cause joint destruction if untreated

Clinical Features
- Pain, swelling, stiffness
- Mechanical symptoms (catching, locking)
- Slowly progressive

Diagnosis
- MRI (low signal on T1 and T2 due to hemosiderin)
- Synovial biopsy confirms diagnosis

Treatment
- **Surgical synovectomy** (arthroscopic or open)
- Radiotherapy or targeted molecular therapy in diffuse/recurrent cases

Q29. Explain the role of corticosteroid injections in elbow conditions.

Indications
- *Inflammatory or degenerative conditions including:*
  - Lateral/medial epicondylitis
  - Olecranon bursitis (non-septic)
  - Elbow arthritis
  - Elbow synovitis
  - Distal biceps tendinopathy (with caution)

Mechanism
- Reduces inflammation, pain, and swelling
- Provides temporary symptom relief

Procedure
- Performed under aseptic technique
- Often image-guided for deep/intra-articular targets

Precautions
- Avoid overuse post-injection
- Limit frequency (risk of tendon rupture, skin atrophy)
- Contraindicated in septic conditions

Surgical Procedures and Rehabilitation (Elbow)

Q30. Write a short note on ligament reconstruction in chronic elbow instability.

(JIPMER 2016)

Definition

Surgical repair or reconstruction of collateral ligaments (e.g., **ulnar collateral ligament** in throwers or **lateral ulnar collateral ligament** in posterolateral rotatory instability).

Indications

- Chronic elbow instability
- Failed conservative management
- Recurrent dislocations or subluxations

Procedure

- Autograft (e.g., palmaris longus) or allograft used
- Tensioned and fixed anatomically to restore stability
- Often combined with bony procedures if needed

Q31. Discuss the principles of rehabilitation following elbow surgery.

Goals

- Pain control
- Early mobilization to prevent stiffness
- Gradual strengthening and range of motion (ROM)

Phases

1. *Immediate postoperative (0–2 weeks):* Splinting, edema control, gentle ROM
2. *Early rehabilitation (2–6 weeks):* Passive and active-assisted ROM
3. *Strengthening phase (6–12 weeks):* Light resistance, functional training
4. *Advanced rehabilitation (>3 months):* Sport-specific or occupation-specific training

Considerations

- Close coordination between surgeon and physiotherapist
- Use of hinged braces or continuous passive motion (CPM) devices
- Monitor for signs of heterotopic ossification

Q32. Explain the complications of elbow arthroplasty.

Early

- Infection
- Nerve injury (ulnar neuropathy)
- Wound issues

Late

- Aseptic loosening
- Periprosthetic fracture
- Triceps insufficiency
- Limited ROM or instability
- Polyethylene wear and mechanical failure

Management

Prompt diagnosis and tailored intervention (e.g., antibiotics, revision surgery)

Q33. Write a short note on the use of 3D printing in elbow reconstruction.

Applications
- *Preoperative planning:* Creation of anatomical models from CT scans
- *Patient-specific implants:* Custom plates or prostheses
- *Surgical guides:* For accurate screw/implant placement
- Useful in **complex elbow trauma**, malunions, or congenital deformities

Benefits
- Improves surgical precision
- Reduces operative time
- Enhances outcomes in anatomically challenging cases

Q34. Lateral epicondylitis (tennis tlbow)—pathology, clinical features, and management.

(AIIMS Delhi 2021, MUHS Maharashtra 2022)

Definition

Lateral epicondylitis (Tennis elbow) is an **overuse tendinopathy** involving the **origin of the extensor carpi radialis brevis (ECRB)** muscle at the lateral epicondyle of humerus.

Pathology

Degenerative process:
- **Microtears** at the ECRB origin.
- **Angiofibroblastic hyperplasia** (tendinosis, not true inflammation).
- Histologically shows collagen disorganization, neovascularization.

Risk factors:
- Repetitive wrist extension/supination activities.
- Racquet sports, manual laborers, repetitive computer work.

Clinical Features

Symptoms:
- Gradual onset lateral elbow pain.
- *Pain aggravated by:*
    - Gripping objects.
    - Wrist extension activities (e.g., lifting kettle, opening jar).

Examination:
- Tenderness over lateral epicondyle.
- Pain on resisted wrist extension (Cozen's test positive).
- Pain on resisted middle finger extension (Maudsley's test).
- Full range of elbow motion (differentiates from arthritis).

Diagnosis

Clinical diagnosis mainly.

Imaging:
- X-ray elbow (to rule out arthritis, calcification).
- *MRI/Ultrasound:* Rarely needed; may show ECRB tendon thickening/tears.

Management

Non-Surgical Management of Tennis Elbow

(RGUHS Karnataka 2023, PGI Chandigarh 2022)

Activity modification: Avoid repetitive wrist extension and gripping tasks.

Physiotherapy:
- Eccentric strengthening of wrist extensors.
- Stretching exercises.

Orthotic devices: Counterforce brace (forearm strap) to reduce tension on ECRB.

Medications: NSAIDs for pain relief.

Injections:
- Corticosteroid injection (local infiltration around ECRB)—for short-term symptom relief.
- *Platelet-rich plasma (PRP) injections:* Alternative for chronic cases (promotes tendon healing).

Shockwave therapy: Emerging non-invasive option (stimulates tendon healing).

Surgical Management (Reserved for Persistent Symptoms >6–12 Months)

Procedures:
- Open or arthroscopic **release and debridement of ECRB origin**.
- Removal of degenerated tissue ± lateral epicondylar debridement.

Post-operative care:
- Early mobilization.
- Gradual strengthening.

Exam Tip

When answering Tennis elbow:
- **Mention ECRB tendon involvement and angiofibroblastic degeneration** early.
- Always divide management into **non-surgical (first-line)** and **surgical (for refractory cases)**.
- **Name tests like Cozen's and Maudsley's** clearly for viva points.

Q35. Medial epicondylitis (Golfer's elbow)—clinical features and management.

(Asked in: PGI Chandigarh 2022, RGUHS Karnataka 2023)

Definition

Medial epicondylitis (Golfer's elbow) is an **overuse tendinopathy** affecting the **common flexor-pronator origin** (mainly **flexor carpi radialis** and **pronator teres**) at the **medial epicondyle** of the humerus.

Etiology
- Repetitive wrist flexion and forearm pronation.
- Seen in golfers, throwing athletes, carpenters, and manual laborers.

Clinical Features

Symptoms:
- Pain and tenderness over the medial aspect of the elbow.
- Worsens with activities involving wrist flexion and pronation.
- Decreased grip strength in some cases.

Physical examination:
- Tenderness over medial epicondyle.
- Pain on resisted wrist flexion and pronation.
- Elbow range of motion is usually preserved.

Special tests:

Golfer's elbow test: Pain reproduced by resisted wrist flexion with elbow extended.

Diagnosis

Clinical diagnosis

X-rays (optional): To rule out calcification at the epicondyle or arthritis.

MRI (rarely needed): May show tendinosis or partial tendon tears in chronic cases.

Management

Non-surgical (first line):

- **Rest** and activity modification (avoid provocative activities).
- **NSAIDs** for pain relief.
- **Ice application** over medial elbow.
- *Physiotherapy:*
  - Stretching of flexor-pronator muscles.
  - Eccentric strengthening exercises.
- *Bracing:* Counterforce strap or elbow band over flexor mass.
- *Injections:*
  - Corticosteroid injections for persistent cases.
  - Platelet-rich plasma (PRP) injections (emerging therapy).

Surgical management (reserved for refractory cases after 6–12 months):

- *Medial epicondylar debridement:*
  - Release of degenerative tissue.
  - Repair of flexor-pronator origin if needed.

Post-operative: Early mobilization with strengthening once pain subsides.

Exam Tip

When answering medial epicondylitis:

- **Focus early on flexor carpi radialis + pronator teres involvement.**
- In management, **emphasize conservative therapy first.**
- If mentioning surgery, **state "only after failed non-surgical treatment for 6–12 months."**

Q36. Etiology, diagnosis, and management of cubital tunnel syndrome (ulnar nerve entrapment at elbow).

(Asked in: JIPMER Puducherry 2022, PGI Chandigarh 2021)

Definition

Cubital tunnel syndrome is **compression or irritation of the ulnar nerve** at the **elbow**, specifically in the **cubital tunnel** (posterior to the medial epicondyle).

Etiology

Intrinsic causes:

- Thickening of the Osborne's ligament (roof of cubital tunnel).
- Osteophytes (degenerative arthritis).
- Ganglion cysts.
- Heterotopic ossification (post-trauma).

Extrinsic causes:

- Prolonged elbow flexion (desk jobs, sleeping with bent elbows).
- Valgus instability.
- Direct trauma (contusion or fractures).

Clinical Features

Symptoms:

- Numbness and tingling along the **ulnar distribution** (little finger, half of ring finger).
- Worsening symptoms with elbow flexion.
- Weakness of hand muscles (grip weakness, clumsiness).
- Nocturnal symptoms common.

Signs:

- Positive **Tinel's sign** at cubital tunnel (tap over nerve → tingling).
- Positive **Elbow flexion test** (symptoms worsen on elbow flexion for 60 seconds).
- Wasting of hypothenar eminence and interossei muscles.
- Ulnar claw hand (advanced cases).

Diagnosis

Clinical: History + physical examination.

Nerve conduction studies (NCS)/Electromyography (EMG):

- Gold standard.
- Shows slowed conduction velocity across the elbow.

Imaging:

- X-ray elbow to rule out bony causes (osteophytes, deformities).
- MRI/Ultrasound if soft tissue mass suspected.

Management

Conservative:

- Indicated for mild to moderate symptoms.
- *Activity modification:*
    - Avoid prolonged elbow flexion.
    - Use night-time elbow extension splint.
- NSAIDs for pain.
- Physiotherapy (nerve gliding exercises).

Q37. Describe surgical options for cubital tunnel syndrome.

(MUHS Maharashtra 2023)

Indications for Surgery

- Persistent symptoms despite 3–6 months of conservative management.
- Progressive motor weakness.
- Severe nerve conduction block.

Surgical Procedures

1. *Simple decompression*:
    - Release the roof of the cubital tunnel (Osborne's ligament).
    - No transposition of the nerve.
2. *Anterior transposition*:
    - **Subcutaneous**, **submuscular**, or **subfascial** relocation of ulnar nerve anteriorly.
    - Done to reduce nerve stretch during elbow flexion.
    - Preferred if nerve instability or significant compression.
3. *Medial epicondylectomy*:
    - Resection of a part of the medial epicondyle to decompress the nerve.

Postoperative Care
- Early mobilization encouraged.
- Splinting based on procedure type.
- Gradual strengthening exercises.

Exam Tip
When answering cubital tunnel syndrome:
- **First mention ulnar nerve entrapment behind medial epicondyle.**
- In diagnosis, **always highlight NCS/EMG**.
- In surgical options, **mention simple decompression versus anterior transposition clearly**.

Q38. Olecranon bursitis (non-infective and infective)—causes and management of olecranon bursitis.

(RGUHS Karnataka 2022, AIIMS Delhi 2022)

Definition
Olecranon bursitis is inflammation of the **bursa** overlying the olecranon process of the ulna at the posterior aspect of the elbow.

Etiology
Non-infective (aseptic) causes:
- **Repetitive trauma** or pressure ("student's elbow", "miner's elbow").
- **Inflammatory diseases** (gout, rheumatoid arthritis, pseudogout).
- **Post-traumatic hemorrhagic bursitis** (after direct blow to elbow).

Infective (septic) causes:
- Bacterial infection (commonly Staphylococcus aureus) following:
  - Skin abrasion.
  - Direct inoculation (e.g., injections).
  - Secondary to contiguous infection.

Clinical Features
Symptoms:
- Swelling over posterior elbow.
- Pain (more in septic bursitis).
- Warmth and erythema (suggestive of infection).

Signs:
- Fluctuant swelling at olecranon.
- Tenderness.
- Reduced elbow motion (severe cases).

Key differentiators:
- *In aseptic bursitis:* Swelling is non-tender, non-warm.
- *In septic bursitis:* Swelling is tender, warm, red, sometimes systemic symptoms (fever).

Diagnosis
Clinical examination. Aspiration (if infection suspected):
- *Analyze bursal fluid:* Cell count, Gram stain, culture, crystals (for gout).

X-ray: To rule out underlying fracture, arthritis, or osteomyelitis if chronic.

Management
Non-infective olecranon bursitis:
Conservative:
- Rest and activity modification.
- NSAIDs for pain and inflammation.
- Elbow padding/protection to avoid repeated trauma.
- Aspiration (optional) if large swelling causes discomfort.

Persistent or recurrent cases: Steroid injection into bursa (if infection ruled out).

Rarely surgery: Bursectomy (surgical excision of bursa) if refractory.

Infective (Septic) Olecranon Bursitis
Initial:
- Aspiration for diagnostic confirmation.
- Start empirical antibiotics (e.g., anti-staphylococcal cover like cefazolin).

Further management:
- Repeat aspiration if fluid reaccumulates.
- *Surgical drainage if*:
  - Pus collection,
  - Failure to respond to antibiotics,
  - Overlying skin threatened.

Post-infection care:
- Mobilization once infection resolves.
- Elbow protection during healing phase.

Exam Tip
When answering olecranon bursitis:
- **Always separate non-infective versus infective clearly**.
- **Mention aspiration and analysis** as crucial in diagnosis.
- In management, **start conservatively; escalate to surgery if persistent or septic.**

Elbow Arthritis (Inflammatory and Osteoarthritis)

Q39. Write a note on rheumatoid arthritis of the elbow including clinical features and management.

(PGI Chandigarh 2022, MUHS Maharashtra 2023)

Definition
Rheumatoid arthritis (RA) is a **chronic systemic autoimmune disease** characterized by **synovial inflammation and joint destruction**, commonly affecting small joints including the elbow.

Clinical Features
Symptoms:
- Gradual onset pain and stiffness in elbow.
- Morning stiffness (>30 minutes).
- Swelling and warmth over the joint.
- Decreased range of motion (especially extension).

Signs:
- Effusion, synovial thickening (boggy swelling).
- Tenderness over joint line.

- Progressive loss of motion → Flexion contracture.
- Rheumatoid nodules over extensor surface.
- Instability (late-stage due to ligamentous destruction).

Systemic features:
- Fatigue, anemia, generalized weakness.
- Other joints involved (hands, wrists, knees, etc.)

Diagnosis
Clinical criteria: 2010 ACR/EULAR Rheumatoid Arthritis Classification Criteria.

Investigations:
- Raised ESR, CRP.
- Positive rheumatoid factor (RF) and anti-CCP antibodies.
- *X-ray:* Joint space narrowing, erosions, periarticular osteopenia.

MRI: Early synovitis, bone marrow edema.

Management
Medical (first line):
- *Disease-modifying anti-rheumatic drugs (DMARDs):*
  - Methotrexate (first-line).
  - Leflunomide, Sulfasalazine.
- Biologics (e.g., TNF inhibitors) in refractory cases.
- NSAIDs and corticosteroids for symptomatic relief.

Physiotherapy: ROM exercises to maintain mobility.

Surgical
Indications:
- Pain refractory to medical management.
- Severe functional limitation.

Procedures:
- Synovectomy (early disease with persistent synovitis).
- Total elbow arthroplasty (end-stage joint destruction).
- Arthrodesis (rare; in young manual laborers needing strength over motion).

Q40. Management options in osteoarthritis of the elbow.

(Asked in: AIIMS Delhi 2022)

Definition
- **Osteoarthritis (OA)** of elbow is usually **secondary** to trauma, heavy manual work, or repetitive overuse.
- Primary OA is rare.

Clinical Features
Symptoms:
- Gradual onset pain, stiffness.
- *Mechanical symptoms:* Locking, catching (due to loose bodies).
- Decreased terminal extension initially.

Signs:
- Crepitus on movement.
- Pain at extremes of flexion/extension.

Diagnosis

X-ray:

- Joint space narrowing.
- Osteophyte formation (especially at olecranon and coronoid processes).
- Loose bodies.
- Subchondral sclerosis.

CT scan: Useful to detect small loose bodies and detailed bone assessment.

Management

Non-operative:

- NSAIDs
- Physiotherapy to maintain ROM.
- Activity modification (avoid heavy loading).

Operative:

Early disease:

- *Arthroscopic debridement:*
    - Removal of loose bodies
    - Osteophyte excision (olecranon fossa, coronoid fossa)
    - Capsular release

Advanced disease:

- Open debridement (ulnohumeral arthroplasty/"Outerbridge-Kashiwagi procedure").
- Total elbow arthroplasty (TEA) for severe OA with functional disability (especially elderly, low-demand patients).

Exam Tip

When answering elbow arthritis questions:

- **Mention RA has systemic signs + requires DMARDs.**
- **Osteoarthritis is more mechanical** (pain on activity, loose bodies).
- For both, **early physiotherapy and late surgical options** must be clearly stated.
- **Total Elbow Arthroplasty** is a common final solution in both end-stage RA and OA!

Q41. Causes, prevention, and management of elbow stiffness.

(Asked in: AIIMS Delhi 2022, PGI Chandigarh 2022)

Causes

- Prolonged immobilization.
- Post-traumatic HO formation.
- Intra-articular fractures.
- Poor physiotherapy compliance.

Prevention

- **Early mobilization** (within pain limits).
- Indomethacin post-operative (for HO prevention).
- Radiation therapy in selected cases (rare).

Management

Non-operative:

- Aggressive physiotherapy.
- Static/dynamic splinting.

Surgical:

- *Arthrolysis:* Open or arthroscopic release of adhesions and capsule.

Key Point: Surgery usually delayed until **soft tissue maturation** (~6 months).

Q42. Management of heterotopic ossification.

(MUHS Maharashtra 2023, CMC Vellore 2023).

Prophylaxis
- NSAIDs (Indomethacin) after injury/surgery.
- Radiation therapy (rarely).

Surgical Excision
- After ossification matures (usually after 6 months).
- Followed by aggressive rehabilitation to prevent recurrence.

Heterotopic Ossification Around Elbow (Post-burn, and Neurological)

Q43. Describe heterotopic ossification including etiology, diagnosis, and treatment.

(JIPMER Puducherry 2023, MUHS Maharashtra 2022)

Definition
- *Heterotopic Ossification (HO)*: Abnormal formation of mature lamellar bone in **soft tissues** (muscles, ligaments, joint capsules) **where bone should not normally exist**, especially around joints like **elbow**.

Etiology

Post-traumatic:
- Elbow fractures (supracondylar, distal humerus).
- Elbow dislocations.
- Surgical interventions (ORIF around elbow).

Neurological causes:
- Traumatic brain injury (TBI).
- Spinal cord injury (SCI).

Post-burn injury:
- Severe burns involving upper limbs.
- Prolonged immobilization.

Genetic causes: Fibrodysplasia ossificans progressiva (rare, congenital).

Other factors:
- Prolonged immobilization.
- Aggressive early passive mobilization.

Pathophysiology
- Tissue injury → Mesenchymal cell differentiation → Osteoblast activity → Bone formation within soft tissues.
- Driven by local inflammation, hypoxia, and abnormal signaling (BMP pathway).

Clinical Features

Symptoms:
- Pain, swelling around elbow.
- Stiffness and reduced range of motion (early clue).

Signs:
- Firm, tender swelling (early phase).
- Later hard, palpable mass.
- Decreased flexion-extension arc.
- Possible nerve compression (especially ulnar nerve).

Diagnosis
Clinical suspicion: History of trauma, burns, surgery, or neurological injury.

Imaging:
- *X-ray:*
  - Normal in early stages (first 2–3 weeks).
  - *Later:* Heterotopic bone formation visible after 3–6 weeks.
- *Bone scan (3-phase scintigraphy):*
  - **Earliest method** to detect HO.
  - Increased tracer uptake indicates active bone formation.
- *CT scan:* Detailed anatomical assessment (for surgical planning).

Lab findings:
- Elevated alkaline phosphatase (during active phase).
- Normal calcium and phosphate levels.

Treatment
Prevention (important!):
- **Indomethacin (NSAID)** prophylaxis post-trauma/surgery.
- **Low-dose radiation therapy** (rare nowadays).
- Gentle, controlled ROM exercises (avoid aggressive therapy initially).

Non-operative:
- *Early stage:* Symptomatic treatment with NSAIDs.
- Physiotherapy to maintain available ROM without exacerbating inflammation.

Operative (surgical excision):
- *Indications:*
  - Severe restriction of elbow motion (especially flexion <100°).
  - Nerve compression (e.g., ulnar nerve).
- *Timing:*
  - After **maturation** of HO (around **6 months** post-injury).
  - Radiographic evidence of mature cortical bone and decreased uptake on bone scan.

Post-operative care:
- Indomethacin prophylaxis to prevent recurrence.
- Early mobilization and supervised physiotherapy.

Q44. Role of radiation therapy in preventing heterotopic ossification.

- *HO:* Abnormal bone formation in soft tissues post-trauma/surgery
- *Indications for prophylaxis:* THR, elbow trauma surgery, burns, head injury

Radiation
- *Dose:* 700–800 cGy single dose within 72 hours post-operative
- *Mechanism:* Inhibits mesenchymal cell differentiation into osteoblasts

Alternatives NSAIDs (indomethacin)
Risk: GI upset, delayed bone healing

Exam Tip
When answering HO:
- **Always mention bone scan detects early HO** (important viva point).
- In management, **stress that surgical excision is delayed until maturity (~6 months)** to minimize recurrence risk.
- **Indomethacin prophylaxis** is a must both for prevention and post-excision.

Q45. Cubital tunnel syndrome—diagnosis and management.

(Asked in: JIPMER Puducherry 2022, PGI Chandigarh 2021)

Definition

Compression of **ulnar nerve** at cubital tunnel (around medial elbow).

Clinical Features

- Paresthesias in ulnar distribution (ring and little fingers).
- Hand weakness (especially intrinsic muscles).
- Positive **Tinel's sign** over cubital tunnel.
- Clawing of ulnar fingers in late stages.

Diagnosis

Clinical tests:

- Tinel's sign.
- Elbow flexion test.

Nerve conduction studies (NCS/EMG): Confirm ulnar neuropathy at elbow.

Management

Non-operative:

- Activity modification (avoid elbow flexion >90°).
- Night splinting in extension.
- NSAIDs

Surgical:

- *Indications:* Persistent or progressive symptoms, weakness, EMG changes.
- *Options:*
    - Simple decompression.
    - Anterior transposition of the ulnar nerve (subcutaneous/submuscular).
    - Medial epicondylectomy.

Exam Tip

When answering elbow conditions:

- **Start with clear anatomy → cause → clinical features → diagnosis → management.**
- For trauma topics (olecranon fracture, elbow dislocation), **always mention early mobilization importance**.
- For nerve entrapments (cubital tunnel), **Tinel's sign and NCS confirmation** must be mentioned

Q46. Write a note on synovial plica syndrome of the elbow—diagnosis and treatment.

(Asked in: PGI Chandigarh 2021)

Definition

Synovial plica syndrome refers to **painful mechanical symptoms** caused by **thickened, inflamed remnants of synovial folds** within the elbow joint—particularly in the **radiocapitellar joint**.

Anatomy

- **Synovial plicae** are normal embryological remnants present in ~90% of elbows.
- They become symptomatic when hypertrophied or fibrotic due to repetitive trauma or inflammation.

Etiology

Primary causes:

- Repetitive overuse (throwing athletes, racquet sports).
- Minor trauma leading to synovial irritation and thickening.
- Post-injury or post-surgical scarring inside the elbow joint.

Clinical Features

Symptoms:

- Lateral elbow pain (similar to lateral epicondylitis).
- Clicking, snapping, or catching sensation during elbow motion.
- Pain worsens with elbow extension or pronation-supination movements.

Signs:

- Localized tenderness over the lateral side of elbow (radiocapitellar joint).
- Pain with forearm rotation at 90° elbow flexion.
- Sometimes palpable thickened plica ("snapping" sensation).

Important: Range of motion usually **preserved** (unless associated with chronic fibrosis).

Diagnosis

Clinical diagnosis: Based on characteristic symptoms and examination findings.

Imaging:

- *MRI:*
  - Best investigation.
  - Shows thickened synovial fold interposed between radial head and capitellum.
- *Ultrasound:* Can sometimes detect thickened plica dynamically during movement.

Differential diagnoses:

- Lateral epicondylitis.
- Radial head subluxation.
- Loose bodies.
- Osteochondritis dissecans.

Management

Conservative (first line):

- Rest and activity modification.
- NSAIDs for pain and inflammation.
- Physiotherapy (ROM exercises, strengthening forearm muscles).

Interventional: Local corticosteroid injection into radiocapitellar joint if persistent symptoms.

Surgical (for refractory cases):

- *Arthroscopic resection of synovial plica:*
  - Minimally invasive.
  - Excellent success rates (~85–90% relief).
- Open plica excision is rarely required.

Post-operative care:

- Early ROM exercises.
- Gradual return to sports and full activity over 6–8 weeks.

Exam Tip

When answering about synovial plica syndrome:

- **Emphasize mechanical symptoms (clicking/snapping).**
- **MRI is the investigation of choice.**
- For treatment, **conservative first, arthroscopic resection if persistent.**

Q47. Write a short note on biceps tendon rupture at the elbow.

Definition

- Rupture of the **distal biceps tendon** at radial tuberosity.

Mechanism:
- Sudden eccentric loading of flexed elbow.
- Common in middle-aged males lifting heavy objects.

Clinical Features:
- "Pop" sound, pain, swelling, reverse Popeye sign.
- Weakness in **supination (most affected)** and flexion.

Diagnosis

Hook test, MRI.

Treatment
- **Surgical repair** preferred in active individuals.
- Conservative (non-dominant hand, low-demand patients).

Q48. Explain the clinical features and management of triceps tendon rupture.

Rare but serious injury, often due to trauma or fall on outstretched hand.

Clinical Features
- Posterior elbow pain, swelling.
- Loss of **active extension**.
- Palpable gap above olecranon.

Diagnosis
- X-ray may show avulsion fragment.
- Ultrasound or MRI for tendon integrity.

Management
- **Surgical repair** for complete tears.
- Conservative management for partial tears in low-demand patients (immobilization + rehabilitation).

Q49. Discuss the role of PRP (platelet-rich plasma) in elbow tendinopathies.

Mechanism
- PRP contains concentrated **growth factors (PDGF, TGF-β, VEGF)**.
- Promotes tendon healing via angiogenesis and collagen synthesis.

Indications in Elbow
- **Lateral epicondylitis** (most evidence).
- Medial epicondylitis.
- Adjunct in post-surgical rehabilitation of tendon repairs.

Advantages
- Minimally invasive.
- Avoids steroid side effects.

Limitations
- Mixed evidence.
- Costly and protocol-dependent.

Q50. Tuberculosis of the elbow joint.

Second most common site of TB arthritis in upper limb

Clinical Features
- Insidious pain, swelling
- Gradual loss of motion
- Night cries, constitutional symptoms
- Boggy joint, cold abscess, sinus

Investigations
- *X-ray:* Phemister triad (juxta-articular osteoporosis, marginal erosions, joint space narrowing)
- *MRI:* Early detection
- ESR, CRP elevated
- *Synovial biopsy:* Granulomatous inflammation

Treatment
- ATT (6–12 months)
- Immobilization (initial), followed by gradual mobilization
- *Surgery:* Synovectomy or arthrodesis (rare)

Q51. French osteotomy (short note).

- *Indication:* Correct cubitus varus deformity post supracondylar fracture
- *Technique:* Lateral closing wedge osteotomy (Chevron)
- *Fixation:* Plate/screws or K-wire
- *Advantages:* Simple, effective, restores carrying angle

Q52. Diagnosis and treatment of distal biceps tendinopathy.

Presentation
- Anterior elbow pain, worse with supination/lifting
- Weak supination and flexion

Diagnosis
- Hook test (positive if tendon not palpable)
- MRI/USG confirms tear or tendinosis

Treatment
- *Partial tear/tendinosis:* NSAIDs, rest, physiotherapy, PRP
- *Complete tear:* Surgical repair (single or dual-incision)

Q53. Discuss the anatomical considerations in elbow arthroscopy.

- *Challenges:* Close proximity to neurovascular structures (ulnar, radial, median nerves).
- *Portals:* Anterolateral, anteromedial, posterolateral.
- *Structures at risk:* Ulnar nerve (especially during medial portal).
- *Applications:* Debridement, loose body removal, synovectomy.

Q54. Role of corticosteroid injections in elbow conditions.

Indications
- Lateral epicondylitis (Tennis elbow)
- Medial epicondylitis (Golfer's elbow)
- Olecranon bursitis
- Rheumatoid arthritis synovitis

Mechanism
- Anti-inflammatory
- Breaks pain-spasm cycle

Cautions
- Not for active infection
- Avoid repeated injections (tendon degeneration, rupture risk)

Q55. Radial head excision.

Indications
- Comminuted radial head fracture (Mason Type III) not amenable to fixation.
- Chronic post-traumatic arthritis of radial head.
- Tumor of radial head.
- As salvage in failed fixation or arthroplasty.

Contraindications
- Associated interosseous membrane injury (Essex–Lopresti lesion).
- DRUJ instability.
- Young, active patients.
- Ligamentous elbow instability.

Surgical Approach
- *Lateral (Kocher's approach):*
    - Interval between anconeus and extensor carpi ulnaris.
    - Care to avoid posterior interosseous nerve (PIN).
    - Access radial head and neck for excision.

Q56. Painful elbow—differential diagnosis.

- Lateral epicondylitis (Tennis elbow)
- Medial epicondylitis (Golfer's elbow)
- Olecranon bursitis
- Posterior impingement
- Osteoarthritis or RA
- Radial tunnel syndrome
- Referred pain from cervical spine
- Ligamentous instability (UCL, LCL)
- Ulnar neuritis

Q57. Cubitus valgus.

Definition
Increased carrying angle of elbow >15° (males) or >20° (females).

Causes
- Post-traumatic malunion (especially lateral condyle nonunion).
- Congenital (e.g., Turner syndrome).
- Post-infective sequelae.

Clinical Significance
- May cause tardy ulnar nerve palsy.
- Cosmetic deformity.
- Functional limitation in severe cases.

Management

- Observation if mild.
- Corrective supracondylar osteotomy if functional or cosmetic issues.
- Ulnar nerve transposition in case of palsy.

Q58. Elbow problems in throwing athletes.

Common Issues

- Medial epicondyle apophysitis ("Little League elbow").
- UCL sprain or tear.
- Valgus extension overload syndrome.
- Osteochondritis dissecans of capitellum.
- Posterior impingement.
- Flexor-pronator strain.

Diagnosis

- Clinical exam + valgus stress test.
- MRI/USG for soft tissue injuries.
- X-ray for osteochondral injuries.

Treatment

- Rest, rehabilitation, technique modification.
- PRP or surgical UCL reconstruction (Tommy John surgery) in elite athletes.

Q59. Indications and contraindications of total elbow replacement (TER).

(KMC Manipal 2017)

Indications

- Rheumatoid arthritis with joint destruction.
- Post-traumatic arthritis.
- Non-reconstructible distal humerus fractures in elderly.
- Tumors involving distal humerus.
- Ankylosed or painful elbow affecting quality of life.

Contraindications

- Active infection.
- Inadequate bone stock.
- Young manual laborers (due to lifelong activity restrictions).
- Poor soft tissue envelope.

Q60. Volkmann ischemic contracture (VIC).

Definition

Sequela of untreated or delayed compartment syndrome of forearm, leading to fibrosis and contracture of muscles.

Causes

- Supracondylar fracture of humerus (most common).
- Tight bandages/plaster casts.
- Crush injuries.

Clinical Features

- Flexion contracture of wrist/fingers.
- Clawed hand, weak grip.
- Possible sensory deficits.

Treatment
- Early fasciotomy (acute stage).
- *Late stage:* tendon lengthening, muscle slide procedures (Max Page), osteotomy or functional muscle transfers.

Q61. Radial club hand (radial hemimelia).

Definition
Congenital deficiency of the radius resulting in radial deviation of the hand.

Classification (Bayne and Klug)
Type I–IV based on radial deficiency severity.

Associated Syndromes
- TAR syndrome (thrombocytopenia).
- VACTERL, Fanconi anemia.

Treatment
- Splinting/stretching in early infancy.
- Centralization surgery at 6–12 months.
- Tendon transfers.
- Ulnar lengthening if needed.

7.3 Wrist and Hand Disorders

Rajesh Kapila, Meganath Pawar, Suraydev Aman Singh

Basic Anatomy and Biomechanics of the Hand and Wrist

Q1. Describe the anatomy of the wrist joint in detail.

- *Bones involved:* Distal radius and ulna + 8 carpal bones (scaphoid, lunate, triquetrum, pisiform, trapezium, trapezoid, capitate, hamate)
- *Joints:* Radiocarpal, midcarpal, intercarpal, distal radioulnar
- *Ligaments:* Volar and dorsal radiocarpal, ulnar and radial collateral, TFCC
- *Movements:* Flexion, extension, radial/ulnar deviation, circumduction

Q2. Discuss the biomechanics of wrist motion and stability.

- *Motion:*
  - Flexion (80–90°), extension (70–80°)
  - Radial deviation (~20°), ulnar deviation (~30–40°)
- *Stability:*
  - Provided by bony congruity, ligamentous structures, and TFCC
  - Muscle-tendon units contribute dynamically

Q3. Anatomy of the hand (Key points for theory/viva).

Compartments
- **Thenar** (abductor pollicis brevis, opponens, flexor pollicis brevis)
- **Hypothenar** (abductor/flexor/opponens digiti minimi)
- **Adductor** (adductor pollicis)
- **Central** (lumbricals, tendons of FDP/FDS)
- **Interosseous** (palmar and dorsal interossei)

Blood Supply
- **Superficial palmar arch** (from ulnar artery)
- **Deep palmar arch** (from radial artery)

Nerves
- *Median nerve*: Thenar muscles, lateral two lumbricals, lateral palm sensation
- *Ulnar nerve*: Interossei, medial two lumbricals, hypothenar, medial palm sensation
- *Radial nerve*: No hand muscles, only sensation over dorsum

Flexor Zones (Kanavel's zones)
Used to classify tendon injuries—Zone II is the **"No Man's Land"**

Flexor Tendon Zones (for Fingers II–V)

Zone	*Location*	*Structures involved*	*Clinical significance*
I	From FDS insertion to fingertip	FDP tendon only	Jersey finger injury (FDP avulsion)
II	From FDS insertion to A1 pulley (middle of middle phalanx to distal palmar crease)	FDS and FDP tendons in a tight sheath	"No man's land" – challenging due to high adhesion risk

Continued

Continued

Zone	*Location*	*Structures involved*	*Clinical significance*
III	Palm—from A1 pulley to distal edge of transverse carpal ligament	Tendons + lumbricals	Better prognosis; wide exposure possible
IV	Carpal tunnel region	Tendons + median nerve	Risk of median nerve injury, fibrosis
V	Forearm proximal to wrist crease	Muscle–tendon junctions, multiple tendons	Often associated with nerve/artery injuries

Thumb Flexor Zones

Zone	*Location*	*Structures involved*
TI	Distal to IP joint	FPL
TII	From IP to MCP joint	FPL within tendon sheath
TIII	Thenar region	FPL + thenar muscles

Why It Matters (Clinical Importance)

- *Helps guide surgical approach and prognosis*:
  - **Zone II** has poor prognosis due to narrow space, dual tendons (FDS and FDP), and synovial sheath → prone to **adhesions** and scarring.
- **Post-operative rehabilitation** differs by zone (early mobilization crucial in Zones I–II).
- Understanding helps identify **injured structures** and plan **appropriate tendon repair**.

Mnemonic for Fingers (I–V)

"Find The Palmar Carpal Forearm"

- *F*: Fingertip (Zone I)
- *T*: Tendon sheath area (Zone II - "No man's land")
- *P*: Palmar (Zone III)
- *C*: Carpal tunnel (Zone IV)
- *F*: Forearm (Zone V)

Q4. Write a short note on the intrinsic and extrinsic muscles of the hand.

(Christian Medical College Vellore 2017)

- *Extrinsic muscles:*
  - Originate in forearm
  - Flexor (FDS, FDP, FPL), Extensor (ED, EPL, EPB, EI)
- *Intrinsic muscles:*
  - Thenar (APB, FPB, OP), hypothenar (ADM, FDM, ODM), lumbricals, interossei
  - Fine motor control, precision grip

Q5. Describe the blood supply of the hand and its clinical significance.

- *Main arteries:*
  - Radial artery (forms deep palmar arch)
  - Ulnar artery (forms superficial palmar arch)
- *Clinical note:*
  - Allen's test used before radial artery cannulation
  - Rich collateral supply helps with ischemia resistance

Q6. Discuss the anatomy and function of the flexor and extensor tendons of the hand.

- *Flexor tendons:*
  - FDS (inserts middle phalanx), FDP (distal phalanx)
  - Run through fibrous sheaths with synovial lining

- *Extensor tendons:*
  - ED, EPL, EPB, EI, EDM
  - Pass under extensor retinaculum; dorsal compartments

Q7. Explain the importance of the TFCC in wrist stability.

- *TFCC (triangular fibrocartilage complex):*
  - Composed of fibrocartilage disc, meniscus homologue, radioulnar ligaments
  - Stabilizes distal radioulnar joint (DRUJ)
  - Absorbs axial load across ulnocarpal joint
  - Injury → pain with pronation/supination, DRUJ instability

Q8. Write a short note on the biomechanics of grip and pinch.

(RGUHS)

- *Grip:* Power grip uses extrinsic flexors (FDS, FDP), intrinsic stabilizers (lumbricals, interossei)
- *Pinch:* Precision grip involves thenar muscles (especially FPL, OP) and index finger flexors
- *Key factors:* Wrist extension enhances finger flexion strength (tenodesis effect)

Ligament and Soft Tissue Injuries of the Wrist and Hand

Q9. Surgical anatomy of lower end of radius.

Articular Surfaces

- *Distal end articulates with:*
  - **Scaphoid (lateral facet)**
  - **Lunate (medial facet)**
  - **Ulna (at sigmoid notch)**

Important Landmarks

- *Lister's tubercle*: Dorsal bony prominence, separates EPL and ECRB tendons
- *Radial styloid*: Lateral projection
- *Volar tilt:* ~11°
- *Radial inclination:* ~22°
- *Length difference with ulna:* ~11 mm (ulnar variance)

Tendon Relations

- *Dorsally:* Extensor tendons (in 6 compartments)
- *Ventrally:* Flexor tendons, FCR and FPL

Q10. Write a short note on anatomy of the deep palmar space.

The **deep palmar space** is one of the **three major palmar spaces** of the hand.

Location

Lies **deep to the flexor tendons** of the fingers and **superficial to the metacarpals** and interossei.

Boundaries

- *Anterior (volar):* Flexor tendons and lumbricals
- *Posterior (dorsal):* Metacarpal bones and interossei
- *Lateral:* Mid-palmar septum (extends from palmar aponeurosis to 3rd metacarpal)
- *Medial:* Hypothenar septum

Contents
- Tendons of **flexor digitorum profundus (FDP)**
- 3rd and 4th **lumbricals**
- **Deep palmar arch**
- **Metacarpal bones**

Clinical Significance
- Common site for **deep space infections** (e.g., from spread of infected tendon sheaths)
- Presents with **swelling on dorsum of hand**, pain with finger movements

Q11. Describe potential spaces of the hand.

These are **normally collapsed spaces** that can expand with infection or fluid collection.

Palmar Spaces
1. *Thenar space*:
   - Between thenar muscles and adductor pollicis
   - Infected from index finger synovial sheath
2. *Mid-palmar space*:
   - Between flexor tendons and interossei of 3rd–5th fingers
   - Infected from middle/ring/little fingers
3. *Parona's space (forearm)*:
   - Between pronator quadratus and FDP
   - Continuation of flexor tendon sheath infections

Dorsal Spaces
- *Dorsal subaponeurotic space:* Between extensor tendons and metacarpals
- *Dorsal subcutaneous space:* Just under the skin

Q12. Describe intrinsic and extrinsic muscles of the hand.

(KEM 2015)

Intrinsic Muscles (Origin and Insertion Within the Hand)
- *Thenar muscles:* Abductor pollicis brevis, flexor pollicis brevis, opponens pollicis
- *Hypothenar muscles:* Abductor digiti minimi, flexor digiti minimi, opponens digiti minimi
- *Lumbricals:* Flex MCP, extend PIP and DIP (via extensor expansion)
- *Interossei:*
  - *Palmar (3):* Adduct fingers (PAD)
  - *Dorsal (4):* Abduct fingers (DAB)
- **Adductor pollicis**

Extrinsic Muscles (Originate in Forearm, Insert into Hand)
- *Flexors:* FDS, FDP, FPL
- *Extensors:* EDC, EPL, EPB, APL, EI, EDM

Function
- *Intrinsic:* Fine motor control, precision grip
- *Extrinsic:* Power grip, gross movement

Q13. Describe blood supply of the hand and clinical significance.

Main Arteries
- **Ulnar artery** → Superficial palmar arch
- **Radial artery** → Deep palmar arch

Branches
- **Superficial arch** → Common palmar digital arteries → Proper digital arteries
- **Deep arch** → Palmar metacarpal arteries

Clinical Significance
- *Allen's test:* Assesses patency of radial/ulnar arteries before cannulation/surgery
- *Vascular injury:* Can lead to ischemia or Volkmann's contracture
- *Replantation surgery:* Requires microsurgical identification of arterial supply

Q14. Describe anatomy and function of flexor and extensor tendons.

Flexor Tendons
- **FDS**: Inserts into middle phalanx → flexes PIP
- **FDP**: Inserts into distal phalanx → flexes DIP
- **FPL**: Inserts into distal thumb phalanx

Zones (Verdan's Classification)
Zone II: "No man's land" (FDS + FDP within flexor sheath)

Extensor Tendons
- *EDC*: Inserts via extensor expansion into middle and distal phalanges
- *EPL/EPB/APL*: Thumb extensors/abductors

Dorsal Compartments (6)
For example 1st: APL, EPB (De Quervain's)

Function
- *Flexors:* Gripping and grasping
- *Extensors:* Releasing, fine control

Q15. Describe biomechanics of grip and pinch.

Grip Types
1. *Power grip*:
   - Whole hand grasps object (e.g., hammer)
   - Uses extrinsic muscles + wrist stabilizers
2. *Precision grip*:
   - Thumb + fingertips (e.g., writing)
   - Involves intrinsic muscles

Pinch Types
- *Key pinch:* Thumb + lateral index
- *Tip pinch:* Tip of thumb + index
- *Palmar pinch:* 3-finger pinch

Key Biomechanics
- Requires intact thumb opposition
- Balanced flexor–extensor activity
- Normal wrist extension enhances grip via **tenodesis effect**

Q16. Describe significance of carpal arch and flexor retinaculum.

(AIMS Kochi 2019)

Carpal Arch
- Concavity formed by **carpal bones**
- Roofed by **flexor retinaculum (transverse carpal ligament)**
- Forms **carpal tunnel**

Contents of Carpal Tunnel

- **Median nerve**
- **9 tendons**: FDS (4), FDP (4), FPL (1)

Flexor Retinaculum

- Prevents bowstringing of flexor tendons
- Acts as pulley system

Clinical Relevance

- *Carpal tunnel syndrome:* Compression of median nerve under retinaculum
- Surgical release involves cutting the retinaculum

Q17. Describe distal radioulnar joint (DRUJ) anatomy.

Structure

- *Formed by:*
  - **Ulnar notch of radius**
  - **Head of ulna**
- *Joint type:* **Pivot synovial joint**
- *Allows:* **Pronation-supination of forearm**

Stabilizers

- *Primary:* **Triangular fibrocartilage complex (TFCC)**
- *Secondary:*
  - Interosseous membrane (distal part)
  - Extensor carpi ulnaris (ECU) subsheath

TFCC Components

- Articular disc
- Meniscus homologue
- Dorsal/volar radioulnar ligaments
- Ulnar collateral ligament
- ECU sheath

Q18. Describe functions of the hand.

Function	*Structures involved*
Power grip	Long flexors, extensors, intrinsic muscles
Precision/Pinch	Thumb opposition, index/middle fingers
Sensation	Dense mechanoreceptors (especially fingertips)
Expression	Gestures, sign language
Manipulation	Fine movements, writing, tools use

Thumb is responsible for ~40% of hand function.

Q19. Importance of triangular fibrocartilage complex (TFCC) in wrist stability.

(DYPU Pune 2019)

Components

- Articular disc (main TFCC)
- Dorsal/volar radioulnar ligaments
- Ulnar collateral ligament
- Meniscus homologue
- ECU tendon sheath

Function

- Stabilizes **DRUJ**
- Cushions between **ulna and carpus**
- Transmits load (20% of axial load through ulna)

Clinical Relevance

- **TFCC injury** → ulnar-sided wrist pain
- Seen in trauma, repetitive strain (e.g., gymnastics)
- Diagnosed via **MRI or wrist arthroscopy**
- Treated with splinting or arthroscopic debridement/repair

Q20. Explain the pathophysiology and treatment of TFCC injuries.

- *Pathophysiology:*
  - Triangular fibrocartilage complex (TFCC) stabilizes the distal radioulnar joint (DRUJ) and ulnar carpus.
  - Injuries may result from trauma (FOOSH) or degenerative wear.
- *Symptoms:* Ulnar-sided wrist pain, clicking, decreased grip strength
- *Diagnosis:* MRI, wrist arthroscopy (gold standard)
- *Treatment:*
  - *Conservative:* Splinting, NSAIDs, steroid injection
  - *Surgical:* Arthroscopic debridement or repair (for central/ulnar tears)

Q21. Write a short note on scapholunate ligament injuries.

- *Mechanism:* FOOSH injury with wrist extension and ulnar deviation
- *Findings:*
  - Pain over dorsal wrist
  - Watson's test is positive
  - Widened scapholunate interval on X-ray (>3 mm = Terry Thomas sign)
- *Management:*
  - *Early:* Casting
  - *Late/Chronic:* Ligament repair, tendon graft, or partial wrist fusion

Q22. Discuss the clinical presentation and management of lunotriquetral ligament injuries.

(MUHS 2012)

- *Presentation:*
  - Ulnar-sided wrist pain
  - Pain exacerbated by ulnar deviation or grip
- *Diagnosis:*
  - MRI or wrist arthroscopy
  - Ballottement (Reagan's) test may reproduce symptoms
- *Management:*
  - Immobilization for minor tears
  - Arthroscopic or open repair for complete tears
  - Fusion in chronic instability

Q23. Carpal instability—midcarpal instability (MCI).

Definition

Abnormal movement between **proximal and distal carpal rows**, especially at **capitate–lunate interface**

Causes
- Ligamentous laxity
- Wrist trauma (e.g., perilunate injury)
- Repetitive loading (gymnasts, weightlifters)

Types
- *Volar intercalated segment instability (VISI):* Lunate tilts volarly (often after lunotriquetral ligament injury)
- *Dorsal intercalated segment instability (DISI)*: Lunate tilts dorsally (after scapholunate ligament injury)

Signs
- **"Clunk" during ulnar to radial deviation**
- Pain, reduced grip strength

Treatment
- Wrist splints, proprioceptive therapy (early)
- Surgery for chronic/failed cases—ligament reconstruction or partial arthrodesis

Q24. Describe scapholunate ligament injuries—short note.

Function
Connects **scaphoid** and **lunate**; stabilizes carpal mechanics

Injury Mechanism
- Fall on outstretched hand
- Causes **rotational instability**, leading to **DISI**

Clinical
- Dorsal wrist pain
- Clicking
- Positive **Watson test**

Radiology
- SL gap >3 mm ("**Terry Thomas sign**")
- DISI (dorsal tilt of lunate)
- "Ring sign" of flexed scaphoid

Treatment
- *Acute:* Direct ligament repair
- *Chronic:*
  - Partial wrist arthrodesis (e.g., 4-corner)
  - Proximal row carpectomy
  - SLAC wrist requires salvage surgery

Q25. Lunotriquetral ligament injuries—clinical and management.

Function
Links **lunate** and **triquetrum**, maintaining **VISI** stability

Mechanism
- FOOSH (fall on outstretched hand)
- Ulnar deviation injury

Clinical
- Ulnar-sided wrist pain
- Pain during ulnar deviation and grip

- Clicking/Snapping
- Positive **Ballottement test**

Radiology
- Often normal on plain X-rays
- VISI pattern on lateral view (lunate tilted volarly)
- MRI or arthrogram confirms diagnosis

Management
- *Acute:* Cast immobilization (6 weeks)
- *Persistent:* Arthroscopic repair or open ligament reconstruction
- *Chronic:* Ulnar-side fusion (LT fusion or lunate replacement)

Q26. Role of arthroscopy in wrist ligament injuries.

(GGMC 2018)

Advantages
- Minimally invasive
- **Diagnostic + therapeutic** in same setting
- Visualize TFCC, SL, and LT ligaments directly
- Classify injury severity (e.g., Palmer classification for TFCC)

Procedures
- **Debridement** of tears (e.g., TFCC)
- **Thermal shrinkage** or repair of SL/LT ligaments
- Synovectomy in inflammatory conditions

Indications
- Chronic ulnar wrist pain
- Unexplained mechanical symptoms
- Post-traumatic instability (TFCC, SL, LT)
- Diagnostic aid when MRI is inconclusive

Q27. Carpal instability—midcarpal instability (MCI).

Definition
Abnormal movement between **proximal and distal carpal rows**, especially at **capitate–lunate interface**.

Causes
- Ligamentous laxity
- Wrist trauma (e.g., perilunate injury)
- Repetitive loading (gymnasts, weightlifters)

Types
- *Volar intercalated segment instability (VISI)*: Lunate tilts volarly (often after lunotriquetral ligament injury)
- *Dorsal intercalated segment instability (DISI):* Lunate tilts dorsally (after scapholunate ligament injury)

Signs
- **"Clunk" during ulnar to radial deviation**
- Pain, reduced grip strength

Treatment
- Wrist splints, proprioceptive therapy (early)
- Surgery for chronic/failed cases—ligament reconstruction or partial arthrodesis

Q28. De Quervain's tenosynovitis.

Q. Decribe diagnosis and management of De Quervain's disease.

(Asked in: PGI Chandigarh 2022, RGUHS Karnataka 2023)

Definition
- **De Quervain's Tenosynovitis**: **Stenosing tenosynovitis** of the **first dorsal compartment** of the wrist, involving the:
  - **Abductor pollicis longus (APL)**
  - **Extensor pollicis brevis (EPB)** tendons.

Etiology

Overuse injury: Repetitive thumb abduction and extension movements (lifting babies, golfers, racquet sports).

Inflammation and thickening: Of the extensor retinaculum → tendon entrapment → pain and limited thumb motion.

Risk factors:
- Middle-aged women.
- Pregnancy and postpartum period (fluid retention and repetitive lifting).

Clinical Features

Symptoms:
- Pain over **radial side** of wrist.
- *Pain aggravated by:*
  - Thumb movement (especially abduction and extension).
  - Grasping and lifting objects.

Signs:
- Tenderness over radial styloid.
- Swelling/thickening palpable at the first dorsal compartment.

Key diagnostic test:
- **Finkelstein Test** (see below).

Diagnosis

Clinical diagnosis: Based on symptoms, examination, and positive Finkelstein test.

Imaging:
- Not routinely needed.
- Ultrasound: May show thickened tendons and sheath.
- *MRI*: Only in doubtful or atypical cases.

Management

Conservative (first line):
- Rest and activity modification.
- Thumb spica splint (immobilizing wrist and thumb).
- NSAIDs for pain and inflammation.
- *Local corticosteroid injection into first dorsal compartment:* High success rate (~80–90% with single injection).

Surgical (Indications: Failure of conservative therapy after 3–6 months):
- *First dorsal compartment release:*
  - Longitudinal incision over the radial styloid.
  - Open the extensor retinaculum.
  - Release entrapped tendons.
- Care must be taken to protect **superficial radial nerve** branches.

Postoperative care:
- Early mobilization encouraged to prevent stiffness.
- Gradual return to activities.

Exam Tip

When answering De Quervain's disease:
- **Always highlight APL and EPB involvement.**
- **Clearly describe Finkelstein test procedure and positivity.**
- Management is **conservative first, surgery for resistant cases.**

Q29. Describe Finkelstein test and its significance.

(Asked in: MUHS Maharashtra 2022).

Procedure:
- Patient flexes the thumb into the palm.
- Fingers are closed over the thumb (making a fist).
- Examiner ulnarly deviates the wrist.

Positive Test

Sharp pain along the radial aspect of the wrist.

Significance
- Highly sensitive for **De Quervain's tenosynovitis.**
- Indicates entrapment and inflammation of APL and EPB tendons.

Q30. Pathology, clinical features, and management of Dupuytren's contracture.

(Asked in: AIIMS Delhi 2021, MUHS Maharashtra 2023)

Definition

Dupuytren's contracture is a **progressive fibrosing disorder** of the **palmar fascia**, leading to **fixed flexion deformities** of the fingers.

Pathology

Key mechanism: Abnormal proliferation of **fibroblasts** and **myofibroblasts** → collagen deposition (mainly type III collagen) → nodule and cord formation.

Structures involved:
- Pretendinous bands.
- Spiral bands.
- Natatory ligaments (in severe cases).

Risk factors:
- Genetic predisposition (autosomal dominant).
- Male sex (common after 40 years).
- Northern European ancestry ("Viking disease").
- Diabetes mellitus.
- Chronic alcohol intake.
- Epilepsy (long-term phenytoin use).

Clinical Features

Symptoms:
- Painless nodules on the palmar side of hand.
- Gradual flexion contracture of fingers.

Common sites:
- **Ring finger** (most common) > Little finger > Middle finger.
- Bilateral in up to 45% cases.

Signs:
- Palpable firm cords along flexor surfaces.
- Inability to fully extend affected fingers (measured using Hueston's tabletop test—positive if hand can not lay flat on table).

Associated conditions:
- Plantar fibromatosis (Ledderhose disease).
- Penile fibromatosis (Peyronie's disease).

Diagnosis
Clinical diagnosis:
- Based on examination.
- No imaging usually needed.

Special tests:
- *Hueston's tabletop test:* Patient cannot place palm flat on the table—contracture significant.

Management
Conservative:
- *Early nodules without contracture:* Observation only.
- Splinting or stretching has limited success; not routinely recommended.

Indications for surgery:
- MCP joint flexion contracture >30°.
- Any functional PIP joint contracture.

Surgical Options *(Asked in: PGI Chandigarh 2022)*
1. *Needle aponeurotomy*:
   - Percutaneous division of cords using a needle.
   - Minimally invasive, high recurrence.
2. *Collagenase injection (Xiaflex)*:
   - Enzyme injection to dissolve cords.
   - Followed by manipulation after 24–48 hours.
3. *Limited fasciectomy (most common)*:
   - Excision of diseased fascia only.
   - Preferred for moderate disease.
   - Care to protect digital neurovascular bundles.
4. *Dermofasciectomy*:
   - Excision of skin and fascia, followed by skin grafting.
   - Indicated for recurrent or aggressive disease.
5. *Amputation*: Rare, reserved for severe recurrent deformities in elderly non-functional hands.

Postoperative Care
- Hand therapy with splints.
- Regular stretching exercises.

Exam Tip
When writing about Dupuytren's contracture:
- **Start with palmar fascia fibrosis and collagen type III deposition.**
- **Mention Hueston's tabletop test for diagnosis.**
- In surgery, **differentiate needle aponeurotomy, limited fasciectomy, and dermofasciectomy** clearly.

Q31. Pathophysiology and treatment of trigger finger (stenosing tenosynovitis).

(Asked in: JIPMER Puducherry 2022, RGUHS Karnataka 2022)

Definition

Trigger finger is a **stenosing tenosynovitis** of the **flexor tendon sheath**, leading to **painful catching, clicking, or locking** during finger movement.

Pathophysiology

Anatomy:
- Tendons of flexor digitorum superficialis (FDS) and flexor digitorum profundus (FDP) glide through a fibro-osseous tunnel supported by pulley systems.
- **A1 pulley** (at the level of the MCP joint) is most commonly involved.

Mechanism:
- Chronic inflammation → Thickening of A1 pulley.
- Tendon nodule formation → Disruption of smooth tendon gliding.

Cycle: Repeated trauma/inflammation → Fibrosis and narrowing of pulley → Tendon catches or locks on attempting flexion-extension.

Risk factors:
- Diabetes mellitus (most important).
- Rheumatoid arthritis.
- Repetitive gripping activities.
- Female sex (middle-aged women).

Clinical Features

Symptoms:
- Pain and tenderness over the A1 pulley (palmar MCP region).
- Clicking, popping, or locking sensation while flexing the finger.
- Morning stiffness.
- Inability to extend the finger (in severe cases).

Signs:
- Palpable nodule at A1 pulley.
- Active/passive snapping during finger motion.
- In late stages, fixed flexion contracture.

Most commonly involved: Ring finger > Thumb > Middle finger > Little finger > Index finger.

Diagnosis

Clinical diagnosis:
- Based on history and physical examination.
- No imaging required unless atypical.

Treatment

A. Conservative Management:

First line for mild to moderate cases:
- Activity modification (reduce repetitive gripping).
- NSAIDs for pain relief.
- **Splinting** (MCP joint in extension) to rest the tendon.

Corticosteroid injection:
- Into the flexor sheath at A1 pulley.
- High success rate (up to 70–80%).
- Especially effective in early-stage and non-diabetic patients.

B. Surgical Management

Indications:

- Failed conservative management after 2 steroid injections.
- Persistent locking or fixed deformity.
- Diabetics (less responsive to injections).

Procedures:

1. *Percutaneous release*:
   - Needle used to divide A1 pulley.
   - Minimally invasive; quicker recovery.
2. *Open surgical release*:
   - Direct incision over A1 pulley.
   - Complete release under vision.
   - Preferred in recurrent cases, diabetics, or multiple digit involvement.

Post-operative Care

- Early mobilization encouraged.
- Full functional recovery usually within 2–4 weeks.

Exam Tip

When answering Trigger Finger:

- **Clearly mention A1 pulley involvement** early.
- **Explain pathology as "tendon nodule + pulley narrowing"**.
- Treatment starts conservatively; surgery is definitive for resistant cases.

Peripheral Nerve Injuries and Compression Syndromes

Q32. Carpal tunnel syndrome (CTS)—clinical features, diagnosis, and management.

(Asked in: AIIMS Delhi 2022, PGI Chandigarh 2021)

Definition

Carpal tunnel syndrome: **Compression of the median nerve** at the level of the carpal tunnel (wrist).

Anatomy

- *Carpal tunnel formed by:*
  - *Floor and sides:* Carpal bones.
  - *Roof:* Flexor retinaculum (transverse carpal ligament).
- *Structures inside:*
  - Median nerve,
  - 9 flexor tendons (FDS, FDP, FPL).

Etiology

Idiopathic (most common).

Secondary causes:

- Rheumatoid arthritis.
- Diabetes mellitus.
- Hypothyroidism.
- Pregnancy (fluid retention).
- Obesity.
- Repetitive wrist flexion activities.

Clinical Features

Symptoms:

- Numbness, tingling (paresthesia) in **median nerve distribution**:
  - Thumb, index, middle, and radial half of ring finger.
- Nocturnal worsening (patients may shake hand for relief—"flick sign").
- Weakness in thumb opposition (thenar muscles).
- Clumsiness (dropping objects).

Signs:

- *Tinel's sign:* Tapping over carpal tunnel reproduces tingling.
- *Phalen's test:* Wrist flexion for 60 seconds reproduces symptoms.
- Thenar muscle atrophy (late stage).
- Decreased two-point discrimination (>5 mm abnormal).

Diagnosis

Clinical examination: Primary method.

Electrodiagnostic studies:

- *Nerve conduction velocity (NCV):* Slowing across carpal tunnel.
- *Electromyography (EMG):* Denervation of thenar muscles (advanced disease).

Ultrasound/MRI:

- Rarely needed.
- May show median nerve swelling.

Q33. Carpal tunnel syndrome versus pronator syndrome.

Feature	CTS	Pronator syndrome
Nerve	Median	Median
Site	Wrist	Proximal forearm
Symptoms	Night symptoms common	Daytime symptoms
Sensory loss	Thenar area spared (palmar branch unaffected)	Thenar area affected
Tinel's sign	Positive at wrist	Negative
Treatment	Wrist splint, surgery	Stretching, rare surgery

Q34. Clinical tests for diagnosing carpal tunnel syndrome (CTS).

CTS is compression of the **median nerve** at the **carpal tunnel**.

Common Clinical Tests

Test	Description	Positive sign
Tinel's sign	Tapping over carpal tunnel	Tingling in median nerve distribution
Phalen's test	Wrist flexion for 60 seconds	Numbness/tingling in thumb, index, middle
Durkan's test	Direct pressure over carpal tunnel	Reproduces symptoms
Thenar atrophy	Wasting of thenar eminence	Late sign of chronic compression
Nerve conduction study	Measures motor/sensory conduction	Reduced velocity across wrist

Q35. Differences between carpal tunnel syndrome versus pronator syndrome.

Feature	Carpal tunnel syndrome (CTS)	Pronator syndrome
Compression site	Under flexor retinaculum (carpal tunnel)	At pronator teres or proximal forearm
Sensory loss	Thenar area spared (palmar cutaneous nerve bypasses tunnel)	Palmar and dorsal median distribution affected
Nocturnal symptoms	Common	Rare
Phalen's/Tinel's	Positive	Negative
Forearm pain	Uncommon	Common

Q36. Compare conservative versus surgical treatment of CTS.

(Asked in: MUHS Maharashtra 2022, JIPMER Puducherry 2022)

Conservative Treatment (First-line for Mild to Moderate CTS)
Lifestyle modification: Activity modification (avoid repetitive wrist movements).

Splinting: Night-time wrist splint in neutral position.

Medications:
- NSAIDs for pain relief.
- Short course of oral steroids.

Steroid injections:
- Local corticosteroid injection into carpal tunnel.
- Good short-term relief but recurrence common.

Indications:
- Mild symptoms.
- Early-stage disease.
- Pregnancy-related CTS (usually resolves postpartum).

Surgical Treatment
Indications:
- Failed conservative management (after 6 weeks to 3 months).
- Severe symptoms (thenar wasting, motor weakness).
- Positive electrodiagnostic studies showing severe compression.

Surgical options:
- *Open carpal tunnel release:* Division of transverse carpal ligament.
- *Endoscopic carpal tunnel release:*
  - Minimally invasive.
  - Faster recovery, less scar tenderness.

Postoperative Care
- Early finger motion.
- Wrist splinting (briefly).
- Physiotherapy if stiffness develops.

Comparison Summary

Feature	Conservative	Surgical
Indication	Mild-moderate CTS	Severe or refractory CTS
Methods	Splint, NSAIDs, steroid injection	Open or endoscopic ligament release

Continued

Continued

Feature	Conservative	Surgical
Success rate	30–70% temporary relief	>90% long-term relief
Risk	Recurrence common	Surgical complications (scar, pillar pain, nerve injury rare)

Exam Tip

When answering CTS:

- **First describe anatomy, symptoms, and two clinical tests.**
- Always **mention NCV/EMG as diagnostic confirmation.**
- Clearly **compare conservative versus surgical**, including indications and success rates.

Q37. Radial nerve palsy affecting the hand—management.

- *Types:*
  - High lesion (e.g., spiral groove) → wrist drop, sensory loss on dorsum of hand.
  - Posterior interosseous nerve (PIN) → motor only (finger extension loss).
- *Management:*
  - *Conservative:* Splinting, PT.
  - *Surgery:* Tendon transfers (e.g., for wrist extension).

Q38. Wartenberg's syndrome (superficial radial nerve entrapment).

- *Cause:* Compression between brachioradialis and ECRL tendons.
- *Symptoms:* Burning, tingling over dorsoradial hand.
- *Aggravating factors:* Watch strap, tight cuffs.
- *Treatment:* Avoid compression, NSAIDs, surgical release if persistent.

Q39. Ulnar nerve entrapment at Guyon's canal.

- *Location:* Wrist-level compression (cyclist's palsy).
- *Zones:*
  - *Zone 1:* Mixed (motor + sensory)
  - *Zone 2:* Motor only
  - *Zone 3:* Sensory only
- *Symptoms:* Sensory loss in little finger + weakness in intrinsic hand muscles.
- *Treatment:* Splinting, activity modification, decompression surgery if needed.

Arthritis and Degenerative Conditions of the Hand and Wrist

Q40. Wrist osteoarthritis—classification and management.

- *Types:*
  - Primary OA (rare)
  - *Secondary OA (common)*: Post-traumatic (e.g. SLAC, SNAC wrist)
- *Stages:*
  - *SLAC wrist:* Scapholunate advanced collapse (due to SL ligament injury)
  - *SNAC wrist:* Scaphoid nonunion advanced collapse
- *Management:*
  - *Conservative:* NSAIDs, splints, corticosteroid injections.

- *Surgical:*
  - Proximal row carpectomy
  - Four-corner fusion
  - Total wrist arthrodesis/arthroplasty

Q41. Rheumatoid hand deformities.

(Asked in: PGI Chandigarh 2022, MUHS Maharashtra 2023)

Overview

- Rheumatoid arthritis (RA) causes **progressive synovitis** and **ligamentous laxity**, leading to **hand deformities** due to:
  - Joint instability
  - Tendon rupture
  - Soft tissue imbalance

Common Hand Deformities

1. *Swan neck deformity*:
   - **Hyperextension of PIP joint + flexion of DIP joint.**
   - *Causes:*
     - Volar plate attenuation
     - FDS tendon imbalance
     - Tight intrinsic muscles
2. *Boutonniere deformity*:
   - **Flexion of PIP joint + hyperextension of DIP joint.**
   - *Causes:*
     - Central slip rupture,
     - Volar migration of lateral bands.
3. *Ulnar deviation and subluxation at MCP joints*: Due to synovitis, radial collateral ligament weakening, volar subluxation of proximal phalanges.
4. *Z deformity of thumb*: Flexion of MCP joint + hyperextension of IP joint.
5. *Mutilans deformity (arthritis mutilans)*: Severe destruction leading to "**telescoping fingers**" (opera glass hand).
6. *Tendon ruptures*: *Vaughan-Jackson syndrome:* sequential extensor tendon ruptures from ulnar to radial side.

Q42. Boutonnière deformity.

Non-surgical (Early, Reducible Deformity)

- PIP joint splint in extension (6 weeks)
- Allow DIP joint movement
- Start active/passive mobilization after splinting

Surgical

Persistent deformity:

- Central slip reconstruction
- Dorsal repositioning of lateral bands

Advanced deformity: PIP joint arthrodesis.

General Principles

- Early management with **DMARDs** is crucial to prevent deformities.
- In late-stage deformities, **function > cosmetic correction.**
- **Fusion (arthrodesis)** is often the best choice for **severe fixed deformities.**

Exam Tip

- **List Swan Neck → Boutonnière → Ulnar Deviation → Z Deformity → Mutilans** sequentially.
- In treatment, **always divide early versus late management**.
- Emphasize **fusion for late-stage fixed joints**.

Q43. Management of swan neck.

(Asked in: AIIMS Delhi 2022)

Swan Neck Deformity

- *Non-surgical (early, flexible deformity)*:
  - Silver ring splints/custom splints to block PIP hyperextension.
  - Physiotherapy to maintain mobility.
  - **Surgical**
- *Mild/early stage*:
  - Intrinsic release
  - Volar plate advancement.
- *Late stage (fixed deformity)*:
  - PIP joint arthrodesis (~30° flexion position)
  - Rarely PIP joint arthroplasty.

Q44. Thumb CMC arthritis—pathophysiology and treatment.

- *Pathophysiology:* Degeneration of trapeziometacarpal joint → instability, subluxation
- *Symptoms:* Pain at base of thumb, worsened by pinch/grip
- *Treatment:*
  - *Conservative:* NSAIDs, splints, steroid injections
  - *Surgical:*
    - Trapeziectomy ± ligament reconstruction/tendon interposition (LRTI)
    - CMC arthrodesis or implant arthroplasty

Q45. Psoriatic arthritis of the hand—clinical features and treatment.

- *Features:*
  - Asymmetric oligoarthritis
  - DIP joint involvement
  - Dactylitis (sausage digits)
  - *Nail changes:* pitting, onycholysis
- *Treatment:*
  - NSAIDs
  - DMARDs (methotrexate, sulfasalazine)
  - Biologics (TNF inhibitors) in severe cases
  - Surgery for advanced deformity or joint destruction

Congenital and Developmental Disorders of the Hand

Q46. Syndactyly—classification and management.

Definition

Failure of separation of fingers during development.

Classification
- *Simple:* Only soft tissue fusion
- *Complex:* Involves bone/cartilage fusion
- *Complete:* Full length of digit
- *Incomplete:* Partial fusion

Surgical Indications
- Functional impairment (e.g., border digits involved)
- Aesthetic concern
- *Age:* Usually done at **1–2 years** of age

Surgical Principles
- Z-plasty incisions to avoid contracture
- Grafting (e.g., full-thickness skin) may be required

Q47. Polydactyly—overview and surgical correction.

Definition
Presence of supernumerary digits

Types
- *Preaxial (radial)*: Thumb side
- *Postaxial (ulnar)*: Little finger side
- *Central:* Rare (middle digits)

Surgical Management
- *Age:* **Usually 6–12 months**
- *Involves:*
  - Excision of the extra digit
  - Tendon and soft tissue balancing
  - Reconstruction of joint capsule if needed

Infections and Soft Tissue Conditions

Q48. Pyogenic flexor tenosynovitis—management.

Definition
Bacterial infection of the flexor tendon sheath (commonly *Staphylococcus aureus*)

Symptoms
Pain, swelling, and stiffness of finger

Treatment
- *Early:* IV antibiotics, splinting, elevation
- *Delayed/severe:*
  - Surgical drainage (longitudinal incision along the sheath)
  - Irrigation and debridement

Q49. Kanavel's signs (flexor tendon sheath infections).

- *Four Cardinal Signs*:
  1. Fusiform swelling of the finger
  2. Finger held in slight flexion

3. Pain on passive extension
4. Tenderness along flexor sheath

- *Clinical relevance:* Highly specific for **infectious tenosynovitis**, requiring **urgent surgical intervention**

Q50. Felon.

Definition
Abscess or infection of the **pulp space of the fingertip**, usually due to penetrating trauma.

Causative Organism
Staphylococcus aureus

Features
- Severe throbbing pain
- Swollen, tense, red distal finger pad
- Often fluctuant

Management:
- *Early:* Oral antibiotics, elevation
- *Late/Abscess:* **Incision and drainage (I&D)** via lateral or volar approach

Q51. Paronychia.

Definition
Infection of the **nail fold**, usually from nail biting, manicuring, or hangnails.

Acute Paronychia
- Painful, red, swollen nail margin
- Pus may form
- *Causative organism: Staphylococcus aureus*
- *Tx:* Antibiotics, I&D if pus present

Chronic Paronychia
- Common in wet workers (e.g., housekeepers)
- Candida involvement
- *Tx:* avoid moisture, topical antifungals/steroids

Q52. Difference between felon and paronychia.

Feature	*Felon*	*Paronychia*
Location	Finger pulp (fleshy tip)	Nail fold (around the nail)
Cause	Penetrating injury, trauma	Nail biting, manicure, moisture
Main organism	Staph aureus	*Staphylococcus aureus*, *candida* (chronic)
Symptoms	Throbbing pain, tense swelling	Swelling/redness near nail
Treatment	Incision and drainage	Antibiotics, drainage if needed

Miscellaneous Conditions of the Hand and Wrist

Q53. Intersection syndrome—short note.

Definition
Overuse inflammatory condition involving crossing of **1st and 2nd extensor compartments**

Symptoms

- Pain ~4–6 cm proximal to wrist, dorsal radial side
- Swelling, crepitus on movement

Management

- Rest, NSAIDs, splinting
- Steroid injection or surgical release if persistent

Q54. Raynaud's phenomenon—diagnosis and treatment.

Definition

Vasospastic response to cold/emotion → color changes (white → blue → red)

Types

- *Primary:* Idiopathic, benign
- *Secondary:* Associated with connective tissue disorders (e.g., SLE, scleroderma)

Diagnosis

Clinical, cold provocation test, ANA (if suspected autoimmune cause)

Treatment

- *Lifestyle:* Avoid cold, stress
- *Medications:* **Calcium channel blockers** (e.g., nifedipine)
- Treat underlying cause if secondary

Q55. Steroid injections—role in wrist and hand conditions.

- *Uses:*
    - De Quervain's tenosynovitis
    - Trigger finger
    - Carpal tunnel syndrome (temporary relief)
    - Intersection syndrome
    - Inflammatory arthritis
- *Mechanism:* Anti-inflammatory, reduces swelling and pain
- *Considerations:*
    - Use ultrasound guidance for accuracy
    - Limit repeated use to prevent tendon weakening or atrophy

Surgical Procedures and Rehabilitation—Hand and Wrist

Q56. Tendon repair in the hand—principles and techniques.

(RGUHS 2012)

- *Principles:*
    - Preserve tendon length and tension
    - Minimize handling and preserve vascularity
    - Early mobilization post-repair to prevent adhesions
- *Techniques:*
    - **Core suture techniques** (e.g., Modified Kessler, 4-strand)
    - Use of **epitendinous sutures** for smooth gliding
    - Choice of technique depends on zone of injury (Zones I–V for flexors)

Q57. Wrist fusion (arthrodesis) in arthritis.

- *Indications:*
    - End-stage wrist arthritis (RA, post-traumatic, SLAC)
    - Painful instability
- *Techniques:*
    - **Total wrist fusion** for pain relief and stability
    - **Partial fusion** (e.g., 4-corner fusion) to preserve some motion
- *Drawback:* Loss of motion but high pain relief

Q58. Rehabilitation after flexor tendon repair.

- *Protocols:*
    - *Early passive mobilization:* Kleinert protocol
    - *Early active mobilization:* Duran protocol
    - Splinting in flexed position for tendon protection
- *Goals:*
    - Prevent adhesions
    - Preserve tendon glide
    - Restore strength and function gradually over 8–12 weeks

Q59. Nerve repair and grafting in the hand—short note.

- **Direct repair** (neurorrhaphy) if tension-free ends
- **Nerve grafting** (e.g., sural nerve) for defects >1–2 cm
- **Microsurgical technique** essential
- *Post-operative care:* Splinting, sensory re-education

Q60. Wrist arthroplasty—indications and complications.

(CMC Vellore 2019)

- *Indications:*
    - RA or OA with pain and motion loss
    - Low demand elderly patients
- *Complications:*
    - Loosening
    - Implant failure
    - Infection
    - Reduced grip strength
- *Alternative:* Fusion if high-demand patient

Q61. 3D printing in hand and wrist reconstruction.

- *Applications:*
    - Patient-specific implants and guides
    - Pre-operative planning (complex fractures, deformities)
    - Prosthetic limb and splint fabrication
- *Advantages:*
    - Customization
    - Better anatomical fit
    - Cost-effective long-term in complex cases

Q62. Ganglion cyst of wrist—diagnosis and treatment.

(Asked in: JIPMER Puducherry 2023, RGUHS Karnataka 2023)

Definition

A **ganglion cyst** is a **benign, mucin-filled cystic swelling** arising from a joint capsule or tendon sheath, most commonly around the **wrist**.

Etiology and Pathogenesis

Origin: Outpouching/herniation of synovial tissue from a joint or tendon sheath.

Pathogenesis: Myxoid degeneration of connective tissue → production of gelatinous fluid → cyst formation.

Risk factors:
- Repetitive wrist activities.
- Minor trauma.
- More common in females (3:1), aged 20–40 years.

Common Sites

Wrist (most common):
- **Dorsal wrist** (70%)—originates from scapholunate joint.
- **Volar wrist**—arises from radioscaphoid or scaphotrapezial joint.

Other sites: Dorsum of foot, ankle, knee, fingers (retinacular cysts).

Clinical Features

Symptoms:
- Painless or mildly painful swelling.
- Size may fluctuate.
- Cosmetic concern is often the presenting complaint.
- Sometimes discomfort during wrist movements.

Signs:
- Smooth, soft, fluctuant to firm swelling.
- Mobile transverse to plane of underlying joint.
- Positive **transillumination** (mucinous fluid inside).

Diagnosis

Clinical examination is usually sufficient.

Investigations (in doubtful cases):
- *Ultrasound:*
  - Confirms cystic nature.
  - Differentiates from solid tumors.
- *MRI:* Only if atypical presentation or deep ganglia suspected.
- *Needle aspiration:* Clear, gelatinous fluid confirms diagnosis.

Differential diagnoses:
- Synovial cyst
- Lipoma
- Tenosynovitis
- Giant cell tumor of tendon sheath.

Treatment

Conservative (first line):
- *Observation:* Many cysts resolve spontaneously.
- *Aspiration:*
  - Removal of gelatinous fluid using a needle.

- May combine with corticosteroid injection.
- Recurrence common (~50%).

Surgical Management

Indications:
- Symptomatic cyst (pain, restricted motion).
- Cosmetic concern.
- Recurrence after aspiration.

Procedure:
- **Complete surgical excision** of ganglion cyst including its stalk and part of capsule/joint capsule.
- Dorsal ganglion excision requires careful protection of radial artery (in volar ganglion).

Recurrence rate: ~5–15% even after proper surgical removal.

Newer Techniques

Arthroscopic ganglionectomy—minimally invasive, quicker recovery.

Exam Tip

When answering about ganglion cyst:
- **Mention dorsal wrist > scapholunate joint origin** clearly.
- **Always highlight transillumination test.**
- Treatment is **conservative first, surgery for recurrence or symptomatic cases.**

Q63. Madelung's deformity.

(Asked in: AIIMS Delhi 2021, PGI Chandigarh 2022)

Definition

Madelung's deformity is a **developmental abnormality of the distal radius**, caused by **growth disturbance of the volar-ulnar portion of the distal radial physis**, leading to **wrist deformity** and **functional limitation**.

Etiology

Congenital/Developmental: Premature closure or dysplasia of the **ulnar-volar part** of the distal radial growth plate.

Associated conditions:
- **Leri–Weill dyschondrosteosis** (short stature, mesomelia)
- **Turner's syndrome**
- **Post-traumatic** physeal injury

Pathophysiology

Disturbed growth of distal radius → relative overgrowth of ulna → volar subluxation of the carpus → wrist deformity.

Clinical Features

Symptoms:
- Cosmetic deformity (prominent ulnar head)
- Pain with wrist movement
- Weak grip strength
- Decreased range of motion (pronation, supination, dorsiflexion)

Signs:
- Dorsal bowing of distal radius
- Increased prominence of ulnar head
- Volar and ulnar tilt of distal radius
- Palmar subluxation of the carpus

Deformity appearance: **Radial and palmar deviation of hand** relative to forearm.

Radiological Features

X-ray (PA and lateral views):

- Increased volar tilt (>15°)
- Increased radial inclination
- Positive ulnar variance
- Triangularization of the carpus ("V-shaped carpal bones")

MRI: Useful in early detection of physeal abnormalities before deformity becomes clinically apparent.

Management

Non-surgical (mild cases):

- Observation for asymptomatic or mild deformities
- Wrist splinting for pain relief
- Activity modification

Surgical (indications):

- Significant pain
- Progressive deformity
- Functional impairment

Surgical options:

1. *Epiphysiodesis*: For early detected cases to prevent progression.
2. *Corrective osteotomy*: Radial dome osteotomy to correct alignment.
3. *Ulnar procedures*: Ulnar shortening osteotomy for significant positive variance.
4. *Darrach procedure (rarely used today)*: Distal ulna excision in adults with painful ulnar head prominence.

Timing

Ideally after skeletal maturity unless deformity is severe and progressive.

Postoperative Care

- Immobilization,
- Gradual physiotherapy and mobilization.

Exam Tip

- Always **mention volar-ulnar physeal growth disturbance** early.
- *Describe clinical deformity:* **radial + palmar hand deviation**.
- Differentiate clearly between **early (observation)** and **late (osteotomy/ulnar shortening)** management.

Q64. Wrist arthrodesis.

Definition

Surgical fusion of wrist joint bones to eliminate pain and provide stability, usually at the expense of mobility.

Indications

- Advanced arthritis (e.g., rheumatoid, post-traumatic)
- Post-infective damage
- Brachial plexus palsy (to stabilize the hand)
- Irreparable instability
- Painful wrist deformity

Procedure

- *Bones typically fused:* **radius, lunate, capitate, and 3rd metacarpal.**
- *Position of fusion:* ~10–15° extension, slight ulnar deviation, and pronation.

Pros
- Pain relief
- Increased grip strength
- Stable hand for function

Cons
- Loss of wrist motion
- Adjacent joint arthritis over time

Q65. Scaphoid non-union.

Definition
Failure of healing of a scaphoid fracture beyond 6 months.

Why It Happens?
- Poor blood supply (especially to proximal pole)
- Late diagnosis
- Inadequate immobilization
- Smoking

Complications
- Scaphoid nonunion advanced collapse (SNAC) wrist
- Osteoarthritis

Treatment
- Bone grafting (vascular or non-vascular)
- ORIF with Herbert screw
- *In some cases:* Scaphoid excision + limited wrist fusion

Q66. Claw hand versus ulnar claw hand.

Claw Hand (True/Complete Claw Hand)

Definition
Hyperextension of MCP joints + flexion at IP joints of **all fingers**, due to **combined median and ulnar nerve palsy**.

Causes
- Leprosy (common in India)
- Advanced combined nerve injuries

Ulnar Claw Hand

Definition
Clawing of only **ring and little fingers** due to **ulnar nerve palsy** (especially at wrist level).

Mechanism:
Loss of intrinsic muscles (lumbricals and interossei) → imbalance → clawing

Feature	*True claw hand*	*Ulnar claw hand*
Nerves involved	Ulnar + Median	Ulnar only
Fingers affected	All digits	4th and 5th fingers
Common cause	Leprosy, severe trauma	Ulnar nerve lesion at wrist
Muscle loss	Lumbricals of all fingers	Medial two lumbricals only
MCP/IP pattern	MCP hyperextension, IP flexion	Same (but only ring/little fingers)

Q67. Intrinsic plus hand (safe position hand).

Definition

A hand posture where the **MCP joints are flexed** and **IP joints are extended** due to dominance of **intrinsic muscles** (lumbricals/interossei).

Causes

- Rheumatoid arthritis
- Burns
- Early intrinsic muscle contracture

Significance

- Opposite of claw hand
- **Functional position**, often used as **immobilization posture** in hand splinting.

Q68. Ulnar paradox.

Definition

The paradox where **higher (proximal) ulnar nerve lesions cause less clawing**, while **lower (distal) lesions cause more severe clawing**.

Why?

- In proximal lesion → both FDP (flexor digitorum profundus) and lumbricals are paralyzed → no strong IP joint flexion → less clawing.
- In distal lesion → FDP intact (causing flexion) but lumbricals lost → severe clawing.

"The closer the lesion to the paw, the worse the claw."

Q69. Zancolli's capsulodesis.

Indication

- **Ulnar claw hand** due to intrinsic muscle loss
- To prevent MCP hyperextension and improve IP extension

Principle

- **Tightens volar MCP joint capsule** to limit hyperextension, mimicking lumbrical action

Method

- Incision over volar MCP joint
- Volar plate tightened and sutured to prevent MCP hyperextension
- Often done along with tendon transfers (e.g., Brand or FDS transfers)

Q70. Various flaps for hand reconstruction.

Local Flaps

- *Cross-finger flap*: For dorsal finger defects
- *Thenar flap*: For fingertip pulp loss
- *V-Y advancement flap*: For fingertip injuries

Regional Flaps

- *Groin flap*: Based on superficial circumflex iliac artery
- *Abdominal flap*: For major palmar defects

Free Flaps
- Radial forearm flap
- Anterolateral thigh (ALT) flap
- Toe-to-thumb transfer

Q71. Scapholunate advanced collapse (SLAC) wrist.

Definition
A progressive wrist arthritis resulting from **scapholunate ligament injury**.

Stages
1. Radioscaphoid arthritis
2. Capitate-lunate joint involvement
3. Pancarpal arthritis

Causes
- Chronic untreated SL dissociation
- Trauma, degenerative arthritis

Treatment
- *Early:* radial styloidectomy
- *Intermediate:* **proximal row carpectomy** or **four-corner fusion**
- *Advanced:* total wrist fusion

Q72. Ulnar styloid impingement syndrome.

Definition
Pain and restricted motion due to **impingement of the ulnar styloid** on the triquetrum or TFCC (triangular fibrocartilage complex).

Symptoms
- Ulnar-sided wrist pain
- Pain during ulnar deviation/pronation
- Positive **ulnocarpal stress test**

Diagnosis
- X-ray may show prominent ulnar styloid
- *MRI:* TFCC pathology

Treatment
- NSAIDs
- Ulnar styloid excision or arthroscopic TFCC repair if conservative measures fail

Q73. Kapandji procedure (for DRUJ instability).

Indications
- DRUJ arthritis or instability
- Failed conservative management
- Rheumatoid arthritis
- Post-traumatic derangement (e.g., after distal radius fracture)

Principle
Create pseudarthrosis in distal ulna to eliminate pain from DRUJ while preserving forearm rotation.

Technique
- **Distal subcapital resection** of ulna (~1 cm)
- Avoid damaging surrounding soft tissues
- Leave the ulnar shaft intact to prevent instability

Pros
- Preserves rotation
- Simpler than full ulnar head resection

Cons
- May cause instability, impingement
- Often replaced by **Darrach's or Sauvé–Kapandji** procedures

Q74. Kienböck's disease (avascular necrosis of lunate).

Pathophysiology
Repetitive trauma or ulnar negative variance → **compromised lunate vascularity** → necrosis

Lichtman's Staging
1. Normal X-ray; MRI shows necrosis
2. Sclerosis of lunate

3A. Collapse without carpal instability
3B. Collapse **with fixed scaphoid rotation**
4. Generalized arthritis

Symptoms
- Dorsal wrist pain
- Decreased grip strength
- Decreased ROM

Treatment
- *Stage I–II:* Immobilization, revascularization
- *Stage III:* Joint leveling (radial shortening, ulnar lengthening)
- *Stage IV:* Proximal row carpectomy or wrist arthrodesis

Q75. Pinch in quadriplegics (tendon transfers).

Problem
Quadriplegics with C6-C7 injuries have **no hand grip or finger function**, but often have **wrist extensors intact**

Solution Tendon Transfers
- *Use tenodesis effect*: Wrist extension → passive finger flexion
- *Tendon transfer (Brand's technique)*:
    - **BR (brachioradialis)** or **wrist extensors** transferred to **FPL** and **FDP**
- Achieves **key pinch (thumb-index pinch)**

Prerequisite
- Functional wrist extensors
- Motivated patient with good rehabilitation potential

Post-operative
Splinting and extensive rehabilitation are critical

Q76. Infection of the hand—overview.

Common Infections

Type	*Description*
Felon	Abscess in pulp of fingertip
Paronychia	Infection around nail fold
Tenosynovitis	Infection of synovial sheath of flexor tendons
Deep space infection	Involves thenar/midpalmar spaces
Septic arthritis	Infected MCP/IP joint
Cellulitis	Superficial skin infection
Osteomyelitis	Usually from open injury or extension from soft tissue

Causative Organisms
- *Staphylococcus aureus* (most common)
- *Streptococcus* species
- MRSA (in hospital/IV drug use)
- Anaerobes (in bite injuries)
- Mycobacteria/fungi (chronic)

Kanavel's Signs (Flexor tenosynovitis)
1. Finger held in flexion
2. Fusiform swelling
3. Pain on passive extension
4. Tenderness along the flexor sheath

Principles of Treatment
- Early → IV antibiotics, immobilization
- Abscess or spread → **surgical drainage**
- Hand elevation, wound care
- Avoid delay - can lead to **permanent stiffness or deformity**

Q77. Wrist osteoarthritis—classification and management.

(NEIGRIHMS 2009)

Classification
Based on **location and cause**:
1. *Primary OA*: Age-related degeneration (rare in wrist)
2. *Secondary OA*:
    - Scapholunate advanced collapse (SLAC) wrist
    - Scaphoid nonunion advanced collapse (SNAC) wrist
    - **Post-traumatic** (distal radius fracture)
    - **Inflammatory** (RA, PsA)
    - **Kienböck's disease**

Radiological Stages (SLAC wrist)
1. Radioscaphoid arthritis
2. Midcarpal arthritis (capitate-lunate)
3. Pancarpal arthritis

Management
- *Conservative:* NSAIDs, splints, activity modification

- *Surgical:*
  - *Early:* Radial styloidectomy
  - *Mid-stage:* **Proximal row carpectomy** or **4-corner fusion**
  - *End-stage:* **Total wrist fusion or arthroplasty**

Q78. Explain the role of arthroscopy in wrist ligament injuries.

- *Diagnostic:*
  - Direct visualization of TFCC, SL, LT tears
  - Gold standard for small intra-articular ligament evaluation
- *Therapeutic:*
  - Debridement of partial tears
  - Repair/reconstruction of ligaments

It has got advantage of minimal soft tissue disruption, faster recovary

Q79. Describe management of radial nerve palsy affecting the hand.

(WBUHS 2013)

Causes
- Humeral shaft fractures
- Compression (Saturday night palsy)

Clinical Features
- Wrist drop
- Loss of thumb/finger extension
- Sensory loss over dorsum of hand (1st web space)

Management
1. *Conservative*:
   - Splinting (dynamic cock-up splint)
   - Physiotherapy
   - Recovery in 3–6 months
2. *Surgical*:
   - *If no improvement >3 months:*
     - **Tendon transfer** (e.g., pronator teres to ECRB, FCR to EDC)
     - Nerve repair/grafting (if laceration)

Congenital and Developmental Disorders

Q80. Syndactyly—classification and management.

Definition
Failure of separation of digits during development.

Classification

Type	*Details*
Simple	Skin only
Complex	Bone fusion present
Complete	Entire digit joined
Incomplete	Partial fusion
Complicated	With other anomalies (e.g., Apert's)

Management
- Surgery around 1–2 years of age
- Use of skin grafts if needed
- Early intervention for border digits (e.g., thumb-index)

Q81. Polydactyly—short note and surgical correction.

Definition
Supernumerary digits; can be pre-axial (thumb side), post-axial (little finger side), or central

Classification
- **Wassel's classification** for thumb polydactyly (I–VII)
- Type IV most common

Management
- Surgery at **6–12 months**
- Excision of extra digit + ligament/tendon reconstruction
- Preserve the better-developed digit

7.4 Spine

Younis Kamal, Farid Hussain, Agnivesh Tikoo

Anatomy and Biomechanics of the Spine

Q1. Embryology and development of the vertebral column.

(NEIGRIHMS 2019)

- Derived from **sclerotome** (part of somite in paraxial mesoderm).
- **Notochord** contributes to nucleus pulposus.
- *Resegmentation:* Caudal part of one sclerotome fuses with cranial part of the next → vertebral body.
- Ossification begins at 8 weeks gestation → completed by 25 years.

Q2. Anatomical differences between cervical, thoracic, and lumbar vertebrae.

Feature	***Cervical***	***Thoracic***	***Lumbar***
Body size	Small	Heart-shaped	Large, kidney-shaped
Foramina	Transverse foramina	None	None
Spinous process	Bifid	Long, sloping down	Short, horizontal
Articular facet plane	Horizontal (flexible)	Coronal (rotatory)	Sagittal (flex/ext)
Rib articulation	None	Yes (costal facets)	No

Q3. Biomechanics of cervical, thoracic, and lumbar spine.

- *Cervical:* Mobile → rotation (C1-C2), flexion/extension (C3–C7).
- *Thoracic:* Least mobile (rib cage) → mainly rotation.
- *Lumbar:* Supports load → allows flexion/extension, limited rotation.

Q4. Role of intervertebral discs in spinal stability and movement.

- *Made of:*
  - *Nucleus pulposus:* Shock absorber.
  - *Annulus fibrosus:* Provides tensile strength.
  - *Endplates:* Nutrient diffusion.

Functions
- Load distribution.
- Motion between vertebrae.
- Height and curvature maintenance.

Q5. Structure and function of spinal ligaments.

Ligament	***Location***	***Function***
Anterior longitudinal	Anterior to vertebral body	Limits extension
Posterior longitudinal	Posterior to vertebral body	Limits flexion
Ligamentum flavum	Lamina to lamina	Maintains posture, elastic recoil
Interspinous/Supraspinous	Between spinous processes	Limit flexion
Intertransverse	Between transverse processes	Limit lateral flexion

Q6. Arterial supply and venous drainage of spine.

- *Arterial:*
  - Segmental arteries (vertebral, intercostal, lumbar).
  - Anterior and posterior spinal arteries supply cord.
- *Venous:*
  - **Internal vertebral venous plexus** (Batson's plexus – valveless).
  - Routes for **metastasis** (e.g., prostate cancer to spine).

Q7. Describe the vertebral artery course and its importance in cervical spine surgery.

(Asked in: JIPMER 2021)

Course of Vertebral Artery

- *V1 (Pre-foraminal segment):* Originates from subclavian artery to C6 transverse foramen
- *V2 (Foraminal segment):* C6 to C2 transverse foramina
- *V3 (Extradural segment):* From C2 transverse foramen, winds laterally over C1 arch into foramen magnum
- *V4 (Intradural segment):* Inside dura, joins opposite vertebral artery to form basilar artery

Importance in Surgery

- *Risk of injury:* During posterior approaches (e.g., C1-C2 transarticular screw fixation), anterior approaches, decompressions
- *Anatomic variations:* High-riding vertebral artery at C2, aberrant course increases surgical risk
- *Preoperative planning:*
  - CT angiography to delineate vertebral artery course
  - Avoidance of injury during screw placement, drilling
- *Complications of injury:*
  - Massive bleeding
  - Stroke (posterior circulation infarct)
  - Death

Key Surgical Precautions

- Use navigation (intraoperative CT, O-arm)
- Careful dissection near transverse foramina
- Screw trajectory planning based on preoperative imaging

Q8. Functional anatomy of atlantoaxial joint.

- *Composed of:*
  - Median atlanto-dental joint (dens and anterior arch of C1).
  - 2 lateral atlantoaxial joints (C1-C2 facets).
- **Transverse ligament** stabilizes dens.
- Allows **50% of cervical rotation**.

Q9. Role of sacroiliac joint in load transmission.

- Synovial (anterior) and syndesmotic (posterior) joint.
- **Transfers body weight** from spine to lower limbs.
- Limited movement; reinforced by **strong ligaments**.

Q10. Anatomical and biomechanical changes in aging spine.

Change	*Effect*
Disc degeneration	↓ height, ↓ shock absorption
Facet osteoarthritis	↓ mobility, pain
Vertebral osteoporosis	Compression fractures
Ligament calcification	Spinal canal narrowing
Postural kyphosis	Sagittal imbalance

Q11. Concept of spinal balance and sagittal alignment.

- Spinal balance = head over pelvis.
- **Pelvic Incidence (PI)** = Pelvic Tilt (PT) + Sacral Slope (SS)
- *Normal sagittal alignment:*
  - Cervical lordosis
  - Thoracic kyphosis
  - Lumbar lordosis
- Imbalance → fatigue, disability, compensatory changes.

Q12. Role of paraspinal muscles in spine biomechanics.

- **Erector spinae** (extension and posture).
- **Multifidus** (segmental stability).
- **Quadratus lumborum** (lateral flexion, lumbar stability).
- **Psoas** (hip flexion and lumbar stabilization).

Functions

- Resist flexion forces.
- Maintain erect posture.
- Prevent instability.

Q13. Structural composition of intervertebral disc.

Three Components

1. **Annulus Fibrosus**:
   - Outer concentric collagen rings
   - Type I collagen
2. **Nucleus Pulposus**:
   - Gel-like center
   - Rich in proteoglycans, Type II collagen
   - Provides shock absorption
3. **Cartilaginous End Plates**:
   - Interface between disc and vertebral body
   - Nutrient diffusion pathway

- Between vertebral bodies (C2–S1)
- *Function:*
  - Shock absorption
  - Load distribution
  - Allows flexibility

Q14. Neuroanatomy of spinal cord and clinical relevance.

- **Extends from medulla to L1–L2** (conus medullaris).
- *Surrounded by meninges:* Dura, arachnoid, pia.
- Ends as **cauda equina**.
- 31 pairs of spinal nerves.

Level	*Structure affected*	*Clinical relevance*
C5–C6	Common disc herniation	Biceps weakness, reflex ↓
T10	Umbilicus dermatome	Reference point for cord injury
L4–S1	Lumbosacral plexus	Sciatica, foot drop

Congenital and Developmental Disorders of the Spine

Q15. Congenital spine anomalies (spina bifida)—types, clinical presentation, and management.

(Asked in: JIPMER Puducherry 2022, RGUHS Karnataka 2022)

Definition

Spina bifida is a **neural tube defect** resulting from **failure of fusion of posterior vertebral arches**, leading to exposure of meninges and/or spinal cord.

Types

1. *Spina bifida occulta*:
    - Incomplete bony closure without protrusion.
    - Skin usually intact (may have tuft of hair, dimple, or lipoma).
    - Often asymptomatic.
2. *Spina bifida cystica*:
    - *Meningocele:*
        - Herniation of meninges through the defect.
        - No neural elements in sac.
        - Better prognosis.
    - *Myelomeningocele:*
        - Herniation of meninges + spinal cord/neural tissue.
        - Neurological deficits common (paralysis, bladder/bowel dysfunction).
3. *Rachischisis*:
    - Most severe.
    - Open spinal cord exposed without skin or bone covering.

Clinical Presentation

Spina bifida occulta:
- Often silent.
- Sometimes presents later with tethered cord symptoms.

Meningocele:
- Visible swelling over spine.
- Minimal or no neurological deficit.

Myelomeningocele:
- Flaccid paralysis.
- Sensory deficits.
- Bladder and bowel incontinence.
- Orthopedic deformities (clubfoot, scoliosis, hip dislocation).

Management

Prenatal Care:

- Folic acid supplementation (400 mcg/day) to prevent NTDs.
- Prenatal diagnosis via ultrasonography or maternal AFP testing.

Postnatal care:

- Protect the lesion at birth (sterile saline dressing).
- Early neurosurgical closure within 24–48 hours (especially for myelomeningocele).

Associated management:

- Orthopedic interventions (for deformities).
- Urological evaluation (urodynamic studies).
- Long-term physiotherapy and rehabilitation.

Prognosis:

- Depends on the severity and level of neurological involvement.
- Myelomeningocele has poorer prognosis than meningocele.

Q16. Classification of congenital spinal deformities and their management.

Classification (Winter's Classification)

- *Failures of formation:* Hemivertebra, wedge vertebra
- *Failures of segmentation:* Block vertebra
- *Mixed defects:* Complex deformities

Management

- *Observation:* Mild, non-progressive cases
- *Bracing:* Rarely effective
- *Surgical correction:* Indicated in progressive curves
    - **Hemivertebra excision**, **posterior spinal fusion**, **growth-friendly systems** in early-onset

Q17. Klippel–Feil syndrome—clinical features and management.

Features

- Congenital fusion of ≥2 cervical vertebrae
- *Classic triad:*
    - Short neck
    - Low posterior hairline
    - Limited neck motion

Associations

- Sprengel deformity
- Congenital scoliosis
- Renal/cardiac anomalies

Management

- **Observation** if asymptomatic
- **Surgical decompression** in myelopathy
- Address **associated deformities**

Q18. Diastematomyelia—clinical significance.

Definition

Congenital **split spinal cord malformation** by a bony/fibrous/cartilaginous septum.

Types

- *Type I:* Dual dural sacs
- *Type II:* Single dural sac with divided cord

Clinical Features

- Back pain, scoliosis, neurological deficits
- Often associated with tethered cord

Management

- **MRI diagnosis**
- **Surgical excision** of septum and cord untethering

Q19. Congenital spinal stenosis—natural history and management.

Definition

Narrow spinal canal from birth, often due to **short pedicles** (e.g., achondroplasia)

Clinical Course

- Often asymptomatic early
- May develop **neurological symptoms** with minor trauma or disc herniation

Management

- **Activity modification**
- Surgery (laminoplasty or decompression) if symptomatic

Q20. Congenital torticollis—description and management.

Definition

Unilateral **contracture of the sternocleidomastoid (SCM)**, usually due to intrauterine malposition or birth trauma

Features

- Head tilt toward involved side
- Facial asymmetry

Management

- **Physiotherapy** (early)
- **Surgical release** if persistent beyond 1–2 years

Q21. Achondroplasia—genetics and spinal features.

Genetics

- *FGFR3* gene mutation
- Autosomal dominant; most cases are **de novo**

Spinal Manifestations

- **Congenital spinal stenosis** (short pedicles)
- **Kyphosis** at thoracolumbar junction
- **Lordosis**, scoliosis
- Risk of **cord compression**

Management

- Monitor growth and neuro status
- Early decompression if symptomatic
- Avoid forceful neck movements in infancy

Q22. Spinal dysraphism (meningocele, myelomeningocele)—clinical features, diagnosis, and management.

(Source: AIIMS Delhi 2021)

Definition

Spinal dysraphism refers to a spectrum of congenital anomalies resulting from incomplete closure of the neural tube.

Types

- *Meningocele:* Herniation of meninges through a vertebral defect (without neural tissue)
- *Myelomeningocele:* Herniation of meninges and spinal cord tissue

Clinical Features

- Visible cystic swelling over the back (often lumbosacral region)
- *Neurological deficits:*
  - Motor weakness
  - Sensory loss
  - Bladder/bowel dysfunction
- *Orthopedic deformities:*
  - Clubfoot (CTEV)
  - Hip dislocation
  - Scoliosis

Diagnosis

- *Prenatal:* Ultrasound, Elevated maternal AFP levels
- *Postnatal:*
  - MRI spine (to assess extent)
  - CT scan (bony defects)

Management

Neonatal period: Early surgical closure (preferably within 24–48 hours) to prevent infection and further damage

Long-term management:

- Physiotherapy for motor recovery
- Orthotic support (e.g., ankle-foot orthosis)
- Urological management (urodynamic studies, CIC - clean intermittent catheterization)

Quick Table

Condition	Defect
Meningocele	Meninges only
Myelomeningocele	Meninges + Neural tissue

Crisp Flowchart

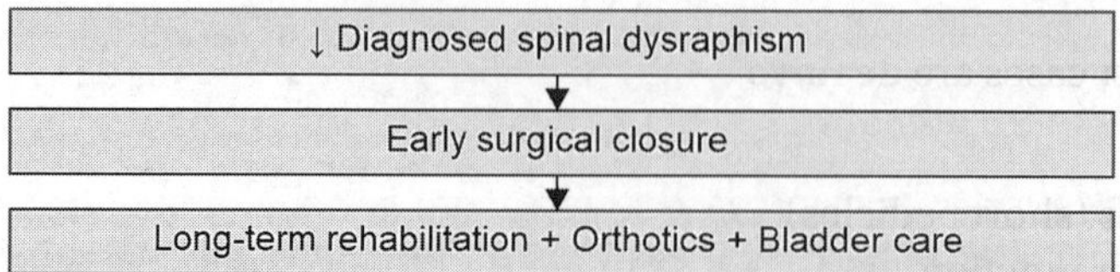

Q23. Tethered cord syndrome—diagnosis and surgical management.

(Source: JIPMER Puducherry 2022)

Definition

Tethered cord syndrome (TCS) is a condition where the spinal cord is abnormally attached (tethered) to surrounding tissues, restricting its movement.

Causes
- Congenital (thickened filum terminale, lipomas)
- Post-surgical (after repair of myelomeningocele)

Clinical Features
- *Progressive neurological deterioration:*
    - Motor weakness (foot drop, leg weakness)
    - Sensory disturbances
    - Bladder/bowel incontinence
- *Orthopedic deformities:*
    - Scoliosis
    - Foot deformities

Diagnosis
- *MRI lumbosacral spine:*
    - Low-lying conus (below L2)
    - Thickened filum terminale (>2 mm)

Management

Surgical management:
- *Detethering surgery:*
    - Release of the tethered cord
    - Microsurgical technique to prevent further neurological decline

Timing: Early surgery preferred before irreversible deficits develop

Quick Table

Feature	*Key point*
Diagnosis	MRI (low conus)
Management	Microsurgical detethering

Crisp Flowchart

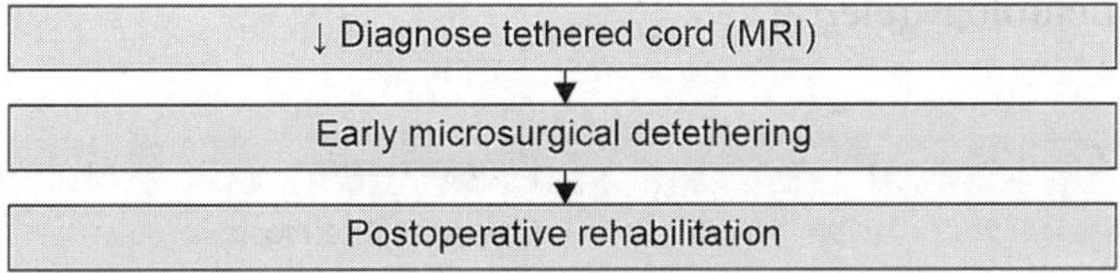

Q24. Vertebral anomalies—types and orthopedic significance.

(Source: RGUHS Karnataka 2023)

Definition

Congenital vertebral anomalies result from defective formation or segmentation of vertebrae during embryogenesis.

Types

Anomaly type	*Example*
Failure of formation	Hemivertebra
Failure of segmentation	Block vertebra
Combined defects	Mixed anomalies

Orthopedic Significance

- *Hemivertebra:* Leads to congenital scoliosis
- *Block vertebra:* May cause short neck, torticollis (e.g., Klippel–Feil syndrome)
- *Mixed defects:* Severe scoliosis/kyphoscoliosis

Associated Conditions

- Congenital scoliosis
- Spinal deformities
- Neurological deficits (if associated spinal cord anomalies)

Management

- *Observation:* Mild deformities without progression
- *Surgical correction:* Progressive curves (early hemivertebra excision, spinal fusion)

Q25. Sacral agenesis—orthopedic implications.

Definition

Partial/complete absence of the sacrum

Clinical Features

- Seen in **caudal regression syndrome**
- Motor/sensory deficits, bladder/bowel dysfunction
- Associated with **diabetes in pregnancy**

Orthopedic Issues

- Hip/knee flexion contractures
- Foot deformities
- Spinal instability

Management

- Orthotic support
- **Soft tissue/bony corrections**
- Bladder management and neurology referral

Quick Table

Defect type	*Clinical result*
Hemivertebra	Congenital scoliosis
Block vertebra	Reduced neck mobility (e.g., Klippel–Feil)

Crisp Flowchart

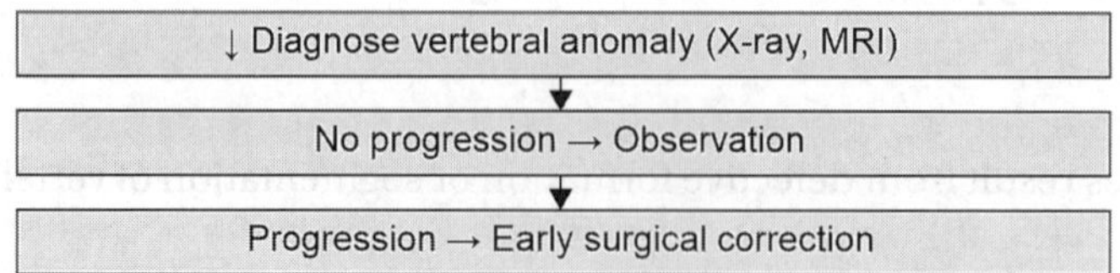

Ultra-crisp Final Memory Markers

Topic	*1-liner recall*
Spinal dysraphism	Early surgical closure
Tethered cord syndrome	MRI → Microsurgical detethering
Vertebral anomalies	Hemivertebra → Scoliosis, Block Vertebra → Klippel–Feil

Degenerative Disorders of the Spine

Q26. Natural history and progression of cervical spondylosis.

- Common after age 40
- *Progresses from:*
  - **Disc degeneration** → osteophytes
  - **Radiculopathy** → myelopathy
- Some patients remain asymptomatic; others develop **gradual neurological decline**
- Surgery may halt progression but does not reverse damage

Q27. Conservative versus surgical management in degenerative spine disease.

Aspect	*Conservative*	*Surgical*
Indications	Mild/moderate symptoms	Severe radiculopathy/myelopathy, failed non-op
Components	NSAIDs, PT, lifestyle changes, injections	Decompression, discectomy, fusion
Advantages	Non-invasive, cost-effective	Quick relief, definitive in severe cases
Limitations	Slower results, may not stop progression	Surgical risks, cost

Q28. Cervical spondylotic myelopathy (CSM)—clinical features, diagnosis, and management.

(Source: AIIMS Delhi 2021, MUHS Maharashtra 2022)

Definition

CSM is spinal cord dysfunction caused by chronic degenerative changes of the cervical spine (discs, vertebrae, ligaments).

Clinical Features

- Neck pain, stiffness
- Upper limb numbness, clumsiness (difficulty buttoning, writing)
- Gait disturbances (spastic gait)
- Bowel/bladder dysfunction (late)

Diagnosis

- *MRI cervical spine:* Gold standard (cord compression, T2 hyperintensity)
- *X-rays:* Disc space narrowing, osteophytes
- *CT scan:* Bony canal narrowing

Management

Conservative:

- *Mild symptoms:* Analgesics, neck physiotherapy

Surgical:

- *Indications:* Progressive neurological deficit, significant cord compression
- *Procedures:*
  - *Anterior:* ACDF (1–2 levels)
  - *Posterior:* Laminectomy + fusion or Laminoplasty (multilevel compression)

Quick Table

Management type	*Indications*
Conservative	Mild symptoms
Surgery	Progressive signs/MRI cord compression

Crisp Flowchart

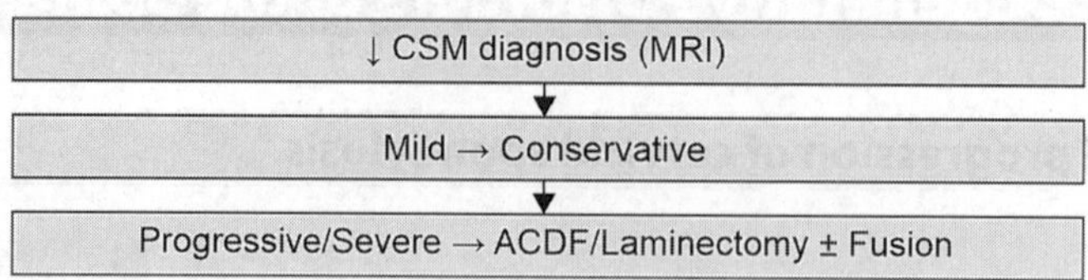

Q29. Discuss the classification and management of lumbar disc herniations.

(Asked in: RGUHS Karnataka 2022, MUHS 2021)

Definition

Lumbar disc herniation is the protrusion or extrusion of nucleus pulposus through a weakened annulus fibrosus, causing nerve root compression.

Common Levels Affected

- L4–L5 (L5 root)
- L5–S1 (S1 root)

Classification

- *By morphology:*
    - *Protrusion:* Base wider than herniation
    - *Extrusion:* Herniation wider than base
    - *Sequestration:* Free fragment detached
- *By location:*
    - Central
    - Paracentral (most common)
    - Foraminal
    - Extraforaminal

Clinical Features

- Radicular pain (sciatica)
- Sensory disturbances (numbness, tingling)
- Motor weakness
- Reflex changes (SLR positive)

Investigations

- **MRI lumbar spine**—gold standard
- *X-ray:* Rule out other causes

Management

Conservative:

- 90% improve without surgery
- Bed rest (short duration)
- Analgesics, NSAIDs, physiotherapy
- Epidural steroid injections (selected cases)

Surgical:

- *Indications:*
    - Cauda equina syndrome
    - Severe/progressive motor weakness
    - Failed conservative therapy (>6 weeks)
- *Procedures:*
    - Microdiscectomy (gold standard)
    - Endoscopic discectomy (minimally invasive)

Quick Revision Table

Aspect	*Details*
Common levels	L4–L5, L5–S1
Morphology	Protrusion, extrusion, sequestration
First-line management	Conservative
Surgical indications	Neurological deficit, cauda equina, failure of conservative

FLOWCHART: Lumbar disc herniation management

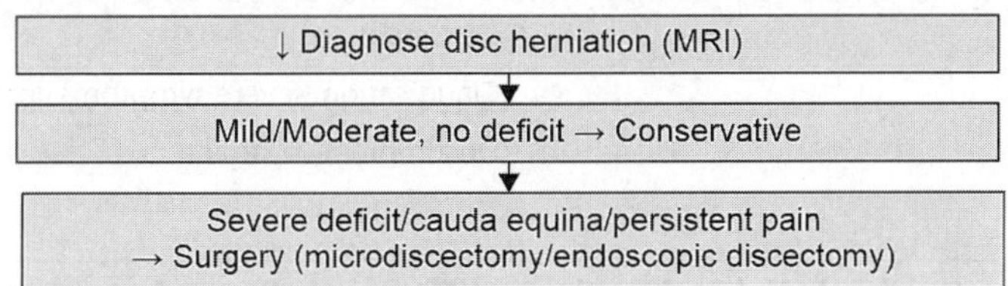

Q30. Pathophysiology of degenerative disc disease (DDD).

- **Aging + biomechanical stress** → degeneration of intervertebral discs.
- ↓ Proteoglycans → ↓ hydration of nucleus pulposus
- ↑ Collagen → fibrosis → loss of disc height
- Annular fissures form → disc bulging/herniation
- **Endplate changes** and **osteophyte formation**
- May cause nerve compression or segmental instability

Q31. Management strategies for lumbar canal stenosis.

(Asked in: PGI Chandigarh 2023)

Definition

Narrowing of the spinal canal causing compression of neural structures.

Causes

- Degenerative changes (disc bulge, facet hypertrophy)
- Ligamentum flavum hypertrophy
- Spondylolisthesis
- Congenital stenosis

Clinical Features

- Neurogenic claudication (pain while walking, relieved by sitting/flexion)
- Radicular pain
- Weakness, numbness

Investigations

- MRI lumbar spine—best modality
- CT for bony anatomy

Management

Conservative:

- Mild to moderate symptoms
- NSAIDs, physical therapy (flexion-based exercises)
- Epidural steroid injections

Surgical:
- *Indications:*
    - Persistent claudication
    - Severe neurogenic symptoms
    - Bladder/bowel dysfunction
- *Procedure:* Decompressive laminectomy ± fusion if instability

Quick Revision Table

Management step	*Details*
First line	Conservative
Surgery indications	Claudication, severe symptoms, instability
Surgery done	Decompressive lamine

Q32. Mechanical versus radicular low back pain—differentiate and treatment.

(Source: TNMGR Chennai 2021)

Feature	*Mechanical pain*	*Radicular pain*
Cause	Muscular, ligamentous strain	Nerve root compression
Pain character	Dull, aching	Sharp, shooting
Radiation	Localized to back	Down the leg (sciatica)
Neurological signs	Absent	May be present
Aggravating factors	Activity-related	Coughing, sneezing

Management
- *Mechanical pain:* Rest, physiotherapy, NSAIDs
- *Radicular pain:*
    - MRI spine
    - Conservative initially → Surgery if persistent or progressive deficits

Quick Table

Pain type	*Initial management*
Mechanical	NSAIDs + Physiotherapy
Radicular	MRI + Conservative → Surgery if needed

Q33. Prolapsed intervertebral disc (PIVD)—diagnosis and microdiscectomy technique.

(Source: JIPMER Puducherry 2023)

Diagnosis
- MRI lumbar spine
- Positive SLR test (straight leg raise)

Microdiscectomy Technique

Steps:
- Small posterior incision
- Paraspinal muscle dissection
- Laminotomy if needed
- Removal of herniated disc fragment
- Minimal damage to normal tissues

Advantages:

- Less postoperative pain
- Early mobilization
- Better cosmetic outcome

Quick Table

Technique feature	*Detail*
Incision	Small (2–3 cm)
Recovery	Early mobilization

Crisp Flowchart

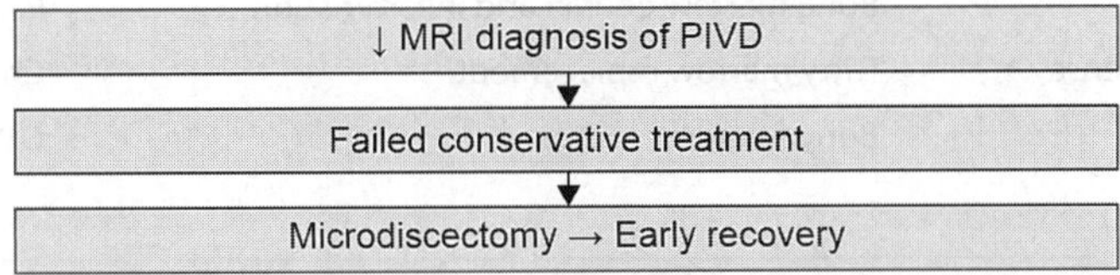

Topic	*1-liner recall*
CSM	MRI cord compression → Surgery if deficit
Lumbar disc herniation	90% recover conservatively
Lumbar stenosis	Claudication + MRI diagnosis
Spondylolisthesis	Meyerding grading guides management
Mechanical vs. radicular pain	Local back pain vs. radiating pain
PIVD microdiscectomy	Minimally invasive, early recovery

Q34. Cauda equina syndrome—red flag and immediate imaging.

Introduction

Cauda equina syndrome (CES) is a neurosurgical emergency caused by compression of lumbosacral nerve roots. Early recognition and MRI are crucial to prevent irreversible neurological damage.

FLOWCHART: Approach to suspected cauda equina syndrome

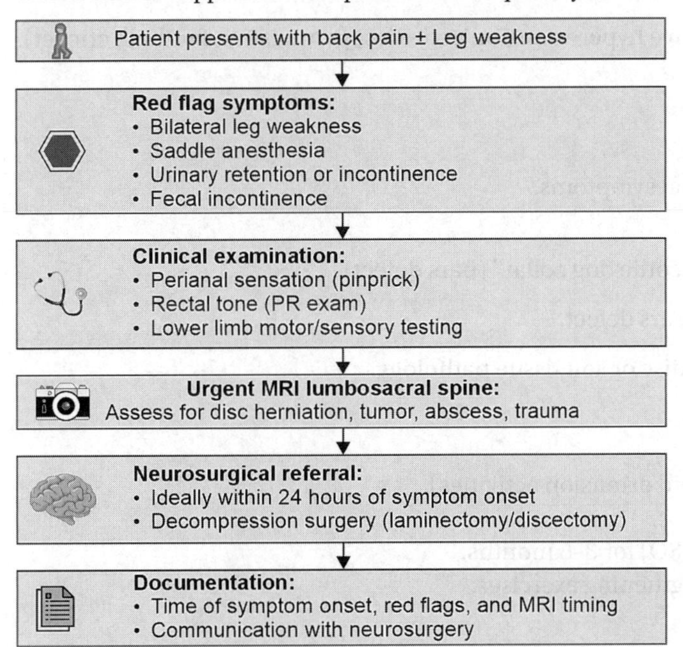

Key Points

- Saddle anesthesia and urinary retention are hallmark signs.
- MRI is the investigation of choice and should not be delayed.
- Early surgical decompression improves neurological outcomes.
- Always perform and document PR and sensory exam.

Q35. Modic changes—types and significance.

Seen on MRI adjacent to endplates in DDD

Type	*Mri signal*	*Histology*	*Clinical relevance*
I	T1 ↓/T2 ↑	Bone marrow edema and inflammation	Painful, active inflammation
II	T1 ↑/T2 isointense	Fatty marrow replacement	Chronic, less painful
III	T1 ↓/T2 ↓	Bony sclerosis	Often asymptomatic

Q36. Role of imaging in degenerative spine disorders.

Modality	*Use*
X-ray	Alignment, spondylolisthesis, disc space, osteophytes
MRI	Gold standard—disc herniation, stenosis, Modic changes
CT	Bony anatomy, foraminal stenosis, OPLL
Dynamic X-ray	Instability (flexion-extension views)

Q37. Describe spondylolysis and its treatment options.

(Asked in: RGUHS Karnataka 2023, MUHS Maharashtra 2022)

Definition

- **Spondylolysis = Defect or fracture in the pars interarticularis** (between superior and inferior articular processes).
- Commonly at **L5**.

Etiology

Stress fractures due to repetitive hyperextension activities (gymnastics, football, cricket).

Clinical Features

- Adolescent low back pain.
- Activity-related pain.
- Minimal or no neurological symptoms.

Diagnosis

X-ray: Oblique view shows "Scottie dog collar" (pars defect).

CT scan: Best for confirming pars defect.

MRI: Evaluate for associated disc or soft tissue pathology.

Treatment Options

Conservative (first line):

- Activity modification (avoid extension activities).
- NSAIDs.
- Brace immobilization (TLSO) for 3–6 months.
- *Physiotherapy:* Core strengthening exercises.

Surgical (rare, if persistent symptoms or instability):
- Direct pars repair (Buck's repair—screw across pars defect).
- Fusion surgery if associated slip or instability.

Q38. Describe spondylolisthesis—classification, clinical features, and management.

(Asked in: AIIMS Delhi 2022, JIPMER 2023)

Definition
Spondylolisthesis refers to anterior (forward) slippage of one vertebra over another.

Common Levels
- L5–S1 (most common)
- L4–L5

Classifications
Etiological (Wiltse classification):
- Dysplastic (congenital)
- Isthmic (pars defect)
- Degenerative (facet arthropathy)
- Traumatic
- Pathological (tumor, infection)
- Post-surgical

Severity (Meyerding grading):
- *Grade I:* 0–25% slip
- *Grade II:* 25–50%
- *Grade III:* 50–75%
- *Grade IV:* 75–100%

Clinical Features
- Low back pain
- Radiculopathy (if nerve root compression)
- "Step-off" deformity on palpation
- Tight hamstring syndrome
- Postural changes (hyperlordosis)

Investigations
- X-ray lumbar spine (standing lateral)
- MRI if radiculopathy present
- CT for bony anatomy

Management
Conservative:
- Indicated for Grade I–II without significant symptoms
- Bracing
- Activity modification
- Physiotherapy

Surgical:
- *Indications:*
  - High-grade slips (Grade III/IV)
  - Progressive slip
  - Neurological deficit
- *Procedures:*
  - Posterior lumbar interbody fusion (PLIF)
  - Transforaminal lumbar interbody fusion (TLIF)

Quick Revision Table

Aspect	*Details*
Most common type	Isthmic (adolescents), degenerative (elderly)
Meyerding grades	I–IV based on % slippage
Surgery indications	High-grade, deficit, pain

FLOWCHART: Spondylolisthesis management

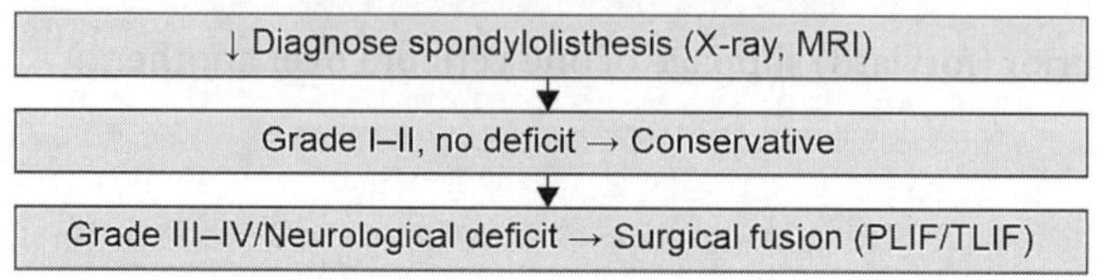

Q39. Describe the management of atlantoaxial instability.

(Asked in: RGUHS Karnataka 2023, TNMGR 2022)

Definition

Atlantoaxial instability (AAI) refers to excessive movement between the atlas (C1) and the axis (C2) due to disruption of the ligaments and/or bony structures maintaining stability.

Etiology

- Congenital (Down syndrome, Os odontoideum)
- Traumatic (fractures, ligament injuries)
- Inflammatory (rheumatoid arthritis)
- Neoplastic, infectious (tuberculosis)

Clinical Features

- Neck pain, restricted movements
- *Neurological signs:* Myelopathy (clumsiness, gait disturbance), lower cranial nerve palsies (severe cases)

Investigations

- *Dynamic X-rays (flexion-extension views)*: Measure anterior atlantodental interval (ADI). ADI >3mm abnormal in adults.
- *MRI:* Cord compression, ligament integrity
- *CT scan:* Bony anatomy

Management

Conservative management:

- *For reducible, stable injuries without neurological deficits:*
  - Cervical collar/halo vest immobilization

Surgical management:

- *Indications:* Neurological deficit, irreducible instability, progressive deformity
- *Procedures:*
  - *Posterior C1-C2 fusion:* Gallie, Brooks, or Harms technique
  - *Transarticular screw fixation:* High fusion rate but requires precise technique
  - *Occipitocervical fusion:* In cases involving occiput or severe instability

Postoperative Care

- Immobilization with cervical collar or halo
- Physiotherapy for neck mobility (after fusion consolidation)

Q40. Role of spinal injections in degenerative spine disorders.

Types

- **Epidural steroid injection**—disc herniation, spinal stenosis
- **Facet joint injections**—facet arthropathy
- **Medial branch blocks**—diagnostic for facet-mediated pain
- **Sacroiliac joint injections**

Benefits

- Short-term relief
- Diagnostic and therapeutic
- Helps defer or determine need for surgery

Q41. Role of anterior decompression in thoracic disc herniations.

(Asked in: PGI Chandigarh 2021)

Definition

Thoracic disc herniation (TDH) is rare but can cause severe neurological impairment due to the narrow thoracic spinal canal.

Clinical Features

- Mid-back pain
- Myelopathy (spastic paraparesis)
- Radicular pain (intercostal neuralgia)
- Bowel/bladder dysfunction

Diagnosis

- MRI thoracic spine (preferred)
- CT scan to detect calcified discs

Why Anterior Decompression?

- Most thoracic discs herniate anteriorly
- Posterior approaches (laminectomy) risk cord injury
- Direct anterior access allows safe removal

Surgical Techniques for Anterior Decompression

Transthoracic approach:

- Via thoracotomy
- Direct visualization and removal of herniated disc

Video-assisted thoracoscopic surgery (VATS):

- Minimally invasive option
- Less morbidity compared to open thoracotomy

Costotransversectomy or lateral extracavitary approach: Alternative to anterior approaches for lateralized herniations

Complications of Anterior Approach

- Pulmonary complications (pneumothorax, atelectasis)
- Injury to great vessels, thoracic duct
- Postoperative pain

Quick Revision Table

Approach	*Usefulness*
Transthoracic	Best for central discs
VATS	Minimally invasive alternative
Costotransversectomy	Lateral discs

FLOWCHART: Thoracic disc herniation management

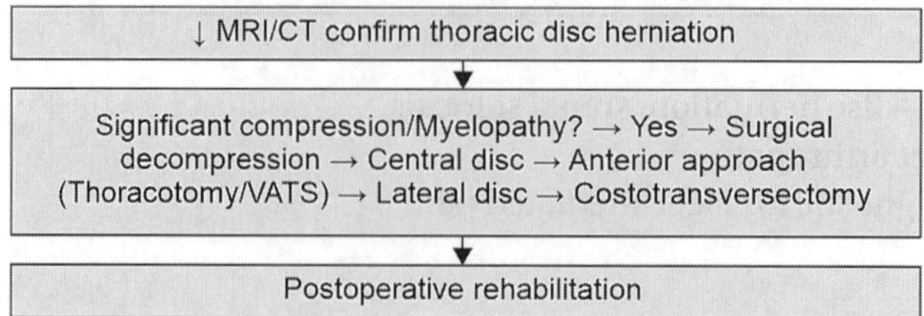

Infections of the Spine

Q42. Pathogenesis and management of pyogenic spondylodiscitis.

Pathogenesis

- Hematogenous spread (most common)
- Direct inoculation (e.g., surgery, injections)
- *Common organisms: Staphylococcus aureus*, Streptococcus, Gram-negative bacilli

Pathology

- Infection starts at **endplates**, spreads to disc and adjacent vertebrae
- May form **paravertebral/epidural abscess**

Management

- **Rest**, immobilization
- **IV antibiotics** (6 weeks), then oral (6 more weeks)
- *Surgical intervention if*:
  - Neurological deficit
  - Instability
  - Abscess
  - Failure of conservative management

Q43. Complications of untreated spinal infections.

- **Neurological deficit** (cord compression)
- **Spinal deformity** (kyphosis, scoliosis)
- **Paraspinal/epidural abscess**
- **Sepsis/systemic spread**
- **Chronic osteomyelitis**
- **Instability → pathological fractures**

Q44. Role of MRI and CT in diagnosing spinal infections.

Imaging	*Utility*
MRI	Gold standard—early marrow changes, disc involvement, epidural/paravertebral abscess, cord compression
CT	Better for detecting bony destruction, sequestrum, surgical planning
CT-guided biopsy	Diagnostic for organism identification

Q45. Role of biopsy in diagnosis of spinal infections.

- *Indications:*
  - Unclear etiology
  - Atypical presentation
  - Non-responsiveness to empirical antibiotics

- *Techniques:*
    - **CT-guided needle biopsy**—minimally invasive, preferred
    - Open biopsy if needle fails
- *Utility:*
    - Confirms diagnosis
    - Microbiological culture and sensitivity
    - Histopathology (TB granulomas, fungal elements, etc.)

Q46. Management of spinal epidural abscess (SEA).

Definition

Accumulation of pus in the **epidural space** causing **cord compression**

Etiology

- Hematogenous spread, trauma, IV drug use
- *Organism: Staphylococcus aureus*

Clinical Features

- *Triad:* **Back pain, fever, neurological deficit**
- Rapidly progressive paraplegia if not treated

Diagnosis

MRI with contrast: Loculated epidural collection

Treatment

- **Emergency decompressive laminectomy** + drainage
- **IV antibiotics** for 6 weeks
- **Steroids** in some cases for cord edema

Spinal Tuberculosis (Pott's Spine)

Q47. Clinical features, diagnosis, and management of spinal tuberculosis.

(Asked in: AIIMS Delhi 2021, RGUHS Karnataka 2022)

Introduction

- **Spinal tuberculosis (Pott's spine)** is the **most common form of skeletal TB** (~50% cases).
- Caused by *Mycobacterium tuberculosis* reaching the spine via hematogenous spread.

Clinical Features

Constitutional symptoms: Fever, night sweats, weight loss, malaise.

Local symptoms:

- Back pain—insidious onset, progressive.
- Paraspinal muscle spasm.
- Gibbus deformity (localized kyphosis).

Neurological deficits (in ~30% cases):

- Paraparesis or paraplegia (spinal cord compression).
- Sensory deficits, bladder-bowel involvement in advanced cases.

Diagnosis

Imaging:

- *MRI spine*: Investigation of choice.
  - Shows vertebral destruction, disc involvement, abscess formation, spinal cord compression.

X-rays:

Late findings: Vertebral body destruction, disc space narrowing, kyphotic deformity.

CT scan: Bony details, sequestrum identification.

Microbiological tests: Needle aspiration or biopsy → GeneXpert, AFB staining, culture.

Blood tests:

- Raised ESR, CRP.
- Positive Mantoux/IGRA supportive.

Management

1. *Antitubercular therapy (ATT)*:
   - Mainstay.
   - *Regimen:* 4-drug therapy (HRZE) for 2 months, followed by two drugs (HR) for 10–12 months total.
2. *Immobilization*: Spinal brace (TLSO) to reduce pain and prevent deformity progression.
3. **Surgical indications** (remember "**Medical treatment is primary—Surgery only when needed**"):

Indications for Surgery

- Neurological deficit not improving with ATT.
- Large abscess causing compression.
- Severe kyphotic deformity (>40–50°).
- Instability or progressive vertebral collapse.
- Failure of conservative management.

Surgical Options

- Anterior decompression and fusion.
- Posterior decompression and instrumentation (especially in cervico-thoracic or thoracolumbar junction).
- Combined approaches in severe cases.

Q48. Classification of spinal TB.

GATA Classification

- *Type I:* No deformity/neurology → ATT only
- *Type II:* Neurological deficit without deformity → ATT ± surgery
- *Type III:* Kyphosis, instability, abscess, neuro deficit → surgery required

Q49. Pathogenesis and classification of Pott's spine.

(Asked in: MUHS Maharashtra 2022, PGI Chandigarh 2022)

Pathogenesis

Initial infection: Typically begins in **vertebral metaphysis** near subchondral bone.

Spread:

- Infection spreads beneath anterior longitudinal ligament → contiguous vertebrae involved.
- Leads to **paradiscal involvement** (most common), destroying intervertebral discs secondarily.

Abscess formation: Cold abscess tracks along fascial planes (e.g., psoas abscess in lumbar TB).

Sequelae:
- Vertebral collapse → gibbus deformity.
- Cord compression → neurological deficits.

Types of Spinal TB Based on Location

Type	*Description*
Paradiscal	Infection around vertebral endplates; most common type
Central	Involves vertebral body center; risk of vertebral collapse
Anterior	Infection under anterior longitudinal ligament; multiple vertebrae involved
Posterior	Involves posterior elements (rare)

Classification Based on Severity

Modified Kumar's classification or GATA classification (used to guide treatment): Presence/absence of deformity, neurological deficit, extent of bone involvement.

Exam Tip

When writing about spinal TB:
- **Mention paradiscal involvement and MRI as investigation of choice** early.
- **Emphasize ATT as first-line**, and **surgery only for specific indications.**
- For pathogenesis, **show the sequence: Metaphysis → spread → collapse → abscess.**

Q50. Define Pott's disease. Discuss its stages.

Definition

Pott's disease (spinal tuberculosis) is a form of extrapulmonary TB affecting the spine, leading to vertebral destruction, deformity, and possible neurological compromise.

Stages (Tuli's Classification)
- **Stage I**: Early discitis without bone involvement
- **Stage II**: Vertebral body involvement, kyphosis begins
- **Stage III**: Paravertebral abscess, caseation
- **Stage IV**: Neurological deficit (Pott's paraplegia)

Q51. Clinical features of Pott's disease.

- **Back pain** (insidious onset)
- *Spinal deformity:* Gibbus (hump) in thoracic region
- *Constitutional symptoms:* Fever, weight loss, night sweats
- *Neurological signs (30–50%):* Pott's paraplegia (delayed/early onset)
- *Cold abscess:* Paravertebral or psoas
- **Restricted spinal motion**

Q52. Radiological findings in Pott's spine.

Modality	*Findings*
X-ray	Anterior vertebral body destruction, disc space narrowing, kyphosis
MRI	Best modality—bone marrow edema, abscess, cord compression
CT scan	Bone destruction, calcification in abscess, sequestra
USG	Detection of psoas abscess (guides aspiration)

Q53. Short note on classification of Pott's spine.

Tuli's Clinicoradiological Classification

- *Paradiscal (most common)*: Starts near endplates
- *Central:* Whole body collapse
- *Anterior:* Subperiosteal spread
- *Posterior:* Rare, pedicle/lamina
- *Nonosseous:* Only soft tissue/paraspinal abscess

Q54. Describe the pathophysiology, clinical features, and management of Pott's paraplegia.

(Asked in: RGUHS Karnataka 2022)

Definition

Pott's paraplegia refers to neurological deficit resulting from spinal tuberculosis (TB).

Pathophysiology

- Mechanical compression (abscess, granulation tissue, sequestra, bony fragments)
- Ischemia (due to endarteritis obliterans)
- Cord edema
- Late-stage fibrosis and myelomalacia

Types

- *Early onset paraplegia:* Occurs during active disease (within 2 years)—better prognosis
- *Late onset paraplegia:* Occurs after healed disease (fibrosis, deformity)—worse prognosis

Clinical Features

- Gradual onset weakness of lower limbs
- Spasticity, exaggerated reflexes (UMN signs)
- Sensory disturbances
- Bladder/bowel dysfunction (late)

Investigations

- *MRI spine:* Best for cord compression and soft tissue detail
- *X-ray spine:* Kyphosis, vertebral collapse
- ESR, CRP elevated

Management

Medical management:

- Anti-tubercular therapy (ATT)—minimum 12–18 months
- Bed rest (initial phase) + immobilization (bracing)

Surgical management:

- *Indications:*
  - Progressive neurological deficit
  - Severe kyphotic deformity
- *Procedures:*
  - Anterior decompression (corpectomy + fusion)
  - Posterior instrumentation in case of instability

Quick Revision Table

Aspect	*Details*
Pathophysiology	Compression + Ischemia
Early vs. late onset	Early: Active disease; Late: Healed disease
Management	ATT + Surgery if deficit/progression

FLOWCHART: Pott's paraplegia management

↓ Diagnose TB spine (MRI, X-ray)

↓

No Deficit → ATT + Observation
Neurological deficit → ATT + Surgical decompression + Stabilization

Q55. Kyphosis following tubercular spine—evaluation and management.

(Asked in: TNMGR 2022)

Definition

Kyphosis is the most common sequelae following spinal tuberculosis, especially in the thoracic spine.

Causes of Kyphosis in TB

- Vertebral body collapse
- Anterior column destruction
- Healing with fibrous tissue rather than bone

Evaluation

- *Clinical:*
  - Visible deformity (gibbus)
  - Neurological examination (late onset paraplegia)
- *Radiological:*
  - *X-rays:* Kyphotic angle measurement (Cobb's angle)
  - *MRI:* Cord compression, healed versus active disease
  - *CT:* Extent of bony destruction

Severity of Kyphosis (Rajasekaran Classification)

- Mild (<30°)
- Moderate (30–60°)
- Severe (>60°)

Management

Mild-to-moderate kyphosis (<60°) with no neurological deficit:

- Observation
- Bracing (during healing phase)
- ATT to ensure healing

Severe kyphosis (>60°) or with neurological deficit: Surgical Correction

Surgical Principles

- Correction of deformity
- Decompression of spinal cord
- Stabilization with instrumentation

Surgical Techniques

- Anterior decompression + Strut grafting
- Posterior instrumentation with osteotomy (pedicle subtraction osteotomy)
- Combined anterior + Posterior approach

Quick Revision Table

Aspect	*Details*
Main cause	Vertebral body collapse
Clinical evaluation	Deformity, neurology

Continued

Continued

Aspect	***Details***
Radiological evaluation	Cobb's angle, MRI for cord status
Mild/Moderate (<60°)	Observation, brace
Severe (>60°)	Surgical correction

FLOWCHART: Kyphosis after TB management

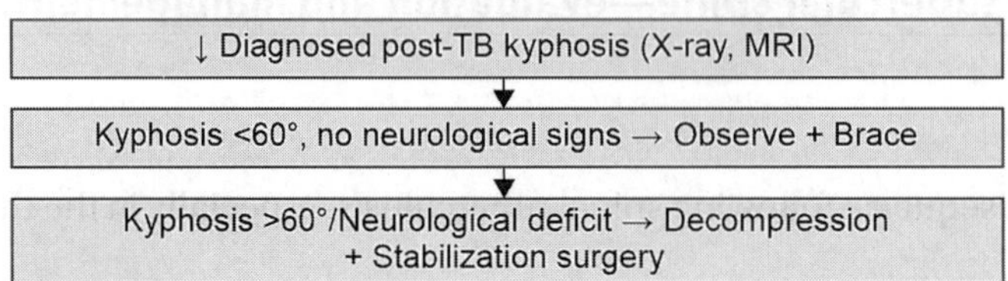

Q56. Indications for surgical management in Pott's disease.

- **Neurological deficit** (progressive/late-onset)
- **Failure of conservative treatment**
- **Large abscesses** not responding to aspiration
- **Kyphotic deformity >40° or progression**
- **Spinal instability** or collapse
- **Diagnostic uncertainty**

Q57. Short notes—paradiscal and central types of Pott's spine.

Type	***Features***
Paradiscal	Involves adjacent vertebral bodies near disc → disc space narrowing early
Central	Central vertebral body involvement → vertebra collapses into "vertebra plana"

Q58. Role of anti-tubercular therapy (ATT) in spinal TB.

- **Cornerstone of treatment**
- *Standard WHO regimen*:
  - *2 months:* HRZE (Intensive phase)
  - *10–16 months:* HR (Continuation phase)
- Continue for **12–18 months** total
- Monitor with ESR/CRP, clinical and radiological assessment
- ATT is **mandatory even post-surgery**

Q59. Complications of spinal tuberculosis.

- Kyphotic deformity
- Paraplegia (early or late onset)
- Cold abscess (psoas, paraspinal)
- Chronic instability
- Spinal canal stenosis
- Drug resistance (MDR-TB/XDR-TB)
- Recurrence or sinus formation

Q60. Posterior versus anterior decompression in spinal tuberculosis.

Approach	*Indication*	*Advantages*	*Limitations*
Anterior	Classical approach for kyphosis, vertebral body disease	Direct decompression, abscess removal	Morbidity, lung exposure
Posterior	Preferred today for many cases	Familiar to spine surgeons, easier fusion	May not address anterior disease fully
Combined	Severe kyphosis or instability	360° decompression and stabilization	Technically demanding

Q61. Differential diagnosis and management of infective spondylitis.

(Asked in: PGI Chandigarh 2021)

Definition

Infective spondylitis refers to infection involving the vertebral body, intervertebral disc, and surrounding soft tissues.

Types and Differentials

Condition	*Features*
Tubercular spondylitis	Gradual onset, anterior vertebral destruction, paravertebral abscess
Pyogenic spondylitis	Acute onset, severe pain, fever, single vertebral involvement
Fungal spondylitis	Immunocompromised patients, slow progressive
Brucellar spondylitis	Endemic areas, systemic features
Neoplastic pathologize	Severe localized severe pain, contitutional symptoms, history of primary maligancy in case of metastasis, and may be assocaited neurological deficit
Non-ifective modic changes	Chronic pain without systematic features

Clinical Features
- Back pain
- Fever (more common in pyogenic)
- Weight loss (TB)
- Neurological deficits (late in TB, early in pyogenic)

Investigations
- MRI spine (best imaging modality)
- *Blood tests:* ESR, CRP, CBC
- Blood cultures (pyogenic)
- TB PCR, GeneXpert from biopsy/aspiration

Management

Medical treatment:
- Empirical antibiotics (after cultures) for pyogenic
- ATT for tubercular
- Antifungal therapy for fungal

Surgical treatment:
- *Indications:*
  - Neurological deficits
  - Failure of medical therapy
  - Instability or severe deformity
- *Procedures:*
  - Anterior debridement and fusion
  - Posterior stabilization if instability present

Quick Revision Table

Infection type	*Key features*
Tubercular	Insidious, cold abscess
Pyogenic	Acute, high fever
Fungal/Brucellar	Immunosuppressed, endemic area

FLOWCHART: Infective spondylitis approach

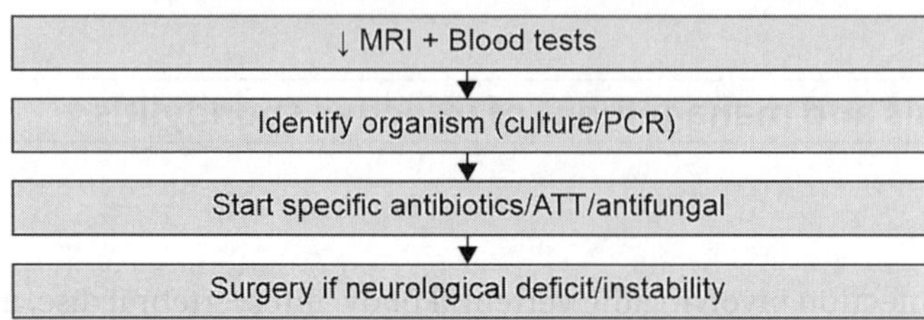

Q62. Multidrug resistant (MDR) TB of spine—management principles.

(Source: MUHS Maharashtra 2023)

Definition

Resistance to at least **isoniazid and rifampicin** in spinal TB.

Management Principles

Second-line ATT: WHO category IV drugs (fluoroquinolones, injectable agents like amikacin, newer agents like bedaquiline)

Duration of treatment: Longer duration (18–24 months)

Surgical indications:
- Neurological deficit
- Instability
- Failure to respond to second-line drugs

Follow-up:
- Regular imaging (MRI/X-rays)
- Monitoring side effects of second-line drugs

Quick Table

Aspect	*Details*
Drugs	Second-line (FQs, amikacin, linezolid)
Treatment duration	18–24 months
Surgery	If neurological deficit/instability

Q63. Prognostic factors in TB spine.

- *Favorable:*
  - Early diagnosis
  - No neurological deficit
  - Minimal vertebral destruction
  - Responsive to ATT
- *Unfavorable:*
  - Kyphosis >60°
  - Late-onset paraplegia

- Multilevel disease
- Drug resistance

Q64. Diagnostic MRI features in TB spine.

- T2 hyperintense paravertebral abscess
- Hypointense vertebral body lesions (T1)
- Disc sparing (initially) or involvement (later)
- "Cold abscess" with smooth walls
- Gibbus deformity or vertebral collapse

Q65. Causes of late-onset Pott's paraplegia.

- Internal gibbus compression
- Kyphotic deformity progression
- Residual abscess or granulation tissue
- Vertebral instability
- Dural fibrosis or arachnoiditis

Q66. Use of metallic implants in TB spine—recent rationale.

- Modern ATT reduces infection risk around implants
- *Implants:*
  - Provide early stabilization
  - Allow deformity correction
  - Enable early mobilization
- Titanium preferred (biocompatible, MRI-safe)

Q67. Paralytic bladder.

- Bladder dysfunction due to **lower motor neuron lesion**
- Areflexic bladder → retention, overflow incontinence
- *Causes:* Cauda equina injury, spinal trauma
- *Tx:* Intermittent catheterization, cholinergic agents

Q68. Neurogenic bladder.

- Bladder dysfunction due to **neurological disease**
- *Types:*
  - Spastic (UMN)
  - Flaccid (LMN)
- *Symptoms:* Urgency, retention, incontinence
- *Tx:* Anticholinergics, catheterization, bladder training

Q69. Autonomous bladder.

- Seen in **complete spinal cord transection (above S2–S4)**
- No voluntary control, but bladder empties reflexively
- Risk of incontinence and UTI

Q70. Automatic bladder.

- Similar to autonomous bladder; caused by **UMN lesion**
- Reflexive voiding occurs once bladder fills
- No cortical control

Q71. Nerve supply of bladder and autonomic bladder management.

Nerve Supply

- **Parasympathetic (S2–S4)** → Detrusor contraction
- **Sympathetic (T11–L2)** → Internal sphincter control
- **Somatic (pudendal, S2–S4)** → External sphincter

Autonomic Bladder

- Disruption of spinal control → reflex bladder activity
- *Management:*
    - Bladder training
    - Anticholinergics
    - Catheterization
    - Surgical options if needed

Q72. Cold abscess—etiopathogenesis and clinical features.

Etiopathogenesis

- Caused by *Mycobacterium tuberculosis*
- *Spread via:*
    - Hematogenous route (common)
    - Direct spread from spinal TB
- *Cold*: Absence of signs of acute inflammation (no warmth, erythema)

Clinical Features

- Painless swelling
- *Common sites:* Paravertebral, psoas, retropharyngeal
- May cause pressure effects (e.g., dysphagia, bladder dysfunction)
- Fluctuant on palpation

Q73. Early versus late-onset paraplegia in spinal TB.

Feature	*Early-onset*	*Late-onset*
Timing	Within 2 years of disease onset	After healing (often >2 years)
Cause	Active inflammation, abscess, granulation	Internal gibbus, kyphotic deformity
Prognosis	Better with ATT and decompression	Poorer; often requires surgery

Q74. Staging of Pott's paraplegia (Girdlestone and Griffith).

(CMC Vellore 2018)

- *Stage I*: Signs of cord irritation (hyperreflexia, clonus).
- *Stage II*: Motor weakness with spasticity
- *Stage III*: Complete motor paralysis (no voluntary movement)
- *Stage IV*: Complete motor + sensory loss ± bladder/bowel involvement

Q75. TB D12–L1 with paraparesis + urinary retention.

Classification (Modified Tuli)

- *Stage I:* Signs of irritation
- *Stage II:* Motor weakness
- *Stage III:* Complete motor loss
- *Stage IV:* Motor + sensory + bladder involvement

Investigations

- MRI spine with contrast
- ESR, CRP
- GeneXpert/biopsy if needed

Treatment Options

- *Medical:* Full course of ATT (RIPE regimen)
- *Surgical:*
    - *Indicated in:*
        - Abscess
        - Kyphotic deformity
        - No improvement with ATT
    - **Anterior decompression** ± instrumentation (D12–L1)

Crisp Flowchart

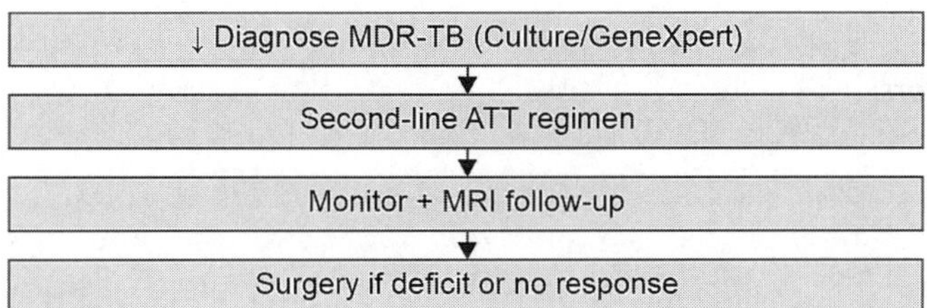

Ultra-crisp Final Memory Markers

Topic	*1-Liner recall*
Pott's spine	ATT first, surgery if deficit
Kyphotic deformity	>60° needs surgical correction
Infective spondylodiscitis	MRI + Biopsy + Specific antibiotics
MDR-TB	Second-line ATT, prolonged treatment

Q76. Tuberculoma.

- **Granulomatous mass** in CNS caused by TB.
- In the spine, may form in **epidural space** or compress spinal cord.
- Seen in **intradural or intramedullary locations**.
- *MRI:* Iso-hypointense on T1, ring-enhancing lesion on contrast.
- *Treatment:* ATT ± steroids; surgery if causing cord compression.

Q77. Routes of TB spinal abscess/cold abscess spread.

1. **Psoas abscess** → groin/thigh
2. **Paravertebral** → chest wall/flank
3. **Retropharyngeal** (cervical TB) → neck swelling
4. **Intercostal space** (dorsal spine)
5. **Gluteal** (through sciatic notch)

Q78. Radiological features of TB spine.

- Vertebral body destruction (anterior)
- Disc space narrowing
- Paravertebral shadows (abscess)
- Gibbus deformity/kyphosis
- *MRI:* T2 hyperintense abscess, vertebral edema

Spinal Tumors

Q79. Describe the staging and surgical management of primary spine tumors.

(Asked in: TNMGR 2022)

Definition

Primary spine tumors originate from vertebral elements (bone, cartilage, soft tissue) and include benign and malignant types.

Examples of Primary Tumors

- *Benign:* Osteoid osteoma, Giant cell tumor (GCT)
- *Malignant:* Chordoma, chondrosarcoma, osteosarcoma, Ewing's sarcoma

Staging

Enneking staging for spine tumors:

- *Benign tumors:*
  - *Stage 1:* Latent
  - *Stage 2:* Active
  - *Stage 3:* Aggressive
- *Malignant tumors:*
  - Low grade versus High grade
  - Intracompartmental versus extracompartmental

Weinstein–Boriani–Biagini (WBB) classification:

- Clock-face system (12 zones + layers A–E)
- Helps in surgical planning

Management Principles

Benign tumors:

- Curettage with/without bone grafting (for latent tumors)
- Wide excision for aggressive tumors (e.g., GCT)

Malignant tumors:

- En bloc resection whenever feasible
- Adjuvant radiotherapy and/or chemotherapy (depending on histology)

Surgical techniques:

- Total en bloc spondylectomy (TES)
- Posterior stabilization with instrumentation

Quick Revision Table

Tumor type	*Treatment*
Benign	Curettage/Marginal Excision
Malignant	En bloc resection + Adjuvant therapy

FLOWCHART: Primary spine tumor management

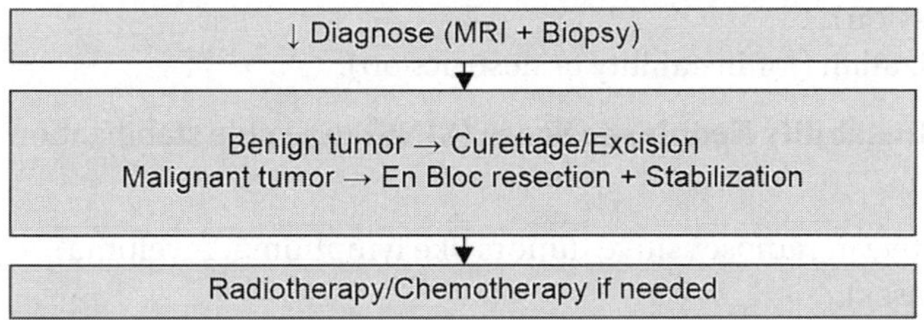

Ultra-crisp Final Memory Markers

Topic	*1-liner memory tip*
Spinal metastasis	NOMS framework guides management
Infective spondylitis	MRI + Culture = Diagnosis
Primary spine tumors	Enneking and WBB staging used

Q80. Classification and management of spinal tumors.

(Asked in: PGI Chandigarh 2022, MUHS Maharashtra 2023)

Introduction

- Spinal tumors may be **primary** (originating in the spine) or **secondary** (metastatic).
- They cause symptoms through **mass effect, instability, and neurological compression**.

Classification (By Location)

1. *Extradural (most common, ~60%)*:
    - Metastases (breast, lung, prostate)
    - Lymphoma
    - Myeloma
2. *Intradural extramedullary*:
    - Meningioma
    - Schwannoma
    - Neurofibroma
3. *Intramedullary*:
    - Astrocytoma
    - Ependymoma
    - Hemangioblastoma

Clinical Presentation

- Localized spinal pain (worsens at night).
- Radiculopathy (nerve root compression).
- Progressive myelopathy (cord compression → weakness, spasticity, bowel/bladder involvement).

Diagnosis

- *MRI spine with contrast*: Investigation of choice.
- *CT scan:* Bone involvement.
- *Biopsy:* Confirm histological diagnosis (especially in primary tumors or unknown secondaries).

Management

Benign tumors:

- Small, asymptomatic → observation.
- Symptomatic → Surgical excision.

Malignant tumors:

- Combination of surgery, radiotherapy, chemotherapy depending on histology.
- *Aim:* Decompress cord, stabilize spine, relieve pain.

Surgical options:
- **Laminectomy** (decompression).
- **Vertebrectomy** and stabilization (for instability or destruction).

Spinal instability: Use **Spinal Instability Neoplastic Score (SINS)** to decide stabilization needs.

Adjuvant therapy:
- Radiotherapy (highly effective in radiosensitive tumors like lymphoma, myeloma).
- Chemotherapy (selected cases).

Key Points
- Primary aim: **Preserve/improve neurological function**.
- Pain control and stabilization equally important.

Q81. Spinal metastasis—evaluation and management options.

(Source: AIIMS Delhi 2023)

Common Primary Sites

Breast, prostate, lung, kidney, thyroid

Clinical Features
- Persistent localized pain (night pain)
- Neurological deficits (weakness, sensory loss)
- Pathological fractures

Evaluation
- X-ray/CT spine (bone destruction)
- MRI (cord compression, soft tissue mass)
- PET-CT (whole body metastasis evaluation)
- Biopsy (confirm histology if diagnosis unclear)

Management Options

Non-surgical (first-line in many cases):
- Radiotherapy (especially radiosensitive tumors like lymphoma, myeloma)
- Chemotherapy/Hormonal therapy (e.g., prostate cancer)

Surgical indications:
- Neurological deficit
- Spinal instability
- Intractable pain

Surgical options:
- Posterior decompression and stabilization (pedicle screw fixation)
- Vertebroplasty/Kyphoplasty (for painful vertebral collapse without instability)

Framework for decision:
- *NOMS:* Neurologic, Oncologic, Mechanical, Systemic assessment

Management Approach

General principles:
- *Multidisciplinary approach:* Oncologist + Spine surgeon + Radiation oncologist.
- Assess patient's life expectancy, tumor sensitivity, neurological status.

Radiotherapy:
- **Stereotactic radiosurgery (SRS)** increasingly used for localized lesions.
- Traditional external beam radiotherapy (EBRT) for palliation.

Minimally invasive techniques:
- *Vertebroplasty/Kyphoplasty:*
    - Cement injection into vertebral body.
    - Relieves pain in vertebral metastasis without significant instability.

Systemic therapy:
- Chemotherapy, hormonal therapy depending on primary.
- Bisphosphonates/Denosumab to strengthen bone.

Quick Table

Treatment modality	*Indications*
Radiotherapy	Radiosensitive tumors
Surgery	Instability/Deficit/Intractable Pain

Crisp Flowchart

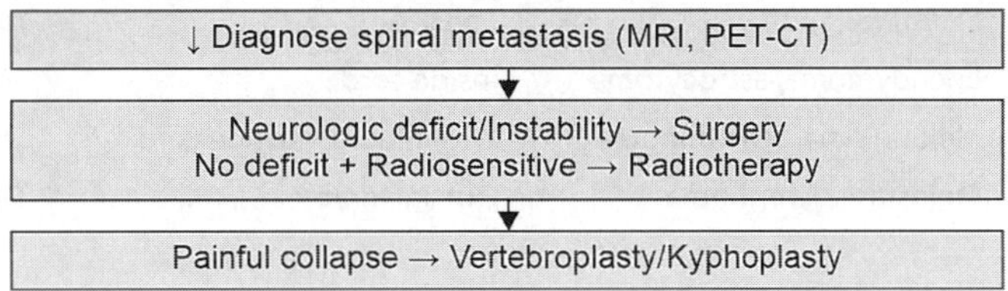

Q82. Spinal instability neoplastic score (SINS).

Factor	*Score*
Location (junctional vs. mobile)	0–3
Pain (mechanical)	0–3
Bone lesion quality (lytic/blastic/mixed)	0–3
Alignment (subluxation/kyphosis)	0–4
Vertebral body collapse	0–3
Posterolateral involvement	0–3

SINS Interpretation
- *0–6*: Stable
- *7–12*: Indeterminate (consider surgery)
- *13–18*: Unstable → Surgical stabilization recommended.

Exam Tip
When writing about spinal tumors:
- **Start with extradural > intradural > intramedullary** classification.
- **Always mention MRI as investigation of choice.**
- For metastatic spine, **state SINS score application clearly**.
- *Emphasize goal:* **Neurological preservation, pain control, mechanical stability**.

Q83. Role of vertebroplasty/kyphoplasty in metastatic spine disease.

(Source: MUHS Maharashtra 2023)

Definitions
- *Vertebroplasty:* Percutaneous injection of bone cement (PMMA) into collapsed vertebral body
- Kyphoplasty: Balloon inserted into vertebral body → inflated to restore height → cement injected

Indications in Metastatic Spine Disease
- Painful osteolytic vertebral body collapse without spinal instability
- Vertebral compression fractures due to metastasis

Advantages
- Immediate pain relief
- Improved mobility
- Minimally invasive

Contraindications
- Spinal instability
- Cord compression needing surgical decompression

Q84. Spinal cord tumors—types and management.

Type	*Examples*	*Location*	*Management*
Intramedullary	Ependymoma, astrocytoma	Inside cord	Microsurgical excision ± RT
Intradural-extramedullary	Meningioma, schwannoma	Within dura, outside cord	Surgical excision
Extradural	Metastasis, lymphoma	Outside dura	Decompression, RT, chemotherapy

Diagnosis
- MRI with contrast
- Neurological exam + spinal level localization

Quick Table

Procedure	*Main indication*
Vertebroplasty	Painful, stable vertebral body collapse
Kyphoplasty	Same + restores vertebral height

Crisp Flowchart

↓ Painful vertebral metastasis

↓

Stable, no instability → Vertebroplasty/Kyphoplasty
Instability/Cord compression → Decompression + Fixation

Ultra-crisp Final Memory Markers

Topic	*1-liner recall*
Primary spine tumor	MRI + Biopsy → En bloc resection
Spine metastasis	NOMS framework guides treatment
Vertebroplasty/Kyphoplasty	Stable fractures → Cement augmentation

Inflammatory and Rheumatological Disorders of the Spine

Q85. Pathophysiology and classification of ankylosing spondylitis (AS).

Pathophysiology
- Chronic inflammatory disease, **HLA-B27 associated**
- Inflammation begins at **entheses** (enthesitis) → bone erosion → repair → syndesmophyte formation → spinal ankylosis
- **Autoimmune + mechanical** factors

Classification

- *Based on assessment of spondyloarthritis international society (ASAS):*
  - **Radiographic axial SpA** → visible sacroiliitis on X-ray (traditional AS)
  - **Non-radiographic axial SpA** → clinical + MRI findings

Q86. Radiological features of ankylosing spondylitis.

(JIPMER 2011)

Sacroiliac Joint

- **Earliest site** involved
- Bilateral and symmetrical **sclerosis** → **erosions** → **fusion**
- Graded I–IV (Modified New York Criteria)

Spine

- **Shiny corners** (Romanus lesions)
- **Syndesmophytes** (marginal, vertical ossification of annulus fibrosus)
- **Bamboo spine** (late stage, fused vertebrae with thin syndesmophytes)
- **Anderson lesions**—discovertebral erosions

Q87. Medical and surgical management of ankylosing spondylitis.

Medical

- *NSAIDs:* First-line (e.g., indomethacin)
- *DMARDs:* Sulfasalazine (for peripheral involvement)
- *Biologics:* Anti-TNF agents (etanercept, infliximab)
- *Physical therapy:* Posture, mobility

Surgical

- *Spinal osteotomy:* For severe kyphosis
- *Hip arthroplasty:* For ankylosed hips
- *Atlantoaxial fixation:* For instability

Q88. Classification and management of seronegative spondyloarthropathies.

Types (HLA-B27 associated, RF negative)

- Ankylosing spondylitis
- Psoriatic arthritis
- Reactive arthritis (Reiter's syndrome)
- Enteropathic arthritis (Crohn's/UC)
- Undifferentiated SpA

Management

- NSAIDs, DMARDs, biologics (anti-TNF, IL-17 inhibitors)
- Physical therapy
- Treat underlying GI/skin conditions
- Surgery if deformity or neurological compromise

Q89. Spinal manifestations of rheumatoid arthritis (RA).

- Mainly affects **cervical spine**

Level affected	*Pathology*
Atlantoaxial	Transverse ligament laxity → instability, pannus
Subaxial	Facet erosion → subluxation (staircase pattern)
Cervicomedullary	Cord compression, myelopathy

- *Symptoms:* Neck pain, stiffness, neurological deficit

Q90. Atlantoaxial instability in rheumatoid arthritis.

- Caused by **pannus formation**, erosion of dens, and ligament laxity
- May lead to **cord compression**

Diagnosis

- *Flexion-extension lateral X-rays:* Atlanto-dental interval (ADI >3mm = instability)
- *MRI:* Pannus, cord compression

Management

- **Cervical collar** (temporary)
- **Posterior C1–C2 fusion** (definitive)
- Avoid flexion maneuvers during intubation

Q91. Diffuse idiopathic skeletal hyperostosis (DISH) and its management.

Definition

Non-inflammatory ossification of ligaments and entheses, especially **anterior longitudinal ligament**

Features

- Flowing **anterior vertebral osteophytes** over ≥4 vertebrae
- Preserved disc height
- No sacroiliitis

Clinical

- Stiffness, dysphagia (cervical involvement)
- Risk of **unstable spinal fractures**

Management

- *Conservative:* NSAIDs, physiotherapy
- Surgery for dysphagia, fractures, cord compression

Q92. Role of biologics in inflammatory spine disorders.

(WBUHS 2019)

- Target **cytokines** (TNF-α, IL-17, IL-23)

Drug class	Example	Indications
Anti-TNF	Infliximab, adalimumab	AS, PsA, IBD-associated SpA
IL-17 inhibitors	Secukinumab	Refractory axial SpA
JAK inhibitors	Tofacitinib	Used in refractory RA

- Reduce inflammation, pain, progression
- Screen for **latent TB** before initiation

Q93. Surgical options for advanced ankylosing spondylitis.

Indications

- Severe spinal deformity (chin-on-chest deformity)
- Non-ambulatory due to kyphosis
- Ankylosed hips
- Neurological deficit from AAI or fracture

Surgical Options

- **Smith–Petersen osteotomy (SPO)**
- **Pedicle subtraction osteotomy (PSO)**—more angular correction

- **Cervical fusion** for instability
- Total hip arthroplasty (THA) for ankylosed hips
- **Spinal stabilization** post fracture in fused spine

Spinal Deformities

Q94. Management of adolescent idiopathic scoliosis (AIS).

(Asked in: AIIMS Delhi 2023, PGI 2022)

Definition

Adolescent idiopathic scoliosis (AIS) is a structural lateral curvature of the spine >10° with unknown cause, presenting between 10 years till skeletal maturity.

Clinical Features

- Asymmetry of shoulders
- Prominent scapula ("rib hump" on forward bending—Adams test)
- Waist asymmetry

Radiological Evaluation

- X-ray spine (PA and lateral)
- **Cobb's Angle** measurement
- Risser sign (skeletal maturity assessment)

Management Principles

Observation: Cobb's angle <20° in skeletally immature patients

Bracing:

- Cobb's angle 20–40°
- Skeletally immature
- *Common brace:* Boston brace (underarm brace)

Surgery:

- Cobb's angle >40–45°
- Rapid progression (>5° per year)
- Poor cosmetic appearance

Surgical Techniques

- Posterior spinal fusion with instrumentation (pedicle screw systems)
- Anterior approach (rarely)

Goals of Surgery

- Curve correction
- Spinal balance maintenance
- Fusion of the least number of segments

Quick Revision Table

Cobb's angle	*Management*
<20°	Observation
20–40°	Bracing (Boston brace)
>40–45°	Surgical correction (fusion)

FLOWCHART: AIS management

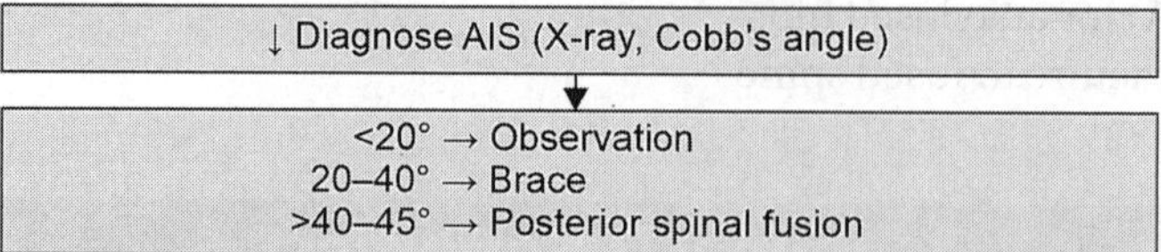

Q95. Describe types and surgical correction methods of Kyphosis.

(Asked in: RGUHS 2023, TNMGR 2022)

Definition

Kyphosis is excessive anterior curvature of the spine in the sagittal plane, usually thoracic spine.

Types of Kyphosis

1. *Postural Kyphosis:*
   - Flexible; improves with posture correction
   - No structural abnormality
2. *Scheuermann's disease*:
   - Juvenile kyphosis
   - Vertebral wedging >5° in at least three consecutive vertebrae
3. *Congenital Kyphosis*: Failure of formation or segmentation of vertebrae
4. *Post-traumatic/Infectious Kyphosis*: After fractures or tuberculosis

Clinical Features

- Visible deformity (humpback)
- Back pain
- Neurological deficits (severe cases)

Surgical Correction Methods

Indications for surgery:

- Kyphotic angle >70–80°
- Pain, progressive deformity
- Neurological deficit

Techniques:

- *Posterior instrumentation and fusion:*
  - Most common
  - Pedicle screw fixation, Rod constructs
- *Osteotomies:*
  - *Smith–Petersen osteotomy:* Flexible deformities
  - *Pedicle subtraction osteotomy (PSO):* Rigid deformities
  - *Vertebral column resection (VCR):* Severe rigid deformities
- *Anterior release + posterior instrumentation:* Combined approach for severe deformities

Quick Revision Table

Kyphosis type	*Features*
Postural	Flexible, no surgery needed
Scheuermann's	Vertebral wedging, Stiff
Congenital	Vertebral anomalies
Post-traumatic/infectious	Secondary

Continued

Continued

Kyphosis type	Features
Postural	Flexible, no surgery needed
Surgical options	***Use***
Posterior fusion	Mild-to-moderate Kyphosis
PSO/VCR	Severe rigid deformity

FLOWCHART: Kyphosis surgical management

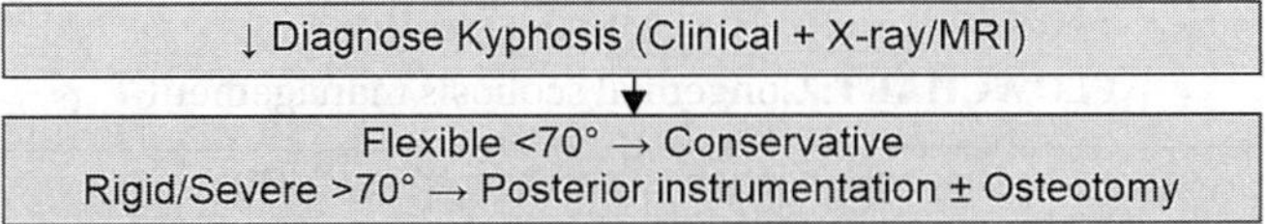

Q96. Management principles in congenital scoliosis.

(Asked in: JIPMER 2021)

Definition

Congenital scoliosis results from anomalous vertebral formation (failure of formation or segmentation) during embryogenesis.

Etiology

- Hemivertebra
- Wedge vertebra
- Unsegmented bar

Clinical Features

- Spinal deformity seen at early age
- *Associated anomalies:*
    - Cardiac defects (VSD, ASD)
    - Genitourinary anomalies
    - Neurological deficits

Radiological Evaluation

- X-ray spine AP and lateral views
- MRI spine (to assess for cord anomalies like tethered cord, diastematomyelia)
- CT for detailed bony assessment

Management Principles

Observation: Mild non-progressive curves

Surgical management:

- Early surgery for progressive deformity
- Prevent further worsening with growth

Surgical options:

- *Hemivertebra excision:* Best for isolated hemivertebra causing progressive scoliosis
- *In-situ fusion:* Fusion without correction for minor curves
- *Growth-friendly procedures:*
    - Growing rods
    - Vertical expandable prosthetic titanium ribs (VEPTR)
- *Definitive spinal fusion:* Older children/adolescents

Quick Revision Table

Anomaly	*Example*
Failure of formation	Hemivertebra
Failure of segmentation	Unsegmented bar
Management	***Indication***
Observation	Mild curve
Hemivertebra excision	Progressive scoliosis
Growing rods/VEPTR	Young children

FLOWCHART: Congenital scoliosis management

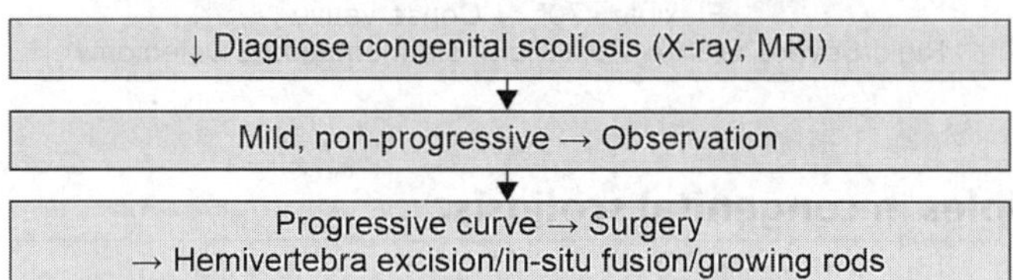

Ultra-crisp Final Memory Markers

Topic	*1-liner memory tip*
AIS	Cobb's >40° → Surgery
Kyphosis	>70° needs correction with osteotomy if rigid
Congenital scoliosis	Early surgery if progressive

Q97. Management of congenital kyphosis.

Types

- *Failure of formation (Type I)*: Wedge vertebra
- *Failure of segmentation (Type II)*: Block vertebra
- Mixed

Management

- **Early diagnosis critical** (progresses rapidly)
- *Surgery:*
  - **Posterior spinal fusion** (early stages)
  - **Vertebral column resection (VCR)** in severe deformity

Q98. Surgical options for scoliosis correction.

Indications

- Cobb angle >45–50°
- Curve progression despite bracing
- Cosmetic/psychological concern
- Respiratory compromise (rare)

Procedures

- **Posterior spinal fusion** (gold standard)
- **Pedicle screw instrumentation**
- **Anterior approach** (less common today)
- **Growth modulation** (growing rods, VEPTR) for early-onset scoliosis

Q99. Kyphosis—causes, classification, and management.

Causes
- Postural
- Scheuermann's disease
- Infective (TB)
- Congenital kyphosis
- Traumatic
- Degenerative

Classification
- *Flexible:* Corrects on bending
- *Fixed/Structural:* Requires intervention

Management
- *Postural:* Physiotherapy
- *Scheuermann's:* Brace if <70°
- *Severe/Rigid kyphosis:* Surgery – osteotomy + posterior fusion

Q100. Role of osteotomies in spinal deformity correction.

Type of osteotomy	*Used for*	*Correction potential*
Smith–Petersen osteotomy (SPO)	Flexible kyphosis	~10° per level
Pedicle subtraction osteotomy (PSO)	Fixed sagittal imbalance	~30–35° per level
Vertebral column resection (VCR)	Severe rigid curves	>45°, 3D correction

Used in **kyphotic deformities, ankylosing spondylitis, post-infective deformities**

Q101. Scheuermann's kyphosis and its management.

Definition
Structural hyperkyphosis (>45°) due to anterior vertebral wedging in ≥3 consecutive vertebrae.

Features
- Adolescents, thoracic spine
- Pain, poor posture, rigid kyphosis

Radiology
- Schmorl's nodes
- Irregular endplates

Management
- *<70°*: Physiotherapy ± bracing (Milwaukee)
- *70° or progressive*: **Posterior fusion ± osteotomy**

Q102. Natural history and management of degenerative scoliosis.

Definition
Adult-onset scoliosis due to **asymmetric disc degeneration and facet arthropathy**

Features
- Back pain
- Neurogenic claudication
- Leg radiculopathy

Management

- *Conservative:* NSAIDs, physiotherapy, epidural injections
- *Surgical:*
  - **Decompression + fusion** if neurological symptoms
  - **Long-segment fusion** if curve >30°, instability

Q103. Role of pedicle screws in deformity correction.

- **Anchor system** for 3-column spinal control
- **Biomechanically superior** to hooks/wires
- Allow **segmental fixation** → better curve correction
- **Improved derotation and translation**
- Enable **shorter fusion segments**

Used in:

- AIS
- Spondylolisthesis
- Kyphotic deformities
- Tumors, trauma

Q104. Concept of selective spinal fusion in scoliosis surgery.

Definition

Fusion of **only the structural curve**, leaving compensatory curves unfused

Principle

- **Non-structural curves** correct spontaneously post-operative
- Prevents unnecessary fusion → maintains mobility

Indications

- Based on **Lenke classification**
- *Example:* Lenke 1A → fuse only thoracic curve

Q105. Neuromuscular scoliosis—principles of treatment.

(Source: PGI Chandigarh 2023)

Definition

Scoliosis arising secondary to neuromuscular diseases like cerebral palsy, muscular dystrophy, or spinal muscular atrophy.

Features

- Long, C-shaped curves
- Pelvic obliquity common
- Poor sitting balance
- High risk of respiratory complications

Management Principles

Non-surgical: Wheelchair support, seating aids, braces (limited role)

Surgical:

- *Indications:*
  - Progressive curve >40–50°
  - Loss of sitting balance

- *Goals:*
  - Correct scoliosis
  - Balance the head, trunk, and pelvis
- *Procedures:* Posterior spinal fusion (extending to pelvis if needed)
- *Preoperative optimization:* Pulmonary function, cardiac assessment, nutrition status

Quick Table

Feature	*Detail*
Curve pattern	Long C-shaped
Management	Surgery if >50° or poor sitting

Crisp Flowchart

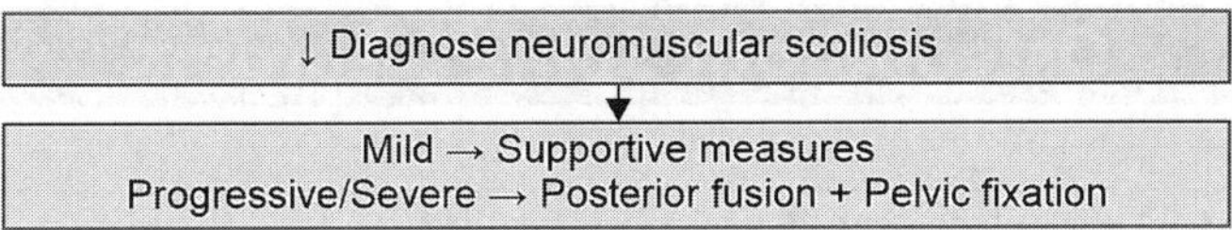

Q106. Non-structural scoliosis.

Definition
Curvature of spine without vertebral rotation or permanent structural change.

Types
1. Postural
2. Leg-length discrepancy
3. Painful scoliosis (e.g., disc prolapse)
4. Hysterical scoliosis
5. Inflammatory (e.g., appendicitis)

Features
- Curve disappears in recumbency or forward flexion
- No vertebral body wedging
- Corrects with cause removal

Ultra-crisp Final Memory Markers

Topic	*1-liner recall*
AIS	Cobb's >40° → Surgery
Kyphotic deformity	>70° → Surgical correction
Congenital scoliosis	Hemivertebra excision if progressive
Neuromuscular scoliosis	Fusion to pelvis often needed

Q107. End vertebra and apical vertebra in scoliosis.

- *End vertebra:* Upper/lower vertebrae at the ends of the curve (max tilt)
- *Apical vertebra:* Most rotated/displaced vertebra at curve apex

Q108. Factors affecting congenital scoliosis progression.

- Type of anomaly (e.g., hemivertebra, bar)
- Location (thoracic worse)
- Number of vertebrae involved

- Age of diagnosis (younger = higher risk)
- Associated anomalies (cardiac, renal)

Q109. Indications for surgery in scoliosis.

- Cobb angle >45–50°
- Progressive curve
- Cosmetic deformity
- Respiratory compromise
- Failure of bracing

Osteoporotic Spine Disorders

Q110. Indications and techniques of vertebroplasty and kyphoplasty.

(DYPU Pune 2016)

Indications

- **Painful osteoporotic vertebral compression fractures (VCFs)** not responding to conservative treatment (typically >2–3 weeks)
- Painful **vertebral metastasis or myeloma**
- **Vertebral hemangioma** (symptomatic)
- **Vertebra plana** (in kyphoplasty)

Contraindications

- Asymptomatic fractures
- Spinal canal compromise/neural compression
- Active infection
- Coagulopathy

Techniques

Procedure	*Description*
Vertebroplasty	Percutaneous injection of polymethylmethacrylate (PMMA) into collapsed vertebral body to stabilize fracture
Kyphoplasty	Involves balloon tamp insertion to restore height, then cavity is filled with cement

Access

Transpedicular or extrapedicular under fluoroscopic/CT guidance

Complications

Cement leakage (higher in vertebroplasty), embolism, infection

Q111. Differential diagnosis of osteoporotic vertebral fractures.

Condition	*Distinguishing features*
Osteoporotic fracture	Elderly, minimal trauma, wedge/compression pattern, multiple levels
Pathological fracture (metastasis)	Lytic lesion, posterior wall involvement, younger age possible
Multiple myeloma	Pancake vertebrae, punched-out skull lesions, M-protein spike
Infective spondylitis (TB/pyogenic)	Endplate destruction, disc involvement, paravertebral abscess
Traumatic fracture (high-energy)	Younger patients, trauma history, retropulsion fragments
Scheuermann's disease	Adolescents, wedged vertebrae with Schmorl's nodes

Imaging Tools
- *X-ray:* Wedge/Pancake deformity
- *MRI:* STIR hyperintensity is suggestive of acute fracture
- *Bone scan:* Differentiates acute versus chronic

Miscellaneous Spinal Disorders

Q112. Baastrup's disease—etiology and management.

Definition
Also called "kissing spine syndrome," Baastrup's disease refers to **hypertrophy and approximation of adjacent spinous processes**, usually in the **lumbar spine**.

Etiology
- Repetitive lumbar extension
- Degenerative changes → collapse of disc space → approximation of spinous processes
- Common in elderly, especially L4–L5 level

Symptoms
- Midline back pain worsened by extension and relieved by flexion
- Palpable tenderness over spinous processes

Management
- *Conservative:* NSAIDs, PT, posture correction
- Interspinous bursa steroid injection
- *Surgery:* Excision of spinous process tip (if refractory)

Q113. Syringomyelia—pathogenesis and treatment.

Definition
Cystic cavitation (syrinx) in the spinal cord, often in **cervical region**

Pathogenesis
- Disruption of CSF flow → accumulation inside central canal
- *Causes:* **Chiari I malformation**, trauma, tumor, arachnoiditis

Symptoms
- Cape-like sensory loss (pain/temperature)
- Weakness, scoliosis, bladder issues

Treatment
- *For Chiari I:* **Posterior fossa decompression**
- Syrinx shunting (syringoperitoneal or syringosubarachnoid)
- Treat underlying lesion

Q114. Spinal AV malformations—classification and management.

(AIIMS JPR 2018)

Types (Oldfield Classification)
- *Type I*: Dural AV fistula (most common)
- *Type II*: Intramedullary glomus
- *Type III*: Juvenile AVM
- *Type IV*: Perimedullary fistula

Symptoms
- Gradual myelopathy
- Back pain, spasticity, bladder dysfunction

Diagnosis
- *MRI:* Flow voids
- *Digital subtraction angiography (DSA):* Gold standard

Management
- Endovascular embolization (Type I, IV)
- Surgical resection (Type II, III)

Q115. Principles of spinal fusion surgery.

Definition
Surgical procedure to **achieve bony union between two or more vertebrae** to eliminate motion at a painful segment.

Principles
- Adequate **decortication** of bone surfaces
- **Bone grafting** (autograft, allograft, synthetic)
- **Stability** via instrumentation (screws, rods)
- Achieve **solid arthrodesis** over time (4–12 months)

Indications
Instability, spondylolisthesis, deformity, infection, tumor

Q116. Indications and complications of spinal instrumentation.

Indications
- Spinal instability
- Deformity correction
- Fractures
- Tumor reconstruction
- Fusion support

Complications
- Hardware failure (screw pullout, breakage)
- Pseudoarthrosis
- Neurological injury
- Infection
- Adjacent segment disease

Q117. Role of artificial disc replacement (ADR) in degenerative spine disease.

Concept
Motion-preserving alternative to fusion in **cervical/lumbar DDD**

Indications
Single-level disc degeneration with radiculopathy (without instability)

Advantages
- Preserves motion
- Reduces adjacent segment disease

Limitations
- Contraindicated in osteoporosis, instability, facet arthritis
- Technically demanding, cost

Q118. Role of intraoperative electrophysiological monitoring in spine surgery.

(RUHS 2018)

Purpose
Monitor spinal cord and nerve root function during high-risk spine procedures

Modalities
- *SSEPs:* Sensory pathway monitoring
- *MEPs:* Motor tracts (corticospinal)
- *EMG:* Root irritation or damage
- *Trigger EMG:* Screw breach detection

Uses
- Deformity correction
- Tumor excision
- Cervical/lumbar instrumentation
- Reduces postoperative neurological deficits

Q119. Role of endoscopic spine surgery in modern practice.

Definition
Minimally invasive spine procedure using **endoscope** via small incision

Indications
- Lumbar disc herniation
- Foraminal stenosis
- Discectomy, rhizotomy

Advantages
- Less tissue disruption
- Less blood loss
- Day care procedure
- Early mobilization, reduced infection risk

Limitations
- Steep learning curve
- Limited by anatomical access (compared to open surgery)

Q120. Principles of rehabilitation in spinal disorders.

Goals
- Pain control
- Restore mobility and function
- Prevent complications and recurrence

Components
- *Physical therapy:* Core strengthening, gait training
- *Occupational therapy:* ADL (activities of daily living) support
- *Pain management:* Meds, injections

- *Psychological support:* Chronic pain coping
- *Assistive devices:* Braces, walkers

Q121. Differentiate between mechanical instability and neurological instability in spine.

(Asked in: TNMGR 2023)

Definitions

- *Mechanical instability:*
  - Failure of spine to maintain alignment under physiological loads
  - Leads to progressive deformity, pain, or structural collapse
- Neurological instability: Dynamic or potential risk to the spinal cord or nerve roots due to abnormal spine movement or alignment

Differences

Feature	*Mechanical instability*	*Neurological instability*
Main problem	Structural support loss	Risk of cord/nerve damage
Presentation	Deformity, mechanical pain	Neurological deficits
Evaluation	X-ray (dynamic views), CT	MRI (cord compression)
Treatment focus	Stabilization (fusion, instrumentation)	Decompression + Stabilization

Quick Revision Table

Instability type	*Key feature*
Mechanical	Pain, deformity
Neurological	Cord/Nerve compression

FLOWCHART: Instability evaluation

↓ Evaluate spine (Imaging)

↓

Mechanical instability → Stabilization surgery
Neurological instability → Decompression + Stabilization

Q122. Posterior spinal decompression and fusion—indications, steps, and complications.

(Source: PGI Chandigarh 2022)

Definition

Posterior spinal decompression and fusion involves removal of compressive structures (lamina, ligamentum flavum) and stabilization using pedicle screws and rods.

Indications

- Spinal cord or nerve root compression (e.g., stenosis, tumors)
- Instability (fractures, deformity correction)
- Failed conservative management

Steps

1. Prone positioning on radiolucent table
2. Midline posterior incision
3. Paraspinal muscle dissection (subperiosteal)
4. Laminectomy/Laminotomy to decompress spinal canal
5. Pedicle screw placement and rod fixation

6. Bone grafting for fusion
7. Wound closure

Complications

- Dural tear (CSF leak)
- Infection
- Pedicle screw misplacement
- Adjacent segment degeneration
- Pseudoarthrosis (nonunion)

Quick Table

Step	*Key point*
Decompression	Laminectomy
Stabilization	Pedicle screws and rods

Crisp Flowchart

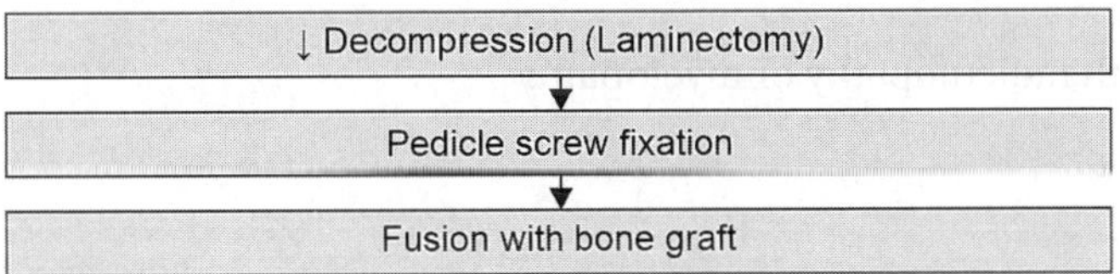

Q123. Pedicle screw fixation—technique and complications.

(Source: MUHS Maharashtra 2022)

Definition

Pedicle screw fixation is a method of spinal stabilization where screws are inserted through the pedicles into the vertebral body.

Technique

1. *Entry point*:
   - *Thoracic:* Junction of lateral facet and transverse process
   - *Lumbar:* Pars interarticularis
2. *Trajectory*:
   - 10–15° medial angulation in lumbar
   - Slight caudal angulation in thoracic
3. Drilling and tapping pedicle track
4. Screw insertion
5. Rods attached and locked

Complications

- Screw malposition (nerve root injury, dural tear)
- Vascular injury (e.g., aorta in thoracic spine)
- Hardware failure (loosening, breakage)
- Infection

Quick Table

Complication	*Example*
Neural injury	Root compression
Vascular injury	Aortic injury (thoracic)
Mechanical failure	Screw loosening

Crisp Flowchart

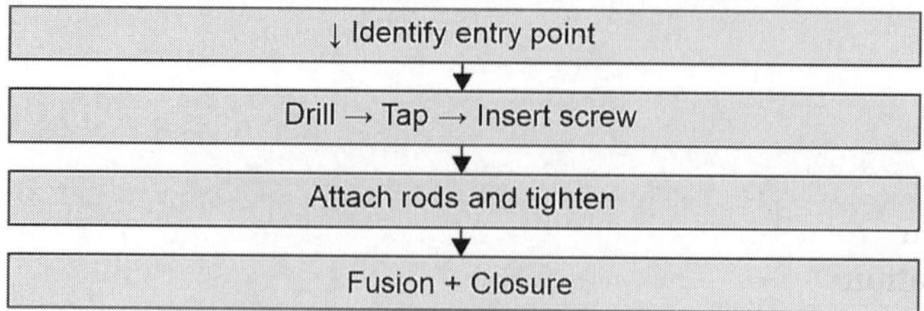

Q124. Anterior cervical discectomy and fusion (ACDF)—indications and steps.

(Source: AIIMS Delhi 2022)

Definition

ACDF involves anterior approach to cervical spine, removal of disc herniation, and fusion with cage/graft.

Indications

- Cervical disc herniation with radiculopathy or myelopathy
- Degenerative disc disease
- Instability

Surgical Steps

1. Supine position with neck extension
2. Horizontal skin incision (transverse)
3. Dissection through platysma, retract carotid sheath laterally
4. Identification of correct disc level (fluoroscopy)
5. *Discectomy*: Removal of disc, osteophytes
6. Endplate preparation
7. Interbody cage insertion ± anterior plate fixation
8. Layered closure

Complications

- Recurrent laryngeal nerve palsy (hoarseness)
- Dysphagia
- CSF leak
- Pseudarthrosis (fusion failure)

Quick Table

Step	***Key point***
Approach	Anterior neck
Fusion device	Interbody cage ± Plate

Crisp Flowchart

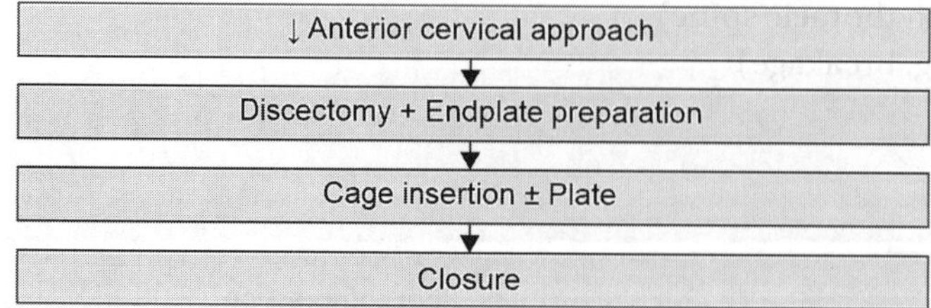

Q125. Minimally invasive spine surgery (MISS)—indications, advantages, and disadvantages.

(Source: JIPMER Puducherry 2023)

Definition

Minimally invasive spine surgery (MISS) refers to spinal procedures performed with smaller incisions, using tubular retractors or endoscopic systems, reducing soft tissue disruption.

Indications

- Lumbar disc herniation
- Spinal stenosis
- Spinal fractures (stable)
- Spondylolisthesis (selected cases)

Advantages

- Less blood loss
- Smaller incision, less muscle damage
- Faster recovery and rehabilitation
- Reduced hospital stay

Disadvantages

- Steep learning curve
- Limited visualization
- Increased radiation exposure (fluoroscopy)

Common MISS Procedures

- Microdiscectomy
- Percutaneous pedicle screw fixation
- Endoscopic lumbar discectomy

Quick Table

Aspect	*Advantage/disadvantage*
Advantage	Less pain, quicker recovery
Disadvantage	Technically demanding

Crisp Flowchart

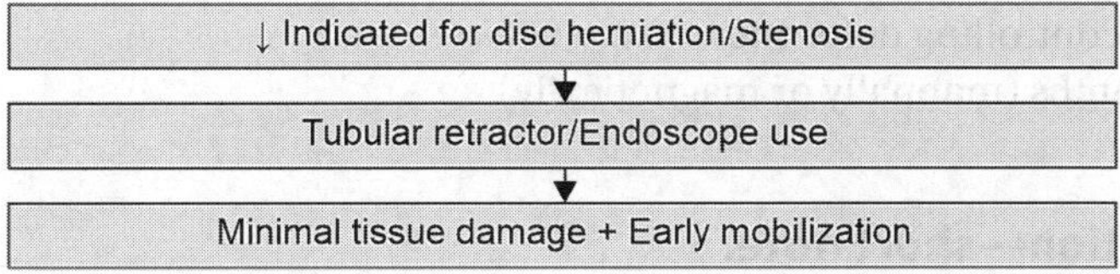

Ultra-crisp Final Memory Markers

Topic	*1-liner recall*
Posterior decompression fusion	Laminectomy + Pedicle Screws
Pedicle screw fixation	Entry point + Trajectory critical
ACDF	Anterior approach + Cage fusion
MISS	Less invasive, technically demanding

Q126. Cauda equina syndrome—short note.

- Compression of **cauda equina nerve roots** (L2–S5)
- *Causes:* Prolapsed disc, tumor, trauma

- *Features:*
    - Bilateral leg weakness
    - Saddle anesthesia
    - Bladder/Bowel dysfunction
- Emergency MRI and decompression

Q127. Costoplasty.

- **Rib excision** done to correct rib hump in scoliosis
- Improves cosmetic appearance
- Often combined with spinal fusion
- Can reduce thoracic stiffness

Q128. Spinal osteotomy.

- Surgical resection of vertebral elements to correct deformities
- *Types:*
    - Smith–Petersen
    - Pedicle subtraction osteotomy (PSO)
    - Vertebral column resection (VCR)
- *Used for:* Kyphosis, scoliosis, ankylosing spondylitis

Q129. Risser's sign—short note.

- **Iliac apophysis ossification grading** (0–5)
- Indicates **skeletal maturity**
- Used in **scoliosis** progression risk assessment
- *Higher grade*: Less growth potential

Q130. Growing Rods—short note.

- Used in **early-onset scoliosis**
- Rods span multiple segments
- Allow spinal growth while controlling deformity
- Lengthened every 6–12 months (manually or magnetically)

Q131. Halopelvic distraction—short note.

- *Gradual correction of severe spinal deformity using:*
    - **Halo ring** (skull)
    - **Pelvic fixation**
- Indicated in rigid kyphoscoliosis
- Risk of neurological complications

Q132. Kyphoplasty—short note.

- Minimally invasive procedure for **vertebral compression fractures**
- Balloon inserted → expands vertebra → cement injected
- Restores height, reduces pain
- Used in **osteoporotic fractures**

Q133. Vertebroplasty—short note.

- Cement injection into collapsed vertebra (without balloon)
- Stabilizes fracture
- Reduces pain, does **not restore height**
- For osteoporotic or metastatic fractures

Q134. Vesselplasty—short note.

- Advanced alternative to vertebroplasty
- Uses **expandable mesh container** to control cement spread
- Prevents leakage
- Reduces risk of spinal cord compression

Q135. Coccydynia.

- Pain in coccyx (tailbone)
- *Causes:* Trauma, prolonged sitting, childbirth
- *Management:*
    - Cushioning
    - NSAIDs
    - Local injection
    - Rarely coccygectomy

Q136. Myelomeningocele.

- *Neural tube defect:* Herniation of meninges + spinal cord
- Common in **lumbosacral** region
- *Associated with:*
    - Hydrocephalus
    - Paralysis, bladder dysfunction
- Requires early surgical closure + supportive care

Q137. Neurogenic versus vascular claudication—differences and causes.

Feature	***Neurogenic claudication***	***Vascular claudication***
Cause	Spinal stenosis	Peripheral arterial disease
Pain relief	Sitting, bending forward	Rest
Walking pattern	Variable distance	Fixed distance
Pain location	Back, buttocks, thighs	Calves
Pulse	Normal	Reduced/Absent

Etiologies

Neurogenic:

- Lumbar canal stenosis
- Cauda equina compression

Vascular:

- Atherosclerosis
- Thromboangiitis obliterans

Q138. Spino-pelvic sagittal balance—clinical and radiological features.

Clinical Features

- Stooped posture
- Horizontal gaze disturbed
- Back pain, fatigue
- Difficulty standing upright

Radiological Parameters

1. *Pelvic incidence (PI)*: Fixed anatomic angle between sacrum and pelvis
2. *Pelvic tilt (PT)*: Angle indicating retroversion of pelvis
3. *Sacral slope (SS)*: Complementary to PT
   - **PI = PT + SS**
4. *Sagittal vertical axis (SVA)*:
   - Distance between C7 plumb line and posterior-superior corner of S1
   - Normal <5 cm

Imbalance: Increased SVA, Mismatch between PI and Lumbar Lordosis

Q139. Navigation in spine surgery.

Definition

Real-time 3D computer-assisted guidance during spine surgery using intraoperative imaging and tracking systems.

Components

- Intraoperative CT/O-arm
- Infrared camera for tracking
- Navigation software

Uses

- Accurate pedicle screw placement
- Deformity correction
- Tumor resection
- Revision spine surgeries

Advantages

- Improved precision
- Reduces risk of neurovascular injury
- Decreases need for fluoroscopy

Q140. Straight leg raise test interpretation in acute LBA.

- *Positive between 30–70°*: **Lumbar disc herniation** (usually L5/S1)
- Pain down posterior thigh/leg (radicular)
- *Crossed SLR positive*: Highly specific for disc herniation
- Differentiates nerve root irritation versus hamstring tightness

Q141. DDx and investigation in 60-year-old with multiple compressed vertebrae.

Differential Diagnosis

1. Osteoporosis
2. Multiple myeloma
3. Metastatic disease

4. Vertebral TB
5. Lymphoma or leukemia

Investigations

- *X-ray spine:* Vertebral collapse, lytic/blastic lesions
- *MRI:* Marrow oedema, soft tissue
- *Blood tests:*
  - CBC, ESR, CRP
  - Calcium, ALP, Vitamin D
  - Serum/urine electrophoresis (myeloma)
- Bone scan or PET-CT (for metastases)
- Biopsy if suspicious

Q142. Various spinal cord syndromes.

1. *Central cord syndrome*: More motor loss in upper limbs
2. *Anterior cord syndrome*: Loss of motor + pain/temperature
3. *Posterior cord syndrome*: Loss of proprioception/vibration
4. *Brown–Sequard*: Ipsilateral motor loss + contralateral pain/temperature loss
5. *Conus medullaris syndrome*: Saddle anesthesia, bladder dysfunction
6. *Cauda equina syndrome*: LMN signs, urinary retention

Q143. Sacral nutation and low back pain.

- *Nutation:* Sacrum tilts anteriorly (relative to ilium)
- Affects **sacroiliac joint stability**
- Abnormal nutation/hypermobility → **SI joint pain**, low backache

Q144. Lumbar root anomalies.

- Conjoined nerve root
- Split nerve root
- Transitional lumbosacral vertebra
- *Clinical relevance:* Confusing MRI findings, surgical risk

Q145. Complications of disc surgery.

- Dural tear
- Nerve root injury
- Infection
- Reherniation
- Failed back syndrome
- CSF leak
- Epidural hematoma

Q146. Wake-up test.

- Intraoperative test during spine surgery
- Wake patient under light anesthesia to move legs → assess **neurological integrity**
- Used in scoliosis/deformity surgery

Q147. Lateral mass fixation.

- Common in **cervical spine stabilization**
- Screws placed into **lateral mass of vertebra (C3–C7)**
- *Technique:* **Magerl** or **Anderson**

Q148. Filum terminale syndrome.

- Tight or thickened filum terminale → tethered cord
- *Causes:* Back pain, neurogenic bladder, foot deformities
- *Tx:* **Surgical release**

Q149. Laminoplasty.

- Posterior decompression while preserving lamina
- Indicated in **cervical myelopathy**, OPLL
- *Types:* **Open-door, double-door**
- Preserves spinal motion versus laminectomy

Q150. Video-assisted thoracoscopy (VAT).

- Minimally invasive approach to anterior thoracic spine
- *Used in:*
  - TB spine (D5–D10)
  - Discectomy, corpectomy
- Reduces morbidity versus thoracotomy

Q151. Dural tear.

- Unintended tear during spine surgery
- Presents with **CSF leak**
- Can cause headache, pseudomeningocele
- *Managed with:*
  - **Primary repair**
  - Dural sealants
  - Lumbar drain (post-operative)

Q152. Nerve root block versus epidural injection.

Feature	*Nerve root block*	*Epidural injection*
Site	Near specific nerve root	Epidural space
Purpose	Diagnostic + therapeutic	Therapeutic (pain relief)
Used in	Radiculopathy	Spinal stenosis, discogenic pain
Medication	Steroid + anesthetic	Steroid + anesthetic

Q153. Spinal fusion methods.

- *Posterior fusion:* PLIF, TLIF
- *Anterior fusion:* ALIF

- *Lateral:* XLIF, DLIF
- *Fusion materials:* Autograft, allograft, cages, bone substitutes
- *Indicated in:* Instability, spondylolisthesis, deformity correction

Q154. Role of physiotherapy in back pain.

- Core strengthening
- Posture correction
- Flexibility exercises
- McKenzie technique

Q155. Failed back syndrome (FBS).

Also called: Failed Back Surgery Syndrome (FBSS)

Definition

A condition where a patient continues to experience **chronic back or leg pain** after spinal surgery, especially **lumbar spine decompression or fusion**.

Causes

- Inadequate decompression of nerve root
- Recurrent disc herniation
- Epidural fibrosis or scar tissue
- Spinal instability
- Arachnoiditis
- Psychosocial factors (e.g., depression, unrealistic expectations)

Clinical Features

- Persistent or recurrent pain post-surgery
- May involve radiculopathy or mechanical back pain
- Often worsens with activity

Investigations

- *MRI with contrast:* Evaluate scar versus recurrent disc
- *CT scan:* Check for fusion status
- *EMG/NCV:* Assess nerve function
- Psychological assessment

Management

- *Conservative:*
  - Physical therapy, pain management (NSAIDs, neuropathic drugs)
  - Psychosocial counseling
- *Interventional:*
  - Epidural steroid injections
  - Nerve root blocks
  - Spinal cord stimulation
- *Surgical:* Only if specific pathology identified (e.g., instability, disc)

Q156. Coccydynia.

Definition

Pain in the **coccyx (tailbone)** region, especially when sitting or rising from a seated position.

Etiology
- Trauma (fall on buttocks)
- Childbirth (especially instrumental delivery)
- Repetitive microtrauma (cycling, prolonged sitting)
- Idiopathic
- *Rare:* Infection or tumor

Clinical Features
- Localized pain at coccyx
- Worse on sitting, bending, or rising from a chair
- Tenderness over coccyx on rectal exam

Diagnosis
- Clinical; confirmed by **dynamic X-ray of coccyx**
- Rule out pilonidal sinus, rectal causes, or neoplasm

Treatment
- *Conservative:*
  - Cushioned seat (donut pillow)
  - NSAIDs
  - Local steroid + anesthetic injection
  - Physical therapy
- *Surgical:*
  - **Coccygectomy** (for chronic, refractory cases)

Q157. What are the indications of surgery in prolapsed intervertebral disc (PIVD)?

(DYPU Pune 2011)

Surgical intervention in PIVD is indicated when conservative treatment fails or when there are red flag signs. The indications can be grouped as follows:

Absolute Indications
1. Cauda equina syndrome
   - Saddle anesthesia
   - Bladder/bowel dysfunction
   - Bilateral leg weakness
2. *Progressive neurological deficit:* Increasing motor weakness despite conservative treatment

Relative Indications
1. *Failed conservative management:* Persistent disabling pain >6 weeks not responding to medication and physiotherapy
2. *Recurrent disc herniation:* Symptomatic recurrence after initial relief
3. *Severe radicular pain*: Not controlled with adequate analgesia, affecting quality of life
4. *Occupational or functional demand:* Early return to work in individuals with high physical demands

Common Surgical Options
- Microdiscectomy
- Laminectomy with discectomy
- Endoscopic discectomy

7.5 Hip

Ashish Jaiman, Abhishek Mahajan

Basic Anatomy and Biomechanics

Q1. Describe the anatomy of the hip joint.

Type
Synovial **ball-and-socket** joint

Articulating Surfaces
- **Acetabulum** of pelvis (formed by ilium, ischium, pubis)
- **Head of femur** (2/3rd sphere, covered by articular cartilage except at fovea)

Key Structures
- *Joint capsule:* Thick and strong; attaches from acetabular rim to intertrochanteric line (anteriorly) and crest (posteriorly)
- *Labrum:* Fibrocartilaginous rim deepening the acetabulum
- *Ligaments:*
  - Iliofemoral (Y-shaped, strongest)
  - Pubofemoral
  - Ischiofemoral
- *Muscles:* Gluteals, iliopsoas, adductors, hamstrings, etc.

Hip flexors: Iliopsoas, rectus femoris, sartorius, pectineus, iliacus

Hip adductors: Adductor longus,brevis and magnus, adductor minimus,gracilis

External rotators: Gluteus maximus, piriformis, obturator externus, obturator internis, superior and inferior gamellus, quadratus femoris

Abductors: Gluteus medius, gluteus minimus, tensor fascia lata

Hip extensors: Gluteus maximus, hamstrings and adductor magnus

Q2. Surgical anatomy of the hip.

Understanding the **hip's complex anatomy** is critical for surgeries like arthroscopy, total hip arthroplasty, and surgical dislocation.

Key Structures
- *Bones:* Femoral head, neck, acetabulum (ilium, ischium, pubis)
- *Capsule and ligaments:*
  - Iliofemoral (strongest)
  - Pubofemoral
  - Ischiofemoral
- *Blood supply:*
  - **Medial femoral circumflex artery** (main for femoral head)
  - Retinacular vessels
- *Nerves:*
  - Femoral nerve (anterior)
  - Sciatic nerve (posterior)
  - Obturator nerve (medial)

Surgical Relevance
- Avoiding avascular necrosis during dislocation
- Safe portals in arthroscopy
- Avoiding nerve injury

Q3. Trabecular pattern of the proximal femur and its importance.

Definition
The **trabecular pattern** in the **proximal femur** represents the internal spongy bone architecture aligned according to the **mechanical stresses** across the hip joint.

Types of Trabecular Systems
1. *Principal compressive trabeculae*:
   - From **medial cortex of shaft → superior femoral head**
   - Resist **compressive forces** during weight-bearing
2. *Principal tensile trabeculae*:
   - From lateral cortex → inferior femoral head
   - Resist **tensile stress**
3. *Secondary compressive trabeculae*: From **calcar femorale** to lesser trochanter
4. *Secondary tensile trabeculae*: Below the greater trochanter; less dense
5. *Ward's triangle*:
   - Area of **relative radiolucency** between principal trabeculae
   - Site of weakness and common in osteoporotic fractures

Clinical Importance
- **Helps absorb stress** during gait and loading
- *Changes in trabecular pattern seen in:*
  - **Osteoporosis** → loss of tensile trabeculae
  - **Fracture risk** assessment
  - **Hip joint diseases** (AVN, arthritis)
- Guides **implant positioning** in arthroplasty

Q4. Short notes on the capsular ligaments of the hip joint.

The **hip joint capsule** is reinforced by **three main ligaments** that contribute to its strength and stability.
1. *Iliofemoral ligament (of Bigelow):*
   - **Y-shaped**; from **AIIS to intertrochanteric line**
   - **Strongest ligament in the body**
   - Prevents **hyperextension** and helps maintain erect posture
2. *Pubofemoral ligament:*
   - From **pubic ramus to intertrochanteric line**
   - Limits **excessive abduction and extension**
3. *Ischiofemoral ligament:*
   - From **ischium to greater trochanter**
   - Lies **posteriorly**
   - Prevents **excessive internal rotation**
4. *Zona orbicularis:*
   - Circular fibers around the **femoral neck**
   - Acts like a **collar**, providing passive stability

Functions of Capsular Ligaments
- Resist excessive extension, abduction, and rotation
- Maintain **hip joint congruency and stability**
- Guide safe ranges of motion

Q5. Development and ossification of the hip joint.

Development

- Begins around **4th–6th week of intrauterine life** as a **mesenchymal condensation**
- Becomes a **ball-and-socket synovial joint** by 12 weeks, gestation
- Formed from the **lateral plate mesoderm**

Ossification Centers

Bone	*Primary ossification*	*Secondary centers*
Ilium	~8th fetal week	Iliac crest
Ischium	~3rd fetal month	Ischial tuberosity
Pubis	~5th fetal month	Pubic symphysis
Femoral shaft	~7th fetal week	Femoral head (~1 year), GT, LT

- *Triradiate cartilage:* Joins ilium, ischium, and pubis; closes around **16–18 years**

Fusion Timeline

- *Femoral head epiphysis fuses with shaft*: **~16–18 years**
- *Acetabular growth depends on*:
  - Proper congruency of femoral head
  - Closure of triradiate cartilage

Clinical Relevance

- Disorders like **developmental dysplasia of the hip (DDH)** arise from faulty joint formation
- Knowledge of ossification centers helps in **age estimation** and diagnosis of **pediatric hip disorders**

Q6. Blood supply of the femoral head and clinical significance.

Main supply

- *Medial circumflex femoral artery (MCFA):* Branch of profunda femoris, supplies most of the head via **retinacular arteries**
- **Lateral circumflex femoral artery (LCFA)**
- *Artery of ligamentum teres (branch of obturator artery)*: Minor role in adults

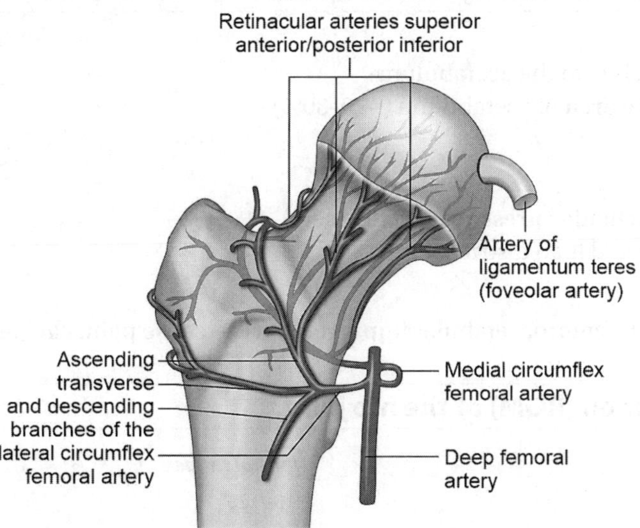

- **Displaced femoral neck fractures** → disrupt retinacular arteries → risk of **AVN**
- Preservation of MCFA is crucial in surgical approaches

Posterior approach to hip must avoid damage to MCFA.
Note: Blood supply of femoral head varies according to age

In Children

- *Primary blood supply:*
  - **Medial and lateral circumflex femoral arteries** (via **retinacular vessels**).
  - **Artery of the ligamentum teres (from the obturator artery)** contributes significantly in early childhood.
  - **Metaphyseal vessels** also contribute before physeal closure.
- *Key point:* The **epiphyseal vessels** (from retinacular arteries) are **separated by the physis (growth plate)** from metaphyseal vessels, making the femoral head vulnerable to ischemia if epiphyseal supply is compromised.

Adolescents

- The **physis is still open**, so the **retinacular vessels** remain the dominant supply.
- The **artery of the ligamentum teres** becomes less significant.
- Still at **high risk** of AVN if trauma disrupts the retinacular vessels.

Adults

- After **physeal closure**, the **retinacular arteries** (branches of the **medial circumflex femoral artery**) become the **primary source**.
- **Posterior superior retinacular arteries** are especially critical.
- **Artery of ligamentum teres** is usually small and has minimal functional contribution in adults.
- The **lateral circumflex femoral artery** contributes to a lesser extent.

Q7. Biomechanics of the hip joint.

Function

Load transmission, stability, and mobility

Forces and Mechanics

- Hip sustains **2.5–5× body weight** during walking/running
- *Abductor mechanism (gluteus medius/minimus + TFL)*: Maintains pelvic stability
- *Lever-arm principle:* Short femoral neck reduces torque for abductors
- Line of force runs from femoral head → acetabulum → sacroiliac joints

Trendelenburg gait occurs with weak abductors.

Q8. Role of the labrum in hip stability and function.

Anatomy

- Fibrocartilaginous rim attached to the acetabulum
- Increases **depth** and **surface area** of acetabulum (~20–30%)

Functions

- Enhances **joint stability**
- Maintains **negative intra-articular pressure** (suction seal)
- Improves **joint lubrication** and load distribution
- Provides **proprioception**

Labral tears → common in FAI (femoroacetabular impingement) → cause pain, clicking

Q9. Normal range of motion (ROM) of the hip joint.

Motion	*Normal range*
Flexion	110–120°
Extension	10–15°
Abduction	30–50°
Adduction	20–30°
Internal rotation	30–40°
External rotation	40–60°

Factors affecting ROM

- Age, gender, muscle tightness, joint pathology (OA, FAI)

ROM is assessed during hip examination and post-operative rehabilitation.

Q10. Hip arthrography.

Definition

A **diagnostic imaging** procedure where contrast dye is injected into the hip joint to evaluate intra-articular structures.

Best used with: MRI (MR arthrogram)

Indications

- **Labral tears**
- Cartilage damage
- Hip instability
- Pre-arthroscopy planning

Procedure

- Fluoroscopic-guided needle insertion
- Injection of contrast dye
- MRI or CT imaging performed

Advantages

- Enhanced visualization of labrum and cartilage
- Higher sensitivity than standard MRI for labral tears

Avascular Necrosis (AVN) of Femoral Head in Adults

Q11. Describe etiology and staging of AVN of femoral head.

(Asked in: AIIMS Delhi 2022, MUHS Maharashtra 2023)

Definition

Avascular necrosis (AVN) is **ischemic death of the bone** and **marrow components** due to disruption of blood supply, leading to **collapse of the femoral head** and secondary **osteoarthritis**.

Etiology

- *Traumatic causes:*
  - Femoral neck fractures
  - Hip dislocations
- *Non-traumatic causes*:
  - Chronic steroid use (most common non-traumatic cause)
  - Alcoholism
  - Sickle cell disease
  - Systemic lupus erythematosus (SLE)
  - Post-radiation therapy
  - Decompression sickness (Caisson disease)
- *Idiopathic*: 20–30% cases have no identifiable cause.

Pathophysiology

Interruption of blood supply → ischemia → death of osteocytes and marrow cells → collapse of subchondral bone → joint incongruity → secondary degenerative arthritis.

Clinical Features

Symptoms:

- Groin pain, often referred to knee
- Limping
- Pain worsened by weight-bearing activities
- Decreased range of motion (especially internal rotation)

Signs:

- Antalgic gait
- Decreased hip abduction and internal rotation

Diagnosis

X-ray (AP and Frog-leg lateral views):

- Early stages normal
- Later stages show sclerosis, cysts, crescent sign (subchondral fracture), femoral head collapse

MRI (gold standard for early detection):

- High sensitivity (~90%)
- Shows double line sign (hypointense outer line, hyperintense inner line)

Bone scan: Cold spot initially (early ischemia).

Q12. Ficat and Arlet classification of AVN hip.

(Asked in: RGUHS Karnataka 2022, PGI Chandigarh 2021)

Ficat and Arlet Staging

Stage	*Findings*
0	Normal X-ray and MRI, asymptomatic
I	Normal X-ray; MRI or bone scan positive (edema)
II	*X-ray*: Sclerosis, cysts; no femoral head collapse
III	Crescent sign (subchondral fracture); early collapse
IV	Flattened femoral head with secondary osteoarthritis (joint space narrowing, acetabular changes)

Q13. Role of MRI in diagnosis of AVN.

MRI is the **gold standard** for early diagnosis.

Findings

- *Double line sign:* Hyperintense inner line (granulation tissue) and hypointense outer line (sclerosis) on T2
- Bone marrow edema (T1 ↓, T2 ↑)
- Crescent sign (early subchondral fracture)

Advantages

- Detects AVN **before X-ray changes**
- Bilateral assessment
- Quantifies lesion size (important for prognosis)

Q14. Management of AVN.

Early Stages (Stage 0–II)

Conservative:

- Restricted weight-bearing
- NSAIDs for pain relief

- Physiotherapy
- Pharmacotherapy (bisphosphonates—limited evidence)

Surgical:
- *Core decompression:* Drilling into femoral head to reduce intraosseous pressure and promote revascularization.
- **Stem cell therapy** (adjunct to core decompression).

Intermediate Stage (Stage II–III)
- *Osteotomies:* Rotational osteotomy to redistribute load-bearing forces away from necrotic area (rarely used now).
- *Bone grafting*: Non-vascularized or vascularized fibular grafts.

Late Stage (Stage III–IV)
Total hip arthroplasty (THA):
- Best option for collapsed femoral heads and secondary osteoarthritis.
- Long-term durable results.

Summary of Surgical Options Based on Stage

Stage	*Management*
I	Core decompression ± medical therapy
II	Core decompression ± bone grafting
III	Core decompression ± bone grafting/THA
IV	Total hip arthroplasty (THA)

Q15. Principles of non-operative and operative management of AVN.

Non-operative (Early AVN—Ficat I or II)
- Restricted weight-bearing
- Bisphosphonates (inhibit osteoclasts)
- Statins (protect vascular endothelium)
- Anticoagulants (for coagulopathy-related AVN)
- Hyperbaric oxygen (limited evidence)

Non-operative is **adjunctive**, not curative in most

Operative Principles
- **Preserve femoral head** in early AVN (I–II)
- **Replace** femoral head in late AVN (III–IV)

Stage	*Surgery*
I–II	Core decompression ± bone grafting/biologics
II–III	Osteotomy (rotational, valgus)
III–IV	Total hip replacement (THR)
Any stage	Stem cell injection (experimental)

Q16. Surgical options for AVN of the hip.

Procedure	*Indication*
Core decompression	Early AVN (Stage I/II)
Bone grafting (non-vascularized or vascularized)	Stage II/III with large lesions
Osteotomy (e.g., valgus intertrochanteric)	Young adults with segmental collapse
THR	End-stage AVN with arthritic changes
Stem cell therapy	Adjunct with decompression (early AVN)

Q17. Core decompression in AVN—discussion.

Definition

A surgical technique involving drilling into the necrotic femoral head to **relieve intraosseous pressure**, promote revascularization and healing.

Indications

- **Ficat stage I or II**
- Symptomatic early AVN
- Small to medium-sized lesions (<30%)

Procedure

- Drill tract from lateral femoral cortex to necrotic area
- Can be done percutaneously
- *May be combined with:*
  - Autologous cancellous graft
  - Bone marrow aspirate concentrate (BMAC)
  - Stem cells/BMPs

Outcomes

- Pain relief
- Delay or prevent collapse
- Better results when done **before collapse (Stage III)**

Best results in patients **<40 years**, small lesions, early stage

Exam Tip

When answering AVN:

- **Mention trauma versus non-traumatic causes** clearly.
- **Always quote Ficat and Arlet stages** with X-ray findings.
- **Management must be stage-specific** (early → decompression, late → THA).

FLOWCHART: AVN of femoral head—diagnosis and management

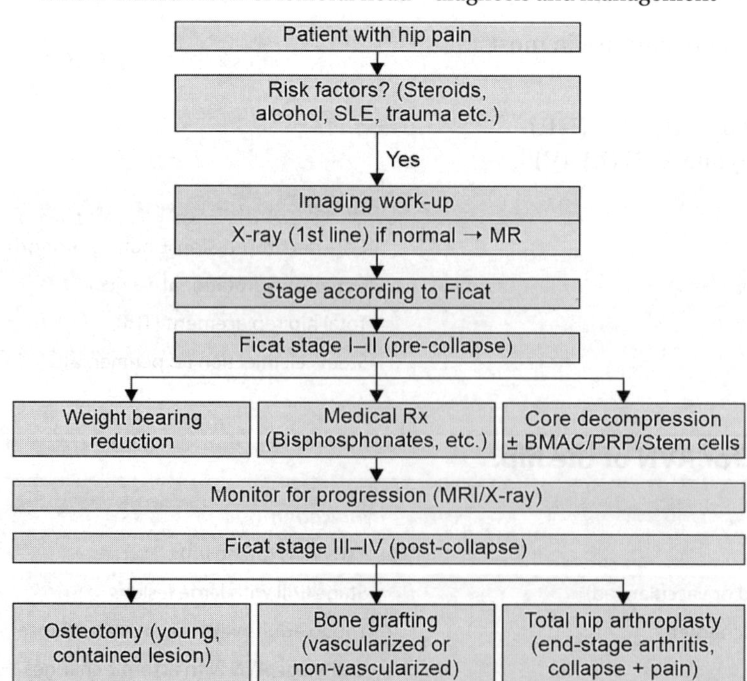

Key Points

- **MRI is the gold standard** for early detection.
- Best results for **core decompression** when done **before collapse**.
- **THR** is definitive for pain relief in late stages.
- *Staging guides treatment:* Ficat I–II (joint preserving), III–IV (joint replacing)

Transient Synovitis of Hip (Toxic Synovitis)

Q18. Describe features and differentiation from septic arthritis.

(Asked in: PGI Chandigarh 2021, RGUHS Karnataka 2023)

Definition

Transient synovitis (also called **toxic synovitis**) is a **self-limiting, non-infectious inflammation of the synovium** of the hip joint in children, causing **hip pain and limp**.

Etiology

Unknown (exact cause), but commonly follows:

- Recent viral infection (upper respiratory tract infection)
- Minor trauma
- Allergic reactions

Age group:
Peak: 3–8 years (boys > girls).

Clinical Features

Symptoms:

- Acute or subacute onset of hip pain
- Limp (painless or mild pain)
- May complain of groin, thigh, or knee pain (referred pain)

Signs:

- Mild restriction of hip movement, especially internal rotation
- No or minimal fever
- Generally well-appearing child
- Able to bear some weight (important differentiator)

Systemic features: Absent or mild (important to differentiate from septic arthritis).

Diagnosis

Clinical diagnosis, supported by:

- *X-ray*: Usually normal; may show mild joint space widening (effusion).
- *Ultrasound hip*: Best initial investigation → shows **joint effusion** (hypoechoic fluid in joint capsule).
- *Laboratory tests*:
    - CBC, CRP, ESR usually **normal or mildly elevated**.
    - Blood cultures **negative**.

Differentiation from Septic Arthritis

Feature	*Transient synovitis*	*Septic arthritis*
Onset	Gradual	Sudden, acute
Fever	None or mild (<38°C)	High-grade fever (>38.5°C)
General condition	Well-appearing	Toxic, sick child
Pain severity	Mild-moderate	Severe, unable to move joint

Continued

Continued

Feature	*Transient synovitis*	*Septic arthritis*
Weight-bearing	Possible with limp	Unable to bear weight
Blood tests (CRP/ESR)	Normal or slightly raised	Markedly elevated
Joint aspiration	Clear or mildly turbid	Purulent fluid

Kocher's Criteria (To Differentiate Septic Arthritis):
- Fever >38.5°C
- Non-weight bearing
- ESR >40 mm/h
- WBC >12,000/mm^3

More criteria positive → higher likelihood of septic arthritis.

Management
Transient synovitis:
- *Conservative:*
  - Bed rest or activity restriction
  - NSAIDs (ibuprofen)
  - Observation (usually resolves within 1–2 weeks)

Follow-up:
- Monitor for improvement within 48–72 hours
- Repeat imaging if symptoms persist (to rule out other pathology)

Warning: If symptoms worsen or no improvement → re-evaluate for septic arthritis.

Exam Tip
When answering transient synovitis:
- **Clearly emphasize child appears well** (vs. toxic in septic arthritis).
- **Always mention ultrasound for joint effusion.**
- **Kocher's criteria** should be quoted to differentiate septic arthritis.

Q19. Osteoarthritis (OA) of the hip—etiology, pathogenesis, and management.

Etiology

Primary	*Secondary*
Age-related degeneration	AVN, DDH, Perthes, SCFE
Genetic predisposition	Trauma, infection, inflammatory arthritis
Obesity, mechanical overload	Acetabular dysplasia, FAI, osteochondritis

Pathogenesis
- Cartilage breakdown → joint space narrowing
- Subchondral bone sclerosis and cysts
- Osteophyte formation
- Synovial inflammation

Management

Non-operative	*Operative*
NSAIDs, physiotherapy	Total hip arthroplasty (THA)
Weight reduction	Hip resurfacing (selective)
Walking aids, intra-articular steroids	Osteotomy (young, pre-arthritic stage)

THA is definitive for end-stage OA.

Q20. Rheumatoid arthritis (RA) of the hip—short note.

- **Chronic autoimmune disease** affecting synovium → pannus formation
- **Bilateral, symmetric** hip involvement common in late RA
- Leads to **joint space loss, protrusio acetabuli**, and **osteopenia**

Ortho Relevance
- *Early symptoms:* Pain, stiffness
- May cause rapid joint destruction
- THA is often required earlier than in OA

Cementless THA preferred due to osteopenia; cervical stem sometimes used.

Q21. Surgical options for secondary OA of the hip.

Cause	*Surgical option*
AVN, DDH, SCFE, trauma	Total Hip Replacement (THR)
Early collapse without arthritis	Osteotomy (VDRO, periacetabular)
Post-infective OA	THR (after quiescent period and negative labs)
Protrusio acetabuli (RA)	THR with medial wall reconstruction

In young adults: Hip preservation surgery is considered first.

Q22. Hip osteotomy—indications, techniques, and outcomes.

Indications
- **Young patients** with pre-arthritic or early arthritis
- AVN, DDH, acetabular dysplasia
- FAI with structural deformity

Techniques

Type	*Use*
Periacetabular osteotomy (PAO)	For acetabular dysplasia
Valgus/Varus femoral osteotomy	To unload necrotic segments (AVN)
Shelf or Chiari osteotomy	Salvage in poor acetabular coverage

Outcomes
- Good pain relief and function in properly selected patients
- **Delays THR** by years
- Requires good cartilage and joint congruity

Q23. Femoroacetabular impingement (FAI)—short note.

Definition
Abnormal contact between femoral head-neck junction and acetabulum → labral injury → OA

Types
- *Cam:* Aspherical femoral head
- *Pincer:* Overcoverage of acetabulum
- *Mixed:* Most common

Symptoms
- Groin pain, clicking, stiffness
- Positive **FADIR** test
- Positive drehmann s sign

Diagnosis
- *X-ray:* Cam bump, crossover sign
- *MRI:* Labral tear

Treatment
- Activity modification
- Arthroscopic/mini-open osteoplasty
- Labral repair if torn

Q24. Snapping hip syndrome—causes.

(DYPU Pune 2011)

Definition
Audible or palpable "snap" around hip during motion

Types and Causes

Type	*Structures involved*
External	IT band or gluteus maximus snapping over greater trochanter
Internal	Iliopsoas tendon snapping over iliopectineal eminence
Intra-articular	Labral tear, loose bodies

Management
- Stretching and physiotherapy
- NSAIDs
- Corticosteroid injection(if persistent, painful snapping interferes with activity of daily living)
- Surgical release (rarely indicated)

Distinguishing type is key to treatment.

Q25. Coxa vara—causes and management.

Definition
Coxa vara: **Femoral neck-shaft angle <120°**

Causes

Congenital/developmental	*Acquired*
Developmental coxa vara	Rickets, fibrous dysplasia
Congenital short femur	Slipped capital femoral epiphysis (SCFE)
Proximal femoral focal deficiency	Post-traumatic malunion

Clinical Features
- Limp, limb length discrepancy
- Decreased hip abduction and internal rotation
- Positive Trendelenburg sign

Management
- *<10 years + deformity <15°:* Observation
- *Progressive or >15° deformity:* **Corrective valgus osteotomy**

Goal: Restore mechanical axis and abductor efficiency.

Difference between Coxa Vara and Coxa Valga

These refer to **abnormal neck-shaft angles** of the femur:

Condition	*Definition*	*Neck-shaft angle*	*Causes*	*Effects*
Coxa Vara	Decreased angle	< 120°	Congenital, rickets, trauma	Limping, leg length discrepancy
Coxa Valga	Increased angle	> 135°	Neuromuscular conditions (e.g., CP)	Instability, hip dislocation risk

Normal neck-shaft angle: ~125–135°

Management

- *Mild cases:* Observation
- *Severe/Symptomatic:* **Corrective osteotomy**

Q26. Femoral anteversion.

Definition

Femoral anteversion is the **angular difference** between the axis of the **femoral neck** and the **transcondylar axis** of the distal femur, in the transverse plane.

- *Normal anteversion:*
  - *Infants:* ~30–40°
  - *Adults:* ~10–15°
- **Increased anteversion** → Internal rotation gait ("in-toeing")
- **Decreased anteversion or retroversion** → External rotation gait ("out-toeing")

Clinical Measurement

1. *Craig's test (trochanteric prominence test)*:
   - Patient prone, knee flexed to 90°
   - Examiner palpates greater trochanter and rotates hip until the trochanter is most prominent laterally
   - The angle of the **tibia to vertical** represents the **anteversion angle**
2. *Observational gait analysis*:
   - Increased anteversion → **in-toeing gait**, knees pointing inward
   - Often seen in children; may resolve spontaneously

Radiological Measurement

1. *Ct scan (gold standard)*:
   - Measures **angle between femoral neck axis and condylar axis** in axial plane
   - Accurate and reproducible
2. *MRI*:
   - Radiation-free alternative to CT
   - Useful in pediatrics
3. *X-ray (less accurate)*:
   - **Dunn view** or biplanar radiographs can give rough estimation
   - Not routinely used for precise anteversion measurement

Orthopedic Importance of Femoral Anteversion

- **Gait abnormalities** in children (e.g., intoeing)
- **Patellofemoral instability** (increased anteversion alters patellar tracking)
- *Total hip arthroplasty:* Anteversion of femoral component must be carefully planned (usually ~15°) to prevent **dislocation**
- *Femoral derotation osteotomy:* Performed in symptomatic excessive anteversion or retroversion

Q27. Non-union of fracture neck of femur.

Definition

Non-union is **failure of fracture healing** within **6–9 months**, with **no progression** toward union.

Etiology (Causes)

1. *Biological factors*:
    - Poor blood supply (femoral head has precarious supply)
    - Osteoporosis (elderly)
    - Infection (rare)
    - Inadequate reduction or fixation
2. *Mechanical factors*:
    - Inadequate stability
    - Delayed surgery
    - Improper implant placement
3. *Patient factors*:
    - Smoking
    - Malnutrition
    - Comorbidities (e.g., diabetes)

Clinical Presentation

- **Persistent pain** in groin or hip
- **Limping or inability to bear weight**
- Leg **shortening** and external rotation deformity
- **Muscle wasting** in chronic cases

Diagnosis

1. *X-ray*:
    - Persistent fracture line
    - Sclerosis at fracture ends
    - Absence of callus
    - Varus collapse or femoral head resorption
2. *CT scan*: Assess for degree of non-union and femoral head integrity
3. *MRI*:
    - To assess **vascularity of the femoral head**
    - Helps differentiate **non-union versus AVN**

Management

Depends on **age**, **bone quality**, and **vascularity of the femoral head**.

1. *In young adults (<60 years):*
    - *Head is viable:*
        - **Pauwel's osteotomy** (valgus intertrochanteric osteotomy)
        - **Open reduction and internal fixation (ORIF)** with bone grafting
    - *Head non-viable:*
        - **Vascularized fibular grafting**
        - **Girdlestone procedure** (excision arthroplasty as salvage)
2. *In elderly (>60 years):*
    - High risk of AVN and poor healing
    - *Preferred treatment:*
        - **Hemiarthroplasty** (unipolar or bipolar), or
        - **Total hip arthroplasty (THA)** if acetabulum is arthritic

Q28. Trendelenburg gait—explanation and causes.

Definition
Waddling or dropping of pelvis on contralateral side during stance phase of gait.

Causes

Neurological	*Musculoskeletal*
Superior gluteal nerve palsy	DDH, Perthes, post-THR
Polio	Coxa vara, abductor insufficiency
Muscular dystrophies	Post-operative gluteus medius dysfunction

Test
Patient stands on one leg → pelvis drops on opposite side if positive

Indicates weakness of **gluteus medius/minimus**

Q29. Hip preservation surgery in young adults.

Objective
Delay or prevent THR by preserving native joint.

Indications
- Pre-arthritic or early arthritis
- DDH, FAI, Perthes disease, AVN
- Chondral defects

Surgical Options

Procedure	*Indication*
Periacetabular osteotomy	Acetabular dysplasia
Surgical dislocation	Cam/pincer impingement (FAI)
Core decompression ± BMAC	Early AVN
Osteochondral autograft	Chondral lesions
Mini-open/arthroscopy	Labral tears, loose bodies

Success depends on preserved cartilage and joint congruency.

Q30. Approaches to the hip joint and posterior approach anatomy.

(GGMC 2019)

Approaches to Hip *(Briefly)*
- *Anterior (Smith-Petersen):* Between sartorius and TFL; used in arthroplasty, pediatric hip surgery
- *Anterolateral (Watson-Jones):* Between TFL and gluteus medius
- *Lateral (Hardinge):* Through gluteus medius; total hip replacement
- *Posterior (Moore/Southern):* Most commonly used for THR and dislocation management

Posterior Approach (Detailed Anatomy)
- *Incision:* Posterior to greater trochanter
- *Interval:* Gluteus maximus split → short external rotators (piriformis, obturator internus, gemelli)
- *Structures at risk:*
  - **Sciatic nerve** (medial to external rotators)
  - **Inferior gluteal artery**

- *Steps:*
  - Detach short external rotators
  - Reflect posterior capsule → expose joint
- *Advantage:* Good exposure, preserves abductor mechanism
- *Disadvantage:* Higher risk of posterior dislocation

Q31. Anatomy of the hip joint in relation to posterior approaches.

Overview of the Hip Joint Anatomy

The **hip joint** is a **ball-and-socket synovial joint**, formed by:

- **Acetabulum** (socket) of the pelvis
- **Femoral head** (ball)

Key Structures in Posterior Approaches

When accessing the hip from the **posterior (posterolateral) side**, the following structures are encountered:

1. *Skin and subcutaneous tissue:*
   - *Standard skin incision:* Posterior or posterolateral line over greater trochanter.
2. *Muscles and tendons:* Posterior approaches require **splitting or detachment** of these muscles:

Muscle	*Relation*	*Handling in surgery*
Gluteus maximus	Superficial and largest gluteal muscle	Split along fibers
Short external rotators	Deep to gluteus maximus	Detached from femur and later repaired
• Piriformis	Posterior-superior to joint	Cut or retracted
• Obturator internus, gemelli	Just posterior to capsule	Cut near insertion
Quadratus femoris	Inferior to other rotators	Identified and protected

3. *Sciatic nerve*:
   - Runs **posterior to the hip joint** and lateral to ischial tuberosity.
   - Lies **deep to piriformis**, at risk during dissection.
   - Protected by **gentle retraction** and staying lateral during dissection.
4. *Hip joint capsule*:
   - Posterior capsule is **incised** to enter the joint.
   - This exposes the **posterior acetabulum and femoral head.**
5. *Blood supply*:
   - The **medial femoral circumflex artery (MFCA)** is critical.
   - Supplies the **posterior-superior femoral head** through retinacular vessels.
   - Posterior approaches **preserve MFCA** if dissection is careful.

Advantages of Posterior Approach

- Wide exposure
- Preservation of abductor mechanism
- Easier positioning

Risks

- **Posterior dislocation** (most common complication)
- **Sciatic nerve injury**
- Need for meticulous **capsule and rotator repair**

Q32. Hardinge approach (direct lateral approach).

Also known as the **Hardinge approach**, this is a **direct lateral approach** used for **total hip arthroplasty** and certain hip fracture surgeries.

Steps and Anatomy

1. *Patient position*: Lateral decubitus position.
2. *Incision*:
    - Centered over the **greater trochanter**.
    - About 10–15 cm, aligned along the femoral shaft.
3. *Muscle exposure*:
    - **Split the fascia lata (IT band)** in line with skin incision.
    - Expose the **gluteus medius**.
4. *Gluteus medius handling*:
    - Anterior third to half of the **gluteus medius** is **detached** from greater trochanter.
    - Also detach **gluteus minimus** and **vastus lateralis** (as a single flap if needed).
5. *Capsule*:
    - Joint capsule is exposed and incised **vertically or T-shaped.**
    - Provides **direct access to femoral head and acetabulum.**

Advantages

- Good exposure of both acetabulum and proximal femur
- Lower dislocation rates than posterior approach
- Useful in **obese patients**

Disadvantages

- *Detachment of abductor muscles can lead to*:
    - **Abductor weakness**
    - **Trendelenburg gait** (limp due to gluteus medius dysfunction)
- Risk to **superior gluteal nerve** if dissection is too superior

Q33. Safe surgical dislocation of the hip.

(AIIMS JPR 2019)

Definition

A surgical technique that allows **full access to the femoral head and acetabulum** (hip socket) while preserving the **blood supply**, especially from the **medial femoral circumflex artery.**

Indications

- Femoroacetabular impingement (FAI)
- Acetabular labral tears (when open access is needed)
- Correction of deformities (e.g. Perthes disease, slipped capital femoral epiphysis)
- Tumor excision

Key Features

- Developed by **Ganz et al.**
- Involves a **trochanteric flip osteotomy** to mobilize the greater trochanter
- The **Z-shaped capsulotomy** allows safe exposure
- Preserves the **retinacular vessels** to avoid **avascular necrosis**

Pros

- 360° visualization of the femoral head and acetabulum
- Allows direct repair of labrum and reshaping of bone
- Safer than previous open techniques

Cons

- Invasive
- Risk of trochanteric nonunion or heterotopic ossification

Q34. Hip arthroscopy.

Definition

A **minimally invasive** surgical procedure using a camera and instruments inserted through small portals to diagnose and treat **intra-articular hip problems.**

Indications

- Labral tears
- Femoroacetabular impingement (FAI)
- Loose bodies
- Synovitis
- Chondral lesions

Procedures done Arthroscopically

- **Labral repair or debridement**
- **Cam and pincer resection** in FAI
- **Chondroplasty**
- Synovectomy or removal of loose bodies

Pros

- Minimally invasive
- Faster recovery than open techniques
- Low complication rates

Cons

- Limited view compared to open dislocation
- Technically demanding
- Not suitable for advanced arthritis

Q35. Differential diagnosis of painful hip in a 30-year-old female and management.

Differential Diagnosis

Category	*Conditions*
Inflammatory	Early rheumatoid arthritis, seronegative spondyloarthropathy
Mechanical	Femoroacetabular impingement (FAI), labral tear
Infective	Tuberculous arthritis, subacute septic arthritis
Avascular necrosis	Idiopathic or steroid/alcohol-related
Traumatic	Occult femoral neck fracture, stress fracture
Neoplastic	Benign tumors (osteoid osteoma), metastasis (rare)
Referred pain	Lumbosacral radiculopathy, sacroiliitis
Metabolic	Osteomalacia, transient osteoporosis of hip (TOH)

Evaluation

- *History:* Pain nature (mechanical/inflammatory), systemic symptoms
- *Examination:* Trendelenburg test, impingement tests
- *Investigations:*
    - X-ray pelvis
    - MRI hip (AVN, labral tears)
    - *Blood tests:* ESR, CRP, RF, ANA, Vit D, calcium
- **Joint aspiration** if infection suspected

Management
- *Inflammatory:* DMARDs, NSAIDs, physiotherapy
- *AVN:* Bisphosphonates, core decompression, THR if advanced
- *Infective:* Anti-TB therapy (if TB), antibiotics
- *FAI/Labral tear:* Arthroscopic debridement/repair
- *TOH:* Conservative—rest, calcium/Vit D

Q36. Limp in a child.

I. Causes of Limp in a Child

Limping in children can be **painful (antalgic)** or **painless**. Causes vary by **age group**:

Age group	*Common causes*
0–3 years	Developmental dysplasia of hip (DDH), toddler's fracture, septic arthritis
3–10 years	Transient synovitis, Legg–Calvé–Perthes disease, juvenile idiopathic arthritis
>10 years	Slipped capital femoral epiphysis (SCFE), trauma, osteomyelitis
Any age	Trauma, infection (septic arthritis, TB), tumors, neuromuscular disorders

II. Tuberculosis (TB) of the Hip

1. *Clinical features*:
    - Insidious onset of **hip/groin pain**
    - **Limping**, limited weight bearing
    - **Night sweats, fever**, weight loss (constitutional signs)
    - Restricted **range of motion**, especially **abduction and internal rotation**
    - **Muscle wasting** around the hip
    - May present with **flexion, adduction, internal rotation deformity**
2. *Diagnosis*:
    - *Blood tests:* ESR ↑, CRP ↑, leukocytes mild ↑
    - *X-ray:*
        - *Early:* Osteopenia around joint, joint space narrowing
        - *Late:* Bone erosion, subluxation, "wandering acetabulum"
    - *MRI:* Detects early joint and soft tissue involvement
    - *Ultrasound:* Detects effusion or abscess
    - *Synovial fluid analysis:* AFB staining, culture
    - **GeneXpert or TB PCR**, biopsy (for confirmation)
3. *Management*:
    - *Conservative (mainstay):*
        - **ATT (anti-tubercular therapy)** for 12–18 months
            - *Intensive phase:* 4 drugs (HRZE)
            - *Continuation phase:* 2 drugs (HR)
        - **Rest, traction, splinting** during active disease
        - Gradual mobilization and physiotherapy
    - *Surgical (if failure of conservative or late sequelae)*:
        - Abscess drainage
        - Synovectomy
        - Corrective osteotomy
        - Arthrodesis or total hip replacement (in adults with advanced disease)

Q37. A 37-year-old boy with fever and pain in left proximal thigh for 10 days.

Most Likely Diagnosis

Acute Osteomyelitis or Septic Arthritis of the Hip

Approach to Management

1. *History and clinical evaluation:*
   - Fever, pain, refusal to bear weight
   - Localized tenderness
   - Limited hip motion or pseudoparalysis
   - Swelling, redness, warmth (if superficial)
   - Look for toxic features (irritability, lethargy)
2. *Immediate investigations:*
   - *CBC:* Elevated WBC count
   - *ESR/CRP:* Significantly raised
   - Blood cultures
   - *X-ray:* Often normal early, may show soft tissue swelling
   - *Ultrasound:* Detects joint effusion or abscess
   - *MRI:* Best for early diagnosis of osteomyelitis or septic arthritis
3. *Emergency management:*
   - *If septic arthritis is suspected (especially in hip)*:
     - Surgical emergency

   Steps:
   - Urgent **joint aspiration** → send for Gram stain, culture, cell count, AFB (if TB suspected)
   - If positive → **urgent arthrotomy or arthroscopic washout**
   - Start **IV antibiotics empirically**, adjust according to culture

   Empirical IV antibiotics:
   - **Ceftriaxone** or **Cefazolin** ± **Vancomycin** (for MRSA coverage)
   - *Duration:* IV for 2–3 weeks → oral antibiotics for 3–4 weeks
4. *Supportive measures:*
   - Analgesia
   - Immobilization (splint)
   - Monitor temperature, inflammatory markers
   - Regular follow-up with repeat imaging and labs

Miscellaneous Topics: Hip

Q38. Acetabular labral tear.

(BJ Medical College Ahmedabad 2011)

Definition

A tear of the **fibrocartilaginous labrum** that lines the rim of the **acetabulum** (hip socket), often due to trauma or **femoroacetabular impingement** (FAI).

Symptoms

- Groin pain or deep hip pain
- Clicking, catching, or locking of the hip
- Stiffness or decreased range of motion

Diagnosis

- **MRI arthrogram** is the gold standard
- *Physical exam:* Positive FADIR or FABER test
- Confirmed during arthroscopy

Management

- *Conservative:* Rest, physiotherapy, NSAIDs
- *Surgical:*
  - **Labral repair** (preferred over debridement)
  - Arthroscopic versus open (surgical dislocation if more extensive correction is needed)

Q39. Hip pointers.

Definition

A **contusion** (bruise) of the **iliac crest** (top rim of the pelvis), usually from a direct blow.

Common in: Contact sports (football, hockey)

Symptoms

- Localized pain over iliac crest
- Swelling, bruising
- Pain with trunk movement

Treatment

- Rest, ice, NSAIDs
- Return to play when asymptomatic

Q40. Athletic pubalgia (sports hernia).

Definition

A condition causing **chronic groin pain** due to injury or weakness in the **posterior inguinal wall**, but without a true hernia.

Causes

- Repetitive twisting and turning at high speed (soccer, hockey)
- Imbalance between abdominal and thigh muscles

Symptoms

- Groin pain aggravated by sports
- No visible hernia
- Pain with sit-ups or resisted hip adduction

Treatment

- Physical therapy
- Surgery (inguinal repair or adductor release if conservative fails)

Q41. Trochanteric bursitis.

Definition

Inflammation of the **bursa** overlying the **greater trochanter** (outer part of the hip).

Symptoms
- Lateral hip pain (worse with lying on the side)
- Pain with climbing stairs or prolonged standing
- Tenderness over greater trochanter

Causes
- Overuse
- Trauma
- Associated with IT band tightness

Treatment
- NSAIDs, physical therapy
- Corticosteroid injections
- *Rarely:* Bursectomy if refractory

Q42. Heuter's interval.

Definition
Heuter's interval (also called the **Hueter interval**) is an **anatomic intermuscular plane** used in the **anterior approach to the hip** (e.g., Smith–Petersen approach).

Boundaries
- *Medial:* Sartorius muscle (femoral nerve)
- *Lateral:* Tensor fascia lata (TFL) muscle (superior gluteal nerve)
- Lies between **two muscles innervated by different nerves**, which makes it a **safe surgical plane.**

Surgical Importance
- Used in **direct anterior hip arthroplasty**
- Minimizes muscle damage
- Allows access to the hip joint capsule with minimal disruption

Q43. Protrusio acetabuli.

Definition
A condition where the **femoral head** is **medially displaced** and **protrudes into the pelvic cavity**, crossing the **ilioischial (Kohler's) line** on X-ray.

Types
- **Primary (idiopathic)**—often bilateral, slow progression
- **Secondary**—due to:
  - Rheumatoid arthritis
  - Paget's disease
  - Osteomalacia
  - Trauma or infection (e.g., TB)
  - Marfan syndrome

Radiographic Features
- Medial displacement of femoral head
- Femoral head crosses **Kohler's line**

Clinical Significance
- Decreased range of motion
- Pain and early osteoarthritis
- Surgical challenge in hip replacement (need for bone grafting or specialized implants)

Q44. Sonication.

Definition

A **microbiological technique** used to detect **biofilm-associated infections**, especially in **orthopedic implants** (e.g., prosthetic joint infections).

Principle

- The removed implant is placed in a sterile container with fluid.
- **Ultrasonic waves** are applied → **disrupt biofilms** → release bacteria into fluid.
- Fluid is then cultured to detect **low-virulence organisms.**

Advantages

- Increases diagnostic yield compared to conventional cultures
- Particularly useful in **low-grade infections** or when antibiotics have already been given

Applications

- Diagnosis of **periprosthetic joint infections (PJI)**
- Evaluation after revision arthroplasty

Q45. Sacroiliitis.

Definition

Inflammation of the sacroiliac (SI) joint, where the sacrum meets the ilium.

Causes

- **Seronegative spondyloarthropathies** (e.g., ankylosing spondylitis, reactive arthritis)
- Infection (septic sacroiliitis)
- Pregnancy or mechanical stress

Symptoms

- Lower back pain
- Buttock pain (may radiate to thigh)
- Worse with prolonged standing or sitting

Diagnosis

- *Clinical exam:* FABER test, SI joint tenderness
- *Imaging:*
    - *X-ray:* Sclerosis, erosions
    - *MRI:* Early inflammation (most sensitive)
    - HLA-B27 testing (in inflammatory cases)

Treatment

- NSAIDs, physical therapy
- TNF inhibitors in autoimmune cases
- Antibiotics for infection-related sacroiliitis

7.6 Knee Joint

Sumit Banerjee, Mohamad Waseem Dar, Manish Singh

Basic Anatomy and Biomechanics

Q1. Anatomy of the knee joint—including ligaments and menisci.

(GMERS Medical College 2018)

Type
Modified hinge joint (synovial)

Bones
- Femur (condyles)
- Tibia (plateau)
- Patella (articulates with femoral trochlea)

Ligaments
- *Extracapsular:*
  - *Medial collateral ligament (MCL)*: Resists valgus stress
  - *Lateral collateral ligament (LCL)*: Resists varus stress
- *Intracapsular:*
  - *Anterior cruciate ligament (ACL)*: Prevents anterior tibial translation
  - *Posterior cruciate ligament (PCL)*: Prevents posterior tibial translation
- **Patellar ligament**—from patella to tibial tuberosity

Menisci
- *Medial:* C-shaped, less mobile, attached to MCL
- *Lateral:* O-shaped, more mobile
- *Functions:* Shock absorption, load distribution, stability, joint lubrication

Q2. Biomechanics of knee joint during gait.

Phases
- *Stance phase:*
  - Knee flexes ~15° at heel strike → shock absorption
  - Then extends for mid-stance → support
- *Swing phase:*
  - Flexion (~60°) for foot clearance
  - Extension before heel strike

Muscle Roles
- *Quadriceps:* Control knee flexion during loading
- *Hamstrings:* Control extension during terminal swing

Ground Reaction Force (GRF)
Passes behind knee (flexion moment) → countered by quadriceps

Q3. Screw-home mechanism of the knee.

Definition
Terminal rotation that **locks the knee** in full extension

Mechanism

- *Last 20–30° of extension:*
  - **Tibia externally rotates** on femur (open chain), or
  - **Femur internally rotates** on tibia (closed chain)

Why It Happens?

- Lateral femoral condyle finishes gliding before medial condyle
- Medial condyle continues moving → external tibial rotation

Unlocking

By **popliteus muscle** during flexion

Q4. Blood supply of the knee joint and clinical significance.

Sources

- *Genicular branches of:*
  - Femoral artery
  - Popliteal artery
  - Anterior tibial artery

Anastomotic Network

- Formed around patella and femoral condyles
- Ensures collateral flow

Clinical Significance

- Rich vascularity aids healing
- **Menisci (especially medial)** have peripheral vascular supply only → central tears heal poorly
- Cruciate ligaments have limited vascularity → impacts healing

Q5. Bursae around the knee and clinical importance.

Bursa	*Location*	*Clinical condition*
Prepatellar	Over patella	Housemaid's knee
Infrapatellar (superficial)	Below patellar ligament	Clergyman's knee
Infrapatellar (deep)	Between ligament and tibia	Can get inflamed from overuse
Suprapatellar	Above patella (with joint)	Effusion seen here
Pes anserine bursa	Medial tibia (below joint line)	Anserine bursitis (OA, obesity)
Semimembranosus bursa	Posteromedial joint capsule	Baker's cyst (if enlarged)

Q6. Locking and unlocking mechanism—short note.

Locking

- Occurs in the final **30° of extension**
- **Lateral femoral condyle** completes motion before medial → causes **external rotation** of tibia (open chain)

Unlocking

- Initiated by **popliteus muscle**
- Causes **internal rotation** of tibia → unlocks knee for flexion

Important for energy-efficient standing.

Q7. Role of menisci in knee stability and function.

Function	*Details*
Load transmission	Transmit ~50–70% load in extension
Shock absorption	Distributes joint forces
Joint congruity	Deepen the articular surfaces
Lubrication	Spread synovial fluid
Proprioception	Mechanoreceptors in horns
Stability	Resists anterior translation (especially medial)

Meniscal tears compromise joint longevity → early OA

Q8. Cruciate ligaments in knee biomechanics.

Ligament	*Origin → insertion*	*Function*
ACL	Medial aspect of lateral femoral condyle → anterior tibial plateau	Prevents anterior translation of tibia
PCL	Lateral aspect of medial femoral condyle → posterior tibia	Prevents posterior translation of tibia

Biomechanical Role

- Stabilize knee in **AP direction**
- Guide rotation and pivoting
- *ACL:* Prevents hyperextension
- *PCL:* Critical in weight-bearing flexion

Q9. Q-angle and clinical relevance.

Definition

Angle between line of quadriceps pull and patellar tendon

Normal values

- *Males*: ~12–15°
- *Females*: ~15–18°

Clinical Relevance

- ↑ *Q-angle:* Patellar subluxation, valgus deformity
- ↓ *Q-angle:* Varus deformity
- Measured in **full extension**

High Q-angle is a risk factor for **patellofemoral pain syndrome**

Q10. Factors responsible for knee stability.

Static stabilizers	*Dynamic stabilizers*
Ligaments (ACL, PCL, MCL, LCL)	Quadriceps, hamstrings, popliteus
Joint capsule	Gastrocnemius
Menisci	Iliotibial band

Other Factors

- Geometry of femoral condyles
- Screw-home mechanism
- Joint congruity

Instability occurs with ligament injury or loss of neuromuscular control.

Q11. Embryology and development of the knee joint.

(Rajasthan University of Health Sciences 2019)

- *Limb bud formation:* ~4th week
- Interzone cells → joint cavity and menisci
- *Chondrification:* 6th–8th week
- *Ossification:*
  - *Femoral condyles:* ~9th fetal week
  - *Tibial epiphysis:* Appears ~birth
  - *Patella:* Ossifies ~3–5 years

Developmental Abnormalities

- Congenital dislocation of patella
- Discoid meniscus
- Tibial torsion

Q12. Fabella.

Definition

The **fabella** is a **sesamoid bone** located in the **lateral head of the gastrocnemius muscle**, **posterior to the lateral femoral condyle**.

Prevalence

- Seen in **10–30%** of the population
- More common in **Asians**
- Can be **bilateral**

Clinical Significance

- Usually **asymptomatic**
- Can cause **posterolateral knee pain** (Fabella syndrome)
- May **irritate the common peroneal nerve**
- **Seen on X-ray or MRI** (may be mistaken for loose body or fracture)

Fabella Syndrome

- Pain during knee extension
- Aggravated by activities involving knee flexion-extension
- Caused by **impingement between fabella and femoral condyle**

Management

- *Conservative:* NSAIDs, activity modification
- *Surgical:* **Fabellectomy** if persistent symptoms or nerve compression

Quick Recap

Feature	*Detail*
Location	Posterolateral knee (gastrocnemius)
Bone type	Sesamoid
Symptoms	Posterolateral pain, nerve impingement
Diagnosis	X-ray/MRI
Treatment	Conservative → Fabellectomy

Q13. Special tests for diagnosis of anterior cruciate ligament (ACL) injury.

(Asked in RGUHS Karnataka 2023)

Introduction

Anterior cruciate ligament (ACL) injuries are common among athletes and result in knee instability.

Special Clinical Tests

1. *Lachman test:*
   - ***Most sensitive test.***
   - Knee flexed to 20–30°.
   - Tibia pulled anteriorly; increased anterior translation suggests ACL tear.
2. *Anterior drawer test:*
   - Knee flexed to 90°.
   - Anterior movement of tibia against femur.
   - Less sensitive than Lachman.
3. *Pivot shift test:*
   - Highly specific for ACL tear.
   - Involves valgus stress and internal rotation during knee flexion.
   - Positive test causes sudden reduction ("shift") felt.

Supporting Investigations

- *MRI knee:* Gold standard non-invasive imaging.
- *Arthroscopy:* Direct visualization, definitive diagnosis.

Mnemonic for remembering ACL tests

"LAP" → **L**achman → **A**nterior Drawer → **P**ivot Shift

Gold Standard Clinical Tests

Test	*Technique*	*Interpretation*
Lachman test	20–30° knee flexion; anterior translation	Increased laxity: ACL tear
Anterior drawer test	90° knee flexion; pull tibia anteriorly	Anterior displacement: ACL deficiency
Pivot shift test	Valgus + internal rotation while extending	Clunking: ACL insufficiency

Other Important Points

- *Lachman test*: **Most sensitive** (best screening test).
- *Pivot shift test*: **Most specific** (best confirmatory test).
- *MRI:* Investigation of choice to confirm ACL tear.

Mnemonic for ACL Tests Order

"LAP" → **L**achman → **A**nterior Drawer → **P**ivot Shift

Tips for Answering in an Exam

- Always start with a small 2–3 line **Introduction**.
- Use **headings and bullet points** for clarity.
- **Name-drop important tests** and **classification systems** if relevant.
- Where possible, **draw simple diagrams** of clinical tests (especially Lachman and Pivot Shift).

Q14. Clinical examination of the knee joint—steps.

1. *Inspection*:
   - Swelling, deformity (genu valgum/varum), muscle wasting
   - Patella alignment, scars, skin changes
2. *Palpation*:
   - Joint line tenderness (medial/lateral)
   - *Effusion:* **Patellar tap**, **Fluid shift**
   - Patellar tenderness (PFJ pain)
   - Temperature
3. *Range of motion (ROM)*:
   - *Active and passive:* Flexion (0–135°), extension (0°)
   - Crepitus or restriction

4. *Stability tests*:
   - *Ligamentous:* Lachman, drawer, Valgus/Varus stress
   - *Meniscus:* McMurray, Apley's
5. *Special tests*:
   - Patellar grind (Clarke's), apprehension test
   - Thessaly's test
6. Gait and functional assessment

Q15. Assessment and grading of knee effusion.

Clinical Tests
- *Patellar tap test:* Positive in moderate effusion
- *Fluid displacement test:* Mild effusion
- *Balloon sign:* For large effusion

Grading (subjective)
1. *Mild*: Detectable by bulge test
2. *Moderate*: Positive patellar tap
3. *Severe*: Tense swelling, marked fluctuation

Q16. MRI in meniscal, chondral, and ligamentous knee injuries.

(SRIHER 2011)

Meniscus
- *Normal:* Triangular dark structure on T1/T2
- *Tear:* Linear high signal reaching articular surface
  - Horizontal/Vertical/Radial/Flap tear
  - Bucket-handle tear → displaced fragment in intercondylar notch

Ligaments
- *ACL/PCL:*
  - *Normal:* Low signal (black band)
  - *Tear:* Discontinuity, high signal, non-visualization
- *Collateral ligaments:* Thickened, irregular, or disrupted fibers in tear

Articular Cartilage
- *T2-weighted:* Bright cartilage; defects appear as **irregularity or thinning**
- Graded I–IV (Outerbridge classification)

Sequences
- *T1:* Anatomy, marrow
- *T2/STIR:* Fluid, edema, inflammation
- *PD-weighted with fat suppression:* Menisci and cartilage best visualized

Q17. Differential diagnosis of anterior knee pain.

Cause	*Key features*
Patellofemoral pain syndrome	Pain on stairs, squatting, prolonged sitting
Chondromalacia patella	Softening of patellar cartilage; crepitus, positive grind test
Patellar tendinitis (Jumper's knee)	Tenderness over inferior pole of patella
Osgood-Schlatter disease	Adolescent athletes; pain over tibial tuberosity
Sinding–Larsen–Johansson	Pain at inferior patellar pole (children)
Prepatellar bursitis	Swelling over patella; tenderness
Fat pad impingement	Pain on extension, swelling below patella

Q18. Clinical features and diagnosis of patellofemoral instability.

Causes

- Shallow trochlear groove
- Increased Q angle
- Patella alta
- Generalized ligament laxity

Clinical Features

- Recurrent patellar dislocation/subluxation
- "Giving way" during activity
- Apprehension during lateral movement

Examination Tests

- *Apprehension test:* Lateral push on patella causes fear/tightening
- Patellar tracking test
- Increased Q-angle (>15° females, >10° males)

Imaging

- *X-ray:* Skyline/Merchant view—lateral tilt or subluxation
- *MRI:* MPFL tear, trochlear dysplasia

Congenital and Developmental Knee Disorders

Q19. Congenital dislocation of the knee—classification, diagnosis and management.

Definition

A rare condition characterized by hyperextension and anterior subluxation or dislocation of the tibia at birth.

Classification (Leveuf and Pais)

Type	*Description*
I	Hyperextension, reducible
II	Tibia subluxed anteriorly, partially reducible
III	Tibia completely dislocated, irreducible

Diagnosis

- *Clinical:* Genu recurvatum, inability to flex knee
- *X-ray:* Anterior tibial displacement
- *Associated with:* Arthrogryposis, Larsen syndrome

Management

- *Type I/II:* Gentle stretching + serial casting
- *Type III:* Surgical quadriceps lengthening + capsular release
- *Timing:* Early correction is critical for good ROM

Q20. Blount's disease—pathophysiology and treatment.

Definition

Developmental disorder of the medial proximal tibial physis → progressive **tibia vara**

Pathophysiology

- Disordered endochondral ossification of medial physis
- Increased medial load → growth inhibition
- *Two types:* Infantile (≤3 years), Adolescent (>10 years)

Radiographic Signs
- **Langenskiöld classification** (Stages I–VI)
- Beaking and sloping of medial metaphysis
- Metaphyseal-diaphyseal angle >11° is diagnostic

Treatment

Age/stage	Management
<3 years, early stage	Bracing (KAFO)
>3 years or severe deformity	Proximal tibial valgus osteotomy
Severe cases	External fixation (Ilizarov)

Q21. Discoid meniscus—short note.

Definition
A congenital anomaly where the **lateral meniscus** is disc-shaped instead of crescentic.

Types (Watanabe classification)
- *Type I:* Complete
- *Type II:* Incomplete
- *Type III:* Wrisberg type (unstable)

Clinical
- Snapping, popping, joint line pain
- More common in children, often bilateral

Management
- *Asymptomatic:* Observe
- *Symptomatic:* Saucerization + meniscoplasty ± repair

Ligamentous and Meniscal Injuries

Q22. Anatomy and biomechanics of the anterior cruciate ligament (ACL).

(CMC Vellore 2017)

Anatomy
- *Origin:* Posterior medial aspect of lateral femoral condyle
- *Insertion:* Anterior intercondylar area of tibia
- *Bundles:*
    - **Anteromedial (AM)**—tight in flexion
    - **Posterolateral (PL)**—tight in extension
- *Blood supply:* Middle genicular artery
- *Innervation:* Posterior articular branch of tibial nerve

Biomechanics
- Prevents **anterior tibial translation**
- Secondary restraint to tibial rotation and varus/valgus stress
- Works synergistically with hamstrings

Q23. ACL injuries—classification and management.

Classification
- *Grade I:* Partial tear, no instability
- *Grade II:* Partial tear with laxity
- *Grade III:* Complete rupture

Diagnosis
- *Clinical:* **Lachman test**, anterior drawer test, pivot-shift
- *MRI:* Gold standard for visualizing ACL tears

Management

Non-operative	*Operative*
Low-demand, sedentary	Young, active, athletes
No instability	Associated meniscal or multi-ligament injury
Focus: Rehabilitation and proprioception	ACL reconstruction (arthroscopic)

Indications of Surgery
- Symptomatic instability
- Active individuals
- Associated meniscus or ligament injuries
- Failed conservative management

Techniques
- *Grafts:*
  - Autograft (BTB, hamstring – STG)
  - Allograft (used less often)
- *Approach:* Arthroscopic
- *Tunnel placement:* Anatomic femoral and tibial tunnels

Rehabilitation Protocol

Phase	*Goals*
0–2 weeks	Reduce swelling, achieve full extension
2–6 weeks	ROM exercises, begin closed-chain strength
6–12 weeks	Strengthening, balance
3–6 months	Proprioception, jogging
6–9 months	Return to sports (if strength and control regained)

Q24. ACL injury in a 20-year-old athlete—management and graft comparison.

Management
- *Indication for surgery*: Active athlete with instability
- *Procedure:* Arthroscopic anatomic single-bundle ACL reconstruction

Graft Options

Graft	*Merits*	*Shortcomings*
BTB autograft	High fixation strength, bone-to-bone healing	Anterior knee pain, risk of patellar fracture
Hamstring (STG)	Less donor site morbidity	Soft tissue healing, slower fixation
Quadriceps	Good strength, less pain	Less commonly used, may affect extension
Allograft	No donor site pain, shorter surgery	Delayed incorporation, risk of disease

Fixation Devices
- **Endobutton (suspensory)**
- Interference screws (metal/bioabsorbable)

Q25. Double bundle ACL reconstruction (SN).

- Reconstructs both **AM and PL bundles**
- Better rotational stability

- Technically demanding
- Not routinely done; reserved for high-demand athletes

Q26. Endobutton (SN).

- **Suspensory femoral fixation** device
- Small metallic button flipped on cortical side of femur
- Secures graft loop; used in ACL reconstruction
- Easy and strong fixation

Q27. PCL anatomy, biomechanics, and treatment of chronic PCL injury.

Anatomy

- *Origin:* Lateral aspect of medial femoral condyle
- *Insertion:* Posterior tibial sulcus
- *Bundles:*
  - Anterolateral (tight in flexion)
  - Posteromedial (tight in extension)

Biomechanics

- Prevents **posterior tibial translation**
- Secondary stabilizer for rotation
- Stronger than ACL

Treatment of Chronic Symptomatic PCL Injury

Non-surgical:

- Bracing (posterior tibial support)
- Quadriceps strengthening

Surgical:

- **PCL reconstruction** (arthroscopic)
  - *Grafts:* Hamstring, quadriceps, Achilles allograft
  - Single- or double-bundle

Indications:

- Grade III instability
- Persistent symptoms despite rehabilitation
- Combined ligamentous injuries

Q28. PCL injury—diagnosis and treatment.

Mechanism

- Dashboard injury (posterior tibial blow)
- Hyperflexion or hyperextension with rotation

Diagnosis

- Posterior drawer test, sag sign, quadriceps active test
- *MRI:* Confirms PCL tear, evaluates menisci

Management

Grade i–ii (partial)	*Grade iii (complete)*
Conservative: Physio, brace	PCL reconstruction (autograft or allograft)

Surgery indicated for symptomatic instability or combined injuries.

Classification (Grade I–III based on posterior drawer)

Management

Grade	Treatment
I–II	Non-operative: Brace in extension, rehabilitation
III	Surgical reconstruction (especially with multi-ligament injury)

Surgical Options

- Single versus double bundle PCL reconstruction
- Autograft (hamstring, quadriceps) or allograft

Q29. Posterolateral corner (PLC) injury—short note.

Structures Involved

LCL, popliteus tendon, popliteofibular ligament

Mechanism

- Hyperextension + varus + external rotation
- Often seen with **PCL or ACL injuries**

Diagnosis

- **Dial test**, external rotation recurvatum test
- Varus stress test at 30°

Treatment

- *Grade I–II:* Bracing + rehabilitation
- *Grade III:* **Surgical reconstruction** (autograft)

Missed PLC injuries → graft failure in ACL/PCL reconstructions

Q30. Multi-ligamentous knee injuries—treatment options.

Definition

Injury to ≥2 major ligaments (ACL, PCL, MCL, LCL, posterolateral corner)

Initial Management

- Assess vascular status (check for **popliteal artery injury**)
- Rule out **knee dislocation**
- Stabilize knee (hinged brace or external fixator)

Definitive Treatment

- Surgical reconstruction (usually delayed 2–3 weeks)
  - Combined ACL/PCL reconstruction
  - Repair or reconstruction of MCL, LCL, or PLC
- Consider staged procedures if multiple repairs are needed

Post-operative Rehabilitation

- Slower and more protected than isolated ACL rehabilitation
- Emphasis on ROM, quadriceps activation, and bracing

Q31. Knee instability patterns—ligament-based.

Ligament injured	Instability pattern
ACL	Anterior instability
PCL	Posterior instability

Continued

Continued

Ligament injured	*Instability pattern*
MCL	Valgus + rotational instability
LCL	Varus instability
PLC (posterolateral corner)	External rotation + varus
Combined (ACL + MCL)	Anteromedial rotatory instability (AMRI)
ACL + PLC	Anterolateral rotatory instability (ALRI)

Clinical tests (pivot-shift, dial test, varus/valgus stress) are essential for localization.

Q32. Role of bracing in ligament injury management.

Types of Braces

Brace type	*Use*
Hinged knee brace	MCL, LCL injuries
Functional brace	Post ACL/PCL surgery or rehabilitation
Posterior tibial support brace	For isolated PCL injuries
Offloading brace	To reduce strain on healing ligaments

Roles

- Protect healing ligaments
- Guide joint motion
- Prevent further injury
- Increase proprioception

Limitations

- Should not replace structured rehabilitation
- Prolonged use may cause muscle weakness

Quick Summary Table

Topic	*Key points*
ACL anatomy and biomechanics	AM/PL bundles; prevents anterior tibial translation
ACL reconstruction	Autograft, anatomic tunnel, rehabilitation in five phases
PCL injury management	Grade I–II non-operative; Grade III → surgical
Multi-Ligament injury	Requires vascular check + staged reconstruction
Bracing in ligament injuries	Supports healing, varies by ligament; should complement rehabilitation, not replace it

Q33. Discoid meniscus (SN).

- Congenital thickened, disc-shaped lateral meniscus
- More prone to tearing
- *Clinical:* Snapping knee, pain in children
- *MRI:* Enlarged meniscus
- *Treatment:* Saucerization ± repair

Q34. Meniscal tears—mechanism, features and treatment.

Mechanism

- Twisting injuries on a planted foot (especially in sports)
- Degenerative tears in older adults

Clinical Features
- Joint line tenderness
- Locking, clicking, swelling
- McMurray's or Thessaly test (+ve)

Treatment

Acute/peripheral	*Degenerative/central*
Meniscal repair (if vascular)	Partial meniscectomy
Arthroscopy-assisted	Post-operative rehabilitation

Aim is to **preserve meniscus** wherever possible.

Q35. Meniscal tears—classification.

Classifications
By morphology:
- Longitudinal
- Radial
- Horizontal
- Flap (parrot-beak)
- Bucket-handle
- Complex (degenerative)

By location:
- *Red-red zone:* Peripheral, vascular
- *Red-white zone:* Intermediate
- *White-white zone:* Central, avascular

Q36. Ramp lesion.

Definition
Peripheral longitudinal tear of posterior horn of **medial meniscus**, associated with ACL injuries.

Diagnosis
- Often missed on MRI
- Identified on arthroscopy (posteromedial portal)

Treatment
- All-inside repair using suture devices
- Preserving meniscus critical for knee stability

Q37. Indications and techniques for meniscectomy.

Meniscectomy
- *Indications:*
    - Irreparable tear (degenerative, central, complex)
    - Locked bucket-handle
- *Technique:*
    - **Arthroscopic partial meniscectomy** preferred
    - Preserve as much meniscus as possible

Q38. Meniscal repair—indications and techniques.

Role of Meniscal Repair

Preserves meniscal function (shock absorption, stability)

Indications

- **Young patient**
- Peripheral (red-red or red-white) tear
- Longitudinal or bucket handle tears

Techniques

Type	*Approach*
Inside-out	Most common, strong fixation
Outside-in	For anterior horn tears
All-inside	Minimally invasive, pre-loaded devices

Healing better in **vascular zones**.

Q39. Meniscus transplantation.

- Indicated in young patients with prior **total meniscectomy**
- Allograft (fresh/frozen)
- Helps restore joint biomechanics, delay OA
- Done arthroscopically with suture or bone plug techniques

Q40. Role of MRI in ligament and meniscal injuries.

Utility

- Gold standard non-invasive imaging
- Shows **ligament continuity, edema, bone bruise, meniscal tears**
- Essential for surgical planning

MRI Findings

Structure	*Findings*
ACL	Discontinuity, abnormal orientation, edema
PCL	"Wavy" or disrupted fiber pattern
Menisci	Intra-substance signal reaching articular surface

Can differentiate between **acute versus chronic tears**.

Q41. Autologous chondrocyte implantation (ACI)—role in cartilage defects.

Indications

- Focal full-thickness cartilage defect (grade III–IV)
- *Size:* **>2 cm^2**
- Patient <50 years, high functional demand

Procedure

1. *Stage 1*: Arthroscopic harvest of chondrocytes
2. Cells cultured in lab (~4–6 weeks)
3. *Stage 2*: Implantation under periosteal flap (or collagen membrane)

Outcomes

- Good long-term results in focal chondral lesions
- *Risk:* Periosteal hypertrophy, graft delamination

Evolved Techniques

Matrix-induced ACI (MACI): Scaffold-based

Q42. Microfracture surgery—indications and outcomes.

Indications

- Small, full-thickness cartilage defects (<2–4 cm^2)
- Low-demand patients
- Cost-effective alternative to ACI

Technique

- Arthroscopic
- Debride cartilage → perforate subchondral bone (~3–4 mm depth) → marrow stem cell migration

Outcome

- Stimulates fibrocartilage formation (not hyaline)
- Symptomatic relief, but long-term durability limited

Q43. Osteochondral autograft transfer system (OATS) procedure.

- Transfers **cylindrical osteochondral plugs** from non-weightbearing to defect area
- Indicated in **focal cartilage defects <2–3 cm^2**
- *Advantage:* Transfers **hyaline cartilage**
- Also called **mosaicplasty** when multiple plugs used

Summary Table

Topic	*Highlights*
Meniscal tear management	Repair in red-red zone; meniscectomy if irreparable
Meniscectomy vs. repair	Preserve as much meniscus as possible
OCD knee	Stable: Non-operative; unstable: Surgical fixation
ACI	For large focal cartilage defects in young patients
Microfracture	For small lesions; fibrocartilage outcome
Pivot Shift	Best test for ACL-related rotational instability

Knee Arthritis and Degenerative Conditions

Q44. Spontaneous osteonecrosis of the knee (SPONK) lesion.

Common in: Elderly females, medial femoral condyle

Etiology

Microfractures or vascular compromise

Clinical

- Sudden medial knee pain without trauma
- Local tenderness

MRI

Subchondral hypointense area

Management

- *Early:* Non-weight bearing, NSAIDs
- *Late:* HTO or UKA/TKA

Q45. Osteoarthritis of the knee—etiology, pathogenesis and treatment.

Etiology

- *Primary OA:* Age, obesity, genetic predisposition
- *Secondary OA:* Trauma, inflammatory arthritis, metabolic disorders

Pathogenesis

1. **Cartilage degeneration** → proteoglycan loss
2. **Subchondral bone sclerosis and osteophyte formation**
3. Synovial inflammation + joint space narrowing
4. Muscle weakness and joint deformity (varus/valgus)

Treatment

Non-surgical	*Surgical*
Weight reduction, NSAIDs	Arthroscopic lavage (rare)
Physiotherapy, orthotics	HTO for unicompartmental disease
Viscosupplementation, PRP	UKA or TKA for end-stage disease

Early diagnosis + multimodal management improves long-term outcomes.

Q46. Kellgren and Lawrence grading—knee OA.

Grade	*Radiological features*
0	Normal
1	Doubtful narrowing, possible osteophytes
2	Definite osteophytes, possible narrowing
3	Moderate narrowing, sclerosis, osteophytes
4	Severe narrowing, sclerosis, large osteophytes, deformity

Grade ≥2 is considered **radiographic OA**

Q47. Surgical options—end-stage knee OA.

Procedure	*Indications*	*Drawbacks*
Total knee arthroplasty (TKA)	Multicompartment OA	Major surgery, risk of infection
Unicompartmental knee arthroplasty (UKA)	Isolated medial/lateral OA	Requires ligament integrity
High tibial osteotomy (HTO)	Young active patients with varus OA	Not suitable in advanced arthritis
Arthrodesis	Salvage option (infection, severe trauma)	Loss of mobility

Choice depends on **age, activity level, joint involvement**.

Q48. Unicompartmental knee replacement (UKR)—short note.

Indications

- Isolated medial or lateral OA

- Intact cruciate ligaments
- No patellofemoral symptoms

Outcomes
- Faster recovery
- Less blood loss
- More physiological gait
- Easier revision to TKA

Better suited for **older, low-demand patients.**

Q49. OA of bilateral knees in 45-year-old female.

Pathogenesis
- Early cartilage degeneration → subchondral sclerosis → osteophytes
- *Contributing factors:* Obesity, hormonal changes, malalignment, prior trauma

Management
- *Non-operative:* Weight loss, NSAIDs, physio, bracing, injections
- *Surgical:*
  - HTO (if varus)
  - UKA
  - TKA (if advanced)

Q50. Malaligned knee biomechanics and medial compartment OA treatment.

Biomechanics
- Varus deformity → mechanical axis shifts medially → increased medial compartment loading
- Results in cartilage wear, osteophytes, meniscal extrusion

Treatment Options
- *Conservative:* Unloader braces, physio
- *Surgical:*
  - *HTO:* For young, active patients with varus + medial OA
  - *UKA:* For isolated medial OA
  - *TKA:* For advanced OA

Q51. Rheumatoid arthritis (RA) of the knee—short note.

Pathology
- Autoimmune synovitis → cartilage erosion + joint destruction
- Pannus formation + ligamentous laxity

Clinical Features
- Pain, swelling, morning stiffness
- Instability, valgus deformity

Management
- DMARDs (Methotrexate)
- NSAIDs, steroids
- Synovectomy, TKA in late disease

TKA in RA has good outcomes but **higher infection risk.**

Q52. Intra-articular injections in OA knee.

Injection type	*Mechanism*	*Use case*
Corticosteroids	Anti-inflammatory	Acute flare, severe synovitis
Hyaluronic acid (HA)	Viscosupplementation	Mild–moderate OA, controversial effect
Platelet-rich plasma (PRP)	Anti-inflammatory + chondroprotective	Younger patients, early OA
Stem cell therapy	Regenerative potential (experimental)	Early OA

Always combine with **rehabilitation + lifestyle advice.**

Q53. Hemophilic arthritis of the knee—short note.

Etiology
- Recurrent intra-articular **bleeds** (Factor VIII/IX deficiency)

Features
- Synovial hypertrophy
- Hemosiderin deposition
- Early onset deformities (flexion, valgus)
- *Target joint:* Knee > ankle > elbow

Management
- Factor replacement
- Synovectomy (chemical/radioactive/arthroscopic)
- TKA in late stages

Preventive prophylaxis is key in reducing joint damage.

Q54. Osteochondritis dissecans (OCD) of the knee—short note.

Definition
A condition where a **subchondral bone fragment** and its overlying cartilage become ischemic → may separate and become a loose body.

Common Site
Lateral aspect of medial femoral condyle

Etiology
- Repetitive microtrauma
- Ischemia
- Genetic factors
- Skeletal immaturity (juvenile OCD)

Clinical Features
- Activity-related pain
- Swelling, stiffness
- *Mechanical symptoms:* Catching, locking (if loose fragment)

Imaging
- *X-ray (tunnel view)*: Lucency/fragment
- *MRI:* Best for staging and cartilage integrity

Management

Stable, juvenile	*Unstable/Adult/Loose body*
Activity modification, brace	Arthroscopic drilling, fixation, or debridement
Regular MRI follow-up	Osteochondral autograft ± chondroplasty

Early diagnosis: Better prognosis in skeletally immature patients.

Knee Infections and Tumors

Q55. Pigmented villonodular synovitis (PVNS)—clinical features and management.

(NEIGRIHMS 2014)

Definition

A rare, benign proliferative disorder of the **synovium**, characterized by **hemosiderin-laden villous and nodular overgrowth**

Types

- Localized (intra-articular nodule)
- Diffuse (more aggressive, entire synovium)

Clinical Features

- Chronic, insidious **monoarticular swelling** (commonly **knee**)
- Pain, stiffness, joint effusion
- Possible joint erosion

Imaging

- *MRI:* Hypointense on both T1/T2 (due to hemosiderin)
- "Blooming" on GRE sequences
- May show erosions on X-ray

Management

Localized pvns	*Diffuse pvns*
Arthroscopic excision	Total synovectomy (arthroscopic/open)
Low recurrence	Higher recurrence → adjuvant radiotherapy

Recurrence rate can be up to **30–50%** in diffuse type.

Q56. Synovial chondromatosis of the knee—short note.

Definition

A **benign metaplastic disorder** of synovium → formation of **multiple cartilaginous loose bodies** within the joint.

Etiology

- Primary (idiopathic)
- Secondary (due to OA, trauma)

Clinical Features

- Intermittent swelling
- Mechanical symptoms (locking, clicking)
- Chronic pain with ROM limitation

Radiology

- *X-ray:* Multiple intra-articular **calcified bodies**

- *MRI:* Non-calcified nodules better visualized
- Arthroscopy shows **"rice body"-like** appearance

Management
- **Arthroscopic or open synovectomy** + loose body removal
- Recurrence possible if incomplete excision

Rarely, can undergo malignant transformation to **chondrosarcoma**.

Sports Injuries and Miscellaneous Knee Conditions

Q57. Patellar tendinitis (jumper's knee)—diagnosis and management.

Definition
Chronic overuse injury at the **patellar tendon insertion on the inferior pole** of the patella.

Diagnosis
- Pain localized over inferior patellar pole
- Aggravated by jumping, stairs, squats
- *MRI:* Shows thickened tendon with signal changes

Management
- Rest, activity modification
- Eccentric strengthening exercises
- PRP injections for chronic cases
- Surgery (tendon debridement) in refractory cases

Seen in **basketball, volleyball, and track athletes.**

Q58. Iliotibial band syndrome—short note.

Definition
Lateral knee pain due to friction of the **iliotibial band over the lateral femoral condyle.**

Risk Factors
- Runners, cyclists
- Genu varum, tight ITB

Clinical
- Lateral knee pain during repetitive flexion-extension
- Tenderness over Gerdy's tubercle

Management
- ITB stretching, foam rolling
- NSAIDs
- Corticosteroid injection if needed

Q59. Patellofemoral pain syndrome (PFPS)—biomechanics and management.

Biomechanics
- Patella maltracking due to **Q-angle increase**, muscle imbalance
- Increased contact stress on **lateral facet**

Symptoms
- Anterior knee pain with squatting, sitting, stairs
- "Theater sign"—pain after prolonged sitting

Management
- Strengthen **VMO**, stretch lateral structures
- Patellar taping, orthotics
- *Rarely:* **Lateral release** or realignment procedures

Q60. Patellofemoral overlap syndrome—pathoanatomy and management.

(WBUHS 2017)

Definition

Impingement due to abnormal contact between patella and femoral trochlea, causing anterior knee pain.

Pathoanatomy
- Patella alta
- Lateral tilt
- Dysplastic trochlea
- Tight lateral retinaculum

Management
- *Conservative:* Quad strengthening, taping
- *Surgical:*
  - Lateral release
  - MPFL reconstruction
  - Tibial tubercle distalization if alta
  - Trochleoplasty in severe dysplasia

Q61. Anterior knee pain—causes and management.

Cause	*Management*
Patellofemoral pain syndrome	Rehabilitation, taping, orthoses
Patellar tendinitis	Rest, eccentric exercises, PRP
Osgood–Schlatter disease	Rest, NSAIDs, activity modification
Sinding–Larsen–Johansson syndrome	Similar to OSD
Chondromalacia patellae	Strengthening, arthroscopy (if severe)

Diagnosis is often **clinical + MRI** for structural issues.

Q62. Osgood–Schlatter disease—clinical features and treatment.

Definition

Apophysitis of tibial tubercle due to repetitive traction from **patellar tendon.**

Features
- Adolescent males
- Anterior knee pain + tibial swelling
- Worsens with running, jumping

Management
- Rest, NSAIDs
- Stretching (quadriceps, hamstrings)
- Self-limiting; surgery if painful ossicle persists after skeletal maturity

Q63. Bipartite patella—short note.

Definition

Congenital condition where **patella develops from multiple ossification centers** → failure of fusion.

Types (Saupe classification)

- *Type I:* Inferior pole
- *Type II:* Lateral margin
- *Type III:* Superolateral (most common)

Clinical Significance

- Usually asymptomatic
- May present with anterior knee pain post-trauma
- MRI distinguishes from fracture

Management

- Conservative
- Excision if symptomatic

Q64. Recurrent patellar instability.

Pathoanatomy

- Trochlear dysplasia
- Patella alta
- Increased Q-angle
- Lateralized tibial tuberosity (↑ TT–TG distance)
- MPFL tear or laxity
- Genu valgum

Imaging

- *X-ray:* Merchant (skyline), lateral views
- *CT:* TT–TG distance >20 mm is abnormal
- *MRI:* MPFL tear, trochlear morphology, cartilage

Treatment

- *Conservative:* Bracing, VMO strengthening
- *Surgical (if recurrent/symptomatic)*:
  - MPFL reconstruction
  - Tibial tubercle transfer (Elmslie–Trillat)
  - Trochleoplasty (severe dysplasia)
  - Lateral release (rare)

Q65. Arthroscopy in knee disorders—diagnostic and therapeutic role.

(AIIMS BBSR 2015)

Diagnostic Uses

- Meniscal, cartilage, ligament injuries
- Synovial biopsy
- Evaluation of unexplained pain/swelling

Therapeutic Uses

- Meniscectomy or repair
- ACL/PCL reconstruction

- Chondroplasty
- Synovectomy
- Loose body removal

Minimally invasive with quicker rehabilitation and less morbidity.

Q66. Quadriceps tendon rupture—biomechanics and treatment.

Biomechanics
- Sudden eccentric overload while the foot is fixed
- Typically in older patients with comorbidities (DM, renal failure)

Clinical
- Inability to **extend knee or perform straight leg raise**
- Palpable gap above patella
- High-riding patella (patella baja)

Management
- *Surgical repair (early)*: Transosseous sutures or suture anchors
- Immobilisation in extension post-operative
- Gradual ROM and strengthening

Q67. Indications and methods of osteotomies around the knee.

Indications
- Medial compartment OA with varus deformity (HTO)
- Valgus deformity (DFO—distal femoral osteotomy)
- Genu recurvatum, genu varum/valgum
- Post-traumatic malalignment

Methods
1. *High tibial osteotomy (HTO)*:
    - Opening wedge (medial)
    - Closing wedge (lateral)
    - Dome osteotomy
2. *Distal femoral osteotomy (DFO)*: For valgus deformity
3. *Tibial tuberosity transfer*: For patellar maltracking
4. *Guided growth (epiphysiodesis)*: In skeletally immature patients

Aim
Shift load from degenerated to preserved compartment.

Q68. Treatment of medial compartment arthrosis + high tibial osteotomy (HTO).

Non-operative
- Weight loss, NSAIDs
- Bracing (valgus unloader)
- *Injections:* Steroids, hyaluronic acid

Surgical Options
- *HTO:* Young active patients with varus + medial OA
- *Unicompartmental knee arthroplasty (UKA):* Elderly with isolated medial OA
- *Total knee replacement (TKR):* Advanced OA

Q69. High tibial osteotomy in detail.

Indications
- <60 years, active lifestyle
- Medial OA with varus alignment
- Good ROM

Techniques
- *Opening wedge (medial):* Simpler, no fibular osteotomy
- *Closing wedge (lateral):* Faster healing but more invasive

Complications
- Overcorrection
- Nonunion
- Peroneal nerve injury

Q70. Patellofemoral replacement (PFR).

- Partial knee arthroplasty for **isolated patellofemoral arthritis**
- *Indications:*
  - Isolated PFJ OA (Grade III–IV)
  - Preserved tibiofemoral compartments
- *Contraindications:* Ligament instability, widespread arthritis
- *Advantages:* Bone-sparing, quicker recovery
- May convert to TKR if disease progresses

Q71. Loose bodies in knee.

- Free fragments (cartilage, bone) floating in joint
- *Causes:*
  - Osteochondritis dissecans
  - Trauma
  - Degenerative OA
- *Symptoms:* Locking, catching, pain, effusion
- *Diagnosis:* X-ray, MRI

Classification of Loose Bodies
1. *By origin*:
   - Osteochondral (OCD, trauma)
   - Synovial (RA, synovial chondromatosis)
   - Post-surgical
2. *By composition*:
   - Cartilaginous
   - Bony
   - Fibrous

Treatment: Arthroscopic removal

Q72. Mosaicplasty.

- **Osteochondral autograft transplantation** technique
- Small cylindrical plugs harvested from **non-weight-bearing** areas of femoral condyle

- Implanted into chondral defect
- Best for focal cartilage defects (1–4 cm^2)
- Restores hyaline cartilage surface

Q73. Autologous chondrocyte implantation (ACI).

- *Two-stage procedure:*
  1. Arthroscopic cartilage biopsy
  2. Cultured chondrocytes implanted under a periosteal patch (or collagen membrane)
- *Indications:* Focal full-thickness cartilage defects >2 cm^2
- *Outcome:* Good long-term pain relief and function in select patients

Q74. Arthroscopic management of osteochondral lesions of the knee.

- Used for **OCD**, trauma, or degenerative lesions
- *Procedures include:*
  - **Debridement and lavage**
  - **Microfracture** for small defects
  - **Mosaicplasty or ACI** for larger defects
- Minimally invasive, quicker recovery, allows assessment of cartilage status

Q75. Popliteal cyst (Baker's cyst).

- Fluid-filled swelling in **popliteal fossa**
- Results from communication between knee joint and gastrocnemius-semimembranosus bursa
- *Secondary to intra-articular pathology:* OA, RA, meniscal tear
- *Symptoms:* Posterior knee swelling, tightness, restricted flexion
- *Diagnosis:* Ultrasound, MRI
- *Treatment:* Address underlying cause; cyst may resolve
  - Aspiration + steroid injection
  - Surgical excision (rarely)

Q76. Recurrent versus habitual dislocation of patella.

Feature	*Recurrent*	*Habitual*
Timing	After trauma, starts in adolescence	Since early childhood
Dislocation occurs when	Knee is flexed during activity	Every time knee is flexed
Associated deformity	Trochlear dysplasia ± ligament laxity	Contracted lateral structures
Management	MPFL reconstruction	Realignment procedures + soft tissue release

Q77. Meniscal cyst.

- Fluid-filled swelling along **meniscus margin**, usually lateral
- Associated with **horizontal meniscal tear**
- *Treatment:* **Arthroscopic cyst decompression + meniscectomy**

Q78. Synovial plica syndrome.

- Embryological remnant becomes inflamed/thickened
- Presents as **anterior knee pain**, clicking

- Medial plica most common
- *Treatment:* NSAIDs, stretching; **arthroscopic excision** if persistent

Q79. Morant Baker's cyst (popliteal cyst).

- **Fluid collection** between semimembranosus and medial head of gastrocnemius
- Secondary to intra-articular pathology
- May rupture → mimic DVT
- Treat underlying cause ± aspiration or excision

Q80. Semimembranosus bursitis.

- Posteromedial knee swelling
- May coexist with **Baker's cyst**
- Pain with flexion
- *Treatment:* NSAIDs, aspiration, manage underlying joint disease

Q81. Tibial collateral ligament bursitis/fibrositis.

- Medial knee pain, tenderness along MCL
- *Causes:* Overuse, trauma
- *Treatment:* Rest, NSAIDs, local injection

Q82. Snapping knee.

- Audible or palpable "snap" during motion
- *Causes:*
  - *Lateral:* The iliotibial (IT) band over lateral condyle
  - *Medial:* Semitendinosus over tibia
- Rarely intra-articular
- *Tx:* Stretching, local injection, surgical release if severe

Q83. Closed versus open chain exercises in ACL rehabilitation.

Closed chain	***Open chain***
Foot fixed (e.g., squats)	Foot free (e.g., leg extension)
Safer for ACL graft	Higher shear force on ACL graft
Early rehabilitation	Delayed introduction (6+ weeks)

Q84. Management of post-operative stiffness (knee).

- *Prevention:* Early ROM, pain control
- *Treatment:*
  - Physiotherapy
  - Manipulation under anesthesia (MUA)
  - Arthroscopic adhesiolysis (if >3 months)

Q85. Post-traumatic knee stiffness.

Causes

- Prolonged immobilization
- Arthrofibrosis
- Malunion
- Infection

Prevention

- Early ROM exercises
- Adequate analgesia
- Early physio post-surgery

Management

- *<3 months:* MUA (manipulation under anesthesia)
- *3 months:* Arthroscopic or open release

Q86. Arthroscopic management of osteochondral lesions.

- Debridement
- Microfracture
- Mosaicplasty
- ACI/MACI

Choice depends on **size**, **depth**, and **location**

Q87. Options for focal cartilage defect (medial condyle)

- *<2 cm^2:* Microfracture
- *2–4 cm^2:* Mosaicplasty
- *>4 cm^2:* ACI/MACI
- *Others:* Osteochondral allograft

Q88. Chondroplasty in osteoplasty.

- *Chondroplasty:* Debridement of fibrillated cartilage
- Done arthroscopically
- Often part of **osteoplasty** (bone reshaping)

Q89. Causes of patellar maltracking.

- Increased **Q-angle**
- Shallow trochlear groove (trochlear dysplasia)
- Patella alta
- Lateral retinaculum tightness
- VMO weakness
- Genu valgum

Q90. Genu recurvatum (SN).

Definition

Genu recurvatum is a **hyperextension deformity of the knee**, where the tibia extends beyond the normal range (typically >5–10° beyond neutral extension).

Etiology

- *Neuromuscular:* Poliomyelitis, cerebral palsy
- *Post-traumatic:* Improper healing after fracture or ligament injury
- *Post-surgical:* Over-lengthening of patellar tendon, excessive release in TKA
- *Ligament laxity:* Generalized hypermobility (e.g., Ehlers–Danlos)
- *Growth plate disturbance:* Especially upper tibial physis

Clinical Features

- Visible posterior knee bowing
- Limp, instability, pain on standing
- *Gait:* Hyperextension during stance phase

Management

- *Mild/Early:* Bracing, physiotherapy (hamstring/quads strengthening)
- *Severe/Fixed:* Surgical options:
    - Anterior closing wedge osteotomy of tibia
    - Soft tissue procedures in neuromuscular cases

Q91. Windswept deformity (SN).

Definition

A **combined angular deformity** of the knees where **one knee shows genu valgum** and the **other shows genu varum**, giving a "windswept" appearance.

Etiology

- **Rickets** (most common in children)
- Skeletal dysplasias (e.g., pseudoachondroplasia)
- Juvenile idiopathic arthritis
- Hemophilia
- Cerebral palsy (due to muscle imbalance)
- Post-traumatic or post-infective growth plate damage

Clinical Features

- Asymmetric gait
- Limb length discrepancy
- Joint line obliquity
- Early joint degeneration (especially medial/lateral compartments)

Management

- *Conservative:* In growing children with mild deformity—bracing, vitamin D/calcium
- *Surgical:*
    - Growth modulation (hemiepiphysiodesis)
    - Corrective osteotomies (distal femur/proximal tibia) once growth is complete

Q92. B/L genu valgum in 11-year-old.

Etiology

- Physiologic up to 7 years
- *Pathologic:* Rickets, renal osteodystrophy, trauma, infection

Evaluation

- *Clinical:* Intermalleolar distance
- *X-ray:* Mechanical axis, femoro-tibial angle

Management

- Guided growth (stapling, 8-plate)
- Corrective osteotomy if >13 years or severe deformity

Q93. Genu varum versus genu valgum.

Feature	***Genu varum***	***Genu valgum***
Deformity	Bow-legged	Knock-knee
Axis shift	Medial	Lateral
Causes	Blount's, rickets	Rickets, JIA, trauma
OA risk	Medial compartment	Lateral compartment

7.7 Foot and Ankle

Biswajit Sahu, Zubair Ahmad Lone, Saransh Bahl

Basic Anatomy and Biomechanics

Q1. Anatomy of the ankle joint.

- *Joint type:* Synovial hinge joint
- *Articulations:* Tibia, fibula, and talus
- *Capsule and synovium:* Encloses talocrural joint
- *Ligaments:*
  - *Medial (deltoid):* Resists eversion
  - *Lateral:* ATFL, CFL, PTFL—resist inversion
- *Movements:* Dorsiflexion and plantarflexion
- *Neurovascular:* Supplied by anterior tibial, posterior tibial, and peroneal arteries

Q2. Biomechanics of the foot and ankle.

- *Ankle joint:* Dorsiflexion (20°), plantarflexion (50°)
- *Subtalar joint:* Inversion and eversion
- *Midfoot:* Adaptation and shock absorption
- *Forefoot:* Stability and propulsion during push-off

Q3. Arches of the foot and clinical significance.

- *Medial longitudinal arch:* Talus is the keystone; dynamic and shock-absorbing
- *Lateral longitudinal arch:* Static, weight-bearing
- *Transverse arch:* Maintains foot contour
- *Clinical:*
  - Flatfoot (pes planus) → instability
  - High arch (pes cavus) → stress fractures

Q4. Blood supply of the foot and ankle.

- **Anterior tibial artery** → dorsalis pedis
- **Posterior tibial artery** → medial and lateral plantar arteries
- *Peroneal artery:* Lateral support
- *Relevance:* Essential for wound healing, especially in diabetic feet

Q5. Ligaments stabilising the ankle.

- *Medial:* Deltoid ligament
- *Lateral:*
  - Anterior talofibular ligament (ATFL)
  - Calcaneofibular ligament (CFL)
  - Posterior talofibular ligament (PTFL)
- *Syndesmosis:* Maintains distal tibiofibular joint (AITFL, PITFL, interosseous)

Q6. Subtalar joint and its movements.

- *Articulation:* Talus + calcaneus
- *Type:* Plane synovial
- *Movements:* Inversion (20–30°) and eversion (5–10°)
- *Function:* Allows adaptation on uneven surfaces

Q7. Windlass mechanism of the foot.

- During **toe dorsiflexion**, plantar fascia tightens → elevates medial arch
- Acts like a windlass (winch) to convert the foot into a rigid lever during push-off
- Dysfunction → flatfoot or plantar fasciitis

Q8. Role of plantar fascia in foot biomechanics.

- *Origin:* Medial calcaneal tuberosity → metatarsal heads
- *Function:*
  - Supports medial arch
  - Facilitates the windlass mechanism
- *Pathology:* Plantar fasciitis → heel pain syndrome

Q9. Peroneal tendons—anatomy and function.

- *Muscles:* Peroneus longus and brevis
- *Course:* Posterior to lateral malleolus
- *Function:* Foot eversion and ankle stability
- *Injury:* Tendonitis or subluxation in sports injuries

Q10. Gait cycle and abnormalities.

- *Phases:*
  - *Stance (60%):* Heel strike → foot flat → midstance → toe-off
  - *Swing (40%):* Acceleration → mid-swing → deceleration
- *Abnormalities:*
  - Antalgic gait → pain avoidance
  - Trendelenburg gait → gluteus medius weakness
  - Equinus gait → tight Achilles tendon
  - Foot drop → peroneal nerve palsy

Congenital and Developmental Foot Disorders

Q11. Congenital talipes equinovarus (CTEV)—classification and management.

Definition

CTEV, or clubfoot, is a congenital deformity characterized by four components: cavus, adductus, varus, and equinus.

Classification

- *Idiopathic:* Most common; isolated deformity.
- *Non-idiopathic:* Associated with neuromuscular disorders (e.g., spina bifida, arthrogryposis).

Management

- *Ponseti method:*
  - Serial manipulations and casting.
  - Percutaneous Achilles tenotomy if equinus persists.
  - Bracing with foot abduction orthosis to prevent relapse.
- *Surgical:* Reserved for resistant cases; includes soft tissue release or osteotomies.

Q12. Pathoanatomy of CTEV (Clubfoot).

Components (Mnemonic: CAVE):

1. **C**avus—plantarflexed 1st ray
2. **A**dduction—of forefoot at midfoot
3. **V**arus—of hindfoot
4. **E**quinus—of ankle (tight Achilles)

Pathology

- *Contracture of soft tissues:* Tibialis posterior, Achilles, capsule
- Hypoplastic bones, especially talus

Q13. Ponseti method for clubfoot correction.

Principles

- Gentle manipulation of the foot followed by casting to gradually correct deformity.
- Typically involves 5–7 casts changed weekly.
- Achilles tenotomy performed if necessary.
- Post-correction bracing to maintain alignment.

Outcomes

High success rate with minimal need for extensive surgery.

Q14. Surgical management of CTEV in a 6-month-old.

- *If Ponseti method fails → Surgery:*
  - *Soft tissue release:*
    - Posteromedial release (Turco)
    - Z-lengthening of Achilles
    - Capsulotomy of talonavicular and subtalar joints
  - *Timing:* ~6–9 months ideal

Q15. Congenital vertical talus—etiology and treatment.

Etiology

- Often associated with neuromuscular disorders (e.g., arthrogryposis, spina bifida).
- Characterized by rigid dorsal dislocation of the navicular on the talus.

Treatment

- *Non-operative:* Serial casting to stretch soft tissues.
- *Surgical:* Open reduction of the talonavicular joint with possible tendon lengthening.

Q16. Tarsal coalition—classification and management.

Definition

Abnormal connection between two or more tarsal bones, leading to restricted foot motion.

Classification

- *By tissue type:*
    - Fibrous (syndesmosis)
    - Cartilaginous (synchondrosis)
    - Osseous (synostosis)
- *By location:*
    - Calcaneonavicular (most common)
    - Talocalcaneal

Management

- *Conservative:* Activity modification, orthotics, NSAIDs.
- *Surgical:* Resection of the coalition or arthrodesis in severe cases.

Q17. Metatarsus adductus—short note.

Definition

Medial deviation of the forefoot relative to the hindfoot.

Types

- *Flexible:* Correctable manually.
- *Rigid:* Not passively correctable.

Management

- *Flexible:* Observation and stretching exercises.
- *Rigid:* Serial casting; surgery in refractory cases.

Q18. Congenital Pes cavus—causes and treatment.

Causes

- Often linked to neuromuscular disorders (e.g., Charcot–Marie–Tooth disease).
- Can be idiopathic.

Treatment

- *Conservative:* Orthotics, physical therapy.
- *Surgical:* Soft tissue release, tendon transfers, osteotomies for severe deformities.

Q19. Congenital rocker-bottom foot—pathology and management.

Definition

Also known as congenital vertical talus; characterized by a convex plantar surface

Pathology

- Dorsal dislocation of the navicular bone on the talus.
- Associated with neuromuscular conditions

Management

- *Non-operative:* Serial casting.
- *Surgical:* Open reduction and stabilization of the talonavicular joint

Q20. Postural talipes equinovarus—short note.

(RMLIMS 2016)

Definition

A flexible foot deformity due to intrauterine positioning.

Features

- Foot can be passively corrected to normal position.
- No structural abnormalities.

Management

- Gentle stretching exercises.
- Typically resolves spontaneously.

Q21. Pes planus.

Definition

Pes planus is a condition characterized by **flattening of the medial longitudinal arch** of the foot.

Types and Differentiation

Feature	*Flexible flatfoot*	*Rigid flatfoot*
Arch	Normal in non-weight bearing; flattens on standing	Always absent—both weight bearing and non-weight bearing
Mobility	Hindfoot flexible and reducible	Hindfoot stiff and fixed (valgus deformity)
Pain	Usually asymptomatic or mild	Often painful
Common in	Children, adolescents	Pathological, e.g., tarsal coalition
Tiptoe test (Jack's test)	Arch reappears	No arch reappearance
Associated features	Ligament laxity, obesity	Coalition, vertical talus, inflammatory arthritis

Evaluation

Clinical tests:

- *Jack's test:* Arch reappears when standing on tiptoe (flexible)
- *Heel rise test:* Hindfoot varus indicates flexible deformity
- *Gait analysis:* Check pronation
- Check for **Achilles tightness (Silfverskiöld test)**

Radiology:

- *X-rays (AP and lateral foot):*
  - ↓ Calcaneal pitch (<17°)
  - ↑ Talo–1st metatarsal angle (Meary's angle)
  - Talonavicular subluxation
- *CT/MRI:* Used in rigid flatfoot to assess for **tarsal coalition**

Non-surgical Treatment (First-line)

- *Supportive footwear*: Firm arch and heel support
- *Orthotics*: OTC or custom arch supports
- *Stretching and strengthening*: Focus on Achilles and posterior tibial tendon
- *Weight management*: Reduces stress on feet
- *NSAIDs*: For pain relief
- *Activity modification*: Avoid high-impact sports

Surgical Treatment (For Severe or Rigid Cases)

- **Tendon repair** (e.g., posterior tibial tendon)
- *Osteotomies*: Bone realignment
- *Joint fusion*: In advanced or arthritic cases
- **Lateral column lengthening/Calcaneal osteotomy**

Children

- Usually flexible and painless
- Treat only if symptomatic with **orthotics, stretching, or shoe changes**

Q22. Flexible flatfoot.

- *Asymptomatic:* No treatment needed (reassurance)
- *Symptomatic:*
  - Orthotic arch supports
  - Stretching (Achilles/gastroc), footwear modifications
  - *Surgery (rare):* Calcaneal osteotomy, tendon transfer (e.g., Kidner procedure)

Q23. Rigid flatfoot.

- Treat **underlying cause** (e.g., tarsal coalition)
- *Conservative:*
  - Activity modification
  - Orthotics
- *Surgical:*
  - Resection of coalition ± interposition
  - Triple arthrodesis in severe deformity
  - Medial column lengthening or hindfoot realignment

Q24. Idiopathic toe walking in children—management.

Definition

Persistent toe walking without underlying neurological or orthopedic cause.

Management

- *Observation:* Many cases resolve spontaneously.
- *Physical therapy:* Stretching exercises for calf muscles.
- *Orthotics:* Ankle-foot orthoses to encourage heel strike.
- *Serial casting:* To improve ankle dorsiflexion.
- *Surgical:* Achilles tendon lengthening in refractory cases.

Q25. Corrective osteotomies for congenital foot deformities—indications and techniques.

(IMS-BHU 2015)

Indications

- Persistent deformities unresponsive to conservative treatment.
- Structural abnormalities causing functional impairment.

Techniques

- *Medial cuneiform opening wedge osteotomy:* For metatarsus adductus.
- *Calcaneal osteotomy:* For hindfoot varus or valgus.
- *Dorsiflexion osteotomy of the first metatarsal:* 20.

Indications

- *Persistent structural deformities that:*
  - Affect function
  - Cause pain or gait abnormalities
  - Fail to respond to conservative treatment (e.g., casting, bracing)
- *Associated conditions:* Resistant **CTEV**, **Pes cavus**, **vertical talus**, or **metatarsus adductus**

Techniques (Based on Deformity Type)

Deformity	Osteotomy used	Purpose
Metatarsus adductus	Medial cuneiform opening wedge osteotomy	Realigns the forefoot medially
Pes cavus	Dorsiflexion osteotomy of first metatarsal ± calcaneal cuts	Reduces cavus and balances the foot

Continued

Continued

Deformity	*Osteotomy used*	*Purpose*
Vertical talus	Talonavicular reduction + possible navicular osteotomy	Reconstructs medial column and corrects rocker-bottom foot
Hindfoot varus/valgus	Medial/lateral sliding calcaneal osteotomy	Realigns the hindfoot
Rocker-bottom foot	Calcaneal shortening or midfoot wedge resection	Restores normal longitudinal arch
CTEV (resistant cases)	Dwyer's osteotomy (lateral closing wedge of calcaneus)	Corrects residual hindfoot varus

Post-op Considerations
- Immobilization in cast for 6–8 weeks
- Weight-bearing status depends on the procedure type
- Physical therapy to restore ROM and function

Summary Flowchart

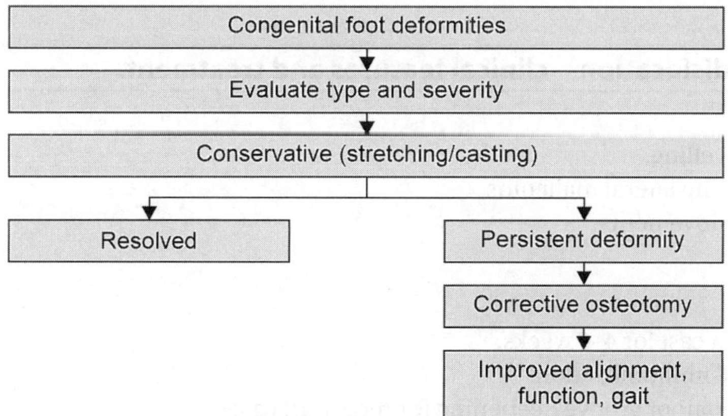

Ligamentous and Tendon Injuries of the Ankle

Q26. Diagnosis and management of ankle sprains.

Classification
- *Grade I:* Mild stretching of ligaments.
- *Grade II:* Partial ligament tear.
- *Grade III:* Complete ligament rupture.

Diagnosis
- *Clinical evaluation:* Swelling, bruising, pain, and instability.
- Imaging (X-ray, MRI) to rule out fractures or assess ligament damage.

Management
- *Grade I and II:*
  - RICE protocol (*R*est, *I*ce, *C*ompression, *E*levation).
  - Functional rehabilitation exercises.
- *Grade III:*
  - Immobilization with a brace or cast.
  - Physical therapy.
  - Surgical intervention in cases of chronic instability.

Q27. High ankle sprains (syndesmotic injuries).

Definition
Injury to the distal tibiofibular syndesmosis ligaments.

Mechanism
External rotation or dorsiflexion of the foot.

Diagnosis
- Pain above the ankle.
- Positive squeeze test.
- MRI for definitive assessment.

Management
- *Stable injuries:* Immobilization and physical therapy.
- *Unstable injuries:* Surgical fixation with screws or suture-button devices.

Q28. Peroneal tendon dislocation—clinical features and treatment.

Clinical Features
- Lateral ankle pain and swelling.
- Snapping sensation over the lateral malleolus.
- Instability during ankle movements.

Treatment
- *Conservative:*
  - Immobilization with a cast for 4–6 weeks.
  - Physical therapy post-immobilization.
- *Surgical:* Retinaculum repair or groove deepening for recurrent cases.

Q29. Achilles tendinopathy—classification and management.

Classification
- *Insertional:* At the tendon's attachment to the calcaneus.
- *Non-insertional:* Mid-portion of the tendon.

Management
- *Conservative:*
  - Eccentric loading exercises.
  - NSAIDs and activity modification.
- *Surgical:*
  - Debridement of degenerative tissue.
  - Tendon repair or augmentation in severe cases.

Q30. Posterior tibial tendon dysfunction (PTTD).

Definition
Progressive flattening of the foot due to posterior tibial tendon insufficiency.

Stages
- *Stage I:* Tendon inflammation without deformity.
- *Stage II:* Flexible flatfoot deformity.
- *Stage III:* Rigid flatfoot deformity.
- *Stage IV:* Ankle involvement with valgus tilt.

Management

- *Early stages:* Orthotics, physical therapy, and NSAIDs.
- *Advanced stages:* Surgical intervention including tendon transfer or osteotomies.

Q31. Role of physical therapy in chronic ankle instability.

Goals

- Restore proprioception and neuromuscular control.
- Strengthen peroneal muscles.
- Improve balance and coordination.

Interventions

- Balance training (e.g., wobble boards).
- Resistance exercises for ankle stabilizers.
- Functional movement retraining.

Q32. Lateral ankle ligament reconstruction—indications and techniques.

Indications

Chronic lateral ankle instability unresponsive to conservative treatment.

Techniques

- *Modified broström procedure:* Direct repair of the anterior talofibular and calcaneofibular ligaments.
- *Anatomic reconstruction:* Using tendon grafts for ligament augmentation.

Q33. Plantar plate injuries—biomechanics and treatment.

Biomechanics

- Plantar plate stabilizes the metatarsophalangeal joints.
- Injury leads to toe deformities and forefoot pain.

Treatment

- *Conservative:*
  - Taping and orthotics.
  - Activity modification.
- *Surgical:*
  - Direct repair of the plantar plate.
  - Osteotomies for realignment in severe cases.

Q34. Flexor hallucis longus (FHL) tendonitis.

Definition

Inflammation of the FHL tendon, common in dancers and athletes.

Symptoms

- Pain along the posteromedial ankle.
- Pain exacerbated by toe flexion.

Management

- *Conservative:*
  - Rest and NSAIDs.
  - Physical therapy focusing on stretching and strengthening.
- *Surgical:* Tendon release or debridement in refractory cases.

Q35. Old achilles tendon rupture—clinical features and management.

(PGIMER 2014)

Clinical Features

- Missed >4 weeks post-injury
- Weak plantar flexion, limp
- Positive **Thompson's test**
- Palpable gap, muscle wasting
- Difficulty toe-walking

Management

- *Non-operative:* For low-demand or elderly
    - Heel lift, bracing, physiotherapy
- *Surgical:* Preferred for active patients
    - V-Y advancement

Foot and Ankle Arthritis and Degenerative Conditions

Q36. Ankle osteoarthritis.

Causes

- *Post-traumatic (most common)*: Fractures, ligament injuries
- Primary OA (rare)
- *Inflammatory:* RA, hemophilia
- Neuropathic (Charcot)
- Septic arthritis sequelae

Clinical Presentation

- Deep **ankle pain**, worsens with walking
- Swelling, stiffness, reduced ROM
- Antalgic gait, possible varus/valgus deformity

Management Options

Conservative:

- NSAIDs, physiotherapy
- Bracing (AFO)
- Injections (corticosteroids, hyaluronic acid)

Surgical:

1. *Arthrodesis (ankle fusion)*:
    - Gold standard in young, active patients
    - Eliminates pain, but sacrifices motion
    - *Techniques:* Open/arthroscopic, screws/plates
2. *Total ankle replacement (TAR)*:
    - Preserves joint motion
    - Indicated in low-demand, older patients
    - *Contraindications:* Severe deformity, infection, osteoporosis
    - *Risks:* Loosening, infection, implant wear

Q37. Role of total ankle arthroplasty (TAA) in end-stage ankle arthritis.

Indications

End-stage ankle arthritis with preserved bone stock and adequate alignment.

Contraindications
Severe deformity, poor bone quality, active infection, or neuropathy.

Advantages
Preserves ankle motion, leading to more natural gait and potentially less stress on adjacent joints.

Considerations
Requires precise surgical technique and patient selection.

Q38. Total ankle replacement versus ankle arthrodesis.

Aspect	*Total ankle replacement (TAR)*	*Ankle arthrodesis (fusion)*
Motion preservation	Yes	No
Gait mechanics	More natural	Altered
Adjacent joint stress	Less	More
Longevity	Implant lifespan: ~10–15 years	Potentially lifelong
Revision risk	Higher	Lower

Both procedures are effective; choice depends on patient factors and surgeon expertise.

Q39. Treatment options for first metatarsophalangeal (MTP) joint arthritis.

Non-surgical
NSAIDs, shoe modifications (e.g., stiff-soled shoes), orthotics, corticosteroid injections.

Surgical
Cheilectomy (removal of bone spurs), arthrodesis (fusion), or joint replacement.

Q40. Hallux rigidus—short note.

Definition
Degenerative arthritis of the first MTP joint leading to stiffness and pain.

Symptoms
Pain during dorsiflexion, swelling, and limited motion.

Management
- *Conservative:* NSAIDs, shoe modifications.
- *Surgical:* Cheilectomy, arthrodesis, or joint replacement depending on severity.

Q41. Management of post-traumatic arthritis of the foot and ankle.

Approach
- *Conservative:* Physical therapy, NSAIDs, orthotics, activity modification.
- *Surgical:* Arthroscopic debridement, osteotomy, arthrodesis, or joint replacement depending on joint involvement and severity.

Q42. Rheumatoid foot.

Common Deformities
- *Forefoot:*
    - Hallux valgus

    - Subluxed/Dislocated lesser MTPs
    - Hammer/Claw toes
- *Midfoot:* Collapse of longitudinal arch
- *Hindfoot:* Valgus deformity due to tibialis posterior dysfunction

Surgical Interventions

Deformity	*Surgical option*
Hallux valgus	First MTP fusion or osteotomy
Dislocated MTPs	Weil osteotomy, MTP resection arthroplasty
Claw toes	Tendon balancing, PIP arthrodesis
Hindfoot valgus	Triple arthrodesis (ST, TN, CC joints)
Midfoot collapse	Medial column fusion

Postoperative Care
- Protective weight-bearing (6–8 weeks)
- Orthotics/Footwear support
- Disease-modifying antirheumatic drugs (DMARDs) continued
- Physiotherapy for gait retraining

Q43. Gout.

Clinical Features
- Acute monoarthritis, usually **first MTP joint** ("**podagra**")
- Swelling, redness, excruciating pain
- **Tophi** in chronic cases: Ears, fingers, tendons
- May mimic infection or septic arthritis

Diagnosis
- *Joint aspiration:* Monosodium urate crystals (needle-shaped, negatively birefringent)
- *Serum uric acid:* May be normal during acute attack
- *X-ray:* "**Punched-out erosions with overhanging edges**"

Management Strategies

Acute attack:
- NSAIDs (indomethacin), colchicine
- Steroids (oral/intra-articular)

Chronic management:
- **Allopurinol**, febuxostat (xanthine oxidase inhibitors)
- *Lifestyle:* ↓ red meat, alcohol; hydration
- Monitor renal function and urate levels

Surgical:
Rarely needed: Tophi excision or joint debridement

Summary Table

Condition	*Key points*
Ankle OA	Usually post-traumatic; managed by fusion or TAR depending on patient profile
Rheumatoid foot	Multilevel deformities; often require MTP arthroplasty or triple fusion
Gout	Acute monoarthritis; urate crystals diagnostic; managed with NSAIDs + urate-lowering therapy

Foot Deformities and Biomechanical Disorders

Q44. Causes and treatment of cavus foot (Pes cavus).

Definition

Abnormally high **medial longitudinal arch** of the foot

Etiologies

- Often associated with neurological conditions such as Charcot–Marie–Tooth disease, cerebral palsy, or spinal cord tumors.
- It can also be idiopathic or result from muscle imbalances.
- Post-traumatic or compartment syndrome

Clinical Evaluation

- Elevated arch
- **Claw toes**
- Hindfoot varus
- *Coleman block test:* Assess hindfoot flexibility
- Weak peroneals, tight Achilles
- *Gait:* Lateral foot overloading, instability

Radiology

- *Meary's angle:* ↑ arch (midfoot)
- **Calcaneal pitch** >30°
- MRI to rule out neuromuscular cause

Treatment

- *Conservative:*
  - Custom orthotics to redistribute pressure.
  - Physical therapy to improve strength and flexibility.
- *Surgical:*
  - Considered for severe deformities or when conservative treatments fail.
  - Procedures may include tendon transfers, osteotomies, or plantar fascia release.

Q45. Causes, clinical assesment, pathophysiology, and management of hallux valgus.

Contributing factors

- Genetics
- Footwear (narrow-toed shoes)
- Pes planus
- Rheumatoid arthritis

Clinical Assessment

- Medial bony swelling (bunion)
- Lateral drift of hallux
- Decreased first MTP ROM
- Pain over medial eminence
- Overriding of 2nd toe in severe cases

Measurements (on X-ray AP View)

- **HVA** (hallux valgus angle) >15°
- **IMA** (intermetatarsal angle) >9°

Pathophysiology
- Medial deviation of the first metatarsal and lateral deviation of the hallux, leading to a bunion formation.
- Contributing factors include genetic predisposition, improper footwear, and ligamentous laxity.

Management
- *Conservative:*
  - Footwear modifications to reduce pressure on the bunion.
  - Orthotic devices to correct alignment.
- *Surgical:*
  - Indicated for persistent pain or functional impairment.
  - Procedures include osteotomies (e.g., Chevron, Scarf), arthrodesis, or bunionectomy.

Q46. Surgical techniques used in hallux valgus correction.

Common Surgical Techniques
- *Chevron osteotomy:* Distal metatarsal osteotomy for mild to moderate deformities.
- *Scarf osteotomy:* Diaphyseal osteotomy suitable for moderate to severe deformities.
- *Akin osteotomy:* Proximal phalanx osteotomy often combined with other procedures.
- *Lapidus procedure:* Fusion of the first tarsometatarsal joint for hypermobility.
- *Minimally invasive surgery:* Utilizes small incisions, leading to faster recovery.

Surgical Correction
Indicated if:
- Pain, shoe wear issues, or cosmetic concern
- HVA >20°, IMA >10°

Techniques
- **Distal metatarsal osteotomy** (Chevron)
- **Proximal metatarsal osteotomy**
- *Lapidus procedure:* First TMT joint fusion
- *Scarf osteotomy:* For moderate to severe deformity
- *Silver bunionectomy:* For mild, cosmetic cases

Q47. Bunion deformity and its surgical treatment.

Definition
A bunion is a bony prominence at the first metatarsophalangeal (MTP) joint due to hallux valgus deformity.

Surgical Treatment
- *Osteotomy:* Realignment of the first metatarsal bone.
- *Arthrodesis:* Fusion of the MTP joint, typically in severe cases.
- *Exostectomy:* Removal of the bony prominence.
- *Minimally invasive techniques:* Utilize smaller incisions for reduced recovery time.

Q48. Management of adult-acquired flatfoot deformity.

Etiology
Often results from posterior tibial tendon dysfunction, leading to progressive flattening of the arch.

Management
- *Conservative:*
  - Orthotic devices to support the arch.
  - Physical therapy focusing on strengthening the posterior tibial tendon.

- *Surgical:*
  - Indicated for advanced stages or when conservative treatments fail.
  - Procedures may include tendon transfers, osteotomies, or arthrodesis.

Q49. Etiology and treatment of hammer toe and claw toe deformities.

(Baba Farid University of Health Sciences Faridkot Punjab 2015)

Definitions

Deformity	Mtp	Pip	Dip
Claw toe	Hyperextension	Flexion	Flexion
Hammer toe	Normal	Flexion	Normal
Mallet toe	Normal	Normal	Flexion

Causes

- *Neuromuscular:* Charcot–Marie–Tooth, diabetes, CP
- RA, trauma, poorly fitted shoes
- Muscle imbalance between extensors/flexors

Treatment

- *Conservative:*
  - Footwear modifications to accommodate deformities.
  - Orthotic devices and physical therapy.
- *Surgical:*
  - Tendon release or transfer.
  - Joint arthroplasty or fusion in rigid deformities.

Quick Summary Table

Condition	Key features
Hallux valgus	Lateral hallux deviation; chevron/scarf osteotomy; assess HVA, IMA
Claw/Hammer/Mallet toe	Deformity patterns vary by joint; neuromuscular/RA causes
Cavus foot	High arch, hindfoot varus, claw toes; often CMT; Coleman block test for flexibility

Q50. Freiberg's disease-short note.

Definition

Avascular necrosis of the metatarsal head, most commonly affecting the second metatarsal.

Clinical Features

- Pain in the forefoot, especially during weight-bearing activities.
- Swelling and limited joint motion.

Management

- *Conservative:* Activity modification, orthotic devices, and NSAIDs.
- *Surgical:* Debridement, osteotomy, or joint replacement in advanced cases.

Diabetic Foot and Neuropathic Conditions

Q51. Classification and management of diabetic foot ulcers (DFUs).

Classification Systems

- *Wagner classification:*
  - *Grade 0:* Intact skin

- *Grade 1:* Superficial ulcer
- *Grade 2:* Deep ulcer to tendon or joint capsule
- *Grade 3:* Deep ulcer with abscess or osteomyelitis
- *Grade 4:* Partial foot gangrene
- *Grade 5:* Whole foot gangrene

- *University of texas (UT) classification:* Considers depth, infection, and ischemia.

Management

- *Offloading:* Use of total contact cast (TCC) or specialized footwear.
- *Wound care:* Regular debridement and moist dressings.
- *Infection control:* Appropriate antibiotic therapy.
- *Revascularization:* For ischemic ulcers.
- *Glycemic control:* Maintaining optimal blood sugar levels.

Q52. Role of total contact casting (TCC) in diabetic foot management.

- *Purpose:* Offloads pressure from the ulcerated area, promoting healing.
- *Mechanism:* Distributes weight evenly across the foot.
- *Indications:* Non-infected, non-ischemic plantar ulcers.
- *Benefits:* Accelerated healing rates and reduced ulcer recurrence.

Q53. Surgical options for advanced diabetic foot infections.

- *Debridement:* Removal of necrotic tissue.
- *Drainage:* Addressing abscesses or deep infections.
- *Revascularization:* Restoring blood flow in ischemic limbs.
- *Amputation:* Partial or complete, in cases of extensive gangrene or non-viable tissue.

Q54. Role of footwear in preventing diabetic foot complications.

- *Proper footwear:*
  - Reduces pressure points.
  - Prevents callus formation and ulcers.
  - Accommodates foot deformities.
- *Features:*
  - Seamless interiors.
  - Adequate cushioning.
  - Custom orthotics, if necessary.

Q55. Importance of vascular assessment in diabetic foot ulcers.

(BFUHS 2013)

- *Purpose:* Determines blood flow adequacy for healing.
- *Methods:*
  - Ankle-brachial index (ABI).
  - Toe pressures.
  - Transcutaneous oxygen measurements.
- *Implications:*
  - Guides need for revascularization.
  - Predicts healing potential.

Q56. Neuropathic versus Ischemic foot ulcers.

Feature	*Neuropathic ulcers*	*Ischemic ulcers*
Cause	Peripheral neuropathy	Peripheral arterial disease
Location	Plantar surface of foot	Tips of toes, lateral foot
Pain	Often painless	Painful
Appearance	Callused margins	Pale, necrotic tissue
Pulses	Usually present	Diminished or absent
Management focus	Offloading and glycemic control	Revascularization

Q57. Charcot arthropathy.

Definition

Progressive, destructive joint disease due to **neuropathy**, most commonly seen in **diabetics** (foot and ankle).

Pathophysiology

- *Neurotraumatic theory:* Repetitive microtrauma not sensed due to neuropathy
- *Neurovascular theory:* Autonomic dysfunction → hyperemia → osteolysis

Eichenholtz Stages

Stage	*Description*	*Radiology*
0	Pre-radiographic inflammation	Clinical signs only; MRI shows edema
1 (Development)	Fragmentation, subluxation	Joint destruction, debris, periarticular fractures
2 (Coalescence)	Resorption of debris, healing begins	Less fragmentation, sclerosis appears
3 (Reconstruction)	Bone remodeling, stabilization	Stable deformity; rocker-bottom foot

Radiographic Features

- Joint subluxation/dislocation
- Osteolysis, fragmentation
- "**Rocker-bottom deformity**"
- *Later:* Sclerosis, ankylosis

Management in Diabetics

Stage 0–1:

- **Immobilization** with total contact cast (TCC)
- Non-weight bearing

Stage 2–3:

- Protected weight bearing
- Custom footwear/bracing

Surgical (Selected Cases)

- Exostectomy
- Realignment osteotomy or arthrodesis (late deformity)

Q58. Pathophysiology of charcot neuroarthropathy.

(NEIGRIHMS 2013)

Definition

Progressive destruction of bones and joints in neuropathic patients.

Mechanisms
- Peripheral neuropathy leading to loss of protective sensation.
- Repetitive trauma unnoticed by the patient.
- Inflammatory response causing bone resorption.

Q59. Clinical presentation and management of plantar warts.

Cause
Human papillomavirus (HPV) infection.

Presentation
- Painful, thickened lesions on the soles.
- May have black dots (thrombosed capillaries).

Management
- Topical salicylic acid
- Cryotherapy
- Laser therapy
- Surgical removal in refractory cases

Surgical Procedures and Miscellaneous Foot and Ankle Conditions

Q60. Indications and techniques of ankle fusion (ankle arthrodesis).

Indications
- End-stage ankle arthritis (e.g., post-traumatic, rheumatoid).
- Severe deformity or instability unresponsive to conservative treatment.
- Failed total ankle replacement

Techniques
- *Open arthrodesis:*
  - *Approaches:* Anterior, lateral, or posterior.
  - *Fixation methods:* Screws, plates, or external fixators.
- *Arthroscopic arthrodesis:* Minimally invasive; suitable for patients with minimal deformity.

Optimal Positioning
Neutral dorsiflexion, slight valgus (0°–5°), and external rotation.

Q61. Ankle arthroscopy and its applications.

Definition
A minimally invasive surgical procedure using an arthroscope to visualize, diagnose, and treat intra-articular ankle pathologies.

Applications
- Debridement of osteochondral lesions.
- Removal of loose bodies.
- Treatment of anterior impingement syndromes.
- Synovectomy for inflammatory conditions.
- Assessment and management of ligamentous injuries.

Advantages
Reduced postoperative pain, faster recovery, and minimal scarring.

Q62. Role of tendon transfers in foot deformity correction.

Purpose
To restore balance and function in cases of muscle imbalance or paralysis.

Common Tendon Transfers
- *Posterior tibial tendon transfer:* Used in foot drop to restore dorsiflexion.
- *Split tibialis anterior tendon transfer (SPLATT):* Addresses varus deformities in cerebral palsy.
- *Peroneus longus to brevis transfer:* Corrects peroneal tendon dysfunction.

Considerations
Patient selection, donor muscle strength, and postoperative rehabilitation are crucial for successful outcomes.

Q63. Triple arthrodesis.

- Fusion of **Subtalar, talonavicular, calcaneocuboid** joints
- Indicated for hindfoot arthritis, rigid flatfoot, CTEV
- Provides pain relief and correction but sacrifices motion

Q64. Triple arthrodesis—indications and surgical techniques.

(AMC 2013)

Indications
Severe hindfoot arthritis, deformities, or instability unresponsive to conservative treatment.

Procedure
Fusion of the subtalar, talonavicular, and calcaneocuboid joints to provide a stable, pain-free foot.

Considerations
Loss of hindfoot motion; careful patient selection is essential.

Q65. Lambrinudi triple arthrodesis.

- Modified triple arthrodesis with plantarflexion of talus
- Used in **rigid equinus deformity** (e.g., neglected clubfoot)
- Corrects equinus + varus

Q66. Orthotic and prosthetic options for foot and ankle disorders.

Orthotic Devices
- *Ankle-foot orthoses (AFOs):* Provide support and alignment; used in foot drop, spasticity.
- *Supramalleolar orthoses (SMOs):* Offer medial-lateral stability; used in pediatric populations.
- *Custom insoles:* Address specific biomechanical issues like overpronation.

Prosthetic Options
- Partial foot prostheses for transmetatarsal amputations.
- Syme's prosthesis for ankle disarticulations.
- Below-knee prostheses for transtibial amputations.

Q67. Principles of rehabilitation following foot and ankle surgery.

Phases
1. *Immediate postoperative phase*: Pain management, edema control, and protection of surgical site.
2. *Early mobilization phase*: Gradual weight-bearing as tolerated, range-of-motion exercises.

3. *Strengthening phase*: Targeted exercises to restore muscle strength and proprioception.
4. *Functional training phase*: Gait training, balance exercises, and return-to-activity protocols.

Goals

Restore function, prevent complications, and facilitate return to daily activities.

5. *Tendon and soft tissue disorders:*
   - *Achilles tendinopathy:* Compare conservative and surgical management; discuss rehabilitation protocols.
   - *Posterior tibial tendon dysfunction:* Outline stages, diagnostic criteria, and treatment strategies.
   - *Plantar fasciitis:* Describe the etiology, clinical features, and management options.
6. *Neurological and gait disorders:*
   - *Cerebral palsy-related deformities:* Describe various foot and ankle deformities in cerebral palsy and their management.
   - *Gait abnormalities:* Discuss different types of gait patterns and their clinical significance.
     - FHL tendon transfer
     - Turn-down flap or graft (e.g., fascia lata)

Miscellaneous Disorders

Management of heel pain:

- *Causes:* Plantar fasciitis, calcaneal spur, bursitis
- *Tx:*
  - Stretching (Achilles, fascia)
  - Heel cups, orthotics
  - NSAIDs
  - Steroid injection
  - Rarely surgery (fasciotomy)

Retrocalcaneal Bursitis and Haglund's deformity:

- Inflammation of bursa between Achilles and calcaneus
- *Haglund's:* Bony prominence of posterosuperior calcaneus
- Pain with shoe wear, swelling
- *Tx:* Heel lift, NSAIDs, calcaneoplasty if severe

Q68. Haglund's disease (Haglund deformity).

Definition

Bony **prominence of posterosuperior calcaneus** → causes **retrocalcaneal bursitis** and **Achilles impingement**

Clinical

- Posterior heel pain, swelling
- Aggravated by tight shoes ("pump bump")
- Redness, tenderness at Achilles insertion

Treatment

- *Conservative:* Heel lift, NSAIDs, eccentric stretching
- *Surgical:* Excision of bony prominence + bursectomy if persistent

Plantar Fasciitis

- Degeneration of plantar fascia at its calcaneal insertion
- Heel pain, especially first steps in morning
- *Risk:* Obesity, prolonged standing
- *Tx:* Stretching, orthotics, steroid injection, ESWT

Calcaneal Spur

- Osteophyte at plantar fascia insertion
- Often incidental on X-ray

- Not always painful
- *Tx:* Conservative (same as plantar fasciitis)

Sever's Disease
- Apophysitis of calcaneus in growing children (8–13 years)
- Pain with activity, tenderness at heel
- *X-ray:* Sclerotic apophysis
- *Tx:* Activity restriction, heel pads

Q69. Briefly describe metatarsalgia.

[Assam Medical College (affiliated to Srimanta Sankaradeva University of Health Sciences) 2014]

Definition

Metatarsalgia is **pain in the forefoot** localized to the **metatarsal heads**, especially under the **2nd and 3rd MTP joints**, due to **abnormal pressure distribution** or inflammation.

Etiology
- *Mechanical:* Long second metatarsal, cavus foot
- RA or inflammatory arthropathy
- Improper footwear (high heels)
- Fat pad atrophy (elderly)
- Morton's neuroma
- Freiberg's disease (osteochondrosis)

Clinical Features
- Plantar pain under forefoot during walking
- Callosities
- Tenderness over metatarsal heads

Treatment
- *Conservative:* Metatarsal pads, footwear modification, NSAIDs
- *Surgical:* **Weil osteotomy** or **metatarsal head resection** in severe cases

Q70. Stress fracture (March fracture).

- Repetitive microtrauma; common in **second metatarsal**
- Seen in athletes/military
- Local tenderness, swelling
- *X-ray:* Callus seen after 2–3 weeks
- *Tx:* Rest, stiff-soled shoes

Q71. Jaipur foot/SACH foot.

- *Solid ankle cushioned heel (SACH):* Non-articulated prosthesis
- *Jaipur foot:* Indian low-cost SACH foot
- Allows barefoot walking, squatting
- Made of rubber, wood, sponge

Q72. Accessory navicular bone.

- Accessory ossicle medial to navicular
- May cause pain, medial foot swelling
- *Tx:* Shoe modification, excision if symptomatic

Q73. Köhler's disease.

- Osteochondrosis of navicular bone in children (4–7 years)
- Pain, limping
- *X-ray:* Sclerotic, fragmented navicular
- *Tx:* Self-limiting; NSAIDs, rest

Q74. Ingrown toenail.

- Nail margin penetrates soft tissue → inflammation/infection
- *Tx:* Nail trimming, antiseptics
- *Surgery:* Partial/complete nail avulsion ± matrixectomy

Q75. Turf toe.

- Hyperextension injury of **first MTP joint**
- Sprain of plantar plate
- Seen in athletes (football)
- Pain, swelling at base of big toe
- *Tx:* RICE, stiff-soled shoes, taping

Q76. Mallet toe.

- Flexion deformity of **DIP joint**
- *Causes:* Shoe pressure, RA, neuromuscular
- *Tx:* Shoe modification, DIP fusion if fixed

Q77. JESS fixator.

- Joshi's external stabilization system
- Modular, light-weight fixator for **deformity correction**, especially **CTEV, clubfoot**
- Uses percutaneous pins + rods for gradual distraction

Q78. Causes of gangrene.

Classification

1. *Dry gangrene (ischemic)*:
    - Atherosclerosis
    - Buerger's disease
    - Diabetes
    - Embolism/thrombosis
2. *Wet gangrene (infective)*:
    - Diabetic foot ulcers
    - Infected trauma/wounds
    - Fournier's gangrene
3. *Gas gangrene*:
    - Clostridium perfringens (anaerobic)
    - Foul-*smelling, crepitus, rapidly progressive*

4. *Other causes*:
   - Frostbite, burns
   - Snake bite
   - Pressure ulcers (bedridden patients)

Q79. Treatment of Morton's neuroma.

(RGUHS 2012)

Definition

A perineural fibrosis of the common digital nerve, commonly between the third and fourth metatarsals.

Management

- *Conservative:*
  - *Footwear modification:* Wide toe boxes, low heels.
  - Orthotic devices with metatarsal pads.
  - NSAIDs and corticosteroid injections.
- *Surgical:* Neurectomy or decompression in refractory cases.

Q80. Causes and management of foot drop.

Causes

- Common peroneal nerve palsy (trauma, compression)
- L5 radiculopathy
- Neuropathy (diabetes, CMT)

Management

- *Conservative:*
  - AFO (ankle-foot orthosis)
  - Physiotherapy
- *Surgical:*
  - Nerve decompression
  - Tendon transfer (posterior tibialis → dorsum)

Q81. Post-polio residual palsy (PPRP).

Features

- Results from **anterior horn cell damage** (poliomyelitis)
- Affects children <5 years (common)

Deformities

- **Foot drop** (tibialis anterior palsy)
- **Equinus deformity**
- **Knee hyperextension** (quad weakness)
- **Hip instability, Trendelenburg gait**

Management

- Orthosis (KAFO, AFO)
- Tendon transfers (e.g., posterior tibial to dorsum for foot drop)
- *Deformity correction:*
  - **Triple arthrodesis**
  - Supramalleolar osteotomy

- Limb lengthening (ilizarov)
- Muscle balancing surgery (e.g., gluteus maximus transfer for hip)

Q82. Peroneal nerve entrapment.

Site
- **Common peroneal nerve** at **fibular neck** (most common)
- Superficial or deep branches distally

Causes
- Compression by fibular head (tight plaster, trauma)
- Ganglion cysts
- Habitual leg crossing

Clinical
- Foot drop (deep peroneal)
- Loss of dorsiflexion, eversion
- Sensory loss over lateral leg/dorsum foot

Management
- Remove external compression
- Bracing (AFO)
- Nerve decompression if persistent
- Tendon transfer (tibialis posterior) if irreversible

Q83. Clinical features and management of Tarsal tunnel syndrome.

(JIPMER 2012)

Clinical Features
- Pain, burning, tingling, or numbness along the tibial nerve distribution.
- Symptoms aggravated by prolonged standing or walking.
- Positive Tinel's sign over the tarsal tunnel.

Management
- *Conservative:* NSAIDs, orthotic devices, physical therapy.
- *Surgical:* Tarsal tunnel release in cases unresponsive to conservative measures.

Q84. Chronic ankle instability—management.

Types
- *Mechanical:* Ligamentous laxity
- *Functional:* Proprioceptive/motor control deficit

Management
- *Conservative:*
    - Balance training
    - Peroneal strengthening
    - Ankle brace/taping
- *Surgical:*
    - **Broström procedure** (ATFL repair)
    - **Chrisman-Snook** (tendon augmentation)
    - Subtalar arthrodesis (in selected chronic cases)

Q85. Hansen's foot (neuropathic foot in leprosy).

Features

- Loss of pain, temperature, proprioception
- Claw toes, foot drop
- Painless ulcers, deformity
- Collapse of foot arches

Management

- MDT for leprosy (rifampicin, dapsone, clofazimine)
- Protective footwear
- Debridement of ulcers
- Tendo-Achilles lengthening (if needed)
- Reconstructive surgery for deformity

Q86. Talectomy—indications, merits and demerits.

Definition

Surgical excision of talus—also called **astragalectomy**

Indications

- Neglected/recurrent CTEV (rigid)
- Neuromuscular deformities
- Severe post-traumatic talar AVN
- Resistant equinovarus deformities (spina bifida, arthrogryposis)

Merits

- Corrects severe deformity
- Allows plantigrade foot
- Single-stage procedure

Demerits

- Loss of ankle joint—compensatory midfoot mobility required
- Poor cosmetic result
- Limb shortening
- May require later **triple arthrodesis**

CHAPTER 8

Nerve Injury

Arun K Sharma, Subqat Farooq, Akash Narangyal

Q1. Structure and function of peripheral nerves.

Structure

Peripheral nerves consist of axons (nerve fibers), supporting Schwann cells, and connective tissue sheaths:

- *Axons:* Conduct electrical impulses (motor, sensory, autonomic).
- *Myelin sheath (in myelinated nerves):* Produced by Schwann cells, speeds conduction.
- *Connective tissue layers:*
    - *Endoneurium:* Surrounds individual axons.
    - *Perineurium:* Surrounds a bundle (fascicle) of axons.
    - *Epineurium:* Outermost layer, encloses multiple fascicles and vessels.

Functions

- *Motor:* Impulses from CNS to muscles (efferent).
- *Sensory:* Impulses from receptors to CNS (afferent).
- *Autonomic:* Sympathetic and parasympathetic regulation of organs.

Q2. Classification of nerve fibers.

Based on Diameter and Conduction Velocity

Fiber type	*Function*	*Speed*
A fibers	Large, myelinated	Fast
Aα	Motor to skeletal muscle	Very fast
Aβ	Touch and pressure	Fast
Aδ	Pain and temperature	Medium
B fibers	Preganglionic autonomic	Slower
C fibers	Unmyelinated; pain, temp, postganglionic autonomic	Slow

Alternative: Group I–IV (for muscle afferents)

- *Group I (Ia/Ib)*: Muscle spindle/Golgi tendon organs
- *Group II*: Touch, pressure
- *Group III*: Pain and temperature
- *Group IV*: Unmyelinated, nociceptive

Q3. Blood supply of peripheral nerves.

Source
- *Vasa nervorum:* Small branches from adjacent arteries.
- *Three vascular plexuses:*
  1. Epineurial plexus
  2. Perineurial plexus
  3. Endoneurial plexus

Clinical Importance
- **Ischemia** of vasa nervorum → Neuropathy (e.g., in diabetes, vasculitis).
- Good vascularity is essential for **nerve healing and regeneration**.

Q4. Wallerian degeneration.

Definition
Degenerative changes occurring in the **distal segment** of a nerve **after axonal injury**.

Steps
1. **Axonal fragmentation** distal to injury site.
2. **Myelin breakdown** (via Schwann cells and macrophages).
3. **Phagocytosis** of debris.
4. **Schwann cell proliferation** → Form **Bands of Büngner** to guide regrowth.

Timeline
- Begins within 24–48 hours post-injury.
- Complete by 1–2 weeks depending on location and extent.

Q5. Nerve regeneration and its phases.

Timeline
- Begins ~48–72 hours after injury.
- Axonal sprouts grow at **1–3 mm/day**.

Phases of Regeneration
1. **Degeneration** (Wallerian degeneration in distal stump).
2. **Axonal sprouting** from proximal stump.
3. **Schwann cell proliferation** → Bands of Büngner.
4. **Axon elongation** through endoneurial tubes.
5. **Remyelination** by Schwann cells.
6. **Reinnervation** of target muscles/sensory receptors.

Key Molecular Mediators
- *Neurotrophins:* NGF, BDNF, CNTF
- *Cell adhesion molecules:* CAMs, integrins
- *Intracellular pathways:* MAPK, PI3K/Akt

Q6. Factors affecting nerve regeneration.

Positive Factors
- Younger age
- Distal injury (shorter regeneration distance)
- Clean, sharp injury

- Early surgical repair (<6 months)
- Absence of infection or comorbidities

Negative Factors
- Advanced age
- Proximal or crush injury
- Delayed repair (>6 months)
- Scar formation and fibrosis
- Systemic disease (e.g., diabetes, malnutrition)

Q7. Histological changes in transected nerves.

Distal Segment
- *Wallerian degeneration*:
  - Axonal fragmentation
  - Myelin breakdown
  - Schwann cell and macrophage infiltration

Proximal Segment
- *Retrograde degeneration*:
  - Chromatolysis (dispersion of Nissl granules)
  - Nuclear eccentricity
  - Decreased axoplasmic transport

Repair Phase
- Schwann cells align into Bands of Büngner.
- Fibrosis may develop if endoneurial tube is not preserved.

Q8. Classification, clinical features, and management of nerve injuries according to Seddon's and Sunderland's classifications.

(KMC Manipal 2014)

Seddon's Classification (1943)

Type	*Definition*	*Prognosis*
Neurapraxia	Conduction block without axonal damage	Excellent (full recovery)
Axonotmesis	Axonal disruption with intact endoneurium	Fair (slow recovery)
Neurotmesis	Complete severance of nerve including sheath	Poor (requires surgery)

Sunderland's Classification (1951)

Grade	*Injury*	*Corresponds to seddon*	*Recovery*
I	Neurapraxia (conduction block)	Neurapraxia	Complete
II	Axonal disruption, intact endoneurium	Axonotmesis	Good
III	Disruption of endoneurium	Axonotmesis	Moderate
IV	Disruption of perineurium	Axonotmesis	Poor (often needs surgery)
V	Complete transection	Neurotmesis	Requires surgery

Clinical Features (General for Peripheral Nerve Injury)
- *Motor*: Weakness/paralysis of innervated muscles.
- *Sensory*: Numbness or paresthesia in nerve distribution.
- *Autonomic*: Dry skin, loss of sweating, skin color changes.
- Tinel's sign may indicate regeneration.

Investigations

- **EMG** and **nerve conduction studies** (after 3–4 weeks).
- **MRI/Ultrasound** for structural lesions.
- **Clinical observation** of recovery (serial exams).

Management

A. **Neurapraxia:**
  - *Conservative*: Observation, splinting, physiotherapy.
  - Recovery in days to weeks.

B. **Axonotmesis:**
  - Conservative initially.
  - Recovery in months (1–3 mm/day).
  - Surgery if no improvement by 3–6 months.

C. **Neurotmesis:**
  - *Requires surgical repair*:
    - End-to-end repair.
    - Nerve graft (e.g., sural nerve).
    - Neurolysis (external or internal).

Prognosis

- Best for neurapraxia.
- Recovery depends on severity, age, time to intervention, and location.

Q9. Role of electrodiagnostic studies in the evaluation of peripheral nerve injuries.

Purpose

- To localize the lesion.
- Determine severity and type (neurapraxia, axonotmesis, neurotmesis).
- Assess prognosis and guide management.

Types of Electrodiagnostic Studies

A. *Nerve conduction studies (NCS)*:
  - *Measures*:
    - *Latency*: Time taken for impulse to travel.
    - *Amplitude*: Number of functioning axons.
    - *Conduction velocity*: Speed of impulse.
  - Differentiates demyelinating versus axonal injury.

B. *Electromyography (EMG)*:
  - *Needle insertion into muscle*:
    - Denervation changes (fibrillations, positive sharp waves).
    - Voluntary motor unit recruitment.
  - Identifies **chronicity and extent of injury**.

Timeline for Study

- *Initial EMG*: 2–3 weeks after injury (to allow Wallerian degeneration).
- *Serial studies*: At 6–12 weeks to assess regeneration or recovery.

Indications

- Localize site of compression (e.g., carpal vs. Guyon's canal).
- Confirm diagnosis in suspected neuropathy.
- Determine severity in entrapment syndromes.
- Evaluate recovery potential.
- Differentiate nerve versus root lesions.

Interpretation Examples

Condition	*NCS/EMG finding*
Carpal tunnel syndrome	Delayed median sensory and motor latency
Cubital tunnel syndrome	Conduction block/slowing across elbow
Radial nerve palsy	Decreased CMAP amplitude, denervation on EMG
Root lesion	Paraspinal denervation on EMG

Q10. EMG and nerve conduction studies (NCS).

NCS

- *Motor studies*: CMAP (compound muscle action potential).
- *Sensory studies*: SNAP (sensory nerve action potential).

Finding	*Interpretation*
↓ Amplitude	Axonal loss
↓ Conduction velocity	Demyelination
Conduction block	Neurapraxia

EMG

- *Detects spontaneous activity in denervated muscles*:
    - **Fibrillations**, **positive sharp waves**.
- Motor unit potential analysis for reinnervation.

Clinical Applications

- *Carpal tunnel syndrome*: Prolonged distal latency of median nerve.
- *Cubital tunnel*: Conduction block across elbow.
- *Radial nerve injury*: ↓ CMAP amplitude, denervation on EMG.

Q11. Electrophysiological changes in nerve injury.

Acute Phase

- **Conduction block** in neurapraxia.
- ↓ CMAP (compound muscle action potential).
- ↓ SNAP (sensory nerve action potential).

Denervation

- *On EMG (after 10–14 days)*:
    - **Fibrillation potentials**
    - **Positive sharp waves**
    - Decreased motor unit recruitment

Reinnervation

- Polyphasic motor unit potentials (MUPs).
- Increased recruitment with recovery.

Q12. Mri neurography—indications and advantages.

Definition

High-resolution MRI technique to **visualize peripheral nerves** and surrounding tissues.

Indications

- **Nerve entrapment syndromes** (e.g., piriformis syndrome, CTS).
- Localizing **nerve tumors** or **neuromas**.

- Post-surgical scarring.
- Differentiating root versus plexus injury.

Advantages
- Non-invasive
- Provides detailed anatomical mapping.
- Detects **edema**, **scarring**, and **tumors**.
- Helpful in surgical planning.

Limitations
- High cost
- Operator and machine dependent.
- Limited functional data compared to EMG/NCS.

Q13. Provocative tests for compressive neuropathies.

Test	*Purpose*	*Positive finding*
Phalen's test	Carpal tunnel syndrome	Tingling in median nerve distribution
Tinel's sign	Multiple (CTS, cubital tunnel, etc.)	"Electric shock" on percussion
Durkan's test	Direct pressure on carpal tunnel	Paresthesia in median nerve area
Elbow flexion test	Cubital tunnel syndrome	Numbness in ulnar distribution
Spurling's test	Cervical radiculopathy	Radiating neck-to-arm pain
Froment's sign	Ulnar nerve palsy	Thumb IP flexion during pinch grip

Q14. Tinel's sign and its clinical relevance.

Definition
Percussion over a nerve elicits **tingling or electric-shock sensation** in its sensory distribution.

Clinical Use
- Carpal tunnel syndrome (median nerve at wrist).
- Cubital tunnel syndrome (ulnar nerve at elbow).
- Radial tunnel syndrome.
- Assessment of **nerve regeneration** (progressive distal migration of positive Tinel's indicates axonal regrowth).

Interpretation
- *Positive*: **Irritable or regenerating nerve.**
- Used to **localize entrapment** or **monitor recovery**.

Mechanism of Injury Bases Nerve Injuries

Q15. High-velocity nerve injuries.

- Typically associated with motor vehicle accidents, gunshot wounds, or industrial trauma.
- Often cause traction or avulsion of peripheral nerves, especially in the brachial plexus.
- May result in root avulsion (preganglionic) or postganglionic rupture.
- Require imaging (MRI or CT myelogram) and usually surgical exploration.
- High risk of neurotmesis; surgical repair or nerve transfer often needed.

Q16. Stretch injuries of peripheral nerves.

- Occur due to elongation of nerves beyond physiological limits.
- Seen in birth injuries, sports trauma, or falls.
- May result in varying severity—neurapraxia to axonotmesis.
- Recovery depends on extent of axonal damage and length of stretch.
- Initial management is conservative; surgery if no recovery by 3–6 months.

Q17. Nerve injuries associated with fractures.

- Direct trauma or entrapment of nerve at fracture site.
- *Common examples*:
  - Radial nerve in midshaft humerus fracture (Holstein–Lewis lesion)
  - Ulnar nerve in medial epicondyle fracture
  - Axillary nerve in shoulder dislocation
- Requires careful neurovascular examination pre- and post-reduction.
- May resolve spontaneously or need surgical exploration.

Surgical Principles

Q18. Nerve grafting—indications and techniques.

- Indicated when direct end-to-end repair is not possible without tension.
- *Common indications*: Nerve gap >2 cm, neuroma excision, trauma with segment loss.
- *Common donor grafts*: Sural nerve, medial cutaneous nerve of forearm.
- *Types*:
  - Cable grafts (multiple strands)
  - Grouped fascicular matching (sensory to sensory, motor to motor)
- Sutured without tension using 8-0 or 9-0 nylon.
- Fibrin glue may be used for reinforcement.

Q19. Nerve transfers (e.g., Oberlin, spinal accessory).

- Indicated in root avulsion injuries, irreparable proximal injuries.
- *Principle*: Reinnervate distal targets using expendable nearby motor branches.
- *Common transfers*:
  - *Oberlin transfer*: Ulnar nerve fascicle → biceps branch
  - Intercostal nerves → musculocutaneous
  - Spinal accessory nerve → suprascapular nerve
  - Median nerve fascicle → brachialis branch
- *Advantages*: Shorter distance for regeneration, early reinnervation, avoids grafts.

Q20. Surgical approaches for nerve repair.

- *Varies based on anatomical site*:
  - *Upper limb*: Deltopectoral, posterior shoulder (axillary nerve), medial arm (ulnar nerve)
  - *Brachial plexus*: Supraclavicular, infraclavicular, axillary approach
  - *Lower limb*: Posterior thigh (sciatic), fibular neck (common peroneal)
- *Goal*: Adequate exposure without further nerve injury.

Q21. Delayed versus immediate nerve repair.

Parameter	*Immediate repair*	*Delayed repair*
Timing	Within hours–days	Weeks to months later
Indications	Clean lacerations, fresh injury	Crush injury, infection, unclear extent
Advantages	Faster reinnervation	Better wound evaluation
Drawbacks	High risk in contaminated wounds	Axonal atrophy if delayed too long

Q22. Complications of nerve repair.

- Neuroma formation
- Scar formation and fibrosis
- Misdirection of regenerating axons
- Tension at repair site causing ischemia
- Infection, graft rejection (if allograft)
- Incomplete functional recovery

Q23. Recent advances in nerve repair.

- Fibrin glue for coaptation
- Bioengineered nerve conduits (e.g., collagen tubes)
- Stem cell therapy and growth factor delivery
- Functional electrical stimulation
- Intraoperative nerve stimulation for fascicle identification

Q24. Describe the steps of nerve repair technique.

(RGUHS)

1. Debridement of damaged nerve ends until healthy fascicles seen
2. Aligning fascicles under microscopy
3. Coaptation using epineurial or perineurial sutures (8-0 or 9-0 nylon)
4. Avoid tension at the repair site
5. Reinforcement with fibrin glue
6. Immobilization and soft tissue coverage
7. Post-operative physiotherapy and monitoring

Q25. Methods of closing nerve gaps.

- Direct suturing (if no tension)
- Nerve grafting (autograft preferred – e.g., sural nerve)
- Nerve conduits (synthetic or biological)
- Nerve transfers as an alternative in long gaps
- Vascularized nerve grafts for scarred beds

Q26. Endoneurolysis (internal neurolysis).

- Dissection within the nerve fascicles to release internal scar or adhesions
- Indicated when there is intraneural fibrosis with incomplete recovery
- Requires intraoperative nerve stimulation to preserve motor units
- Risk of fascicular injury; done under microscopy

Q27. Partial and complete neurorrhaphy.

- *Neurorrhaphy*: Suturing of transected nerve ends
  - *Partial*: Only some fascicles aligned and sutured (useful in nerve transfer)
  - *Complete*: Full coaptation of epineurium or perineurium
- *Techniques*: Epineural, perineural, or group fascicular repair
- Must minimize tension and preserve vascularity

Q28. Indications and difficulties in fascicular repair.

- *Indications*:
  - Mixed nerves with identifiable motor/sensory fascicles
  - Need for precise motor to motor, sensory to sensory alignment
- *Difficulties*:
  - Fascicle identification requires expertise and staining
  - Time-consuming, requires high magnification
  - Risk of fascicle mismatch
  - Risk of fibrosis with multiple sutures

Q29. Clinical examination of brachial plexus injury.

Inspection
- Muscle wasting (deltoid, supraspinatus, biceps, forearm)
- Abnormal limb position (e.g., "waiter's tip" posture in Erb's palsy)
- Shoulder subluxation

Palpation
- Tinel's sign (tap along plexus to assess regeneration)
- Tenderness/swelling (clavicle, supraclavicular fossa)

Motor Testing (Root-wise)
- *C5*: Shoulder abduction (deltoid), elbow flexion (biceps)
- *C6*: Wrist extension (ECRL/ECRB)
- *C7*: Elbow extension (triceps)
- *C8–T1*: Finger flexion, intrinsic hand muscles

Sensory Examination
Dermatomal loss (C5–T1 distribution)

Special Tests
- Horner's syndrome (suggests root avulsion)
- Cross-chest adduction test (SC joint dislocation)
- Diaphragm movement (phrenic nerve, C3–C5)

Q30. Brachial plexus birth palsy — types, clinical features, and management.

(Asked in AIIMS Delhi 2022, PGI Chandigarh 2022)

Definition
Brachial plexus birth palsy (BPBP) refers to **injury to the brachial plexus** occurring during **birth** due to traction forces, leading to **motor and sensory deficits** in the upper limb.

Types

Type	Nerve roots involved	Features
Erb's palsy	C5–C6	"Waiter's tip" posture (adduction, internal rotation, extension of elbow, pronation)
Klumpke's palsy	C8–T1	Hand claw deformity, weak intrinsic hand muscles
Total plexus palsy	C5–T1	Complete flaccid paralysis of the limb

Clinical Features

- *Erb's palsy (most common)*:
  - Weak shoulder abduction (deltoid), external rotation (infraspinatus), elbow flexion (biceps).
  - Limb hangs limply at side, internally rotated.
- *Klumpke's palsy*:
  - Weakness of hand muscles.
  - May be associated with Horner's syndrome (ptosis, miosis, anhidrosis).

Diagnosis

- *Clinical examination*: Moro reflex absent on affected side.
- *Imaging*: MRI brachial plexus if severe.

Management

Age/Severity	Management strategy
Mild (early spontaneous recovery)	Physiotherapy, observation
No improvement by 3–6 months	Surgical exploration and nerve repair (nerve grafting, nerve transfers)

Surgical Options

- Neurolysis
- Nerve grafting (sural nerve)
- Nerve transfers (e.g., spinal accessory to suprascapular nerve)

Important Tip

Early passive ROM exercises are crucial to prevent shoulder contractures

Q31. Adult brachial plexus injuries—classification and surgical options.

Causes

Trauma (road traffic accidents, falls, penetrating injuries).

Classification

Type of injury	Description
Preganglionic (root avulsion)	Injury proximal to dorsal root ganglion; poor prognosis
Postganglionic (rupture)	Injury distal to dorsal root ganglion; better prognosis

Clinical Presentation

- Weakness or paralysis of affected muscles.
- Sensory loss in corresponding dermatomes.
- Horner's syndrome if T1 root involved.

Diagnosis

- MRI or CT myelography
- Nerve conduction studies and EMG

Surgical Options

- *Nerve transfers*:
  - Spinal accessory nerve to suprascapular nerve.
  - Intercostal nerves to musculocutaneous nerve.

- *Nerve grafting*: Using sural nerve grafts.
- *Muscle transfers*: Free functioning muscle transfer (e.g., gracilis muscle transfer).
- *Tendon transfers*: Late-stage cases for functional improvement.

Prognostic Factors
- Time to surgery (early better).
- Type of injury (preganglionic worse prognosis).
- Patient's age.

Quick Tips for Theory and Viva
- For **BPBP**, always describe **Erb's versus Klumpke's** clearly.
- In adult brachial plexus injury, **differentiate pre- and post-ganglionic injuries**.
- In **cerebral palsy**, always highlight **multidisciplinary management** and **early intervention**.

Q32. Difference between preganglionic and postganglionic injuries.

Feature	*Preganglionic injury*	*Postganglionic injury*
Site	Proximal to dorsal root ganglion	Distal to dorsal root ganglion
Root avulsion	Common	Absent
Surgical repair	Not possible (no distal stump)	Possible
Sensory neuron cell body	Destroyed	Preserved
Tinel's sign	Absent	Present and progresses distally
Horner's syndrome	May be present	Absent

Q33. Mechanism of injury in brachial plexus.

- *Common mechanisms*:
  - Traction (e.g., head pulled from shoulder—Erb's palsy)
  - Falls or MVAs causing root avulsion
  - Penetrating trauma (e.g., stab or gunshot wounds)
  - Birth trauma (obstetric palsy)
- May involve upper trunk (C5–C6), lower trunk (C8–T1), or total plexus.
- Clinical presentation depends on roots involved.
- *Imaging*: MRI or CT myelogram, especially in suspected avulsion.
- *Surgical options*: Nerve grafting, neurotization, or muscle transfers.

Q34. Indications for surgery, neurolysis, and neurotization.

Surgical Indications
- No recovery in **3–6 months** (especially root avulsions)
- Confirmed **rupture** or **neuroma-in-continuity**
- Total palsy (global BPI)
- Root avulsion on imaging (MRI/CT myelogram)

Neurolysis
- Indicated when intraoperative stimulation shows **intact distal conduction**
- Removes scar tissue from around intact nerve

Neurotization (Nerve Transfer)
- When **proximal root is avulsed or non-repairable**
- *Donor nerves*:
  - Spinal accessory → suprascapular
  - Intercostals → musculocutaneous

- ○ Ulnar fascicles → biceps (Oberlin transfer)
- ○ Contralateral C7

Q35. Mallet score (used in OBPI).

Used to grade upper limb function after **obstetric brachial plexus injury (OBPI)**.

Function	***Score 1–5* (higher is better)**
Global abduction	0° to >160°
External rotation	None to hand to head
Hand to neck	None to full
Hand to spine	None to full
Hand to mouth	None to smooth

- Total score = 25 (Excellent), <15 (Poor)

Q36. Clarke's transfer.

- Used in **C5–C6 BPI** to restore **shoulder abduction** and **external rotation**
- **Transfer of levator scapulae** or **trapezius** to **deltoid insertion**
- Indicated in **late presentations** when primary nerve surgery is not feasible

Q37. Steindler flexorplasty (Steindler transfer).

- **Proximal transfer** of **common flexor origin** (pronator teres, FCR, palmaris longus) to **mid-humerus**
- Restores **elbow flexion** in BPI (C5–C6 injury)
- Must have intact wrist flexors and good hand function
- *Risk*: Loss of wrist flexion strength

Q38. Prognosis of nerve injuries—favorable versus unfavorable.

(AIMS Kochi 2013)

Favorable	***Unfavorable***
Clean-cut injury (sharp laceration)	Crush/Traction/Avulsion injury
Young age	Older age
Distal injuries (e.g., wrist level)	Proximal injuries (e.g., axilla)
Early repair	Delayed repair (>6 months)
Intact motor end plates	Muscle fibrosis/atrophy

Q39. Strength-duration curve.

- Tool to assess **nerve and muscle excitability**
- **Plots** stimulus strength versus duration required for response

Findings	***Interpretation***
Normal curve	Healthy nerve
Shifted right (requires more current)	Partial denervation
Flattened curve	Complete denervation (muscle only responds to long-duration stimuli)

Q40. Nerve conduction velocity (NCV).

- Measures **speed of electrical impulse** through a nerve
- *Normal NCV*: 50–60 m/s (motor), 40–50 m/s (sensory)
- *Slowed in*: Demyelination
- *Reduced amplitude*: Axonal damage
- Used for diagnosing **carpal tunnel, BPI, neuropathy**

Q41. Double crush syndrome.

- A nerve compressed at **two sites** shows greater dysfunction
- *Example*: **Cervical radiculopathy + carpal tunnel syndrome**
- Proximal lesion makes the distal nerve more vulnerable
- Requires addressing **both compression sites**

Q42. Parsonage–Turner syndrome (brachial neuritis).

Definition

Idiopathic inflammation of the brachial plexus (C5–C7 common)

Etiology

Post-viral, post-vaccination, idiopathic

Clinical Features

- Sudden severe shoulder/arm pain → followed by weakness (delayed)
- *Muscles affected*: supraspinatus, infraspinatus, serratus anterior

Diagnosis

Clinical, MRI, EMG (denervation)

Management

- NSAIDs, corticosteroids (early)
- Physiotherapy
- Most recover in 6–18 months

Q43. Outline the anatomical course of the axillary nerve and discuss its vulnerability in shoulder dislocations.

Anatomy

- *Origin*: **Posterior cord** of brachial plexus (C5–C6).
- Passes through the **quadrangular space** with posterior circumflex humeral artery.
- Winds around the surgical neck of the humerus.
- *Motor supply*: Deltoid, teres minor.
- *Sensory*: Upper lateral cutaneous nerve of the arm (regimental badge area).

Vulnerability in Shoulder Dislocations

A. *Mechanism*:
   - Anterior shoulder dislocations (most common) → stretch or compress the axillary nerve in the quadrangular space.
   - Iatrogenic injury during shoulder surgeries (e.g., deltoid splitting approach).
   - Proximal humeral fractures (especially surgical neck).

Clinical Features
- *Motor*: Weakness in shoulder abduction (deltoid) and external rotation (teres minor).
- *Sensory*: Loss over the lateral aspect of the shoulder (regimental badge area).
- Atrophy of deltoid may be visible in chronic cases.

Diagnosis
- *Clinical exam*: Impaired abduction from 15–90°.
- Electromyography (EMG) after 3–4 weeks to confirm denervation.

Management

A. *Conservative*:
  - Most are neuropraxia and recover in weeks.
  - Rest, sling for pain, followed by physiotherapy.
  - EMG to monitor recovery.

B. *Surgical*:
  - Exploration and neurolysis if no recovery in 3–6 months.
  - Tendon transfer (posterior deltoid or trapezius) for irreversible palsy.

Q44. Clinical features and management of radial nerve palsy following midshaft humerus fracture.

(DYPU Pune 2013)

Introduction
- Radial nerve is the most commonly injured nerve in humeral shaft fractures.
- Especially vulnerable in fractures at the **spiral groove**.

Pathophysiology
- Radial nerve lies in contact with the posterior humeral shaft (spiral groove) between the lateral and medial heads of the triceps.
- It is susceptible to traction, entrapment in fracture callus, or laceration.

Clinical Features
- *Motor*: Wrist drop, finger drop, and thumb extension loss.
  - Weakness of triceps if lesion is proximal.
- *Sensory*: Loss over dorsum of hand (first web space) and dorsolateral forearm.
- *Reflexes*: Loss of triceps or brachioradialis reflex (depending on level).

Management

A. *Initial evaluation*:
  - Neurovascular examination.
  - Serial assessment—many are neurapraxia (resolve in 6–12 weeks).

B. *Conservative management*:
  - Indicated in closed fractures without nerve entrapment.
  - Functional bracing of fracture + dynamic cock-up splint.
  - Physiotherapy.

C. *Surgical exploration—indications*:
  - Open fracture with nerve transection.
  - No signs of recovery after 3–4 months.
  - Progressive neurological deficit.
  - Entrapment suspected on imaging/EMG.

D. *Surgical options*:
  - Neurolysis/Nerve repair/Nerve grafting.
  - Tendon transfers for irreparable injuries.

Prognosis

- Excellent in neurapraxia.
- Axonotmesis may recover partially.
- Neurotmesis requires surgical repair.

Q45. Clinical features and management of Holstein–Lewis fracture and its association with radial nerve injury.

Definition

Holstein–Lewis fracture: A spiral fracture of the distal third of the humerus, often associated with **radial nerve palsy**.

Anatomical Basis

Radial nerve transitions from posterior to anterior compartment through the **lateral intermuscular septum** near the distal third of the humerus—vulnerable to entrapment at the fracture site.

Clinical Features

- *Radial nerve palsy*:
  - Wrist drop.
  - Inability to extend fingers and thumb.
  - Sensory loss over dorsal hand (first web space).
- Pain, swelling, deformity over the distal arm.

Management

A. *Initial management*:
   - Detailed neurovascular examination.
   - Closed reduction and splinting (if closed fracture).

B. *Conservative management*:
   - **Non-operative treatment** (functional bracing) if fracture is closed and nerve palsy is present on presentation.
   - Monitor for spontaneous nerve recovery (70–90% resolve spontaneously).

C. *Surgical indications*:
   - Open fracture.
   - Nerve palsy develops after manipulation.
   - No improvement in nerve function after 3–4 months.
   - Associated vascular injury.

D. *Surgical procedure*:
   - **ORIF** with plate fixation.
   - Radial nerve exploration and neurolysis/repair if entrapped or lacerated.

Prognosis

- Most nerve palsies recover within 3–6 months.
- Prognosis poorer in cases of complete transection.

Q46. Anatomical basis and clinical implications of saturday night palsy.

(Goa Medical College 2015)

Definition

A form of **transient radial nerve palsy** due to prolonged compression of the radial nerve at the **spiral groove**, typically during deep sleep or intoxication (e.g., falling asleep with arm hanging over a chair).

Anatomical Basis

- Radial nerve lies in the **spiral groove** of the humerus — superficial and unprotected.
- Prolonged pressure compresses the nerve → ischemia and conduction block (neurapraxia).

Clinical Features

A. *Motor*:
- Wrist drop
- Finger drop
- Weak thumb extension
- Triceps usually spared (innervated above spiral groove)

B. *Sensory*:
- Numbness over dorsum of the hand and posterior forearm.

Diagnosis
- Clinical diagnosis
- EMG/NCS helpful if symptoms persist beyond 3–4 weeks.

Management

A. *Conservative*:
- Most cases are **neurapraxia** and recover spontaneously within 6–8 weeks.
- Cock-up splint to prevent contractures.
- Physiotherapy and passive ROM exercises.

B. *Surgical*:
- Rarely needed
- Indicated if no recovery at 3–6 months → nerve exploration or repair.

Q47. Describe the mechanism of injury, clinical features, and treatment options for anterior interosseous nerve (AIN) syndrome.

(AIIMS JPR 2015)

Anatomy
- AIN is a pure motor branch of the median nerve.
- Arises in the forearm ~5–8 cm distal to lateral epicondyle.
- *Supplies*:
  - **Flexor pollicis longus (FPL)**
  - **Lateral half of FDP (to index/middle)**
  - **Pronator quadratus**

Mechanism of Injury
- Compression or neuritis (e.g., Parsonage–Turner syndrome).
- Trauma, fibrous bands, or iatrogenic causes (venipuncture, cast).
- Idiopathic in many cases.

Clinical Features
- *Weakness of pinch grip*:
  - Can't form "O" sign with thumb and index finger (due to FPL and FDP weakness).
- No sensory deficit (AIN is pure motor).
- May have vague forearm pain initially.

Differential Diagnosis
- Tendon rupture (FPL/FDP) → ruled out by tenodesis.
- Cervical radiculopathy (C7-C8).
- Parsonage–Turner syndrome.

Diagnosis
- Clinical exam (pinch test).
- *EMG/NCV*: Denervation in AIN-innervated muscles.

Treatment

A. *Conservative*:
   - Rest, splinting
   - NSAIDs, physiotherapy
   - Majority recover in 3–6 months if neuritis.

B. *Surgical*:
   - *Exploration if*:
     - No recovery in 3–6 months.
     - Entrapment confirmed.
   - **Neurolysis** or decompression.

Q48. Discuss the clinical presentation and management of posterior interosseous nerve (PIN) entrapment.

Anatomy

- The **PIN** is a motor branch of the **radial nerve**.
- Arises at the level of the lateral epicondyle → passes through the **supinator (Arcade of Frohse)** → enters the posterior compartment of the forearm.
- *Innervates*:
  - Extensor carpi ulnaris
  - Extensor digitorum
  - Extensor indicis
  - Extensor pollicis longus and brevis
  - Abductor pollicis longus

Clinical Presentation

A. *Motor deficit*:
   - Weakness/paralysis of finger extension (finger drop).
   - Thumb extension weakness (can mimic radial nerve palsy).
   - Wrist extension preserved due to ECRL innervation (radial nerve branch before bifurcation).
   - No sensory loss (PIN is motor only).

B. *Pain*: Aching pain in the proximal dorsal forearm, often with resisted supination or finger extension.

Causes of Entrapment

- Fibrous bands of **arcade of Frohse** (most common).
- Repetitive forearm use (e.g., athletes, manual workers).
- Space-occupying lesions (e.g., ganglia, lipomas).
- Iatrogenic (e.g., surgery, injections).
- Inflammatory (rheumatoid synovitis).

Management

A. *Conservative*:
   - Activity modification.
   - NSAIDs, splinting (wrist and fingers in extension).
   - Physiotherapy

B. *Surgical*:
   - *Indications*: Persistent symptoms > 3 months, progressive weakness.
   - *Procedure*: **Decompression** at the arcade of Frohse and along the PIN path.

Q49. Course and sites of radial nerve compression.

Course

Arises from posterior cord → spiral groove → lateral intermuscular septum → anterior elbow → divides into superficial and deep branches

Sites of Compression

1. Axilla (crutch palsy)
2. Spiral groove (saturday night palsy)
3. Lateral intermuscular septum
4. Arcade of Frohse (PIN syndrome)
5. Radial tunnel

Q50. Indications, techniques, and outcomes of tendon transfer procedures in radial nerve palsy.

Indication

- **Radial nerve palsy** with no recovery after 6–9 months.
- Irreparable nerve injury (neurotmesis, failed repair/graft).
- Post-traumatic or iatrogenic causes.

Goals of Tendon Transfer

Restore **wrist extension**, **finger extension**, and **thumb extension/abduction**.

Pre-requisites for Tendon Transfer

1. Soft tissue envelope must be stable.
2. Donor muscles must be functional and expendable.
3. Joints must be mobile (no contractures).
4. Patient compliance with postoperative rehab.

Common Tendon Transfer Techniques

Function restored	***Tendon transferred***	***Recipient tendon***
Wrist extension	Pronator teres (PT)	Extensor carpi radialis brevis (ECRB)
Finger extension	Flexor carpi ulnaris (FCU)/FCR	Extensor digitorum communis (EDC)
Thumb extension	Palmaris longus (PL)/FDS ring finger	Extensor pollicis longus (EPL)
Thumb abduction	FDS middle finger	Abductor pollicis longus (APL)

Alternative Techniques

- Boyes transfer (FDS of middle/ring to EDC/EPL).
- *Tsuge's method*: PT to ECRB, FCU to EDC, PL to EPL.

Surgical Considerations

- Avoid transferring to tight tendons.
- Optimize line of pull and tension.
- Single-incision or multiple-incision techniques.

Outcomes

- Good to excellent functional results in most.
- Rehabilitation critical to success.
- Restoration of near-normal hand function.
- *Complications*: Tendon adhesion, weakness, failure of transfer.

Q51. Anatomical course of the ulnar nerve and its clinical significance in cubital tunnel syndrome.

Anatomy

- *Origin*: Medial cord of brachial plexus (C8–T1).
- *Arm*: Runs medial to brachial artery → posterior to medial intermuscular septum → enters **cubital tunnel** behind the medial epicondyle.
- *Forearm*: Between two heads of **flexor carpi ulnaris**, travels with **ulnar artery**.
- *Hand*: Enters **Guyon's canal**, supplies intrinsic hand muscles.

Cubital Tunnel Syndrome

Second most common compressive neuropathy of the upper limb (after CTS).

Sites of Compression

1. Arcade of Struthers.
2. Medial intermuscular septum.
3. Medial epicondyle groove.
4. Osborne's ligament (roof of cubital tunnel).
5. FCU aponeurosis.

Clinical Features

- *Motor*: Weak grip, clawing of 4th and 5th fingers, Wartenberg's sign, Froment's sign.
- *Sensory*: Numbness/tingling over medial 1.5 digits, ulnar border of hand.
- Nocturnal paresthesias common.

Diagnosis

- Tinel's sign over cubital tunnel.
- Elbow flexion test.
- Nerve conduction studies—slowed conduction across elbow.
- EMG to assess denervation.

Management

A. *Non-operative*:
   - Activity modification.
   - Night splinting (30–45° elbow flexion).
   - NSAIDs.

B. *Surgical*:
   - *Indications*: Persistent symptoms, muscle wasting, failed conservative management.
   - *Options*:
     - Simple decompression.
     - Anterior transposition (subcutaneous/intramuscular/submuscular).
     - Medial epicondylectomy.

Q52. Explain the pathophysiology and clinical features of tardy ulnar nerve palsy.

Definition

Tardy ulnar nerve palsy is defined as delayed onset ulnar neuropathy due to **progressive compression/stretching** of the ulnar nerve over time.

Pathophysiology

- **Chronic traction/compression** of the ulnar nerve at the elbow.

- *Often seen in*:
  - **Cubitus valgus deformity** (secondary to non-union lateral condyle humerus).
  - Previous elbow trauma or surgery.
  - Medial epicondyle malunion or exostosis.

Clinical Features

A. *Motor*:
  - Clawing of 4th and 5th fingers.
  - Wasting of hypothenar and interossei muscles.
  - Weak grip and key pinch.
  - Positive Froment's and Wartenberg's signs.

B. *Sensory*:
  - Paresthesia in medial 1½ fingers.
  - Symptoms worsen with elbow flexion.

Investigations

- *Nerve conduction studies*: Conduction block across elbow.
- *X-ray elbow*: Cubitus valgus or other deformity.
- *EMG*: Denervation of ulnar-innervated muscles.

Management

A. *Non-operative*:
  - *In early/mild cases*: Activity modification, elbow padding, night splinting.

B. *Surgical*:
  - **Anterior transposition** of ulnar nerve (subcutaneous, submuscular).
  - **Medial epicondylectomy** (if deformity is prominent).
  - Corrective osteotomy (rare, if valgus is severe and symptomatic).

Q53. Clinical features and treatment options for Guyon's canal syndrome.

Definition

Ulnar nerve compression in Guyon's canal (at the wrist).

Anatomy

- *Guyon's canal*: Tunnel between pisiform and hook of hamate, covered by pisohamate ligament.
- *Contents*:
  - Ulnar nerve
  - Ulnar artery

Etiology

- Ganglion cyst (most common).
- Repetitive trauma (cyclist's palsy).
- Fracture/dislocation of hook of hamate.
- Tumors, vascular lesions.

Clinical Features

Depends on the zone of compression (Shea and McClain classification):

Zone	*Contents*	*Deficit*
1	Motor + sensory	Motor + sensory loss
2	Motor only	Weakness of intrinsic hand muscles
3	Sensory only	Numbness in ring/little fingers

- *Motor*: Clawing of ulnar digits, interossei and hypothenar wasting, Froment's sign.
- *Sensory*: Numbness in ulnar 1½ digits (palmar side only).

Diagnosis
- Tinel's sign over Guyon's canal.
- EMG/NCS to localize compression.
- *MRI/USG*: Mass or ganglion.

Treatment

A. *Conservative*:
   - Activity modification
   - Splinting
   - NSAIDs
   - Aspiration of ganglion (if appropriate).

B. *Surgical*:
   - **Decompression** of Guyon's canal.
   - Excision of ganglion/tumor if present.
   - Ulnar artery aneurysm repair (if vascular cause).

Q54. Clinical features and management of median nerve injury at the elbow.

Anatomy
- Median nerve (C5–T1) lies medial to brachial artery in the arm.
- Passes through the **cubital fossa**, between heads of pronator teres.
- *Branches*:
  - Anterior interosseous nerve.
  - Palmar cutaneous branch (before wrist).

Causes
- Supracondylar humerus fracture (especially in children).
- Elbow dislocation.
- Iatrogenic (ORIF, injections).
- Compression in pronator teres (Pronator syndrome).

Clinical Features

A. *Motor deficits*:
   - Loss of forearm pronation.
   - Weak wrist flexion (especially radial deviation).
   - Inability to flex thumb IP joint (FPL) and index DIP (FDP) → **"Pointing index"**.
   - Weak thumb opposition and abduction (thenar muscles).
   - Ape thumb deformity (due to thenar wasting).

B. *Sensory deficits*:
   - Palmar aspect of lateral 3½ fingers.
   - Thenar eminence (via palmar cutaneous branch).

C. *Special signs*:
   - *Benediction sign*: When trying to make a fist, inability to flex 2nd and 3rd digits.
   - *Pen test*: Inability to oppose thumb to a pen.
   - **O sign defect** (if AIN involved).

Investigations
- EMG/NCS to confirm and localize lesion.
- Imaging (X-ray for fracture; MRI for mass lesions).

Management

A. *Conservative*:
  - *For incomplete lesions, neuropraxia*: Splinting, physiotherapy, observation.
  - Steroids if inflammatory cause suspected (e.g., pronator syndrome).

B. *Surgical*:
  - *Indications*:
    - Neurotmesis or laceration.
    - Failure of recovery in 3–6 months.
  - *Procedures*:
    - **Nerve repair** or **grafting**.
    - **Neurolysis** if entrapment.
    - **Tendon transfers** in chronic cases.

Prognosis
- Depends on level and type of injury.
- Better outcomes with early recognition and timely intervention.

Q55. Carpal tunnel syndrome (CTS).

(GMERS Medical College 2015)

Pathophysiology
- Compression of median nerve in carpal tunnel.
- *Carpal tunnel*: Bounded by carpal bones (floor) and flexor retinaculum (roof).
- Median nerve shares space with nine tendons (FDS, FDP, FPL).

Causes
- Idiopathic (most common)
- Diabetes, hypothyroidism, pregnancy
- Rheumatoid arthritis
- Repetitive strain injury
- Space-occupying lesions (e.g., ganglion, lipoma)

Clinical Presentation
- *Sensory*: Paresthesia in lateral 3½ digits.
- Nocturnal pain, relieved by shaking hands ("flick sign").
- *Motor*: Thenar muscle wasting, weakness of thumb abduction/opposition.

Clinical Tests
- Tinel's sign (percussion)
- Phalen's test (wrist flexion)
- Durkan's test (compression test)
- Tourniquet test

Investigations
- Nerve conduction studies (delayed latency, reduced amplitude).
- Ultrasound/MRI (space-occupying lesion).

Management

A. *Conservative*:
  - Splinting (neutral wrist).
  - NSAIDs, steroids (oral or injection).
  - Treat underlying cause.

B. *Surgical*:
- *Indications*: Failure of conservative measures, severe symptoms, thenar wasting.
- *Procedure*: **Open** or **endoscopic** carpal tunnel release.

Q56. Cubital tunnel syndrome.

Anatomy
Ulnar nerve compressed behind medial epicondyle in cubital tunnel

Clinical Features
Numbness in ring/little fingers, clawing, Froment's sign

Diagnosis
NCS, EMG

Treatment
- Activity modification, splinting
- Surgical decompression or transposition, if severe

Q57. Pronator teres syndrome.

Site
Median nerve compression between humeral and ulnar heads of pronator teres.

Features
- Forearm pain, sensory loss like CTS but includes thenar eminence.
- Weak FPL, FDP to index, pronation weakness.
- No nocturnal symptoms (unlike CTS).

Management
- Activity modification, physiotherapy.
- Surgical decompression if persistent.

Q58. Ulnar nerve palsy (high and low lesions).

High Lesion (Elbow)
Involves FCU, FDP (ulnar half), intrinsic muscles.

Low Lesion (Wrist)
Intrinsic muscles only

Clinical Signs
- Clawing (more in low lesion – "ulnar paradox")
- Weak grip, hypothenar wasting
- Positive Froment's and Wartenberg's signs

Treatment
- Conservative if neurapraxia.
- *Surgery*: Decompression, transposition, nerve repair.
- Tendon transfers for claw correction.

Q59. Froment's sign.

Test
Ask patient to hold paper between thumb and index.

Positive Sign
Flexion at IP joint of thumb (compensation by FPL due to weak adductor pollicis—ulnar nerve palsy).

Indicates
Ulnar nerve palsy

Q60. Wartenberg's sign.

Definition
Inability to adduct the little finger due to interossei weakness (ulnar nerve).

Seen In
Ulnar nerve palsy

Q61. Ulnar paradox.

Definition
Claw hand is more pronounced in distal ulnar nerve lesions than proximal.

Reason
In high lesions, FDP is also paralyzed, reducing flexion at DIP, so less clawing.

Mnemonic
"The closer the lesion to the claw, the less obvious the deformity."

Q62. Ulnar claw hand.

Definition
MCP hyperextension + PIP/DIP flexion of 4th and 5th digits.

Cause
Unopposed long flexors and extensors due to intrinsic muscle palsy (ulnar nerve).

Q63. Benediction hand.

Description
On asking to make a fist, inability to flex index and middle fingers (median nerve injury).

Cause
High median nerve lesion (affecting FDS and lateral FDP).

Q64. Pointing index.

Definition
In median nerve injury, when attempting a fist, index finger remains extended while others flex.

Cause
Paralysis of FDS and FDP to index finger.

Q65. Ape thumb deformity.

Definition
Thumb lies in same plane as fingers due to loss of opposition and abduction.

Cause
Thenar muscle wasting (median nerve lesion).

Q66. Partial and complete claw hand.

(WBUHS 2015)

Definition

Claw hand is a deformity due to paralysis of the **intrinsic hand muscles**, leading to:
- Hyperextension at the MCP joints
- Flexion at the PIP and DIP joints

Pathophysiology
- Caused by **ulnar and/or median nerve palsy**
- Imbalance between extrinsic (long flexors/extensors) and intrinsic (lumbricals/interossei) muscles

Types

Type	*Nerves involved*	*Affected digits*	*Key features*
Partial claw hand	Ulnar nerve	4th and 5th digits	Seen in isolated ulnar nerve palsy
Complete claw hand	Ulnar + Median nerve	All fingers	More severe deformity, seen in combined nerve injuries (e.g., lower brachial plexus palsy, leprosy)

Management
- *Conservative*: Splinting, physiotherapy
- *Surgical*: Tendon transfers (e.g., Zancolli lasso, Brand's procedure)
- Correction of deformity for functional and cosmetic improvement

Q67. Compression neuropathies—upper limb overview.

Common Sites

Nerve	*Syndrome*	*Site of compression*
Median	Carpal tunnel	Wrist (flexor retinaculum)
Median	Pronator teres syndrome	Between heads of pronator teres
Ulnar	Cubital tunnel syndrome	Elbow (cubital tunnel)
Ulnar	Guyon's canal syndrome	Wrist
Radial	Radial tunnel syndrome	Proximal forearm (arcade of Frohse)
Radial	PIN syndrome	Supinator muscle

General Features
- Pain, paresthesia, weakness, muscle wasting depending on severity
- Provocative tests (e.g., Tinel's, Phalen's)
- Confirm with **NCS/EMG**

Management
- *Conservative*: Splints, NSAIDs, activity modification
- *Surgical*: Decompression or neurolysis

Q68. Causes, clinical features, and management of sciatic nerve injury following hip dislocation.

[Government Medical College (GMC) Srinagar 2015]

Anatomy
- The **sciatic nerve** (L4–S3) exits the pelvis via the greater sciatic notch below the piriformis.
- Divides into **tibial** and **common peroneal** components.
- Lies posterior to the hip joint—making it vulnerable during **posterior dislocation** of the hip.

Causes
- **Posterior hip dislocation** (most common).
- Fracture-dislocation of the acetabulum or femoral head.

- *Iatrogenic (hip surgery*: total hip arthroplasty, ORIF).
- Compression by hematoma or heterotopic ossification.

Clinical Features

- Pain, paresthesia in the posterior thigh and leg.
- *Motor weakness*:
    - *Tibial nerve*: Weak plantarflexion.
    - *Peroneal nerve*: Foot drop (more commonly involved).
- *Sensory loss*: Posterior thigh, lateral leg, and dorsum/sole of foot (depends on division involved).

Diagnosis

- Clinical exam.
- Electromyography (EMG) and nerve conduction studies (after 3 weeks).
- *Imaging*: MRI if compressive pathology suspected.

Management

A. *Immediate management of hip dislocation*:
- **Urgent reduction** (<6 hours to prevent AVN).
- Post-reduction neurovascular assessment.

B. *Observation*:
- Most are neuropraxias.
- *Supportive care*: Splints, physiotherapy, ankle-foot orthosis (AFO) for foot drop.

C. *Surgical exploration*:
- *Indicated if*:
    - Open dislocation with nerve entrapment.
    - No recovery after 3–6 months.
    - Progressive neurological deficit.

Q69. Tibial nerve injury.

Anatomy

- Continuation of sciatic nerve (L4–S3)
- *Innervates*: Calf muscles (plantarflexors), intrinsic foot muscles
- *Sensory*: Sole of the foot

Clinical Features

- Loss of plantarflexion and toe flexion
- Sensory loss over sole
- Clawing of toes if intrinsic foot muscles lost
- Positive **Tinel's sign** at tarsal tunnel (if compression there)

Causes

- Tarsal tunnel syndrome
- Posterior knee dislocation
- Laceration in popliteal fossa or ankle

Management

- Conservative if neurapraxia (splinting, physiotherapy)
- Surgical repair/decompression if needed

Q70. Enumerate the causes of foot drop and outline the diagnostic approach and management strategies.

(DYPU Pune 2015)

Definition

Foot drop refers to weakness or paralysis of **ankle dorsiflexion** and toe extension, leading to a steppage gait.

Causes

Level	*Cause*
Central (brain/spinal cord)	Stroke, cerebral palsy, multiple sclerosis, spinal cord injury
Nerve root (L4–L5)	Lumbar disc herniation, foraminal stenosis
Sciatic nerve	Hip dislocation, posterior approach to hip surgery
Common peroneal nerve	Compression at fibular neck, trauma, habitual leg crossing, plaster cast
Peripheral neuropathy	Diabetes mellitus, vasculitis
Muscle	Muscular dystrophy
Functional/Conversion	Non-organic (psychiatric causes)

Diagnostic Approach

A. *Clinical evaluation*:
- *Gait*: Steppage gait, foot slap.
- *Motor*: Weak dorsiflexion, toe extension, and eversion.
- *Sensory*: Over dorsum of foot and lateral leg (superficial peroneal nerve).
- *Reflexes*: Usually intact.

B. *Electrodiagnostics*:
- **Nerve conduction studies (NCS)**.
- *Electromyography (EMG)*: Localize lesion (e.g., root vs. nerve).

C. *Imaging*:
- *MRI lumbar spine*: For radiculopathy.
- *MRI knee/fibular neck*: For compressive lesions.

Management

A. *Conservative*:
- *Remove compression*: Cast relief, avoid leg crossing.
- *Physiotherapy*: Strengthening, gait training.
- *Ankle-foot orthosis (AFO)*: Prevent plantarflexion during swing phase.

B. *Surgical*:
- **Decompression** of common peroneal nerve (if entrapment confirmed).
- *Tendon transfer*:
  - Tibialis posterior transfer to dorsum of foot in long-standing palsy.

Q71. Management of foot drop.

Initial Management
- Identify cause (NCS/EMG, MRI)
- AFO splint for support
- Physiotherapy

If no recovery by 6–12 months: Surgical exploration or tendon transfer

Q72. Surgical management (<1 year).

Indications
- Lack of nerve recovery by 6 months
- Confirmed axonotmesis or neurotmesis

Options
- Nerve decompression (if entrapment)
- Nerve repair or graft
- Nerve transfer (less common)

Q73. Preoperative assessment before tendon transfer.

Checklist

- **Passive range of motion** at ankle
- Fixed deformity ruled out
- Donor tendon strength ≥ grade 4
- Sensation in sole (to aid proprioception)
- No contractures or spasticity

Q74. Named surgical procedures for foot drop (Obers, Barr's, Bridle, Lambrinudi).

Procedure	*Description*
Obers	TA rerouted laterally (obsolete)
Barr's	Tibialis posterior transferred through interosseous membrane to dorsum of foot
Bridle	TP + PL + PB combined and inserted on dorsum (balanced dorsiflexion)
Lambrinudi	Triple arthrodesis in dorsiflexion (used in rigid deformities)

Q75. Tendon transfer for foot drop.

Common Procedures

- *Tibialis posterior transfer*: Most used (transferred anteriorly)
- *Peroneus longus or FHL*: In some cases
- *Bridle procedure*: Dynamic and balanced

Fixation: To cuneiforms or dorsiflexor tendons

Q76. Arthrodesis and bone block procedures for foot drop.

(Jammu University 2015)

Indications

- Fixed deformity
- Failed tendon transfer
- Severe muscle imbalance

Types

- **Tibiotalar arthrodesis** in neutral/dorsiflexion
- *Bone block*: anterior tibia bone graft prevents plantarflexion

Q77. Role of AFO in peripheral neuropathy.

Purpose of AFO (Ankle-Foot Orthosis)

- Maintains foot in **neutral** or **plantigrade** position
- Prevents **foot drop** during swing phase
- Reduces risk of **falls**
- Improves **gait stability**

Types

- *Rigid AFO*: Full support, limits ankle motion
- *Articulated AFO*: Allows dorsiflexion, blocks plantarflexion
- *Ground reaction AFO*: For crouch gait and quad weakness
- *Carbon fiber AFO*: Lightweight, dynamic assistance

Indications
- Peroneal nerve palsy
- Diabetic neuropathy
- Charcot–Marie–Tooth disease
- Post-polio residual paralysis

Q78. Foot drop gait pattern.

- *High stepping gait*: Exaggerated hip and knee flexion
- *Slapping gait*: Forefoot slaps the ground during stance
- *Compensations*: Circumduction or hip hiking

Q79. Diagnosis and management of common peroneal nerve injury at the fibular neck.

(DYPU Pune 2015)

Anatomy
- Common peroneal nerve (L4–S2) is a branch of the **sciatic nerve**.
- Winds around the **neck of fibula**—superficial and prone to injury.
- *Divides into*:
  - **Deep peroneal nerve** → dorsiflexors, toe extensors.
  - **Superficial peroneal nerve** → foot evertors, skin over dorsum of foot.

Causes
- Trauma (e.g., fibular neck fracture).
- Prolonged leg crossing or squatting.
- Compression by tight plaster/casts.
- *Iatrogenic*: Surgery around knee/lateral leg.
- Tumors (schwannoma, ganglion cyst).

Clinical Features
- *Motor*:
  - Foot drop (weak dorsiflexion).
  - Loss of eversion.
- *Sensory*: Numbness over the dorsum of foot and lateral leg.
- Steppage gait.

Diagnosis
- Clinical examination
- Nerve conduction studies (NCS)
- Electromyography (EMG)
- *MRI*: If mass lesion suspected

Management

A. *Conservative*:
   - Ankle-foot orthosis (AFO).
   - Physiotherapy (strengthening/stretching).
   - Remove compressive cause (cast, splint).

B. *Surgical*:
   - *Indications*:
     - Laceration/Entrapment.
     - Failure to recover in 3–6 months.
   - **Neurolysis/Nerve repair**/Decompression.
   - **Tendon transfer** (e.g., posterior tibial tendon → dorsum) in irreversible palsy.

Q80. Peroneal nerve (PEN) test.

Definition

A **clinical test** to assess function of the **common peroneal nerve**, especially after injury or surgery near the fibular neck.

How to Perform

- Ask the patient to **dorsiflex** and **evert** the foot.
- Weakness suggests **peroneal nerve involvement**.

Interpretation

- *Positive PEN Test*: Inability or weakness in dorsiflexion/eversion → indicates **common peroneal nerve palsy**
- Often due to compression at fibular neck (fractures, prolonged pressure)

Relevance

- Useful in trauma, total hip/knee replacement follow-ups, cast-related compression injuries
- Aids in early identification and treatment of **foot drop**

Q81. Thoracic outlet syndrome (TOS).

Definition

Compression of **neurovascular structures** at the thoracic outlet (brachial plexus, subclavian artery/vein)

Types

- **Neurogenic** (most common)
- **Venous**
- **Arterial**

Causes

Cervical rib, fibrous bands, postural issues, trauma

Clinical Tests

Adson's test, Roos test, Wright's test

Symptoms

- Neck/shoulder pain, paresthesia in ulnar digits, weak grip
- *Venous*: edema, cyanosis
- *Arterial*: coldness, pallor

Management

- *Conservative*: Physiotherapy, posture correction
- *Surgical*: Cervical rib resection, scalenectomy (if refractory)

Q82. Radial tunnel syndrome.

Site

Compression of **radial nerve** in radial tunnel (between brachialis and brachioradialis/supinator)

Features

- Deep aching pain in proximal forearm
- Tenderness over radial tunnel (5 cm distal to lateral epicondyle)
- No motor or sensory deficit (unlike PIN syndrome)

Management

- Rest, splints, physiotherapy
- Surgical decompression if persistent

Q83. Tarsal tunnel syndrome.

Site

Compression of **posterior tibial nerve** beneath flexor retinaculum at the ankle.

Features

- Burning pain and paresthesia in sole of foot
- Worse at night or after prolonged standing
- Positive **Tinel's** over tarsal tunnel

Diagnosis

- EMG/NCS
- MRI to rule out mass lesions

Management

- *Conservative*: Orthotics, NSAIDS
- Surgical decompression if unresponsive

Q84. Superior gluteal nerve palsy.

Anatomy

- Arises from L4–S1 (sacral plexus)
- *Innervates*: Gluteus medius, gluteus minimus, tensor fascia lata

Clinical Features

- Weak abduction of hip
- **Trendelenburg sign** positive (pelvis drops on opposite side while standing on affected limb)
- Waddling gait

Causes

- Iatrogenic (hip surgery, intramuscular injection)
- Pelvic fractures
- L5 radiculopathy (differential diagnosis)

Management

- *Conservative*: Physiotherapy, gait training
- Surgical exploration (if traumatic or compressive cause)

Q85. Femoral nerve palsy.

Anatomy

- Originates from L2–L4 (lumbar plexus)
- *Innervates*: Quadriceps, iliacus, sartorius, pectineus
- *Sensory*: Anterior thigh and medial leg (via saphenous nerve)

Clinical Features

- Weakness of hip flexion, knee extension
- Absent **patellar reflex**
- Sensory loss over anterior/medial thigh and medial leg

Causes

- Retroperitoneal hematoma (e.g., post-angiography)
- Psoas abscess

- Pelvic fractures
- Surgical trauma

Management
- Treat underlying cause
- Bracing (knee extension support)
- Physiotherapy
- Rarely surgical exploration

Q86. Obturator nerve injury.

Anatomy
- Originates from L2–L4
- *Innervates*: Adductor muscles (adductor longus, brevis, magnus), gracilis, obturator externus
- *Sensory*: Medial thigh

Clinical Features
- Weak hip adduction
- Difficulty in crossing legs
- Sensory deficit on medial thigh

Causes
- Pelvic surgery (e.g., lymph node dissection)
- Pelvic trauma/fracture
- Obturator hernia

Management
- *Conservative*: Physiotherapy
- Surgical decompression if entrapment/herniation

Q87. Lateral femoral cutaneous nerve entrapment (meralgia paresthetica).

(RUHS 2017)

Anatomy
- Arises from L2–L3
- Purely sensory
- Passes under inguinal ligament near ASIS

Clinical Features
- Burning pain, numbness over anterolateral thigh
- Worse with standing/walking, relieved on sitting
- No motor deficit

Causes
- Obesity, tight clothing, pregnancy, pelvic masses
- Iatrogenic (e.g., ASIS pin placement)

Diagnosis
Clinical, NCS/EMG (to rule out radiculopathy)

Management
- Weight loss, loose clothing
- NSAIDs, local steroid injections
- Surgical neurectomy (rare)

Q88. Principles of splinting in nerve injuries.

Goals

- Prevent deformity
- Maintain joint alignment
- Improve function
- Assist rehabilitation

Principles

- *Position of function*: e.g., **wrist in extension**, MCPs in flexion
- Protect paralyzed muscles
- Allow stretching of antagonists
- Should be lightweight, easy to apply

Common Splints

Injury	*Splint type*
Radial nerve	Cock-up wrist splint
Ulnar nerve	Anti-claw splint
Median nerve	Opponens splint
Peroneal nerve	AFO

Q89. Tendon transfers for nerve palsies.

Indications

- No recovery by 6–12 months
- Intact donor tendons (MRC ≥ 4)
- Mobile joints

Common Transfers

Nerve palsy	*Transfer options*
Radial	PT → ECRB, FCR → EDC, PL → EPL (Brand's transfer)
Median	BR → FPL, EIP → APB (opponensplasty)
Ulnar	Zancolli lasso, FDS → lateral bands
Foot drop	Tibialis posterior transfer, Bridle procedure

Q90. Describe the indications and principles of tendon transfer in peripheral nerve palsy.

Indications

- Irreversible nerve injury with no recovery >6–12 months
- Functional impairment due to muscle loss
- Healthy donor muscles available (MRC ≥4)
- Full passive range at target joint

Principles

- One muscle → one function
- Direct line of pull (no bowstringing)
- Adequate motor power
- Donor must be expendable

Common Examples

Condition	*Tendon transfer*
Radial nerve palsy	PT → ECRB, FCR → EDC, PL → EPL
Ulnar nerve palsy	FDS → lateral bands (Zancolli lasso)
Foot drop (CPN palsy)	Tibialis posterior → dorsum of foot (Barr's or Bridle procedure)

Q91. Physiotherapy in rehabilitation.

Objectives

- Prevent joint stiffness
- Maintain muscle strength
- Improve circulation
- Prevent contractures
- Restore function post-reinnervation or surgery

Techniques

- Passive and active ROM exercises
- Strengthening exercises
- Functional training
- Gait training (with or without AFO)
- Mirror therapy and proprioception training

Q92. Use of nerve stimulators in rehabilitation.

Types

- Transcutaneous electrical nerve stimulation (TENS)
- Functional electrical stimulation (FES)
- Implanted stimulators (less common)

Uses

- Pain relief (TENS)
- Prevent muscle atrophy (FES)
- Promote reinnervation
- Facilitate motor retraining in partial injuries

Caution

- Avoid overuse in denervated muscles
- Contraindicated in certain cardiac conditions

Q93. Artificial nerve conduits in nerve repair.

Purpose

Bridge nerve gaps when direct repair not possible and autograft is not preferred.

Types

- *Biological*: Collagen, vein, muscle, chitosan
- *Synthetic*: Silicone, polyglycolic acid (PGA), polycaprolactone

Advantages
- Avoid donor site morbidity
- Scaffold for axonal regrowth

Limitations
- Effective for small gaps (<3 cm)
- Limited success in motor nerves

Q94. Stem cell therapy in nerve regeneration.

Types Used
- Mesenchymal stem cells (MSC)
- Schwann-like stem cells

Mechanism
- Promote axonal regeneration
- Secrete neurotrophic factors
- May differentiate into supportive cells

Applications
- Adjunct with nerve conduits or grafts
- Under experimental and trial phase

Limitations
- Regulatory and ethical concerns
- Long-term outcomes not yet established

Q95. Nerve biopsy—indications, technique, complications.

Indications
- Vasculitic neuropathy
- Atypical neuropathies (e.g., leprosy, amyloidosis, sarcoidosis)
- Hereditary neuropathy diagnosis (rare now due to genetic tests)

Technique
- Sural nerve (most common site)
- Small segment excised (2–3 cm)
- Usually performed under local anesthesia

Complications
- Permanent sensory loss in distribution
- Neuroma formation
- Wound complications

Q96. Classification of benign peripheral nerve tumors.

Classification

Tumor type	*Description*	*Common site*
Schwannoma (neurilemmoma)	Benign tumor of Schwann cells, encapsulated, eccentric to nerve	Head, neck, extremities
Neurofibroma	Mixed tumor of Schwann cells, fibroblasts, perineural cells; non-encapsulated	Trunk, skin, associated with NF1
Perineurioma	Tumor of perineurial cells, rare	Extremities
Ganglioneuroma	Arises from sympathetic ganglia	Retroperitoneum
Lipoma	Soft tissue tumor compressing nerve, not of neural origin	Variable

Features

- Slow growing
- May cause pain, paresthesia or motor symptoms via compression
- Tinel's sign often positive

Q97. Schwannomas versus neurofibromas.

Feature	*Schwannoma*	*Neurofibroma*
Origin	Schwann cells	Schwann + other nerve sheath cells
Encapsulation	Encapsulated	Non-encapsulated
Location	Eccentric to nerve	Central within nerve
Mobility	Mobile side-to-side	Less mobile
Association with NF1	Rare	Common (especially plexiform type)
Malignant potential	Very low	Higher, especially plexiform neurofibromas
Histology	Antoni A and B areas, Verocay bodies	Interlacing bundles, myxoid areas
Surgery	Enucleation possible	Often requires nerve sacrifice

Q98. Malignant peripheral nerve sheath tumors (MPNSTs).

Definition

Aggressive soft tissue sarcomas arising from peripheral nerve sheaths or pre-existing neurofibromas.

Risk Factors

- **Neurofibromatosis type 1 (NF1)**—major risk
- Radiation exposure
- Pre-existing plexiform neurofibroma

Clinical Features

- Rapidly enlarging mass
- Pain, neurological deficit
- May mimic benign lesions early

Diagnosis

- *MRI*: Heterogeneous, invasive mass
- *Biopsy*: Spindle cell sarcoma
- *IHC*: S-100 (variable), SOX10, loss of H3K27me3 (specific for MPNST)

Management

- Wide surgical excision (primary)
- *Radiotherapy*: Adjuvant or for unresectable tumors
- *Chemotherapy*: Limited role; may be used in metastatic disease

Prognosis

- Poor due to local recurrence and metastasis
- *5-year survival*: ~30–50%

Q99. Phantom limb.

Definition

A phenomenon where **sensation of the amputated limb** persists after amputation—including pain, tingling, or itching.

Types
- *Phantom sensation*: Awareness of the missing limb
- *Phantom pain*: Painful sensation perceived in the absent limb
- *Stump pain*: Pain at the site of amputation

Mechanism (Multifactorial)
- *Central*: Cortical reorganization in the **somatosensory cortex**
- *Peripheral*: Neuroma formation at stump
- Psychological overlay may contribute

Management
- *Medications*: Gabapentin, amitriptyline, opioids
- **Mirror therapy** (visual feedback)
- Transcutaneous electrical nerve stimulation (TENS)
- Desensitization techniques
- Psychological support, CBT
- *Rare*: Surgical excision of neuroma

Q100. Pain management in nerve injury.

Causes of Pain
- Neuropathic pain due to demyelination, axonal degeneration
- Ectopic discharges, central sensitization

Types of Pain
- Burning, tingling, electric shock-like (neuropathic)
- Allodynia, hyperalgesia

Assessment
- Visual analog scale (VAS), DN4 questionnaire
- Neurological exam, nerve conduction studies

Management
- *Pharmacological*:
  - *Anticonvulsants*: Gabapentin, pregabalin
  - *Antidepressants*: Amitriptyline, duloxetine
  - NSAIDs, opioids (limited role)
- *Interventional*:
  - Nerve blocks
  - Epidural steroids (if root-level pathology)
- *Rehabilitation*: TENS, physiotherapy, desensitization therapy

CHAPTER 9

Neuromuscular and Neurological Disorders

Tarkik Thami, Sachin Kudyar, Shubham Pandoh

Q1. Define neuromuscular disorders. Classify them with examples.

(AIIMS Patna 2018)

Definition

Neuromuscular disorders (NMDs) are a group of conditions that affect the function of the **muscle**, **peripheral nerves**, **neuromuscular junction**, or **motor neurons**, resulting in **muscle weakness, contractures, and functional impairments**.

Classification

Level of involvement	*Example*
Upper motor neuron (UMN)	Cerebral palsy, stroke
Lower motor neuron (LMN)	Spinal muscular atrophy, poliomyelitis
Peripheral nerve	Charcot–Marie–Tooth disease, diabetic neuropathy
Neuromuscular junction	Myasthenia gravis, congenital myasthenic syndromes
Muscle	Duchenne muscular dystrophy, Becker muscular dystrophy, congenital myopathies

Q2. Classify neuromuscular disorders affecting children.

Classification of Pediatric Neuromuscular Disorders

Category	*Examples*
Motor neuron diseases	Spinal muscular atrophy (SMA)
Neuropathies	Hereditary: Charcot–Marie–Tooth (CMT); Acquired: Guillain–Barré
Neuromuscular junction disorders	Congenital myasthenic syndrome
Myopathies (muscle disorders)	Duchenne and Becker muscular dystrophy, congenital myopathies, inflammatory myopathies
CNS disorders with neuromuscular features	Cerebral palsy, leukodystrophies

Q3. Enumerate orthopedic manifestations of neuromuscular disorders.

Common Orthopedic Manifestations

1. *Muscle contractures*: For example, equinus, hamstring, hip flexor
2. *Joint deformities*: For example, scoliosis, hip subluxation/dislocation
3. *Gait abnormalities*: For example, crouch gait, scissoring, toe-walking
4. *Foot deformities*: For example, pes cavus, talipes equinovarus
5. Limb length discrepancies

6. *Fractures*: Due to decreased mobility and osteoporosis
7. *Upper limb contractures*: For example, elbow flexion, thumb-in-palm

Q4. Differences between upper and lower motor neuron lesions.

Feature	*Umn lesion*	*LMN lesion*
Muscle tone	Increased (spasticity)	Decreased (flaccid)
Reflexes	Hyperreflexia	Hyporeflexia or absent
Fasciculations	Absent	Present
Muscle bulk	Slight disuse atrophy	Pronounced atrophy
Babinski sign	Positive	Negative
Examples	Cerebral palsy, stroke	Polio, SMA, peripheral neuropathy

Q5. Describe the pathophysiology of muscle contracture formation in neuromuscular disease.

(PMCH Patna)

Pathophysiology

- Imbalance of forces between agonist and antagonist muscles due to weakness or spasticity.
- Unopposed pull of spastic or stronger muscle leads to sustained abnormal joint positioning.
- Immobilization or decreased movement causes:
  - Sarcomere shortening
  - Perimysial and endomysial fibrosis
  - Decreased extensibility
- Structural muscle changes (e.g., fatty infiltration, fibrosis) further reduce elasticity.

Contributing Factors

- Spasticity (e.g., CP)
- Denervation (e.g., polio, SMA)
- Imbalanced growth of bone and soft tissues (children)

Cerebral Palsy

Q6. Types, clinical features, and orthopedic management of cerebral palsy.

(Asked in PGI Chandigarh 2022, AIIMS Delhi 2021)

Definition

Cerebral palsy (CP) is a **group of permanent disorders** of the development of **movement and posture**, causing activity limitation, attributed to **non-progressive disturbances** in the developing fetal or infant brain.

Types of Cerebral Palsy

Type	*Key features*
Spastic CP	Hypertonia, increased deep tendon reflexes, stiffness. Most common (75%)
Dyskinetic CP	Involuntary movements—dystonia, athetosis
Ataxic CP	Poor coordination and balance
Mixed CP	Combination of spastic and dyskinetic types

Clinical Features

- Motor delay (late sitting, crawling, walking).
- Abnormal muscle tone (hypertonia, hypotonia).

- Contractures and joint deformities.
- Gait abnormalities (scissoring, toe-walking).
- Seizures (30–50% cases).
- Intellectual disability (variable).
- Feeding difficulties and drooling (in severe cases).

Orthopedic Manifestations

- Hip dislocation/subluxation.
- Equinus deformity (tight gastrocnemius-soleus).
- Flexion deformities of hip, knee, elbow.
- Scoliosis
- Upper limb spasticity leading to thumb-in-palm deformity.

Orthopedic Management

Goal	Strategy
Prevent deformity	Stretching exercises, bracing
Correct existing deformities	Tendon release surgeries, osteotomies
Improve function	Botulinum toxin injections, orthotics
Maintain ambulatory ability	Selective orthopedic interventions
Pain relief	Surgery for painful dislocated hips or scoliosis

Surgical Procedures

- Tendon lengthenings (e.g., Achilles, hamstrings).
- Osteotomies (femoral derotation osteotomy).
- Hip containment surgery (varus derotation osteotomy + pelvic osteotomy).
- Spinal fusion for scoliosis.

Key Point

Management must be **individualized—focusing on function, not only cosmetic correction**.

Q7. Classify types of cerebral palsy based on motor involvement and anatomical distribution.

By Motor Abnormality

Type	Features
Spastic (most common)	Hypertonia, hyperreflexia, UMN signs
Dyskinetic	Athetosis, dystonia, chorea
Ataxic	Poor balance and coordination
Hypotonic	Floppy tone, delayed milestones
Mixed	Combination of above (commonly spastic + dyskinetic)

By Anatomical Distribution

Type	Description
Monoplegia	One limb
Hemiplegia	One side of the body
Diplegia	Lower limbs > upper limbs
Quadriplegia	All four limbs involved
Triplegia	Three limbs involved
Double hemiplegia	Both sides involved, one more severely

Q8. Enumerate orthopedic manifestations of cerebral palsy.

- *Joint contractures*: Hip flexion, equinus, knee flexion
- Hip subluxation/dislocation
- *Spinal deformities*: Scoliosis, kyphosis
- *Foot deformities*: Equinus, valgus, varus, pes planus
- *Gait abnormalities*: Scissoring, crouch, toe-walking
- *Upper limb deformities*: Elbow flexion, wrist flexion, thumb-in-palm
- Osteopenia and fractures
- Limb length discrepancy

Q9. What are the gait abnormalities seen in cerebral palsy?

Gait type	*Characteristics*
Equinus gait	Tiptoe walking due to gastro-soleus contracture
Jump gait	Equinus, hip and knee flexion, anterior pelvic tilt
Crouch gait	Excessive hip/knee flexion and ankle dorsiflexion
Scissoring gait	Hip adduction → legs cross during swing phase
Stiff-knee gait	Reduced knee flexion during swing
Waddling gait	Seen in hypotonia or hip abductor weakness

Q10. Describe the management of spastic equinus deformity in CP.

Goals
- Achieve plantigrade foot
- Improve gait and balance

Non-surgical
- Physiotherapy, AFOs
- Stretching, night splints
- Botulinum toxin injection

Surgical
- Percutaneous achilles tendon lengthening
- Vulpius procedure (gastro-soleus recession)
- Split anterior tibialis tendon transfer (SPLATT)—if inversion deformity coexists

Q11. Discuss the role of tendon transfers in CP.

Indications
- Dynamic deformity due to muscle imbalance
- Adequate motor control (GMFCS I–III)
- No fixed contracture

Common Transfers
- *SPLATT:* For equinovarus correction
- *Hamstring transfer:* In crouch gait
- *Rectus femoris transfer:* To posterior knee or sartorius in stiff-knee gait
- *Gracilis or adductor transfer:* For scissoring

Goals
- Improve gait mechanics
- Prevent secondary deformities

Q12. Management of hip subluxation in cerebral palsy.

Surveillance

Hip X-ray with Reimer's Migration Index (MI)

Treatment Based on MI

Migration index (%)	*Treatment*
<30	Observation, therapy
30–50	Botulinum toxin injection, adductor/Iliopsoas muscle release
>50	Soft tissue release+ varus derotation osteotomy (VDRO) ± pelvic osteotomy
Dislocated	Salvage procedure: Femoral head resection (Castle procedure)

Q13. Discuss surgical options in spastic hip dysplasia in CP.

Procedure	*Indication*
Adductor + iliopsoas release	Early subluxation
Varus derotation osteotomy (VDRO)	Migration index >50%
Pelvic osteotomy (Dega's/Pemberton's)	Acetabular dysplasia
Salvage (proximal femoral resection)	Painful dislocation in non-ambulatory child

Q14. Discuss principles of rehabilitation in a child with spastic diplegia.

Goals

- Promote ambulation and independence
- Prevent contractures and deformity
- Improve activities of daily living (ADL)

Components

- *Physiotherapy:* Stretching, strengthening
- *Orthoses:* Ankle foot orthosis (AFO), knee-ankle-foot orthosis (KAFO)
- *Spasticity:* Botulinum toxin injections, selective dorsal rhizotomy (SDR)
- Gait training and assistive devices
- *Multidisciplinary approach:* OT, speech therapy, pediatrician

Q15. Classify Crouch gait and discuss its management.

(IMS and SUM Hospital 2015)

Definition

Excessive hip/knee flexion and ankle dorsiflexion during stance

Classification (Rodda's)

- *Mild crouch*: increased knee flexion, plantigrade foot
- *Moderate crouch*: excessive dorsiflexion, calcaneus gait
- *Severe crouch*: loss of extensor mechanism

Management

- Physiotherapy and orthoses (floor reaction AFOs)
- Botulinum injections
- *Surgical:*
    - Hamstring lengthening
    - Rectus femoris transfer
    - Distal femoral extension osteotomy (DFEO)
    - Patellar advancement

Q16. Describe selective dorsal rhizotomy and orthopedic procedures in CP.

(Asked in MUHS Maharashtra 2023, JIPMER Puducherry 2022)

Selective Dorsal Rhizotomy (SDR)

Definition: Neurosurgical procedure involving selective cutting of dorsal (sensory) nerve rootlets to reduce spasticity.

Indications for SDR

- Spastic diplegia (mostly in ambulatory children).
- Good strength but disabling spasticity.
- *Age:* Ideal between 3–7 years.

Procedure

1. Laminectomy at lumbar spine (L1–L2).
2. Intraoperative EMG stimulation of dorsal rootlets is done to identify abnormal hyperactive rootlets.
3. Abnormal hyperactive rootlets are identified and selectively divided (~40–70% of rootlets).

Outcomes

- Reduces spasticity permanently.
- Improves mobility and gait quality.
- Requires intensive postoperative physiotherapy.

Orthopedic Procedures in CP

Deformity	*Surgery*
Equinus deformity	Achilles tendon lengthening
Hip subluxation/dislocation	Varus derotation femoral osteotomy + pelvic osteotomy
Flexion contractures (knee, elbow)	Hamstring or biceps tendon lengthening
Upper limb deformities	Tendon transfers, muscle releases
Scoliosis	Spinal fusion (if >45–50° curve and progressive deformity)

Botulinum Toxin Role

Used preoperatively or as an adjunct to delay need for surgery in dynamic spasticity.

Quick Tips for Theory and Viva

- Always mention **spastic CP** as the most common type (~70–75%).
- Clearly explain that **SDR is selective sensory rootlet division** to decrease spasticity permanently.
- *Surgical goals:* **Function > Deformity correction**.
- Use mnemonics like **"SAFE"** for SDR indications:
  - *S*trong muscles,
  - *A*mbulatory potential,
  - *F*unctional improvement goal,
  - *E*xclude mixed types.

Q17. Discuss the role of botulinum toxin in treating spasticity in neuromuscular disorders.

Mechanism

Botulinum toxin blocks acetylcholine at neuromuscular junctions (NMJs) → temporary muscle relaxation (~3–6 months)

Indications

- Focal spasticity (e.g., adductors, hamstrings, gastro-soleus)
- Early hip subluxation
- Dynamic contractures

Advantages
- Minimally invasive, can be performed as an outpatient procedure
- Reversible, repeatable
- Delays need for surgery

Limitations
- Not effective for fixed deformities (intra-articular deformities)
- Requires repeated injections
- Expensive
- Availability can be an issue

Poliomyelitis and Residual Deformities

Q18. Post-polio syndrome.

Definition
A condition seen in polio survivors years after initial recovery, characterized by **new muscular weakness, fatigue, and pain**.

Clinical Features
- Gradual onset of new muscle weakness
- Muscle pain, joint pain
- Fatigue, cold intolerance
- Breathing/swallowing difficulty in some

Etiology
Thought to result from **overuse and degeneration** of motor units that were previously trying to compensate.

Management
- Lifestyle modification (activity pacing)
- Energy conservation, orthotics
- Pain management
- Physiotherapy (non-fatiguing)
- Psychosocial support

Q19. Describe and management of residual deformities after poliomyelitis.

(Asked in PGI Chandigarh 2021, MUHS Maharashtra 2022)

Definition
Poliomyelitis is a **viral infection** caused by the **poliovirus** leading to **destruction of anterior horn cells** of the spinal cord, resulting in a **flaccid paralysis**. Residual deformities develop due to **muscle imbalance**, **growth disturbances**, and **joint instability**.

Common Residual Deformities

Region	*Deformities*
Hip	Flexion deformity, abduction contracture, subluxation/dislocation
Knee	Genu recurvatum (hyperextension deformity), flexion deformity
Ankle and foot	Equinus, calcaneus, varus, valgus, cavus
Spine	Scoliosis
Upper limb	Shoulder subluxation, elbow flexion contracture (less common)

Mechanism of Deformity Formation

- Paralysis of certain muscle groups → Unopposed action of stronger muscles → Progressive joint deformity.
- Ligamentous laxity due to lack of active muscular support.

Management

Non-surgical:

- Orthotic support (e.g., KAFO, AFO) for weak limbs.
- Physiotherapy to maintain joint range of motion and strengthen remaining muscles.

Surgical:

- *Soft tissue procedures:*
  - Tendon transfers (to substitute paralyzed muscles).
  - Contracture release surgeries.
- *Bony procedures:*
  - Osteotomies (e.g., femoral derotation osteotomy for hip instability).
  - Arthrodesis (joint fusion) in severely unstable joints (e.g., ankle fusion).
- *Limb lengthening:* Ilizarov technique in case of significant limb length discrepancy.

Key Goal

Restore **functional alignment and stability**, NOT necessarily trying to achieve anatomical perfection.

Q20. Surgical principles in post-polio deformities.

(Asked in RGUHS Karnataka 2022)

Principles of Surgery

1. *Assess muscle power carefully:*
   - Use **Medical Research Council (MRC) grading**.
   - Only perform tendon transfers when the donor muscle has ≥ Grade 4 power.
2. *Prioritize function over cosmetic correction:* For example, maintain plantigrade foot even if minor deformity persists.
3. *Correct fixed deformities first:* Contractures (like hip/knee flexion deformity) must be released before tendon transfers.
4. *Stabilize Joints:* Use fusion procedures if necessary to achieve a stable, painless limb (especially ankle).
5. *Energy conservation in walking:* Preserve ability to walk with minimal orthotic support if possible.
6. *Timing of surgery:* Ideally delayed until child is older (6–8 years), and muscle power deficit is stable.

Common Surgical Procedures

- *Tendon transfers:* Tibialis posterior to dorsum of foot (for foot drop correction).
- *Contracture releases:*
  - Hamstring release (for knee flexion deformity).
  - Achilles tendon lengthening (for equinus deformity).
- *Osteotomies:* Femoral varus derotation osteotomy (VDRO) is indicated for hip subluxation/dislocation.
- *Fusions:* Triple arthrodesis in severe foot deformities.

Mnemonic for Surgical Principles "SAFE ST"

- *S*trength assessment
- *A*lign first (deformity correction)
- *F*unction over form
- *E*nergy efficient walking
- *S*tabilize joints if needed
- *T*iming after stabilization of muscle power deficit

Q21. Management of foot drop in post-polio residual paralysis (PPRP).

Goals

- Prevent tripping
- Restore dorsiflexion
- Improve gait efficiency

Management Options

Non-surgical:

- Ankle-foot orthosis (AFO)
- Physiotherapy and gait training

Surgical:

- *Tendon transfer (if passive ROM is preserved)*: **Tibialis posterior transfer** (Barr's or Bridle procedure)
- *Bony procedures (for fixed deformities)*:
  - **Triple arthrodesis**
  - **Lambrinudi fusion**

Q22. What are the principles of tendon transfer in PPRP?

(BJ Medical College 2014)

Principle	*Description*
Donor muscle	Must have strength ≥ MRC Grade 4
Expendability	Donor function should not compromise essential tasks
Joint mobility	Joint must have full passive range
Straight line of pull	To avoid bowstringing or inefficient action
Single function restoration	Each transfer should address one movement
Free from fibrosis	The bed of tissue where tendon transfer is being planned, should be free from excessive scarring or fibrosis due to a previous surgery

Additional Points

- Assess entire limb function (compensatory mechanisms)
- Perform transfers once bony deformities are corrected.
- Post-operative physiotherapy is essential

Q23. Discuss triple arthrodesis and Lambrinudi procedure.

Triple Arthrodesis

- *Fusion of three joints:* Subtalar, talonavicular, calcaneocuboid
- *Indication:* Fixed hindfoot deformities (equinovarus, cavus)
- *Advantages:* Corrects deformity, stabilizes foot
- *Drawbacks:* Loss of hindfoot motion, risk of adjacent joint arthritis

Lambrinudi Procedure

- Modified triple arthrodesis where **foot is fused in dorsiflexion**
- *Indication:* Rigid equinus foot (e.g., PPRP)
- *Goal:* Convert equinus into plantigrade foot to allow walking
- *Precaution:* Ensure adequate calcaneal bone stock

Q24. Outline surgical correction of knee hyperextension deformity in polio.

Cause

Quadriceps weakness with strong gastroc-soleus causing **genu recurvatum**.

Surgical Options
- Posterior capsulotomy of the knee (for fixed deformity)
- Hamstring release (if contributing)
- Anterior wedge osteotomy of tibia
- Use of floor-reaction orthosis (for mild cases)
- Tendon transfer (e.g., hamstrings to anterior tibia) for dynamic correction

Goals
- Prevent further joint damage
- Improve walking efficiency
- Avoid secondary deformities

Quick Tips for Theory and Viva
- Always **differentiate between paralytic deformities (muscle imbalance)** and **fixed contractures (soft tissue shortening)**.
- Mention **gait analysis** and **orthotic planning** as essential parts of management.
- In surgical planning, **strength testing of donor muscles** (minimum Grade 4/5) is critical before any tendon transfer!

Muscular Dystrophies

Q25. Types and clinical features of muscular dystrophies.

(Asked in PGI Chandigarh 2022, MUHS Maharashtra 2023)

Definition
Muscular dystrophies are a group of **genetic, progressive muscle diseases** characterized by **degeneration and weakness of skeletal muscles**.

Common Types of Muscular Dystrophies

Type	*Key features*
Duchenne muscular dystrophy (DMD)	Most common and severe; early onset (<5 years); Gower's sign positive
Becker's muscular dystrophy	Milder than DMD; later onset (after 5 years)
Limb-girdle muscular dystrophy	Weakness of shoulder and pelvic girdle muscles
Facioscapulohumeral dystrophy	Weakness of facial, shoulder girdle muscles; adolescence onset
Myotonic dystrophy	Distal weakness, myotonia (delayed muscle relaxation), systemic involvement
Congenital muscular dystrophy	Hypotonia at birth, delayed milestones
Emery–dreifuss muscular dystrophy	Early contractures (elbow, Achilles tendon), cardiac conduction defects

Clinical Features (General)
- Progressive muscle weakness.
- Gait abnormalities (waddling gait).
- Gower's sign (climbing up on self to stand).
- Calf pseudohypertrophy (especially in DMD).
- Contractures and scoliosis (later stages).
- Cardiomyopathy (especially in DMD and Becker).
- Respiratory complications in advanced cases.

Mnemonic
"Dumb Legs Can Fail Muscles"
(Duchenne, limb-girdle, congenital, facioscapulohumeral, myotonic)

Q26. Duchenne muscular dystrophy—diagnosis and management.

(Asked in AIIMS Delhi 2021, RGUHS Karnataka 2022)

Etiology
- X-linked recessive disorder.
- Mutation in **dystrophin gene** on Xp21.
- Complete absence of dystrophin protein in muscle fibers.

Clinical Presentation
- Symptoms start by **2–5 years** of age.
- Delayed motor milestones (late walking).
- *Progressive proximal muscle weakness:*
  - Waddling gait.
  - Frequent falls.
  - Difficulty in climbing stairs.
- Positive Gower's sign
- Calf pseudohypertrophy
- Progressive scoliosis
- Cardiac and respiratory muscle involvement by teenage years.
- Wheelchair dependence typically starts to set in around adolescence.

Diagnosis

Test	***Findings***
Serum CPK (creatine phosphokinase)	Elevated (>10 times normal)
Genetic testing	Dystrophin gene mutation analysis
Muscle biopsy	Absence of dystrophin on immunohistochemistry
ECG and echocardiography	Cardiomyopathy changes
Pulmonary function tests	Detect early respiratory compromise

Management

Medical:
- *Steroids (prednisolone, deflazacort):* Slow progression of muscle weakness.
- *Cardiac medications:* ACE inhibitors, β-blockers for cardiomyopathy.
- *Respiratory support:* Non-invasive ventilation (NIV) when needed.

Rehabilitation:
- Physiotherapy to prevent contractures.
- Orthotic support (AFOs, KAFOs) to prolong ambulation.
- Nursing care

Surgical:
- Achilles tendon lengthening (for equinus deformity).
- Spinal fusion for severe scoliosis.

Genetic counseling: Crucial for family planning.

Prognosis
- Progressive worsening.
- Life expectancy improved with modern care (~25–30 years).

Newer Therapies
- Exon skipping therapy (Eteplirsen).
- Gene therapy trials ongoing.

Important Tip

Steroid therapy (daily low dose) is the current standard to slow down progression of the disease.

Quick Tips for Theory and Viva

- *Always state*:
  - **Duchenne = Absence of dystrophin**
  - **Becker = Reduced dystrophin.**
- For DMD diagnosis, **mention CPK, genetic testing, and muscle biopsy.**
- *Management focus:* **Multidisciplinary care + steroids.**

Q27. Gower's sign.

Definition

Gower's sign is a classical clinical sign observed when a patient with **proximal muscle weakness**, especially of the **pelvic girdle**, rises from a sitting or supine position by using their hands to "climb up" their own thighs for support.

Clinical Appearance

- The child rolls over onto their abdomen
- Pushes up on all fours
- Then uses hands on knees and thighs to "walk" up to a standing position

Pathophysiology

- Indicates **weakness of proximal lower limb muscles**, particularly **gluteal and quadriceps group.**
- Seen due to inability to raise the trunk without compensatory support

Common Conditions Associated with Gower's Sign

Condition	*Note*
Duchenne muscular dystrophy	Most classic condition
Becker muscular dystrophy	Less severe form
Polymyositis/Dermatomyositis	Inflammatory myopathies
Spinal muscular atrophy	Anterior horn cell disease
Congenital myopathies	Hypotonia and delayed milestones
Cerebral palsy (hypotonic type)	Occasionally seen

Diagnostic Importance

- One of the **early signs of Duchenne MD**
- Should prompt **muscle enzyme testing (CPK)** and **genetic studies**
- Must be differentiated from orthopedic causes of difficulty in rising

Q28. Compare Duchenne and Becker muscular dystrophy.

Feature	*Duchenne MD*	*Becker MD*
Inheritance	X-linked recessive	X-linked recessive
Onset	Early (2–5 years)	Late (after 10 years)
Mutation	*Absent dystrophin*	*Defective or reduced dystrophin*
Progression	Rapid	Slow
Ambulation	Lost by 10–12 years	Retained into adulthood
Cardiac involvement	Common and early	May occur late
Life expectancy	Late teens–20s	40–50 years or more

Q29. Orthopedic manifestations and complications of muscular dystrophies.

- *Lower limb contractures:* Hip flexion, knee flexion, equinus deformity
- *Upper limb contractures:* Elbow, wrist flexion in later stages
- *Scoliosis:* Progressive after loss of ambulation
- Pelvic obliquity
- *Foot deformities:* Equinus, varus
- Joint stiffness
- Osteoporosis and pathological fractures
- Loss of ambulation and wheelchair dependence

Q30. Describe management of contractures in Duchenne muscular dystrophy.

Non-surgical
- Regular **stretching exercises**
- **Night splints** or orthoses (e.g., KAFOs) to delay contracture progression
- Serial casting in early contracture

Surgical
- Indicated if significant functional limitation or fixed deformity
- Heel cord lengthening for equinus
- Hamstring/iliopsoas releases for crouch gait
- Spinal stabilization for scoliosis (after pulmonary assessment)

Q31. Role of corticosteroids and supportive care in DMD.

Corticosteroids
- Prednisolone or deflazacort
- Prolong ambulation (by 2–3 years)
- Reduce scoliosis progression
- Delay respiratory/cardiac decline

Side Effects
Weight gain, osteoporosis, hypertension, behavioral issues

Supportive Care
- Physiotherapy and contracture prevention
- Non-invasive ventilation (NIV)
- Regular cardiac and respiratory monitoring
- Nutritional support and calcium/vitamin D
- Psychosocial and genetic counseling

Q32. Discuss principles of rehabilitation in muscular dystrophies.

Goals
- Maximize functional independence
- Prevent deformities
- Delay progression

Components
- *Physiotherapy:* ROM, strengthening (non-fatiguing), gait training
- *Orthotics:* AFOs/KAFOs to maintain ambulation and prevent deformity

- *Seating aids:* Wheelchairs, cushions for posture
- *Spinal orthosis:* If scoliosis develops before surgery
- *Pulmonary rehabilitation:* Breathing exercises, assisted cough
- *Multidisciplinary team:* Orthopedist, neurologist, physiotherapist, pulmonologist

Q33. Quick mindmap—neuromuscular and neurological disorders.

Neuromuscular and Neurological Disorders

- *Plexus/Nerve injuries*:
  - Brachial plexus (birth/adult)
  - Peripheral nerve injury classifications (Sunderland, Seddon)
- *Cerebral palsy*:
  - Types (spastic, dyskinetic)
  - Orthopedic procedures (release, rhizotomy)
- *Poliomyelitis*: Residual deformities and tendon transfers
- *Muscular dystrophies*:
  - Duchenne (DMD)
  - Becker
- *Spinal muscular atrophy*:
  - Types I, II, III
  - Genetic therapy options

Spinal Muscular Atrophy

Q34. Classify types of spinal muscular atrophy (SMA). Outline clinical features of SMA type I and II.

(GMERS Medical College 2018)

Classification (Based on Age of Onset and Motor Milestones)

Type	*Onset*	*Motor function*	*Survival*
0	Prenatal	Never move	<6 months
I (Werdnig–Hoffmann)	<6 months	Never sit	<2 years (if untreated)
II	6–18 months	Can sit but cannot walk	Survival into adulthood
III (Kugelberg–Welander)	>18 months	Ambulates, may lose later	Normal lifespan
IV	Adult-onset	Mild weakness	Normal lifespan

SMA Type I (Severe) Features

- Generalized hypotonia ("floppy infant")
- Tongue fasciculations
- Absent reflexes
- Paradoxical breathing
- Difficulty feeding, respiratory distress

SMA Type II (Intermediate) Features

- Delay in milestones
- Can sit but not stand/walk unaided
- Scoliosis, contractures, weak cough
- Finger tremors ("polymini-myoclonus")

Q35. Differentiate SMA from DMD.

Feature	*SMA*	*Duchenne muscular dystrophy (DMD)*
Etiology	Anterior horn cell degeneration	Dystrophin gene mutation
Inheritance	Autosomal recessive (SMN1)	X-linked recessive
CK levels	Normal	High (↑ CPK)
Muscle tone	Hypotonia (floppy)	Pseudohypertrophy
Weakness	Proximal symmetric	Proximal, progressive
Reflexes	Absent	Reduced
Contractures	Less common early	Common
EMG	Denervation pattern	Myopathic pattern
Age of onset	Infancy (Type I/II)	2–5 years

Q36. Discuss orthopedic concerns and management in SMA.

Orthopedic Concerns

- **Scoliosis** (most common deformity)
- Hip dislocation/subluxation
- *Contractures:* Knees, hips, ankles
- **Respiratory compromise** from chest wall deformity
- **Fractures** due to osteopenia

Management Principles

Issue	*Management*
Scoliosis	Spinal orthosis, posterior spinal fusion (early if curve >40°)
Hip instability	Rarely painful → conservative unless painful
Contractures	Passive ROM, splints, soft tissue release if interfering with function
Respiratory care	Assisted cough, BiPAP/NIV support
Nutritional support	Feeding aid or PEG if needed
Fracture prevention	Calcium, Vit D, bisphosphonates if osteoporotic

Q37. Role of orthotics and spinal stabilization in SMA.

(PGI Chandigarh 2017)

Orthotics

- *KAFOs:* Maintain standing in SMA Type II/III
- *AFOs:* Prevent equinus deformity
- *Thoraco-lumbar sacral orthosis (TLSO) brace:* For early scoliosis (Boston/ Milwaukee brace), post-operative support
- *Seating aids:* Improve posture, prevent pressure sores

Spinal Stabilization

- *Indication:* Scoliosis >40–50°, rapid progression, respiratory compromise
- *Procedure:* Posterior spinal instrumentation and fusion
- *Timing:* Ideally before puberty, once pulmonary function >40–50% FVC
- *Improves:* Sitting balance, quality of life, pulmonary outcomes

Q38. Explain the role of tendon transfer in neuromuscular disorders.

Introduction

Tendon transfer is a surgical procedure where the **tendon of a functioning muscle** is **relocated to replace the function of a paralyzed or non-functional muscle.** It plays a vital role in improving function, preventing deformity, and enhancing quality of life in patients with neuromuscular disorders such as **cerebral palsy**, **post-polio residual paralysis**, **brachial plexus injuries**, and **peripheral nerve palsies**.

Principles of Tendon Transfer

- The donor muscle should have **adequate strength** (minimum MRC grade 4).
- The joint to be moved should have a **full passive range of motion.**
- The path of transfer should be **in line with the desired vector of movement.**
- One muscle should perform **one primary function** post-transfer.
- Avoid sacrificing essential muscle functions.

Indications in Neuromuscular Disorders

- Irreversible paralysis due to peripheral nerve injury (e.g., radial nerve palsy)
- Muscle imbalance due to upper motor neuron lesions (e.g., spastic cerebral palsy)
- Flail extremity due to poliomyelitis or brachial plexus injury
- Foot drop or claw hand deformities

Q39. Common neuromuscular disorders and relevant transfers.

Disorder	*Deficit*	*Tendon transfers*
Radial nerve palsy	Wrist and finger extension	PT → ECRB, FCR → EDC, PL → EPL
Ulnar nerve palsy	Clawing of ulnar fingers	FDS → lateral bands (Zancolli lasso)
Median nerve palsy	Thumb opposition	EIP or BR → APB (opponensplasty)
Foot drop (CP or CPN palsy)	Dorsiflexion loss	TP transfer to dorsum of foot (Barr's, Bridle)
Post-polio residual paralysis	Weak quadriceps, dorsiflexors	Gluteus maximus or hamstring transfers
Cerebral palsy	Muscle imbalance causing deformities	Multiple: SPLATT, hamstring lengthening, tibialis anterior transfer, etc.

Benefits of Tendon Transfer

- Restores specific lost function (e.g., opposition, wrist extension)
- Improves independence and ADLs
- Reduces compensatory joint stress and deformities
- Prevents secondary complications (e.g., pressure sores, contractures)

Limitations

- Requires **meticulous preoperative planning**
- Function is not identical to the native muscle
- Post-operative physiotherapy is crucial
- May not benefit in severe spasticity or global limb weakness

Postoperative Rehabilitation

- Splinting (initial immobilization)
- Gradual physiotherapy to **retrain the new muscle action**
- Strengthening and functional integration

Conclusion

Tendon transfer is a valuable reconstructive tool in neuromuscular disorders where irreversible paralysis or muscle imbalance affects limb function. **Proper patient selection, surgical technique, and rehabilitation** are critical for optimal outcomes.

Peripheral Neuropathies

Q40. Define and classify peripheral neuropathies.

(RIMS 2016)

Definition

Peripheral neuropathy refers to a **disorder of the peripheral nervous system**, affecting motor, sensory, or autonomic nerves, leading to weakness, sensory disturbances, and functional disability.

Classification

A. *Based on nerve involvement*:
- *Mononeuropathy:* Single nerve (e.g., common peroneal nerve palsy)
- *Mononeuritis multiplex:* Multiple isolated nerves (e.g., vasculitis)
- *Polyneuropathy:* Generalized, symmetric involvement (e.g., diabetic neuropathy)

B. *Based on type of nerve fibers affected*:
- Motor neuropathy
- Sensory neuropathy
- Autonomic neuropathy
- Mixed

C. *Based on pathology*:
- Axonal degeneration (e.g., metabolic, toxic)
- Demyelination (e.g., Guillain–Barré Syndrome, CMT type 1)

D. *Based on cause*:

Type	*Examples*
Metabolic	Diabetic neuropathy
Toxic	Alcohol, chemotherapy
Hereditary	CMT disease
Infectious	Leprosy, HIV
Autoimmune	Guillain–Barré syndrome
Nutritional	Vitamin B1/B12 deficiency

Q41. Describe clinical features and orthopedic manifestations of diabetic neuropathy.

Clinical Features
- Burning, numbness, tingling in distal limbs (stocking-glove distribution)
- Loss of proprioception and vibration sense
- Decreased reflexes
- Motor weakness in advanced cases
- *Autonomic involvement:* Dry skin, sweating abnormalities

Orthopedic Manifestations
- Charcot neuroarthropathy (midfoot collapse, rocker-bottom foot)
- Foot ulcers (due to pressure points, unnoticed trauma)
- Foot drop (if peroneal nerve involved)
- Instability and falls
- Claw toe deformity due to intrinsic muscle imbalance
- Osteomyelitis following ulcers

Pathophysiology
- Hyperglycemia→ Advanced glycated end-products (AGEs) → Microvascular occlusion

- ↑ Sorbitol accumulation (via aldose reductase) → oxidative stress
- Glycation of nerve proteins
- Demyelination and axonal loss

Types
- Symmetrical polyneuropathy (most common)
- Mononeuropathy (e.g., CN III, femoral nerve)
- Autonomic neuropathy
- Diabetic amyotrophy

Management
- Glycemic control
- *Medications:* Pregabalin, duloxetine, amitriptyline
- Foot care education
- Physiotherapy

Q42. Leprosy neuropathy—pathology, diagnosis, and treatment.

Pathology
- *Mycobacterium leprae* infects Schwann cells → granulomatous inflammation
- Segmental demyelination and fibrosis

Diagnosis
- Nerve thickening (ulnar, common peroneal, greater auricular, posterior tibial)
- Sensory loss before motor
- Skin smear + biopsy
- Nerve conduction studies

Treatment
- *Multidrug therapy (MDT):* Rifampicin + Dapsone ± Clofazimine
- Nerve decompression (in neuritis/entrapment)
- Splints for deformity
- Reconstructive surgery (e.g., claw hand correction)

Q43. Alcoholic neuropathy.

Etiology
- Chronic alcohol use → nutritional deficiency (especially B1, B6, B12)
- Direct toxic effect on nerves

Clinical Features
- Symmetrical distal sensory > motor neuropathy
- Burning feet, numbness, ataxia
- Weakness, especially in lower limbs

Management
- Cessation of alcohol
- Vitamin supplementation (especially B-complex)
- Neuropathic pain medications
- Physiotherapy

Hereditary Neuropathies

Q44. Describe Charcot–Marie–Tooth disease and its orthopedic features.

(Jammu University 2018)

Definition

Charcot–Marie–Tooth (CMT) is a group of **hereditary motor and sensory neuropathies** causing **progressive distal muscle wasting, weakness, and foot deformities**.

Etiology

- Genetic disorder involving *PMP22* gene duplication (most common in CMT1A)
- Inherited in **autosomal dominant**, recessive, or X-linked patterns

Pathophysiology

- Primary demyelination (CMT1) or axonal degeneration (CMT2)
- Leads to distal muscle atrophy and sensory loss

Clinical Features

- *Onset:* Childhood or adolescence
- Distal muscle weakness and atrophy (especially peroneal group)
- Inverted champagne bottle legs
- Pes cavus, claw toes
- Steppage gait or foot drop
- Loss of vibration and proprioception
- Diminished ankle reflexes
- *Hand involvement (late):* Intrinsic wasting, weak grip

Q45. Management of pes cavus in CMT disease.

Goal

Achieve a **plantigrade, braceable**, and pain-free foot to improve gait.

Classification

- *Flexible pes cavus:* Correctable manually
- *Rigid pes cavus:* Fixed deformity

Conservative Management

- Shoe modifications (lateral heel wedge)
- *Orthotics:* Custom insoles, AFOs
- Night splinting and stretching

Surgical Management

Procedure	***Indication***
Soft tissue release (e.g., plantar fascia release)	Mild, flexible deformities
Steindler stripping	Recurrent or mild cavus
Tendon transfer (e.g., peroneus longus to brevis)	Dynamic imbalance
Calcaneal osteotomy (e.g., Dwyer lateral closing wedge)	Hindfoot varus
Midfoot osteotomies (Cole or Japas)	Fixed cavus with forefoot component
Triple arthrodesis	Severe, rigid deformity
Fusion procedures	Adults with arthritis or failure of previous correction

Q46. Discuss surgical correction for claw toes in hereditary sensory motor neuropathy.

Cause

- Imbalance between long toe flexors/extensors and weakened intrinsic muscles
- Hyperextension of MTP joint + flexion of PIP and DIP joints

Surgical Options

Procedure	*Indication*
Extensor to flexor tendon transfer	Flexible claw toe
Capsulotomy and extensor lengthening	Mild to moderate fixed deformity
Flexor to extensor transfer	Dynamic correction
PIP joint arthrodesis	Rigid deformities
MTP joint release or Weil osteotomy	For dorsal dislocation or persistent deformity
Multiple toe procedures	Often combined in a staged or single setting

Post-operative care

- Splinting
- Protective footwear
- Monitoring for recurrence

Rehabilitation and Tendon Transfers

Q47. Discuss principles of rehabilitation in neuromuscular diseases.

(GGMC 2014)

Goals

- Maximize function and independence
- Prevent deformities and contractures
- Maintain joint range and muscle strength

Key Components

- *Physiotherapy:* ROM exercises, muscle strengthening, balance and gait training
- *Orthoses:* AFOs, KAFOs, TLSOs to support posture and gait
- *Assistive devices:* Walkers, wheelchairs, seating aids
- *Occupational therapy:* Training for ADLs and upper limb function
- *Respiratory therapy:* For conditions like DMD and SMA
- Nutritional support and counseling
- Multidisciplinary team involvement (orthopedics, physiotherapy, neurology, rehabilitation)

Q48. Indications and types of tendon transfers in upper and lower limb palsies.

Indications

- Irreversible motor loss (>6–12 months post-injury)
- Adequate donor muscles (MRC ≥ 4)
- Full passive joint mobility
- Clear functional goal (grasp, gait, posture)

Types of Transfers

Upper limb:

- *Radial nerve palsy:* PT → ECRB, FCR → EDC
- *Ulnar nerve palsy:* FDS → lateral bands (Zancolli lasso)
- *Median nerve palsy:* EIP/BR → APB (opponensplasty)

Lower limb
- *Foot drop:* Tibialis posterior → dorsum (Barr's/Bridle)
- *Crouch gait:* Hamstring transfer

SPLATT
Two distinct uses in healthcare and medicine:
- *Split tibialis anterior tendon transfer*:
  - A surgical procedure to correct inturned-foot deformity by splitting the tibialis anterior tendon and re-routing part of it to improve foot alignment
  - Common in children with cerebral palsy or adults with certain spastic conditions, with generally positive outcomes (about 83% success in one study)

Q49. Pre-operative assessment before tendon transfer.

Checklist

Parameter	*Assessment*
Donor muscle strength	MRC grade ≥ 4
Joint mobility	Full passive range
Fixed deformity	Must be corrected pre-operative
Sensory status	Sensate limb preferred
Overall limb function	Evaluate compensatory muscle activity
Patient understanding	Realistic expectations, rehabilitation commitment

Q50. Discuss the bridle procedure for foot drop.

Indication
Foot drop due to common peroneal nerve palsy.

Procedure
- *Tibialis posterior (TP) tendon is split*:
  - One slip to **tibialis anterior**
  - One to **extensor hallucis longus (EHL)**
  - One to **extensor digitorum longus (EDL)**
- Performed through interosseous membrane

Goal
Restore **balanced dorsiflexion** and **prevent inversion deformity**

Post-operative
Splinting and physiotherapy to retrain dorsiflexion.

Q51. Outline common tendon transfers for radial nerve palsy.

Brand's Transfer (Most Accepted)

Function	*Donor*	*Recipient*
Wrist extension	Pronator teres (PT)	Extensor carpi radialis brevis (ECRB)
MCP extension	Flexor carpi radialis (FCR)	Extensor digitorum communis (EDC)
Thumb extension	Palmaris longus (PL)	Extensor pollicis longus (EPL)

Alternatives
- Flexor digitorum superficialis (FDS) to EDC (Boyes' transfer)
- Flexor carpi ulnaris (FCU) to EDC (Jones transfer)

Principles
- Restore one function per transfer
- Avoid deforming forces

Q52. Describe Zancolli lasso procedure.

Indication

Claw hand deformity in **ulnar nerve palsy**.

Procedure
- FDS tendon of ring finger is split and looped around the **A1 pulley** of the MCP joint
- Acts as a **static tenodesis** to **flex the MCP joint**, allowing IP extension

Goal

Correct clawing by restoring balance between long extensors and weak intrinsic muscles of the hand.

Advantages
- Reliable, preserves FDS function partially
- Can be done bilaterally

Recent Advances

Q53. Role of stem cell therapy in neuromuscular disorders.

Principle
- Stem cells, particularly **mesenchymal stem cells (MSCs)** or **induced pluripotent stem cells (iPSCs)**, offer regenerative potential via:
    - Differentiation into myogenic or neuronal cells
    - Secretion of **neurotrophic and anti-inflammatory cytokines**
    - **Paracrine signaling** to promote nerve and muscle repair

Applications
- *Spinal muscular atrophy (SMA):* Ongoing trials
- *Duchenne muscular dystrophy:* Myogenic stem cell infusion to delay degeneration
- *Peripheral nerve injury:* Stem-cell seeded conduits to promote axonal regrowth

Challenges
- Ethical concerns (especially embryonic cells)
- Delivery mechanism and survival in host tissue
- Risk of tumor formation
- Limited clinical translation so far

Current Status
- Promising in animal models
- Human trials are in phase I/II for selected conditions

Q54. Artificial nerve conduits in nerve regeneration.

Definition

Tubular structures used to bridge nerve gaps **when direct repair or autograft is not feasible**.

Types

Type	Examples
Biological	Vein grafts, collagen, chitosan
Synthetic	Silicone, polyglycolic acid (PGA), polycaprolactone
Hybrid	Scaffold + Schwann cells or stem cells

Advantages
- Avoid donor site morbidity
- Guide regenerating axons
- Option for short gaps (<3 cm)

Limitations
- Not ideal for **motor nerves** or long defects
- Risk of inflammation or fibrosis (especially synthetic)
- Slower regeneration versus autograft

Indications
Small-caliber sensory nerve gaps (e.g., digital nerves).

Q55. Functional electrical stimulation (FES) in rehabilitation.

Definition
Use of low-level electrical currents to **stimulate muscle contraction** in paralyzed muscles, coordinated with movement.

Mechanism
- Stimulates peripheral nerves via surface or implanted electrodes
- Promotes functional movement and prevents atrophy

Applications in Neuromuscular Disorders

Condition	Benefit
Foot drop (CMT, stroke)	Stimulates dorsiflexors to improve gait
Spinal cord injury	Trunk/bowel/bladder control, hand grasp
Post-polio paralysis	Prevents disuse atrophy
CP	Improve gait and coordination

Advantages
- Enhances neuroplasticity
- Improves strength and ROM
- Promotes motor relearning

Limitations
- Requires patient cooperation and training
- May be uncomfortable

Q56. Short notes and viva-oriented topics.

The Gross Motor Function Classification System (GMFCS)
Classifies gross motor ability in CP (Levels I–V).

Level	Description
I	Walks without limitations
II	Walks with limitations

Continued

Continued

Level	Description
III	Walks using assistive device
IV	Limited self-mobility, uses wheelchair
V	Dependent mobility, needs full assistance

Q57. Ashworth scale for spasticity.

Grade	Description
0	No increase in tone
1	Slight increase, catch and release
1+	Slight increase, catch + minimal resistance
2	Marked increase through most of ROM
3	Considerable increase, passive movement difficult
4	Rigid in flexion/extension

Q58. Vulpius gastrocsoleus recession.

- For **spastic equinus contracture**
- Lengthens **gastroc-soleus aponeurosis**
- Less risk of over-lengthening than Achilles Z-lengthening

Q59. Tibialis posterior transfer.

- Indicated in **foot drop (CPN palsy)**
- Routed through **interosseous membrane** to dorsum of foot
- Helps restore active dorsiflexion

Q60. Obturator nerve block in CP.

- Used to reduce **hip adductor spasticity**
- Indicated in **scissoring gait** or pain
- Temporary diagnostic/therapeutic step before adductor surgery

Q61. Scissoring gait.

- **Seen in spastic diplegia** (CP)
- Characterized by **hip adduction and internal rotation**
- Legs cross over during swing phase due to **hyperactive adductors**
- Treated with **adductor release**, botulinum, physiotherapy

Q62. Clinical features of 'Crouch Gait' and its management.

Clinical Features

- Excessive **hip and knee flexion**
- **Ankle dorsiflexion** during stance
- Increased **energy expenditure**
- Common in **ambulatory CP patients (GMFCS II–III)**
- May develop after **over-lengthening** of Achilles or tight hamstrings

Management
- *Conservative:* AFOs (ground-reaction), strengthening, stretching
- *Surgical:*
  - Hamstring lengthening
  - Rectus femoris transfer
  - Distal femoral extension osteotomy (DFEO)
  - Patellar advancement
  - Multilevel surgery if needed

Q63. Crouch gait versus jump gait.

Feature	*Crouch gait*	*Jump gait*
Hip	Flexed	Flexed
Knee	Excessively flexed	Flexed
Ankle	Dorsiflexed	Equinus
Common in	Older ambulatory CP child	Younger diplegic CP child
Management	DFEO, hamstring lengthening	Gastrocnemius recession, orthotics

Expensive and device-dependent

Q64. Differentiate between spasticity and rigidity. Pharmacological management of spasticity in CP.

(KMC Manipal 2013)

Feature	*Spasticity*	*Rigidity*
Tone	Velocity-dependent ↑	Uniform ↑ (not velocity-dependent)
Reflexes	Hyperreflexia	Normal or ↓
Clasp knife	Present	Absent (lead-pipe/cogwheel)

Pharmacological Options for Spasticity in CP
- *Oral agents:* Baclofen, diazepam, tizanidine, dantrolene
- Botulinum toxin injections
- Intrathecal baclofen pump (for severe generalized spasticity)

Additional Questions – Neuromuscular Disorders in Orthopedics

Q65. Define torticollis. Signs and symptoms of congenital torticollis in a 9-year-old child.

Definition
Torticollis: **Abnormal head tilt and neck rotation** due to contracture of **sternocleidomastoid (SCM)**.

Congenital Torticollis
- Due to **fibrosis or contracture** of SCM
- May be associated with birth trauma or intrauterine positioning

Signs in a 9-year-old
- Head tilted to one side (typically **toward affected SCM**)
- Chin rotated to opposite side
- Palpable mass/fibrotic band (may not be prominent at this age)
- Facial asymmetry, plagiocephaly
- Restricted passive ROM of neck

Q66. Management of spasmodic torticollis in a child.

Definition

Also called **cervical dystonia**—involuntary, sustained contraction of neck muscles.

Management

- *Conservative:*
  - Physiotherapy and stretching
  - Botox injections (SCM, trapezius)
  - Sensory trick training (gestes antagonistes)
- *Surgical (if severe/refractory)*:
  - Selective peripheral denervation
  - Myectomy or release of SCM/trapezius
- *Medications:*
  - Anticholinergics (trihexyphenidyl)
  - Baclofen
  - Benzodiazepines (e.g., clonazepam)

Q67. Fibromyalgia.

Definition

A **chronic pain syndrome** characterized by **widespread musculoskeletal pain** with **tender points**, **fatigue**, and **sleep disturbance**.

Diagnostic Criteria (ACR)

- Widespread pain index (WPI) + symptom severity (SS) score
- Symptoms >3 months
- No other disorder explaining the pain

Features

- Multiple tender points
- Chronic fatigue
- Sleep disturbance
- Anxiety, depression
- Normal labs

Management

- Patient education and reassurance
- Aerobic and strengthening exercises
- Cognitive behavioral therapy (CBT)
- *Medications:*
  - Tricyclic Antidepressants (amitriptyline)
  - Serotonin-norepinephrine reuptake inhibitors (SNRIs)—duloxetine
  - Pregabalin

CHAPTER 10

Pediatric Orthopedics

10.1 Congenital and Developmental Disorders

Rashid Anjum, Kamal Ji Pandit, Kanav Mahajan

Q1. Differences between pediatric and adult bones.

Feature	*Pediatric bone*	*Adult bone*
Composition	More collagen, less mineral	More mineralized
Periosteum	Thicker, more osteogenic	Thinner
Growth plates	Present (physis)	Absent
Healing	Rapid due to high vascularity	Slower
Fracture patterns	Greenstick, torus, plastic deformation	Complete/complex fractures

Q2. Remodeling in children's bones.

Definition

Ability of growing bones to correct angulation over time.

Best In

- Younger children
- Near physis
- In plane of motion

Clinical Implication

Minor angulations often **do not need surgical correction**.

Q3. Physiological and pathological bowing of legs in children.

Physiological Bowing

- **Genu varum** (bow legs) → common till 18–24 months
- Transitions to **genu valgum** (~3–5 years)
- Symmetrical, painless, resolves with age

Pathological Bowing

- Asymmetric, worsening, or persistent beyond normal age

- *Causes*:
  - **Blount disease**
  - **Rickets**
  - Post-traumatic physeal injury

Hip Disorders

Developmental Dysplasia of the Hip (DDH)

Q4. Definition, etiology, classification, and risk factors of DDH.

(Asked in: AIIMS Delhi 2022, PGI Chandigarh 2021)

Definition

A spectrum of developmental abnormalities ranging from **shallow acetabulum to complete dislocation** of the femoral head from the acetabulum.

Etiology

- *Multifactorial*:
  - Mechanical (breech, oligohydramnios)
  - Genetic predisposition
  - Hormonal (maternal relaxin)
  - Positional (tight swaddling)

Risk Factors

- Female (4:1)
- Breech presentation
- Family history
- First-born child
- Associated conditions (torticollis, metatarsus adductus)

Classification (Tönnis, IHDI)

- Subluxable
- Dislocatable
- Dislocated, reducible
- Dislocated, irreducible

Q5. Clinical and radiological evaluation of DDH.

Clinical Tests (Birth to 3 Months)

- *Barlow test*: Dislocate a dislocatable hip
- *Ortolani test*: Reduce a dislocated hip
- *Galeazzi sign*: Shortened thigh (older infants)
- Asymmetric thigh/gluteal folds, limited abduction

Radiological Evaluation

- *Ultrasound (best before 6 months)*: Graf's method → α and β angles
- *X-ray (after 6 months)*:
  - Shenton's line interruption
  - Hilgenreiner's and Perkin's lines
  - Acetabular index (>30° is abnormal)

Q6. Management of DDH at different age groups.

Age	*Management strategy*
0–6 months	Pavlik harness (if reducible)
6–18 months	Closed reduction + hip spica ± adductor tenotomy
18 months–3 years	Open reduction + pelvic osteotomy ± femoral shortening
>3 years	Open reduction + femoral and/or acetabular osteotomy

- Early detection → non-surgical treatment success is high
- Late diagnosis → often requires surgery

Q7. Role of Pavlik Harness and surgical options in DDH.

(Asked in: MUHS Maharashtra 2022, RGUHS Karnataka 2022)

Management Based on Age

A. Newborn to 6 months

Pavlik Harness:
- Dynamic abduction orthosis maintaining hip in flexion and abduction.
- Allows reduction of hip and promotes acetabular development.
- Duration: 6–12 weeks
- *Success rate*: ~90%

B. 6–18 months

Closed Reduction + Hip Spica:
- Under anesthsia, gentle closed reduction.
- Confirmed by arthrogram.
- Hip maintained in flexion-abduction spica cast for 3 months.

C. >18 months or Failed Closed Reduction

Open Reduction:
- Surgical exposure and reduction of femoral head into acetabulum.
- Indicated if soft tissue obstacles prevent closed reduction.

D. >2–3 years or Residual Dysplasia

Osteotomies:
- Femoral shortening osteotomy (decrease tension for reduction)
- Pelvic osteotomy (Salter's, Pemberton's, Dega osteotomy) to improve acetabular coverage.

E. >6 years
- Salvage procedures only (pelvic/femoral osteotomies)
- Higher risk of poor outcomes.

Key Points in Pavlik Harness Use
- Hip flexion at 90–100°, abduction ~45°.
- Weekly ultrasound monitoring.
- *Complications*:
  - Avascular necrosis (if excessive abduction)
  - Femoral nerve palsy

Q8. Complications of untreated DDH.

- Hip instability or dislocation in walking age
- Limb length discrepancy

- Limited abduction and waddling gait
- Early osteoarthritis (secondary OA)
- Pelvic obliquity, scoliosis

Q9. Indications and techniques of surgical management in DDH.

Indications
- Failure of conservative treatment
- Age >6–12 months with dislocation
- Irreducible dislocation
- Residual acetabular dysplasia

Techniques
1. Open reduction (anterior approach—Smith–Peterson)
2. Femoral shortening osteotomy (to reduce tension on femoral head)
3. *Acetabular procedures*:
   - Salter osteotomy (for redirecting acetabulum)
   - Pemberton, Dega osteotomy (for better coverage)
   - Chiari osteotomy (for older children)

Q10. Role of ultrasonography in DDH diagnosis.

- Gold standard <**6 months age**
- No radiation
- *Detects*:
  - Cartilaginous femoral head
  - Acetabular development
  - Hip stability

Graf Classification
- *Type I*: Normal
- *Type IIa*: Immature (<3 months)
- *Type IIb+*: Pathological
- *Type III/IV*: Dislocated

Used for both diagnosis and follow-up during harness treatment

Q11. Open reduction and osteotomies in DDH.

Open Reduction
- For **irreducible dislocations** or failed closed reduction
- Removes soft-tissue blocks (ligamentum teres, pulvinar, transverse ligament)
- Achieve concentric reduction under vision

Osteotomies
- *Femoral shortening osteotomy*: Prevents excessive tension
- *Pelvic osteotomies*:
  - *Salter*: Anterior redirection
  - *Pemberton*: Incomplete transiliac—reshapes acetabulum
  - *Dega*: For severe dysplasia
  - *Chiari*: Last resort in adolescents

Q12. Discuss Salter's osteotomy and its indications in pediatric hip disorders.

Definition

A **single innominate pelvic osteotomy** that redirects the acetabulum to improve anterolateral coverage of the femoral head

Indications

- Developmental Dysplasia of the Hip (DDH) in children **18 months to 6 years**
- Perthes disease (select cases with hinge abduction)
- Residual hip dysplasia after closed/open reduction

Principle

- Hinges at **pubic symphysis**
- Maintains **acetabular shape** and joint congruity

Procedure

- Oblique cut from sciatic notch to anterior inferior iliac spine
- Acetabulum tilted down and out
- Graft inserted to maintain position

Q13. Screening protocols for neonatal hip instability (short note).

Clinical Tests

- Barlow's test (dislocatable hip)
- Ortolani's test (reducible hip)
- Galeazzi sign (limb length discrepancy)
- Asymmetric thigh/gluteal folds

Imaging

- *Ultrasound*: Gold standard before 6 months (Graf method)
- *X-ray*: Useful after 4–6 months (once ossification appears)

Screening Strategy

- Universal clinical exam at birth, 6 weeks
- *Targeted USG at 6 weeks for*:
    - Breech
    - Family history
    - Positive Barlow/Ortolani

Q14. Perthes disease (idiopathic avascular necrosis of femoral head in children)—pathology, clinical features, and treatment.

(Asked in: PGI Chandigarh 2022, MUHS Maharashtra 2022)

Definition

Legg-Calvé-Perthes disease is **idiopathic avascular necrosis of the femoral head epiphysis** in children, typically between **4–10 years**.

Pathophysiology

1. Interruption of blood supply (likely to lateral epiphyseal artery)
2. Ischemic necrosis of the femoral head
3. Resorption and fragmentation
4. Reossification and remodeling

Result

Collapse and deformity of femoral head if not managed properly → early-onset osteoarthritis

Q15. Clinical stages and radiological findings of Perthes disease.

Clinical Stages

1. *Initial/Ischemic*: Hip pain, limp, restricted ROM
2. *Fragmentation*: Collapse of epiphysis
3. *Reossification*: New bone formation
4. *Healing*: Remodeling of femoral head

Radiological Stages (Waldenström classification)

1. *Initial*: Joint space widening, small ossific nucleus
2. *Fragmentation*: Irregular density, epiphyseal fragmentation
3. *Reossification*: New bone appears
4. *Healing*: Spherical or deformed head

MRI detects early ischemia before X-ray

Classification Systems in Perthes Disease

Q16. Catterall and herring classification systems.

(Asked in: AIIMS Delhi 2021)

Catterall Classification (Based on extent of Epiphyseal Involvement)

- *Group I*: Involvement of anterior part only.
- *Group II*: Less than 50% involvement.
- *Group III*: 50–75% involvement.
- *Group IV*: Entire epiphysis involved.

Herring (Lateral Pillar) Classification

- *Group A*: No loss of height of lateral pillar.
- *Group B*: <50% loss of height of lateral pillar.
- *Group C*: >50% loss of height of lateral pillar.

Clinical Relevance

Herring classification correlates better with prognosis and guides treatment decisions.

Q17. Non-surgical and surgical treatment options.

Non-surgical (Preferred in <6 Years with Good Head Sphericity)

- **Activity restriction**
- NSAIDs for pain
- Physiotherapy to maintain ROM
- **Abduction braces** (e.g., Scottish Rite)

Surgical (for >6 Years, Catterall III/IV or Herring B/C)

- *Femoral varus osteotomy*: redirects head into acetabulum
- *Salter innominate osteotomy*: improves acetabular coverage
- Shelf or Chiari osteotomy (rarely)

Q18. Prognosis and complications of Perthes disease.

Prognostic Factors

- *Age*: <6 years = better prognosis
- *Extent*: Less epiphyseal involvement = better
- *Head containment*: Maintained = better remodeling

Complications
- Femoral head flattening/deformity
- Leg length discrepancy
- Hip stiffness
- Premature osteoarthritis

Q19. Containment principle in Perthes disease.

Definition
Treatment strategy aimed at **keeping the femoral head within the acetabulum** to allow:
- Proper remodeling
- Prevention of flattening
- Better long-term outcomes

Methods of Containment
- *Non-operative*: Abduction orthosis (e.g., Scottish Rite)
- *Surgical*:
  - Femoral varus osteotomy
  - Salter pelvic osteotomy

Goal
Maximize **joint congruity** and preserve **hip function**.

Slipped Capital Femoral Epiphysis (SCFE)

Q20. What is SCFE? Pathophysiology and risk factors.

(Asked in: JIPMER Puducherry 2023, BHU Varanasi 2022)

Definition
Slipped capital femoral epiphysis (SCFE) is a **posteroinferior displacement of the proximal femoral epiphysis** relative to the femoral neck through the growth plate (physis), seen in adolescents.

Pathophysiology
- Weakening of the hypertrophic zone of physis due to hormonal or mechanical factors
- Shear forces → **epiphyseal slippage**
- Most common in **adolescents (10–16 years)**

Risk Factors
- Obesity
- Male gender
- Pubertal growth spurt
- Endocrine disorders (hypothyroidism, GH deficiency)
- Down syndrome
- Renal osteodystrophy
- Family history

Q21. Classification of SCFE and clinical implications.

Based on stability (Loder's classification)
- *Stable*: Able to walk (even with crutches) → lower AVN risk
- *Unstable*: Cannot bear weight → ↑ risk of AVN (~50%)

Based on duration
- *Acute*: <3 weeks
- *Chronic*: >3 weeks
- *Acute-on-chronic*: Acute worsening of pre-existing chronic slip

Based on severity (Southwick angle)
- *Mild*: <30°
- *Moderate*: 30–50°
- *Severe*: >50°

Classification guides treatment strategy and prognosis.

Q22. Clinical and radiological diagnosis of SCFE.

Clinical Features
- Limping adolescent
- Thigh/knee pain (referred)
- Limited **internal rotation and abduction**
- *Drehmann's sign*: ER and flexion during passive hip flexion

Radiology
- *X-ray: AP + frog-leg lateral view*:
  - Widened physis, displacement of epiphysis
  - **Klein's line** (line along superior femoral neck doesn't intersect epiphysis in SCFE)
- *Southwick angle*: Measured on frog-leg view to grade severity

Q23. Management options and indications.

Type of SCFE	*Treatment*
Stable, mild–mod.	In-situ fixation with a single cannulated screw
Unstable SCFE	Gentle reduction + fixation (risk of AVN)
Severe SCFE	Subcapital or modified Dunn osteotomy
Bilateral cases	Contralateral prophylactic pinning (in select cases)

Post-operative
Non-weight-bearing initially, gradual progression

Q24. Complications of SCFE.

- **Avascular necrosis (AVN)**
- **Chondrolysis** (joint cartilage damage → stiffness)
- Leg length discrepancy
- **Femoroacetabular impingement (FAI)**
- Early osteoarthritis
- Screw penetration or migration

Q25. Role of prophylactic fixation in SCFE.

Rationale
High risk of **bilateral involvement** (up to 80% in endocrine cases)

Indications
- Endocrinopathies (e.g., hypothyroidism)
- Contralateral symptoms or abnormal radiographs
- Very young age (<10 years)
- Severe unilateral slip

Benefits
- Prevents contralateral slippage
- Reduces long-term morbidity

Risks
- Surgical complications (infection, hardware issues)
- Potential physeal arrest → leg length discrepancy

Q26. Southwick angle and its importance.

(Asked in: PGI Chandigarh 2022)

Definition
The difference between the slip side and the normal side measured on a frog-leg lateral radiograph.

Importance
- Quantifies severity of slip
- Guides treatment decision (mild/moderate → in situ pinning; severe → corrective osteotomy)
- Assesses prognosis (greater the angle, poorer the outcome).

Exam Tip
When answering SCFE:
- Highlight posterior-inferior slippage of femoral epiphysis.
- Always mention Klein's line and Southwick angle for diagnosis.
- Treatment—surgical for all cases (even stable ones).

Q27. Congenital coxa vara—etiology, clinical features, and management.

Definition
A condition where the **neck-shaft angle is <120°** at birth or early childhood.

Etiology
- *Primary (congenital)*: Idiopathic defect in endochondral ossification of femoral neck
- *Secondary*: Trauma, infection, rickets, or metabolic bone diseases

Clinical Features
- Painless **limp**
- **Shortening** of limb
- Restricted **abduction and internal rotation**
- Positive **Trendelenburg sign**

Radiology
- Decreased neck-shaft angle
- Vertical physis
- Inverted-Y appearance

Management
- *Mild (neck-shaft angle >110°)*: Observation
- *Progressive/angle <110°*: **Valgus subtrochanteric osteotomy**

Q28. Increased femoral anteversion.

- Normal = ~15°; ↑ = >30° (seen in toddlers)
- Presents as **in-toeing gait**, W-sitting

Treatment
- Observation—most cases improve by age 8
- *Derotation osteotomy if*:
    - 3 SDs from normal
    - 10–12 years
    - Cosmetic/Functional issues

Clubfoot (Congenital Talipes Equinovarus—CTEV)

Q29. Clinical features, pathoanatomy, and management of CTEV.

(Asked in AIIMS Delhi 2022, PGI Chandigarh 2021)

Definition

CTEV (commonly called "clubfoot") is a **complex congenital deformity** of the foot characterized by **four classical components**:
- *C*avus (high medial arch)
- *A*dduction of forefoot
- *V*arus of hindfoot
- *E*quinus at ankle

Clinical Features
- Birth deformity (may be unilateral or bilateral).
- **The foot is inverted, adducted, and plantarflexed.**
- Tight achilles tendon.
- Medial and posterior skin creases.
- Smaller and shorter foot compared to normal.
- Calf muscle atrophy may be observed.
- In severe cases, walking occurs on lateral foot border ("walking on outer edge").

Pathoanatomy
- *Bone changes*:
    - Talus is small, medially rotated, and plantarflexed.
    - Calcaneus is in equinus and varus position.
- *Soft tissue contractures*:
    - *Tightened structures*: Posteromedial ligaments (deltoid ligament, spring ligament), Achilles tendon, tibialis posterior tendon.
- *Muscle imbalance*:
    - Weak peroneal muscles.
    - Overactive tibialis posterior and Achilles tendon.

Management

A. *Non-surgical methods*:
- *Ponseti method (Gold standard)*:
    - Serial manipulation and casting.
    - Percutaneous achilles tenotomy (if residual equinus).
- *French functional method*: Daily stretching, taping, and splinting (less commonly used today).

B. *Surgical methods*:
- *Soft tissue release (posteromedial release)*: Done if non-operative methods fail.
- *Bony procedures*: Osteotomies or triple arthrodesis (for neglected or relapsed cases).

Golden Rule
Early diagnosis and treatment are critical—**birth to 2 weeks** is ideal starting time!

Q30. Describe the ponseti method for CTEV correction.

(Asked in MUHS Maharashtra 2022, JIPMER Puducherry 2022)

Introduction
The Ponseti method is a **gentle, sequential manipulation and casting technique** to correct CTEV deformity non-surgically.

Steps in Ponseti Method
1. *Correction sequence (CAVE order)*:
   - First correct **cavus** (supinate forefoot and align first metatarsal).
   - Then correct **adduction** and **varus** simultaneously by abducting foot while stabilizing talus.
   - Finally correct **equinus** by dorsiflexing foot (after Achilles tendon release if needed).
2. *Serial casting:*
   - Weekly manipulation followed by plaster cast application.
   - 5–8 casts usually sufficient.
3. *Percutaneous achilles tenotomy*: Indicated in >80% cases to correct residual equinus.
4. *Bracing phase*:
   - Use of foot abduction brace (Dennis–Browne splint).
   - Full-time for 3 months, then night-time till 3–4 years of age.

Advantages of Ponseti Method
- High success rate (>90% if started early).
- Minimally invasive.
- Reduces need for extensive surgeries.

Common Mistakes to Avoid
- *Incorrect technique*: Manipulation must be gentle and specific.
- Skipping bracing phase → High relapse risk.

Mnemonic for Steps
"CAVE + CAST + TENOTOMY + BRACE"

Quick Tips for Theory/Viva
- Always describe the **four components** of deformity first (CAVE).
- For management, always say "**Ponseti is first-line**; surgery reserved only for resistant or relapsed cases."
- For Ponseti method, **highlight manipulation sequence clearly** (correct cavus first, equinus last).

Q31. Kite's method versus Ponseti method.

Feature	*Kite's method*	*Ponseti method*
Principle	Abduction around talus	Abduction around head of talus
Order of correction	Equinus corrected early	Equinus corrected last
Cast interval	Longer intervals	Weekly
Outcome	Higher recurrence, overcorrection	Higher success, minimal relapse

Ponseti is now the gold standard worldwide.

Q32. Surgical options for clubfoot.

Indicated when conservative management fails (e.g., in **neglected or resistant cases**)

Age/Indication	*Surgery*
6–12 months	Posteromedial soft-tissue release
>2 years/relapse	Medial soft-tissue release + tendon transfers (e.g., tibialis anterior transfer)
Severe deformity	Talectomy, triple arthrodesis (in older children/adults)
Resistant deformity	Ilizarov correction (gradual correction in complex or rigid clubfoot)

Q33. Indications for percutaneous achilles tenotomy.

- Equinus **not corrected** after full correction of cavus, adduction, varus using Ponseti
- **Dorsiflexion <10–15°** after serial casting
- Usually done around **6–8 weeks of age** after 4–6 casts

Outpatient procedure, followed by 3-week cast, then bracing.

Q34. Complications of untreated clubfoot.

- Fixed deformity
- Callosities over lateral border
- Painful gait and limb shortening
- Psychosocial issues
- Degenerative arthritis
- Inability to wear normal footwear

Functionally and socially disabling if untreated

Q35. Recurrence and relapse management in clubfoot.

Causes
- Poor brace compliance
- Incomplete correction
- Syndromic association (e.g., arthrogryposis)

Management
- *Mild*: Repeat Ponseti protocol
- *Moderate*: Re-casting + possible tenotomy
- *Severe/stiff*: Surgical intervention (tendon transfer, posteromedial release)

Long-term bracing (till 4–5 years) essential to prevent recurrence

Q36. Idiopathic versus syndromic clubfoot—short note.

Feature	*Idiopathic clubfoot*	*Syndromic clubfoot*
Cause	Unknown	Part of systemic condition (e.g., spina bifida)
Severity	Moderate to severe	Often rigid, resistant
Response to Ponseti	Good	Poor; often needs surgery
Associated anomalies	Rare	Common (e.g., neurogenic, arthrogryposis)

Syndromic clubfoot requires multidisciplinary approach.

Q37. Pirani versus dimeglio scoring systems in CTEV.

Parameter	*Pirani score*	*Dimeglio score*
Introduced	Pirani, 1999	Dimeglio, 1995
Basis	Six clinical signs (three midfoot, three hindfoot)	Four deformities + reducibility
Scoring	0–6	0–20
Use	Monitoring treatment (Ponseti)	Initial assessment and grading severity
Simplicity	Easy and quick	More comprehensive

Summary

- *Pirani*: Useful for serial evaluation, predicting need for tenotomy
- *Dimeglio*: Better for pre-treatment severity classification

Q38. Management of resistant or relapsed clubfoot in older children.

Causes

- Poor compliance with bracing
- Syndromic clubfoot
- Inadequate casting or surgical scarring

Treatment

- Repeat ponseti method (modified)
- Soft tissue release (PMR)
- *Osteotomies*:
    - Dwyer (lateral closing wedge)
    - Medial cuneiform opening wedge
- **Tibialis anterior transfer** (for dynamic supination)
- **Ilizarov** for multiplanar correction

Q39. Parts of a shoe and CTEV modifications.

Parts of a Shoe

- *Upper*: Vamp, quarter
- *Sole*: Insole, midsole, outsole
- Heel
- Toe box
- *Shank*: Provides rigidity to midfoot
- *Counter*: Reinforces heel

CTEV Shoe Modifications

- Straight medial border to prevent forefoot adduction
- Lateral flare to prevent inversion
- Stiff heel counter to control heel
- Thomas heel (medial extension of heel)
- Abduction bar used in Denis–Browne splint for maintenance after correction

Flatfoot and Cavus Foot

Q40. Congenital vertical talus—etiology, classification, and management.

Definition

A rare rigid foot deformity where the **talus is vertically oriented** and the navicular is dorsally dislocated—aka "**rocker bottom foot.**"

Etiology

- Idiopathic (isolated cases)
- *Syndromic*: **Arthrogryposis, myelomeningocele**, DiGeorge, trisomy 18
- Neuromuscular causes

Classification

- **Isolated** versus **syndromic**
- **Rigid** (true vertical talus) versus **oblique talus** (navicular not fully dislocated)

Management

- *Initial*: Serial casting (reverse Ponseti—dorsiflexion and inversion)
- *Definitive (usually after 6–9 months age)*:
    - Open reduction of talonavicular joint
    - K-wire fixation + soft tissue release
    - Recent advances: Minimally invasive correction + percutaneous pinning

Q41. Difference between congenital vertical talus and oblique talus.

Feature	***Vertical talus***	***Oblique talus***
Talonavicular joint	Irreducible dislocation	Reducible
Lateral view (forced plantarflexion)	Talar axis and first metatarsal non-aligned	Become aligned
Rigidity	Rigid	Semi-flexible
Associated conditions	Arthrogryposis, myelomeningocele	Often idiopathic
Treatment	Serial casting + surgery	Often resolves, observe

Q42. Flexible versus rigid flatfoot—diagnosis and management.

Parameter	***Flexible flatfoot***	***Rigid flatfoot***
Arch on standing	Absent	Absent
Arch on tiptoe	Restores (positive "Jack test")	Does not restore
Symptoms	Usually asymptomatic	Pain, stiffness
Cause	Physiological, ligamentous laxity	Tarsal coalition, vertical talus

Management

- *Flexible*:
    - Reassurance (normal variant)
    - **Orthotics** if symptomatic (medial arch support)
    - Stretching for tight Achilles
- *Rigid*:
    - Evaluate for **tarsal coalition** (CT/MRI)
    - *Initial*: Activity modification, orthotics
    - *Surgery*: Coalition resection ± subtalar fusion if refractory

Q43. Outline the differences between congenital and acquired flatfoot and their management.

Feature	***Congenital flatfoot***	***Acquired flatfoot***
Onset	Present at birth	Later in childhood/adolescence
Type	Rigid (e.g., vertical talus, tarsal coalition)	Flexible (often physiologic), or rigid in late stages
Arch	Absent, rigid	Often present during non-weight bearing

Continued

Continued

Feature	*Congenital flatfoot*	*Acquired flatfoot*
Hindfoot	Fixed valgus	Flexible or progressive valgus
Pain	Often painful early	Becomes painful with progression
Associated anomalies	Yes (neuromuscular, syndromic)	Often none
Radiographs	Abnormal talar positioning	Normal in flexible type
Management	Early casting, surgery	Conservative (orthoses), surgery if symptomatic

Management
- *Congenital (e.g., vertical talus)*: Serial casting, surgical release (open reduction of talonavicular joint)
- *Acquired (flexible)*: Observation, arch supports
- *Acquired (rigid/painful)*: Orthoses, corrective osteotomies (e.g., calcaneal lengthening), arthrodesis in adolescents/adults

Q44. Role of orthotics in pediatric flatfoot.

Indications
- Symptomatic flexible flatfoot
- Pain or fatigue with prolonged walking
- Shoe wear issues or instability

Types of Orthotics
- Medial arch support
- Heel cups for valgus correction
- Custom-molded orthotics for neuromuscular cases

Note: Orthotics **do not correct deformity**, but relieve symptoms and improve function

Q45. Causes and treatment of cavus foot in children.

Definition
A high medial longitudinal arch with **hindfoot varus** and **forefoot equinus** (often a neuromuscular etiology).

Causes
- Idiopathic
- *Neurological*:
  - Charcot–Marie–Tooth (CMT) disease
  - Spinal dysraphism
  - Polio, cerebral palsy, Friedrich's ataxia
- Post-traumatic

Treatment
- *Flexible cavus*: Observation ± orthotics
- *Fixed/mild*: Stretching, custom orthoses
- *Severe/rigid*:
  - Soft tissue releases (plantar fascia, Achilles)
  - *Osteotomies*: Dwyer calcaneal, midfoot
  - *Tendon transfers*: Peroneus longus → brevis
  - Triple arthrodesis (end-stage cases)

Q46. Neurological causes of cavus foot.

Cavus foot is often a sign of underlying **neuromuscular disease**.

Common Neurological Causes

Condition	*Key features*
Charcot–Marie–Tooth	Bilateral cavovarus, claw toes, steppage gait
Friedreich's ataxia	Sensory ataxia, scoliosis, cavus foot
Poliomyelitis	Asymmetric cavus deformity due to motor loss
Spinal cord tumor/dysraphism	Segmental weakness, cavus, neuro signs
Cerebral palsy (rare)	May cause spastic cavus

Evaluation

- **Neurological exam**, EMG/NCS
- MRI spine if red flags
- Genetic testing (e.g., for CMT)

Q47. Metatarsus adductus—differentiation from clubfoot.

Metatarsus Adductus (MTA)

- Medial deviation of forefoot
- Normal hindfoot
- Flexible
- Common in infants

Clubfoot (CTEV)

- Forefoot adduction + hindfoot equinus + varus
- Rigid
- Requires serial casting

Feature	*MTA*	*Clubfoot*
Heel	Normal	Equinus and varus
Forefoot	Adducted	Adducted
Flexibility	Often flexible	Rigid
Treatment	Stretching ± shoes	Ponseti method (casting + tenotomy)

Q48. Calcaneovalgus foot.

- Common neonatal deformity where foot is dorsiflexed and everted
- *Cause*: Intrauterine positioning
- **Usually flexible**

Treatment

- **Stretching + observation**
- *Rigid/refractory*: Serial casting
- Surgery rare (tendon transfer)

Q49. Idiopathic toe walking.

- Children >2 years who **walk on toes** without neurological or orthopedic cause
- Normal neuro exam; no tight Achilles in early stage

Treatment

- Observation (most resolve by 5 years)
- Heel cord stretching
- Serial casting or Botox
- Surgery (gastrocnemius recession) in persistent cases

Q50. Enumerate types of limb length discrepancy and their orthopedic management.

Types of LLD

- *Congenital*: Fibular hemimelia, proximal focal femoral deficiency (PFFD), hemihypertrophy
- *Developmental*: Neurofibromatosis, Perthes disease sequelae
- *Acquired*: Trauma, infection (osteomyelitis), tumors, post-surgical

Measurement

- *Clinical*: Tape measure (ASIS to medial malleolus)
- *Radiological*: Scanogram, CT scanogram, EOS imaging

Management

LLD (cm)	*Treatment*
<2 cm	Observation or shoe lift
2–5 cm	Epiphysiodesis (e.g., percutaneous PETS)
5–20 cm	Limb lengthening (Ilizarov, PRECICE nail)
>20 cm	Consider amputation and prosthetic fitting (especially in PFFD)

Q51. Classify congenital limb deficiencies. Discuss principles of management.

(Asked in AIIMS Delhi 2021, PGI Chandigarh 2022)

Definition

Congenital limb deficiencies refer to a **spectrum of developmental abnormalities** resulting in **partial or complete absence or malformation of limbs** at birth.

Classification

Based on Frantz and O'Rahilly classification

Type	*Description*
Transverse deficiency	Limb develops normally up to a certain point, then absent beyond (like amputation)
Longitudinal deficiency	Specific bones are partially or completely absent along the limb's long axis (e.g., fibular hemimelia, radial club hand)

Examples

- *Transverse*: Congenital amputation at the forearm level.
- *Longitudinal*:
  - *Pre-axial (radial side)*: Radial hemimelia.
  - *Post-axial (ulnar side)*: Ulnar hemimelia.
  - *Central*: Absence of central rays (cleft hand/foot).

Principles of Management

- *Multidisciplinary approach*: Ortho surgeon, pediatrician, physiotherapist, prosthetist.
- *Early diagnosis*: Through clinical exam and imaging (X-ray, USG if needed).
- *Functional goal-oriented treatment*: Promote maximum **function and independence**.
- *Prosthetic fitting*: As early as 6–12 months to aid developmental milestones.
- *Surgical reconstruction*: Lengthening procedures (Ilizarov), amputation and fitting prosthesis, joint reconstructions.
- *Family counseling*: Set realistic expectations; address psychosocial aspects.

Important Concept
Focus on **function > form**—achieving usable limb function is prioritized over cosmetic appearance.

Q52. Proximal femoral focal deficiency (PFFD)—classification and management.

Definition
Congenital partial or complete absence of the proximal femur

Classification (Aitken)
- *Type A*: Short femur with intact hip joint
- *Type B*: Varus deformity, abnormal femoral head
- *Type C*: No acetabular contact
- *Type D*: Complete absence of proximal femur

Clinical Presentation
- Shortened thigh
- Absent or unstable hip
- Foot at level of opposite knee
- Limb length discrepancy

Management

Type	*Management*
A/B	Lengthening procedures (Ilizarov)
C/D	Rotationplasty or Syme amputation + prosthesis

Q53. Fibular hemimelia—features and management.

Definition
Congenital **partial or complete absence of the fibula**—most common long bone deficiency

Clinical Features
- Limb shortening
- Equinovalgus foot deformity
- Absent lateral rays of foot
- Knee instability, ligamentous laxity
- Femoral bowing

Management
- *Mild*: Orthosis
- *Moderate*: **Limb lengthening (Ilizarov)**
- *Severe (no functional foot)*: **Amputation (Syme or Boyd) + prosthesis**

Q54. Congenital tibial hemimelia—description and management.

Definition
Rare condition with **partial or complete absence of the tibia**.

Types
Jones classification (type I–IV) based on tibial presence.

Clinical Presentation
- **Severe varus deformity**
- Foot in **equinovarus**
- Absent or deformed patella
- Knee/ankle instability

Management

Severity	Management
Partial tibia	Tibialization of fibula + fixation
Total absence	Knee disarticulation + prosthesis

Q55. Role of limb lengthening in congenital limb deficiencies.

Indications

- Limb length discrepancy >2–3 cm
- Functional joints with adequate musculature
- Motivated family/patient

Methods

- Ilizarov external fixator
- PRECICE magnetic nail (internal lengthening)
- Chondrodiastasis (growth plate distraction in young children)

Considerations

- Rule of 1 mm/day distraction
- Psychological and physical support essential
- *Monitor for*:
  - Joint stiffness
  - Pin tract infections
  - Premature consolidation

Q56. Congenital patellar dislocation—diagnosis and treatment.

Definition

Lateral dislocation of patella, present at birth and **irreducible** manually.

Features

- Flexion contracture of knee
- Laterally dislocated patella
- Extensor lag
- Often bilateral

Diagnosis

Clinical + X-ray + MRI (for soft tissue)

Management

- *Conservative*: Ineffective
- *Surgical*:
  - Early soft tissue realignment (lateral release, medial plication)
  - Quadricepsplasty
  - Distal realignment (tibial tubercle transfer) in older children

Q57. Physiological versus pathological genu varum and genu valgum.

Feature	Physiological	Pathological
Onset	• *Genu varum*: birth → 2 years • *Genu valgum*: 2–7 years	After 3 years (varum) or 7 years (valgum)
Symmetry	Bilateral, symmetrical	Often asymmetrical
Deformity progression	Self-correcting	Worsens with time

Continued

Continued

Feature	Physiological	Pathological
Radiological features	Normal joint space, smooth metaphyseal line	Metaphyseal beaking, abnormal angles
Examples	Physiologic bowlegs/knock-knees	Blount's disease, rickets, skeletal dysplasia

Observation is adequate in physiological cases; intervention is needed in pathological ones.

Q58. Blount's disease—features, classification and management.

[Assam Medical College (affiliated to Srimanta Sankaradeva University of Health Sciences) 2018]

Definition

Developmental **disorder of the medial proximal tibial physis** → progressive genu varum.

Types

1. *Infantile (<4 years)*: More common, bilateral
2. *Adolescent (>10 years)*: Unilateral, obese children

Clinical Features

- Progressive, **asymmetric varus** deformity
- Internal tibial torsion
- Gait disturbance (waddling, intoeing)
- Ligamentous laxity in adolescents

Radiology

- Beaking and sloping of medial proximal tibial physis
- *Langenskiöld classification*: 6 stages based on physeal changes

Management

Age/Stage	Management
Stage I–II (<3 years)	Orthosis or brace (KAFO)
>3 years or stage III+	*Surgical correction*: Proximal tibial osteotomy ± epiphysiodesis
Severe cases	Gradual correction (Ilizarov frame)

Q59. Indications for surgery in genu valgum.

Normal physiological valgus: Intermalleolar distance <8–10 cm

Surgical Indications

- Intermalleolar distance >10–12 cm after 7 years
- Asymmetry
- Worsening deformity
- Pain or instability
- Cosmetic/functional impairment
- Pathological cause (rickets, skeletal dysplasia)

Options

- *Guided growth (temporary hemiepiphysiodesis)*
- *Corrective osteotomy* (in late adolescents/adults)

Q60. Genu recurvatum.

Definition

Hyperextension deformity of the knee (>5–10° beyond normal extension).

Causes
- Polio
- Hemiplegia/Cerebral palsy
- Ligamentous laxity
- Post-traumatic (after tibial plateau fracture)
- Growth disturbances

Clinical Findings
- Hyperextended knee on standing
- Instability
- May cause anterior knee pain

Treatment
- Orthotic support (floor-reaction AFO)
- Physiotherapy
- Soft tissue release or guided growth in children
- Osteotomy in severe deformities

Q61. Rickets—orthopedic manifestations and management.

(MMC 2013)

Definition
Metabolic bone disorder due to **defective mineralization of osteoid**, most commonly due to **vitamin D deficiency**.

Orthopedic Manifestations
- **Genu varum/valgum**
- Frontal bossing
- Widened wrists/ankles
- Delayed walking
- Rachitic rosary (costochondral junction prominence)
- Metaphyseal cupping and fraying (X-ray)

Management

Component	***Management***
Medical	Vitamin D and calcium supplementation
Orthopedic	Bracing for early deformity
	Osteotomy in severe/progressive cases after 7–8 years
Monitoring	X-rays, biochemical markers (ALP ↑, Ca ↓, PO_4 ↓, PTH ↑)

Types
- Nutritional
- Hypophosphatemic
- Renal rickets (vitamin D–resistant)

Q62. Guided growth techniques in pediatric deformities.

Concept
Temporarily halt growth on the convex side of a physis to allow correction via growth on the concave side.

Techniques
- 8-plate tension band (most common)
- Stapling
- Percutaneous epiphysiodesis

Indications
- *Angular deformities*: Genu valgum, varum
- Early stages of Blount's
- Lateral femoral condyle overgrowth (hemophilia, etc.)

Timing critical → requires monitoring every 6 months
Reversible → remove plate after correction

Q63. Management of congenital pseudarthrosis of tibia—discuss latest techniques.

(AIMS Kochi 2012)

Definition
A rare, challenging condition where there is a segmental defect or pseudarthrosis (non-union) in the tibial shaft, often associated with **neurofibromatosis type 1 (NF-1)**.

Pathophysiology
- Dysplastic periosteum and poor osteogenic potential
- Poor vascularity
- Fibrous hamartoma at fracture site

Management

Treatment	Description
Initial bracing	Early bracing to prevent fracture
Excision of pseudarthrosis	Complete resection of fibrous hamartoma
Intramedullary fixation	Telescopic rods or titanium elastic nails
Bone grafting	Autograft ± BMP-2/7
Ilizarov external fixation	Correction + union + limb lengthening
Cross-union technique	Recently advocated—promotes tibia-fibula fusion using bone graft and fixation
Biological enhancement	Bone morphogenetic proteins (BMP), mesenchymal stem cells
Amputation	Reserved for multiple surgical failures or very short limb

Latest Advances
- Induced membrane (Masquelet technique)
- BMPs and bone marrow aspirate
- Telescopic growing nails in young children
- Combined tibia-fibula intramedullary cross-union

Q64. Congenital kyphoscoliotic tibia.

- Anterior and lateral bowing of tibia in neonates
- Associated with **neurofibromatosis** or **fibular hemimelia**
- May develop **pseudarthrosis**

Treatment
- Bracing (early)
- **Intramedullary fixation ± bone grafting** for nonunion
- Ilizarov if deformity + shortening

Q65. Congenital pseudarthrosis of fibula.

- Failure of union at fibular diaphysis
- Often associated with **tibial bowing, neurofibromatosis**

Treatment
- Observation if asymptomatic
- Fixation with graft/IM nail if ankle valgus or progressive deformity

Q66. Congenital constriction bands (Amniotic band syndrome).

- Fibrous bands cause **constriction rings**, distal swelling, or even **autoamputation**
- May involve nerves, vessels

Treatment
- Z-plasty or staged release
- Amputation for non-salvageable distal segment

Q67. Congenital knee dislocation/hyperextension.

- *Rare; classified as*:
  - *Grade I*: Hyperextension
  - *Grade II*: Subluxation
  - *Grade III*: Dislocation

Treatment
- *Early*: Serial casting
- *Surgery*:
  - Quadricepsplasty
  - V-Y plasty
  - ACL/PCL reconstruction if late

Q68. Nail–Patella syndrome (osteo-onychodysplasia).

- Genetic condition (autosomal dominant)
- *Features*:
  - Nail dysplasia (especially thumbs)
  - Absent or hypoplastic **patella**
  - Elbow dysplasia
  - **Iliac horns** (pathognomonic on X-ray)
  - Possible nephropathy (proteinuria)

Treatment
- Mostly symptomatic—bracing, physio
- Patellar stabilization if dislocation

Q69. Principles of transosseous osteosynthesis (Ilizarov method).

Core Concepts
- Based on **distraction osteogenesis**
- Gradual traction leads to **new bone formation** in gap

Principles
1. *Corticotomy*: Metaphyseal zone
2. *Latency period*: 5–7 days
3. *Distraction phase*: 1 mm/day in four increments
4. *Consolidation*: Immobilization till ossification

Applications
- Limb lengthening
- Deformity correction
- Non-union
- Bone defects, pseudarthrosis

Vertebral and Spinal Anomalies

Q70. Management of vertebral segmentation anomalies.

(RGUHS 2012)

Examples
- Hemivertebrae
- Block vertebrae
- Congenital scoliosis/kyphosis

Pathophysiology
Failure of formation or segmentation during embryogenesis

Management
- *Observation*: Small, non-progressive curves
- *Bracing*: Limited role in congenital anomalies
- *Surgery*:
  - Hemivertebra excision
  - Posterior spinal fusion
  - Growth-friendly techniques (e.g., VEPTR, MCGR rods in early-onset deformities)
- Monitor for **neurological compromise**

Q71. Discuss occult spinal dysraphism and its orthopedic implications.

Definition
A spectrum of **closed spinal cord malformations** with skin-covered defects, unlike open spina bifida. May include:
- Lipomyelomeningocele
- Diastematomyelia
- Tethered cord
- Dermal sinus tract

Clinical Signs
- *Cutaneous stigmata*: Hair tuft, lipoma, dermal sinus
- *Neurological*: Weakness, bladder dysfunction
- *Orthopedic*:
  - Foot deformities (cavus, equinovarus)
  - Scoliosis
  - Limb length discrepancy
  - Hip subluxation/dislocation

Investigations
- *MRI spine*: Gold standard
- *Urodynamics*: For bladder involvement

Orthopedic Management
- Early referral for **neurosurgical detethering**

- *Corrective surgery for deformities*:
  - *Foot*: Soft tissue release, osteotomy
  - *Spine*: Bracing or surgical stabilization
- Bladder care and physiotherapy

Q72. Spina bifida—orthopedic management of lower limb deformities.

Types
- Spina bifida occulta (hidden)
- Meningocele
- Myelomeningocele (most severe)

Orthopedic Issues
- Hip dislocation/subluxation
- Equinus/calcaneus foot deformities
- Flexion/extension contractures of knees
- Scoliosis, pelvic obliquity
- Limb length discrepancy

Management

Deformity	*Treatment*
Hip dislocation	Observation if non-functional
Foot deformity	Ponseti, soft tissue releases
Knee contractures	Bracing or quadricepsplasty
Scoliosis	Bracing or posterior fusion
Gait support	KAFO/AFO depending on lesion level

Upper Limb Anomalies

Q73. Management of radial club hand—types and surgical options.

(RIMS 2012)

Types (Bayne and Klug Classification I–IV)
Ranges from mild radial hypoplasia to complete absence.

Management
- **Passive stretching + splinting** in early infancy
- **Centralization** or **radialization** of carpus over ulna
- Tendon transfers for wrist extension
- Lengthening procedures in adolescence (controversial)

Q74. Congenital dislocation of the radial head.

Types
Anterior (most common), posterior, lateral.

Clinical
- Painless limited elbow ROM (especially supination/pronation)
- Often bilateral

Management
- Observation if asymptomatic
- *Surgical*:
    - Radial head resection (after skeletal maturity)
    - Ulnar osteotomy ± annular ligament reconstruction

Q75. Sprengel deformity—classification and treatment.

Definition
Congenital elevation of scapula due to failure of caudal migration.

Classification: Cavendish (Grades I–IV)
Based on cosmetic severity.

Management
- *Mild*: Observation, physiotherapy
- *Moderate-severe*:
    - **Woodward's procedure** (most accepted)
    - Green's procedure (scapular relocation)

Q76. Polydactyly and syndactyly—types and surgical correction.

(WBUHS 2012)

Polydactyly
- *Preaxial (radial/thumb)*: Common in Caucasians
- *Postaxial (ulnar side)*: Common in African descent

Syndactyly
- Simple versus complex (bone involvement)
- Complete versus incomplete

Surgical Management
- *Timing*: 1–2 years of age
- **Z-plasty, skin grafts**
- Avoid simultaneous release of adjacent digits to prevent vascular compromise

Q77. Congenital trigger thumb—management.

Features
- Flexion deformity at IP joint of thumb
- Palpable Notta's nodule at A1 pulley

Management
- **Observation** until age 2–3 (spontaneous resolution in some)
- *Persistent*: **A1 pulley release** under GA
- Avoid aggressive stretching

Q78. Management of camptodactyly and clinodactyly.

Camptodactyly
- Flexion deformity of PIP joint (typically 5th digit)
- Congenital or acquired
- May be associated with syndromes (e.g., Larsen)

Treatment

- *Mild*: Observation, splints
- *Severe*: FDS release, volar plate release

Clinodactyly

- Angular deviation in coronal plane (usually radial deviation of little finger)
- Often bilateral, familial

Treatment

- *Mild*: Observation
- *Severe*: Corrective wedge osteotomy

Q79. Clinical features and management of congenital radioulnar synostosi.

(Asked in: AIIMS Delhi 2021, RGUHS Karnataka 2022)

Definition

- **Congenital radioulnar synostosis** is a **congenital fusion** between the **proximal radius and ulna**, leading to **fixed pronation deformity** of the forearm.
- It results from **failure of longitudinal segmentation** of the cartilaginous anlage during early embryonic development (~7th week, gestation).

Etiology

Congenital (most common). Often **bilateral** (60–80% cases). Can be associated with:

- Congenital hip dislocation.
- Madelung deformity.
- Syndromes like Holt-Oram, Klinefelter's syndrome.

Types (Cleary and Omer Classification)

Type	*Description*
I	Fibrous union between radius and ulna
II	Bony fusion (synostosis) of proximal radius and ulna

Clinical Features

Symptoms:

- *Limited forearm rotation*: Fixed pronation position.
- Child may not notice early; detected when difficulty arises in tasks needing supination (e.g., carrying a tray, receiving coins).

Signs:

- Forearm fixed in **pronation** (usually 20–60°).
- Flexion-extension at elbow usually **normal**.
- No pain.

Functional Impairment:

- *Mild cases*: Well tolerated.
- Severe fixed pronation (>60°) → Functional disability in daily activities.

Diagnosis

Clinical examination: Key to suspect.

Radiology:

- *X-ray (AP and lateral views)*:
  - Bony bridge between proximal radius and ulna.
  - Absent or hypoplastic radial head.
- *CT scan*: Better visualization if diagnosis unclear on X-ray.

Management

Conservative (Majority):

- Indicated for mild pronation deformity (<60°) or if well-compensated functionally.
- Occupational therapy for adaptive techniques.

Surgical (Selected cases)

Indications:

- Severe pronation deformity (>60–70°).
- Bilateral involvement with functional limitation.

Surgical Options:

- *Derotational osteotomy of forearm bones*:
    - *Goal*: Position forearm in more functional neutral or slight pronation (10–20°).
    - Usually performed at midshaft radius and ulna.
- *Timing*:
    - *Ideal age*: 4–6 years (when compensation is not sufficient and disability is clear).

Important

- Synostosis resection alone has **high recurrence**, thus not recommended.
- Derotation better tolerated functionally than trying to "un-fuse" the bones.

Other Pediatric Elbow Conditions

Q80. Diagnosis and treatment of pulled elbow (Nursemaid's elbow).

(AIIMS BBSR 2012)

Definition

Radial head subluxation due to longitudinal traction on the extended and pronated arm.

Age Group

Common in **children <5 years**.

Clinical Features

- Sudden onset refusal to use the limb
- Elbow held in **slight flexion and pronation**
- No swelling or bruising
- Tenderness over radial head

Diagnosis

- Clinical—radiographs usually **normal**
- Rule out fracture if trauma history is unclear

Treatment

- *Reduction technique (either method works well)*:
    - *Supination-flexion method*: Supinate forearm → flex elbow
    - *Hyperpronation method*: Pronate the forearm quickly
- Immediate return of function confirms success

Q81. Differential diagnosis of pediatric elbow pain.

Key Causes

Category	*Conditions*
Traumatic	Supracondylar fracture, lateral condyle fracture, radial neck fracture
Overuse	Little League elbow, Panner's disease, osteochondritis dissecans

Continued

Continued

Category	*Conditions*
Infectious	Septic arthritis, osteomyelitis
Inflammatory	Juvenile idiopathic arthritis
Mechanical	Nursemaid's elbow
Congenital	Congenital radial head dislocation

Q82. Management of Panner's disease.

Definition

- Idiopathic **osteochondrosis of the capitellum**
- Self-limiting AVN-like condition

Age Group

Boys **5–10 years**, often with repetitive stress (throwing, gymnastics)

Clinical Features

- Lateral elbow pain
- Swelling and tenderness over capitellum
- Decreased ROM (especially extension)

Radiology

- Radiolucency, fragmentation of capitellum
- Later reossification

Treatment

- *Conservative*:
  - Rest, activity modification
  - Splinting if severe pain
- *Prognosis*: Excellent with remodeling and resolution in months

Q83. Little league elbow—short note.

Definition

Overuse injury of the medial elbow in young throwing athletes

Pathology

- **Medial epicondylar apophysitis** due to valgus stress
- Can progress to avulsion fracture or ulnar collateral ligament strain

Clinical

- Medial elbow pain after throwing
- Decreased throwing speed, grip weakness

Imaging

- Widening of medial apophysis
- Fragmentation or sclerosis

Management

- **Activity restriction** (throwing) for 4–6 weeks
- Ice, NSAIDs
- Gradual return with supervised rehabilitation
- Emphasize **pitch count limits and technique correction**

Q84. Describe madelung deformity—clinical features and treatment.

(Asked in PGI Chandigarh 2021, MUHS Maharashtra 2023)

Definition

Madelung deformity is a **developmental abnormality** characterized by a **progressive wrist deformity** due to **premature growth arrest of the ulnar and volar (anteromedial) portion of the distal radial physis**.

Clinical Features

- Usually presents in **early adolescence** (10–14 years).
- Prominent ulnar head (ulna appears dorsally subluxated).
- Dorsal and radial bowing of the forearm.
- Ulnar and volar tilt of the distal radial articular surface.
- Wrist pain, especially during activity.
- *Restricted wrist motion*:
  - Decreased extension
  - Decreased supination
- Cosmetic deformity (common reason for presentation).
- May be bilateral (especially in syndromic cases like Turner's syndrome).

Physical Examination

- Volar and ulnar wrist prominence.
- "Bayonet" appearance of the wrist.
- Positive "Vickers ligament" tightness felt (specific to Madelung deformity).

Diagnosis

- *X-ray findings*:
  - Increased volar tilt and radial inclination of distal radius.
  - Triangular-shaped carpus (called **V-shaped carpus**).
  - Dorsal subluxation of ulnar head.

Management

Severity	*Treatment*
Mild/Asymptomatic	Observation and physiotherapy
Symptomatic/Severe deformity	Surgery

- Vickers ligament release (for early stages).
- Radial corrective osteotomy (for angular correction).
- Ulnar shortening osteotomy (if significant ulnar prominence and pain).
- Distal radioulnar joint (DRUJ) reconstruction if instability persists.

Important Point

Early surgical intervention (Vickers ligament release) can prevent progression if detected before complete physeal closure.

Q85. Pathophysiology of Madelung deformity.

(Asked in AIIMS Delhi 2022)

Basic Pathology

- Premature partial closure of the distal radial growth plate (specifically volar-ulnar aspect).
- Continued growth on dorsal and radial sides → progressive radial tilt and bowing.
- The ulna continues to grow normally, leading to dorsal subluxation of the ulna relative to the radius.

Contributing Factors

- *Congenital/Syndromic associations*:
  - Turner's syndrome.
  - Leri–Weill dyschondrosteosis.
  - Madelung deformity may also be sporadic or idiopathic.
- *Vickers Ligament*:
  - An abnormal ligament seen between the lunate bone and distal radius.
  - Thought to tether growth and worsen deformity.

Biomechanical Effects

- Imbalance between radial and ulnar growth.
- Abnormal carpal alignment → "V-shaped" carpus.
- Worsening deformity during growth spurts.

Key Concept

Madelung = Growth disturbance + Ligament tethering + Carpal malalignment.

General Principles and Classifications

Q86. Approach to a child with limping due to developmental causes.

Stepwise Approach

1. *History*:
   - Age of onset
   - Trauma, fever
   - Morning stiffness, night pain
   - Associated developmental milestones
2. *Examination*:
   - Observe gait (Trendelenburg, antalgic)
   - Hip/knee/foot ROM
   - Limb length discrepancy
   - Look for spine or neurological signs
3. *Differential diagnosis by age*:

Age	Likely causes
<3 years	DDH, toddler's fracture, cerebral palsy
3–8 years	Perthes disease, transient synovitis, rickets
>8 years	SCFE, JIA, AVN, Blount's disease

4. *Investigations*:
   - **X-ray pelvis and hips**
   - ESR, CRP (if infection suspected)
   - MRI hip (for Perthes, early SCFE)
5. *Management*: Based on diagnosis (e.g., observation for transient synovitis, surgical for SCFE or DDH)

Q87. Describe general principles of managing congenital limb deformities.

(PGI Chandigarh 2017)

Principles

1. *Early diagnosis*: Antenatal scans, clinical exam at birth

2. *Detailed evaluation*:
   - Radiographs, CT/MRI, 3D reconstruction if needed
   - Look for associated syndromes (VACTERL, amniotic band syndrome)
3. *Classify the deformity*: E.g., Bayne and Klug (radial club hand), Pappas classification
4. *Multidisciplinary team approach*: Ortho, rehabilitation, genetics, pediatrician, physiotherapist
5. *Phased management*:
   - *Initial*: Observation or bracing
   - *Intermediate*: Soft tissue releases
   - *Definitive*: Osteotomy, limb lengthening, reconstruction, or amputation
6. *Functional goals over anatomical perfection*: Emphasize assistive function and gait

Q88. Role of multidisciplinary management in complex congenital deformities.

Examples
- Arthrogryposis
- CTEV with syndromic associations
- Congenital pseudarthrosis of tibia
- Spina bifida
- Larsen syndrome
- Constriction band syndrome

Team Members
- Orthopedic surgeon
- Pediatrician/geneticist
- Neurosurgeon (spine/tethered cord)
- Physiotherapist
- Orthotist
- Social worker and psychologist

Key Principles
- Early diagnosis and family counseling
- Phased treatment (e.g., correction → function → cosmetic)
- *Goal*: Maximize independence, mobility, and quality of life
- Custom orthoses, gait aids, and adapted therapy
- Repeated evaluation and planning as child grows

Q89. Use of external fixators (Ilizarov) in congenital deformity correction.

Applications
- Limb length discrepancy
- Tibial/fibular hemimelia
- Congenital pseudarthrosis of tibia
- Angular deformities (Blount's, genu varum)
- Clubfoot (relapsed)

Techniques
- **Distraction osteogenesis**
- Angular correction
- Bone transport (segmental defects)
- Joint realignment

Advantages
- Multiplanar correction
- Gradual lengthening
- Preserves soft tissues

Complications
- Pin tract infection
- Joint stiffness
- Psychological impact

Q90. Principles of limb lengthening using Ilizarov technique.

Principle
Based on distraction osteogenesis: New bone forms in the gap between bone ends slowly pulled apart.

Key Concepts
- *Corticotomy*: Low-energy osteotomy preserving medullary vessels
- *Latency period*: 5–7 days post-operative
- *Distraction phase*: 1 mm/day (in 4 increments)
- *Consolidation phase*: Until new bone hardens

Components
- Circular fixator rings
- Tensioned wires/pins
- Hinges for angular correction

Applications
- LLD correction
- Angular deformities
- Non-unions, pseudarthrosis
- Bone defects

Q91. Indications for Van Nes rotationplasty.

Definition
- A surgical procedure where the lower leg is **rotated 180°** and reattached to the femur.
- Ankle functions as a **knee joint** when fitted with a below-knee prosthesis.

Indications
- Proximal focal femoral deficiency (PFFD)—most common
- Femoral bone tumors (e.g., osteosarcoma)
- Severe **trauma**, infection, or congenital femoral deficiency where limb salvage is not possible

Advantages
- Functional gait with below-knee prosthesis
- Better energy efficiency versus hip disarticulation
- Preserves proprioception and limb control

Calcaneovalgus Foot
- Common neonatal deformity where foot is dorsiflexed and everted
- *Cause*: Intrauterine positioning
- Usually flexible

Treatment

- **Stretching + observation**
- *Rigid/refractory*: serial casting
- Surgery rare (tendon transfer)

Idiopathic Toe Walking

- Children >2 years who **walk on toes** without neurological or orthopedic cause
- Normal neuro exam; no tight Achilles in early stage

Treatment

- Observation (most resolve by 5 years)
- Heel cord stretching
- Serial casting or Botox
- Surgery (gastrocnemius recession) in persistent cases

Macrodactyly

- Congenital overgrowth of bone/soft tissue in a digit (mostly **2nd or 3rd toe/finger**)
- Often sporadic or part of **Proteus syndrome, neurofibromatosis**

Treatment

- Shoe modification (mild)
- Debulking ± epiphysiodesis
- Amputation in severe cases

Q92. Congenital muscular torticollis.

- Unilateral **contracture of sternocleidomastoid**
- Head tilt to **affected side**, chin rotated to **opposite side**
- Associated with **plagiocephaly**

Treatment

- Stretching (first-line, effective in 90%)
- *Surgery if persistent >1 year*: **SCM release**

Q93. Sprengel's deformity.

- **Congenital elevation of scapula** due to failure of descent
- Often associated with **Klippel–Feil syndrome**

Clinical

- High scapula, restricted shoulder abduction
- **Omovertebral bar** (fibrous/bony bridge)

Treatment

- *Mild*: Physio
- *Moderate–severe*: **Woodward or Green's procedure** (scapular lowering)

Q94. Congenital kyphoscoliotic tibia.

- Anterior and lateral bowing of tibia in neonates
- Associated with **neurofibromatosis** or **fibular hemimelia**
- May develop **pseudarthrosis**

Treatment

- Bracing (early)
- **Intramedullary fixation ± bone grafting** for nonunion
- Ilizarov if deformity + shortening

Q95. Congenital pseudarthrosis of fibula.

- Failure of union at fibular diaphysis
- Often associated with **tibial bowing, neurofibromatosis**

Treatment
- Observation if asymptomatic
- Fixation with graft/IM nail if ankle valgus or progressive deformity

Q96. Congenital constriction bands (Amniotic band syndrome).

- Fibrous bands cause **constriction rings**, distal swelling, or even **autoamputation**
- May involve nerves, vessels

Treatment
- **Z-plasty or staged release**
- Amputation for non-salvageable distal segment

Q97. Increased femoral anteversion.

- Normal = ~15°; ↑ = >30° (seen in toddlers)
- Presents as **in-toeing gait**, W-sitting

Treatment
- *Observation*: Most cases improve by age 8
- *Derotation osteotomy if*:
  - 3 SDs from normal
  - 10–12 years
  - Cosmetic/functional issues

Q98. Congenital knee dislocation/hyperextension.

- *Rare; classified as*:
  - *Grade I*: Hyperextension
  - *Grade II*: Subluxation
  - *Grade III*: Dislocation

Treatment
- *Early*: Serial casting
- *Surgery*:
  - Quadricepsplasty
  - V-Y plasty
  - ACL/PCL reconstruction if late

Q99. Principles of transosseous osteosynthesis (Ilizarov method).

Core Concepts
- Based on **distraction osteogenesis**
- Gradual traction leads to **new bone formation** in gap

Principles
1. *Corticotomy*: Metaphyseal zone
2. *Latency period*: 5–7 days
3. *Distraction phase*: 1 mm/day in 4 increments
4. *Consolidation*: Immobilization till ossification

Applications
- Limb lengthening
- Deformity correction
- Non-union
- Bone defects, pseudarthrosis

Q100. Agenesis of clavicle (cleidocranial dysostosis).

(BFUHS 2017)

Definition

Complete or partial absence of the clavicle; typically bilateral and associated with cleidocranial dysplasia.

Clinical Features
- Shoulder hypermobility (patient can approximate shoulders at midline)
- Drooping shoulders
- Often detected in infancy/childhood

Radiology
- Partial/complete absence of clavicle on X-ray
- Associated skull anomalies, delayed suture closure

Management
- Usually conservative
- Surgical reconstruction rarely required for severe deformity or cosmetic correction

10.2 Genetic Disorders in Orthopedics

Sajal Maingi, Aditya Chaubey, Iram Mir

Q1. Define genetic disorders and classify them based on inheritance patterns.

(AIIMS BBSR 2012)

Genetic disorders are conditions caused by abnormalities in genes or chromosomes. These abnormalities may be inherited or result from new mutations.

Classification by inheritance

- *Autosomal dominant*: Single altered copy of gene (e.g., **achondroplasia**)
- *Autosomal recessive*: Both gene copies affected (e.g., **osteogenesis imperfecta type IIB**)
- *X-linked*: Mutation on X chromosome (e.g., **Duchenne muscular dystrophy**)
- *Mitochondrial*: Inherited maternally via mitochondrial DNA (rare in orthopedics)

Q2. Describe the role of genetics in orthopedic disorders.

Genetics Influences

- Bone formation (e.g., FGFR3 in achondroplasia)
- Collagen structure (e.g., COL1A1 in osteogenesis imperfecta)
- Cartilage growth and skeletal patterning
- Joint laxity, bone density, and muscle integrity

Genetic Mutations can Cause

- Congenital deformities (e.g., **clubfoot**, **scoliosis**)
- Metabolic bone diseases (e.g., **hypophosphatasia**)
- Syndromic conditions with skeletal involvement (e.g., **Marfan syndrome**)

Q3. Explain the molecular basis of genetic bone diseases.

Bone Diseases Arise Due to Mutations Affecting

- *Collagen genes (COL1A1, COL1A2)*: Osteogenesis imperfecta
- *FGFR genes*: Achondroplasia, hypochondroplasia
- *PHEX gene*: X-linked hypophosphatemic rickets
- *RUNX2*: Cleidocranial dysplasia

Molecular disruptions affect bone matrix formation, mineralization, and remodeling.

Q4. Discuss the role of chromosomal abnormalities in skeletal disorders.

Chromosomal Disorders can Lead to

- Skeletal dysplasia (e.g., Trisomy 18—rocker bottom feet, limb abnormalities)
- Short stature syndromes (e.g., Turner syndrome—monosomy X)
- Multiple anomalies due to chromosomal deletions or duplications

Karyotyping and microarray can help identify structural chromosome abnormalities.

Q5. Explain the role of next-generation sequencing (NGS) in diagnosing genetic disorders.

NGS allows rapid sequencing of thousands of genes simultaneously.

Uses
- Diagnose rare skeletal dysplasias
- Identify pathogenic mutations in bone-related genes
- Facilitate personalized treatment
- Improve prenatal or early postnatal diagnosis

Techniques include **whole genome sequencing**, **exome sequencing**, and **gene panels**.

Q6. Discuss genetic counseling and its importance in orthopedic practice.

Genetic counseling provides patients/families with:
- **Risk assessment**
- Information on **inheritance patterns**
- Implications for **family planning**
- Psychosocial support

Vital for conditions with **recurrence risk**, **early onset**, or **multisystem involvement**.

Q7. Explain the role of prenatal screening in genetic skeletal disorders.

Prenatal Screening Techniques
- Ultrasound (detects limb deformities, short femur, bowing)
- Amniocentesis/chorionic villus sampling (CVS) for genetic analysis
- Cell-free fetal DNA (cfDNA) testing (non-invasive)

Helpful in early detection of disorders like:
- Achondroplasia
- Osteogenesis imperfecta
- Thanatophoric dysplasia

Q8. Morquio syndrome and its spinal manifestations.

Also known as: Mucopolysaccharidosis type IV (MPS IV)

Etiology
- *Genetic basis*: Autosomal recessive
- *Enzyme deficiency*:
    - *MPS IVA*: Deficiency of **galactosamine-6-sulfatase**
    - *MPS IVB*: Deficiency of **beta-galactosidase**

Pathophysiology
- Accumulation of glycosaminoglycans (GAGs), especially **keratan sulfate**, in bones and cartilage → abnormal skeletal development.

Orthopedic and Spinal Manifestations

System	*Findings*
Spine	Odontoid hypoplasia → atlantoaxial instability, cervical spinal cord compression
Vertebrae	Platyspondyly (flattened vertebrae), anterior beaking of vertebral bodies
Thorax	Pectus carinatum (pigeon chest)
Limbs	Genu valgum, joint laxity, short stature

Neurological risk

Cervical instability may cause **myelopathy** or **sudden death** if not addressed early.

Management

- **Early cervical spine screening (MRI)**
- **Occipitocervical fusion** for instability
- Enzyme replacement therapy (ERT) to slow progression

Q9. Skeletal involvement in mucopolysaccharidoses (MPS).

MPS Overview

- A group of lysosomal storage disorders due to **deficient degradation of GAGs**, including dermatan sulfate, heparan sulfate, and keratan sulfate.
- *Inheritance*: Autosomal recessive (except MPS II—X-linked)

Common Skeletal Features (Dysostosis Multiplex)

Radiographic signs	*Examples*
Thickened calvarium	Enlarged skull
J-shaped sella turcica	Seen in lateral skull X-ray
Bullet-shaped metacarpals	Tapering and shortening
Beaked vertebral bodies	Anterior vertebral beaking
Shortened long bones	With widened metaphyses
Hip dysplasia	Delayed ossification, acetabular dysplasia
Genu valgum, joint stiffness or laxity	Especially in MPS IV, MPS I

Neurological Concerns

- Spinal stenosis
- Cervical cord compression (especially in MPS I, IV)

Management Principles

- *Orthopedic*: Spinal decompression, joint corrective surgery, physiotherapy
- *Medical*: Enzyme replacement therapy (ERT), hematopoietic stem cell transplant (in MPS I)

Q10. Role of *RUNX2* gene in bone development.

(NEIGRIHMS 2012)

RUNX2 **(Runt-related transcription factor 2)**

- Master regulator of **osteoblast differentiation**
- Located on **chromosome 6p21**

Functions

- *Initiates expression of osteoblast-specific genes*: Osteocalcin, type I collagen
- Controls transition from **mesenchymal stem cells to pre-osteoblasts**

Clinical Relevance

- *Mutation causes cleidocranial dysplasia*:
  - Delayed fontanel closure
  - Hypoplastic clavicles
  - Supernumerary teeth

Research Use

Target in **bone tissue engineering and anabolic therapy**

Q11. Genetic markers in orthopedic oncology (short note).

Definition
Specific **DNA sequences or mutations** used for **diagnosis, prognosis, and therapy guidance** in bone tumors.

Examples
- EWSR1-FLI1 fusion → Ewing sarcoma
- SYT-SSX1/2 → Synovial sarcoma
- MDM2 amplification → Low-grade liposarcomas
- IDH1/IDH2 mutations → Central chondrosarcomas

Applications
- Confirm **tumor subtype**
- Predict **therapy response or prognosis**
- Guide **targeted therapy**

Q12. Role of molecular biology in osteoporosis research.

Applications
- *Study of genes regulating*:
  - Bone remodeling (RANK/RANKL/OPG pathway)
  - Estrogen receptor signaling
  - Wnt/β-catenin pathway (e.g., LRP5 mutations)

Genetic Risk Factors
Polymorphisms in *COL1A1, ESR1, VDR* genes affect BMD

Molecular Tools
- **GWAS** identify SNPs associated with low BMD
- *Transcriptomics*: studies expression of bone-related genes

Clinical Relevance
- *Supports development of targeted therapies like*:
  - Denosumab (RANKL inhibitor)
  - Romosozumab (sclerostin inhibitor)

Q13. Use of CRISPR technology in orthopedic genetic disorders.

CRISPR-Cas9 System
A **genome-editing tool** that uses **guide RNA** to target and cut specific DNA sequences.

Applications in Orthopedics
- *Correct mutations in*:
  - OI (COL1A1/2)
  - Duchenne muscular dystrophy (DMD)
  - Achondroplasia (FGFR3 mutation)

Advantages
- **Precise**, relatively **cost-effective**
- Potential for **permanent gene correction**

Challenges
- Off-target effects
- Ethical concerns
- Delivery method optimization

Q14. Gene therapy in Duchenne muscular dystrophy (short note).

DMD Overview
- X-linked recessive disorder due to **mutation in dystrophin gene (Xp21)**
- Leads to **progressive muscle degeneration**

Gene Therapy Approaches
1. *Exon skipping (e.g., Eteplirsen)*: Restores reading frame
2. Mini-dystrophin gene delivery via AAV vectors
3. *CRISPR-Cas9*: Experimental correction of gene mutations

Goals
- Restore **functional dystrophin expression**
- Improve **muscle strength and survival**

Challenges
- Vector size limitations
- Immune response

Q15. Define osteogenesis imperfecta (OI) and classify its types.

(AMC 2017)

Osteogenesis imperfecta is a group of inherited connective tissue disorders characterized by **bone fragility** due to defective collagen type I synthesis.

Classification (Sillence Classification)
- *Type I*: Mild, most common, blue sclerae, normal stature
- *Type II*: Perinatal lethal, severe deformities, prenatal fractures
- *Type III*: Severe, progressively deforming, short stature, dentinogenesis imperfecta
- *Type IV*: Moderate severity, normal sclerae, variable bone fragility

(Newer types V–VIII are based on other gene mutations and clinical variations)

Q16. Genetic basis of osteogenesis imperfecta (OI).

Overview
Osteogenesis imperfecta (OI) is a **heritable connective tissue disorder** characterized by **bone fragility** and frequent fractures.

Genetic Basis
- *Type I collagen gene mutations*:
  - **Osteogenesis Imperfecta** and *COL1A2* (90% of cases)
  - Affects quality or quantity of collagen

Inheritance
Mostly **autosomal dominant**, some recessive or X-linked variants

Types (Sillence Classification)

Type	*Severity*	*Mutation effect*
I	Mild	Reduced collagen synthesis
II	Perinatal lethal	Abnormal collagen structure
III	Severe	Progressive deformity
IV	Moderate	Variable expression

Molecular Features
Defective collagen → impaired bone matrix formation → low bone mass and fragility.

Q17. Describe the pathophysiology of OI and its genetic basis.

(KMC Manipal 2016)

- Caused by mutations in *COL1A1* or *COL1A2* genes → impaired synthesis or structure of type I collagen.
- *Type I collagen is critical for*:
  - Bone strength
  - Ligament and tendon integrity
  - Dentin and sclera composition
- *Mutations can result in*:
  - Quantitative defect (less collagen—type I)
  - Qualitative defect (abnormal collagen—types II, III, and IV)

Q18. Discuss the clinical features, diagnosis, and treatment of OI.

Clinical Features

- Recurrent fractures with minimal trauma
- Blue sclerae (especially in type I)
- Dentinogenesis imperfecta (brown, brittle teeth)
- Hearing loss (sensorineural or conductive)
- Short stature, scoliosis
- Joint laxity

Diagnosis

- Clinical history and physical examination
- *Radiographs*: multiple fractures, thin cortices, wormian bones
- Genetic testing
- Bone biopsy in uncertain cases

Treatment

- **Bisphosphonates** (e.g., pamidronate)
- Intramedullary rodding
- Physical therapy
- Hearing aids
- Orthodontic and dental care

Q19. Explain the radiological features of OI.

- **Generalized osteopenia**
- Multiple healed fractures at different stages
- Deformities (e.g., bowing of long bones)
- **Wormian bones** in skull
- Thin cortices, broad metaphyses
- Vertebral compression fractures

Q20. Discuss the role of bisphosphonates in the management of OI.

- *Mechanism*: Inhibit osteoclast activity → reduce bone resorption
- *Benefits*:
  - Increase bone mineral density
  - Decrease fracture rate
  - Improve mobility and growth in children

- *Commonly used*: IV pamidronate or oral alendronate
- Administered in cycles under pediatric supervision

Q21. Explain the differential diagnosis of OI versus child abuse fractures.

(Kashmir University 2018)

Feature	*OI*	*Child abuse*
History	Family history, multiple old fractures	Inconsistent history
Fracture pattern	Long bones, multiple, varying healing stages	Rib, metaphyseal corner fractures
Other signs	Blue sclerae, dentinogenesis, hearing loss	Bruises, burns, neglect signs
Radiology	Generalized osteopenia, wormian bones	Localized injuries
Genetic testing	Positive (COL1A1/COL1A2 mutation)	Negative

Q22. Discuss the orthopedic management of fractures in OI.

- *Acute fractures*: Treated with lightweight splints or casts
- *Surgical management*: **Intramedullary rodding** (e.g., Fassier–Duval rods) for long bones to prevent deformities and repeated fractures
- *Physical therapy*: Muscle strengthening, range of motion
- *Mobility aids*: Walkers, braces to reduce fall risk
- **Rehabilitation** is tailored to function, growth, and fracture frequency

Q23. Marfan syndrome—orthopedic manifestations and management.

Definition

A genetic connective tissue disorder caused by mutations in the *FBN1* gene affecting **fibrillin-1**, a major structural component of elastic fibers.

Orthopedic Manifestations

- Tall stature, long limbs (dolichostenomelia)
- Arachnodactyly (long, slender fingers)
- Pectus deformities (excavatum or carinatum)
- Scoliosis (up to 60% of patients)
- Joint hypermobility
- Protrusio acetabuli (deepened acetabulum)
- Flat feet (pes planus)

Systemic Features

- Aortic root dilation (risk of dissection)
- Lens dislocation (ectopia lentis)
- Mitral valve prolapse

Management

- *Orthopedic*:
  - Bracing or surgery for scoliosis
  - Orthotics for flat feet
  - Surgical correction for pectus deformity
- *Multidisciplinary*:
  - Regular cardiac monitoring (echocardiography)
  - Beta-blockers or angiotensin receptor blockers (for aortic dilation)
  - Avoidance of contact sports (due to aortic dissection risk)

Q24. Ehlers–Danlos syndrome (EDS)—orthopedic implications.

Definition

A group of heritable connective tissue disorders primarily affecting **collagen synthesis or structure** (often involving **COL5A1, COL5A2**, etc.).

Orthopedic Features

- Joint hypermobility (Beighton score >5/9)
- Frequent dislocations and subluxations (shoulder, patella, TMJ)
- Chronic joint pain
- Muscle hypotonia
- Delayed motor development
- Foot deformities (e.g., pes planus)

Skin Features (Depending on Subtype)

- Hyperextensible skin
- Fragile skin, easy bruising
- Poor wound healing (atrophic scars)

Complications

- Spontaneous joint dislocations
- Early-onset osteoarthritis
- *Vascular subtype*: Risk of arterial or organ rupture

Management

- *Conservative*: Physiotherapy, joint protection strategies
- Orthoses for joint stability
- Avoid surgery unless essential due to poor healing
- *Multidisciplinary team*: geneticists, orthopedists, physiotherapists

Q25. Stickler syndrome—musculoskeletal features.

Definition

An autosomal dominant disorder caused by mutations in **COL2A1, COL11A1**, etc., affecting **type II and XI collagen**.

Key Musculoskeletal Features

- Joint hypermobility
- Scoliosis and kyphosis
- Early-onset osteoarthritis (especially hips and knees)
- Short stature
- Flattened midface, micrognathia (Pierre Robin sequence)

Other Systemic Features

- *Eye*: High myopia, vitreoretinal degeneration, retinal detachment
- *Ear*: Sensorineural hearing loss
- *Craniofacial*: Cleft palate or small jaw

Orthopedic Management

- Joint protection strategies
- Physiotherapy
- Bracing for spinal deformities
- Surgical correction of severe skeletal abnormalities

Q26. Nail–Patella syndrome (osteo-onychodysplasia).

- Genetic condition (autosomal dominant)
- *Features*:
    - Nail dysplasia (especially thumbs)
    - Absent or hypoplastic **patella**
    - Elbow dysplasia
    - **Iliac horns** (pathognomonic on X-ray)
    - Possible nephropathy (proteinuria)

Treatment
- Mostly symptomatic—bracing, physio
- Patellar stabilization if dislocation

FLOWCHART: Approach to connective tissue disorders in orthopedics

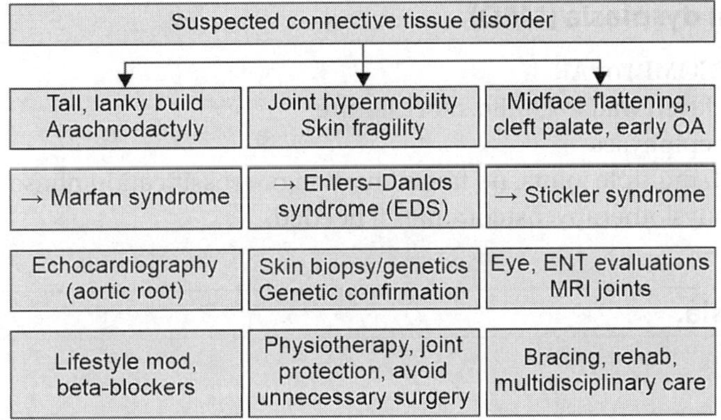

Common Skeletal Dysplasias

Q27. Skeletal dysplasias—classification and ortho relevance.

Definition

A group of **genetic disorders affecting growth and development of bone and cartilage**.

Classification (Based on Molecular/Genetic Basis)
- *Osteochondrodysplasias*: Abnormal development (e.g., achondroplasia)
- *Dysostoses*: Abnormal bone modeling/patterning (e.g., cleidocranial dysplasia)

Examples and Orthopedic Issues

Disorder	***Ortho relevance***
Achondroplasia	Rhizomelia, spinal stenosis
Thanatophoric dysplasia	Lethal neonatal dwarfism
Multiple epiphyseal dysplasia	Early-onset OA, joint pain
Osteopetrosis	Brittle bones, nerve compression

Q28. Thanatophoric dysplasia.

- *Mutation*: Severe FGFR3 mutations
- Lethal perinatal skeletal dysplasia

- *Clinical*: Severe micromelia, narrow thorax, macrocephaly, **"telephone receiver" femora**
- *Outcome*: Respiratory failure due to thoracic insufficiency.

Q29. Spondyloepiphyseal dysplasia (SED).

- *Mutation*: COL2A1 (type II collagen)
- *Features*:
  - Short trunk dwarfism
  - Platyspondyly
  - Delayed ossification of epiphyses
- *Ortho significance*: Kyphoscoliosis, hip dysplasia (early OA), cervical spine instability
- *Management*: Early bracing/spinal fusion, hip preservation procedures.

Q30. Multiple epiphyseal dysplasia (MED).

- *Inheritance*: AD (COL9A1, COMP) or AR
- *Presentation*: Joint pain, delayed walking, mild short stature
- *Radiology*: Small, irregular epiphyses
- *DDx from Perthes*: Bilateral, multiple joints, no fragmentation or reossification phases.
- *Management*: Pain relief, physiotherapy, osteotomies if needed.

Q31. Diastrophic dysplasia.

- *Mutation*: SLC26A2
- *Clinical features*:
  - "Hitchhiker" thumbs
  - Short limbs
  - Cleft palate
  - Joint contractures
  - Cauliflower ears
- *Ortho care*: Corrective surgery for scoliosis, clubfoot, joint stiffness.

Q32. Metaphyseal dysplasia versus rickets.

Feature	***Metaphyseal dysplasia***	***Rickets***
Cause	Genetic (e.g., Schmid type)	Nutritional/vitamin D deficiency
Metaphysis	Irregular, widened metaphysis	Cupping, fraying, splaying
Biochem markers	Normal calcium, phosphate, ALP	↓ Ca^{2+}, ↓ phosphate, ↑ ALP
Systemic findings	Absent	Present (e.g., craniotabes, rickety rosary)
Treatment	Supportive, orthopedic	*Medical*: Vitamin D and calcium

Q33. Management of multiple epiphyseal dysplasia (MED).

Definition

A genetic disorder affecting **ossification of epiphyses** → short stature and joint pain.

Inheritance

Mostly autosomal dominant (e.g., *COMP* gene mutation).

Clinical Features

- Joint pain and stiffness
- Delayed walking
- Genu valgum, coxa vara, flat feet
- Early-onset osteoarthritis

Radiology

- Small, irregular epiphyses
- Delayed ossification
- Hip dysplasia

Management

- *Symptomatic treatment*: Activity modification, analgesics
- Physiotherapy
- **Guided growth** for deformities
- **Osteotomy** for mechanical alignment
- THA in adulthood (for secondary OA)

Q34. Growth modulation in skeletal dysplasias.

Definition

Use of guided growth techniques to correct angular deformities during growth.

Indications

- Genu varum/valgum in achondroplasia, multiple epiphyseal dysplasia
- Disproportionate limb growth

Techniques

- **8-plate hemiepiphysiodesis** (temporary growth arrest)
- Staples
- Can be combined with **lengthening** procedures later

Benefits

- Minimally invasive
- Avoids major osteotomies in growing children
- Reversible and adjustable

Q35. Write a note on arthrogryposis multiplex congenita (AMC).

Etiology:

- Non-progressive contractures in multiple joints at birth
- Due to fetal akinesia (neurogenic or myopathic)

Diagnosis:

- *Clinical features*: Rigid joints, muscle hypoplasia
- Contractures in shoulders, elbows, wrists, hips, knees
- Investigate for CNS anomalies, spinal cord pathologies

Management:

- Early passive stretching and splinting
- **Surgical correction** of deformities (e.g., talipes, knee flexion)
- Physiotherapy for function

Q36. Management of orthopedic deformities in down syndrome.

(RGUHS 2013)

Common Features

- Ligamentous laxity
- Hypotonia
- Atlantoaxial instability
- Hip dislocation
- Foot deformities (flatfoot, hallux valgus)

Management

- **Spinal screening (X-ray cervical spine in flexion/extension)** before sports/surgery
- Observation for hip instability
- Orthotics for pes planus
- Surgery if progressive deformity or instability

Q37. Neurofibromatosis type 1—musculoskeletal manifestations.

(AIMS Kochi 2017)

Orthopedic Features

- Scoliosis (dystrophic or idiopathic)
- Pseudarthrosis of tibia
- Limb overgrowth or undergrowth
- Bone cysts, shortening, subperiosteal erosion

Management

- Regular follow-up for scoliosis progression
- Surgical correction for pseudarthrosis (cross-union, Ilizarov, BMP)
- Monitor limb length discrepancies

Q38. Orthopedic aspects of Larsen syndrome.

Features

- Multiple congenital dislocations (knees, hips, elbows)
- Flattened facies, cervical kyphosis
- Clubfoot, ligamentous laxity

Management

- Early reduction of joint dislocations (especially knees)
- Cervical spine monitoring (risk of instability)
- Foot correction (casting, surgery)
- Bracing and physiotherapy

Q39. Achondroplasia—features and complications.

Cause

Mutation in *FGFR3* gene → inhibited endochondral ossification

Clinical Features

- **Rhizomelic dwarfism** (short proximal limbs)
- Frontal bossing
- Trident hand
- Genu varum

- Thoracolumbar kyphosis
- **Foramen magnum stenosis**, spinal canal narrowing

Orthopedic Complications
- **Genu varum**
- Spinal stenosis → neurologic symptoms
- Recurrent otitis media
- Delayed motor milestones due to hypotonia

Management
- Limb realignment osteotomies
- Decompression (if spinal canal stenosis)
- Supportive rehabilitation and growth monitoring

Q40. Orthopedic management of achondroplasia.

Etiology

FGFR3 gene mutation → impaired endochondral ossification.

Features
- Rhizomelic limb shortening
- Trident hands
- Thoracolumbar kyphosis
- Foramen magnum stenosis
- Genu varum

Management

Problem	*Treatment*
Spinal stenosis	Laminectomy/decompression
Genu varum	Guided growth or osteotomy
Limb length	Controversial (Ilizarov method)
Cervicomedullary compression	MRI surveillance, early decompression if symptomatic

Q41. Radiological features of skeletal dysplasias.

- *Platyspondyly*: Flattened vertebral bodies (e.g., spondyloepiphyseal dysplasia)
- *Delayed ossification*: Seen in epiphyses (e.g., multiple epiphyseal dysplasia)
- *Metaphyseal flaring*: Typical in metaphyseal dysplasia
- *Short long bones*: Rhizomelic (proximal) in achondroplasia
- *Iliac hypoplasia*: Square iliac wings in skeletal dysplasias
- Trident pelvis, champagne glass pelvis, narrow foramen magnum (e.g., achondroplasia)

Q42. Differentiation—achondroplasia versus hypochondroplasia.

Feature	*Achondroplasia*	*Hypochondroplasia*
Inheritance	AD, FGFR3 mutation	AD, FGFR3 mutation
Onset	At birth	Postnatally (2–3 years)
Limb shortening	Rhizomelic, marked	Milder
Skull	Frontal bossing, midface hypoplasia	Normal or mild
Radiology	Trident hand, narrowing of interpedicular distance caudally	Similar but less severe
Intelligence	Normal	Normal

Q43. Marfan syndrome versus homocystinuria (orthopedic context).

Feature	Marfan syndrome	Homocystinuria
Inheritance	AD	AR
Height	Tall, thin	Tall
Lens	Upward dislocation	Downward dislocation
Spine	Scoliosis	Kyphoscoliosis
Chest	Pectus carinatum	Pectus excavatum
Joint	Hypermobile	Hypermobile
Intelligence	Normal	Mental retardation
Thrombosis	No	Common
Management	Aortic monitoring	Low methionine diet, B6

Multiple Hereditary Exostoses (MHE)

Q44. Genetics, clinical features, and complications.

(Jammu University 2013)

- *Genetics*: *AD, EXT1/EXT2* gene mutation
- *Features*:
  - Multiple osteochondromas (metaphysis of long bones)
  - Short stature, limb deformities
  - Genu valgum, forearm bowing, hip subluxation
- *Complications*:
  - Compression neuropathy
  - Limb length discrepancy
  - Malignant transformation (to chondrosarcoma)

Q45. MHE versus solitary osteochondroma.

Feature	MHE	Solitary osteochondroma
Number	Multiple	Single
Inheritance	Genetic (AD)	Sporadic
Deformities	Common	Rare
Malignant risk	Higher	Lower
Growth arrest	Frequent	Rare

Q46. Malignant transformation in MHE.

- *Risk*: ~1–5%
- *Transformation to*: **Secondary chondrosarcoma**
- *Clues*:
  - Rapid growth after skeletal maturity
  - Pain, irregular margins on imaging
- *Imaging*: MRI shows cartilage cap >1.5–2 cm
- *Management*: Wide excision

Other Genetic Bone Disorders

Q47. Fibrous dysplasia and McCune–Albright syndrome.

- *Fibrous dysplasia*:
  - Bone replaced by fibro-osseous tissue
  - "Ground-glass" radiology
  - *Proximal femur*: Shepherd's crook deformity
- *McCune–Albright syndrome*:
  - Polyostotic fibrous dysplasia
  - Café-au-lait spots (coast of Maine)
  - Precocious puberty

Q48. Cleidocranial dysostosis.

- *Features*:
  - Delayed closure of fontanelles
  - **Absent/hypoplastic clavicles**
  - Dental anomalies
  - Short stature
- *Radiology*:
  - Open sutures
  - Wormian bones
  - Hypoplastic clavicles
- *Ortho relevance*: Shoulder hypermobility

Q49. Mucopolysaccharidoses (e.g., Morquio, Hurler).

- *Morquio (MPS IV)*:
  - Severe skeletal dysplasia, normal intellect
  - Atlantoaxial instability
- *Hurler (MPS I)*:
  - Short stature, coarse facies
  - Mental retardation
- *Radiology*: Dysostosis multiplex
- *Treatment*: Enzyme replacement, fusion for instability

Q50. Diaphyseal aclasis.

- Alternative term for MHE
- *Features*: Multiple osteochondromas along diaphyses
- *Ortho significance*: Deformity, compression, malignancy

Q51. Orthopedic manifestations of down syndrome.

- Hypotonia
- Ligamentous laxity
- Atlantoaxial instability
- Hip dislocation
- Genu valgum
- Pes planus

Q52. Management of orthopedic deformities in down syndrome.

Common Issues

- Ligamentous laxity
- Hypotonia
- Atlantoaxial instability
- Hip dislocation
- Flatfoot, genu valgum

Management

- Cervical spine X-rays before sports/surgery
- Observation for hip instability
- Orthotics for foot deformities
- Osteotomy for severe deformities

Q53. Spinal abnormalities in Klippel–Feil syndrome.

(DYPU Pune 2013)

- Congenital fusion of ≥2 cervical vertebrae
- *Triad*: Short neck, low hairline, limited neck motion
- *Associated with*:
  - Sprengel shoulder
  - Scoliosis
  - Renal/cardiac anomalies

Q54. Musculoskeletal manifestations of turner syndrome.

- Short stature
- Cubitus valgus
- Genu valgum
- High arched palate
- Madelung deformity

Q55. Spondyloepiphyseal dysplasia congenita.

- *Mutation*: *COL2A1* gene
- *Features*:
  - Platyspondyly
  - Short trunk dwarfism
  - Cleft palate
  - Retinal detachment
- *Radiology*:
  - Delayed epiphyseal ossification
  - Flattened vertebral bodies

Q56. Camptomelic dysplasia.

- Rare, often lethal skeletal dysplasia
- *Features*:
  - Bowing of long bones (especially tibia/fibula)
  - Hypoplastic scapulae
  - Ambiguous genitalia
  - Respiratory compromise

Q57. Arthrogryposis multiplex congenita (AMC)—etiology, diagnosis, and treatment.

(GGMC 2012)

Etiology

- Non-progressive **congenital joint contractures** in ≥2 areas
- Due to **fetal akinesia**, caused by:
  - Neurogenic disorders (anterior horn cell defects)
  - Myopathies
  - Intrauterine factors (e.g., oligohydramnios)

Diagnosis

- *At birth*: Stiff joints, thin muscles, deformities
- *Most common*: **Amyoplasia** (limb involvement)
- *Investigations*: X-ray, MRI spine, muscle biopsy (if syndromic), genetic tests

Treatment

- Early **physiotherapy**
- Splinting and stretching
- *Surgical*:
  - Clubfoot correction
  - Hip/knee contracture release
  - Tendon transfers
- *Goal*: Maximize function and independence

Q58. Neurofibromatosis type 1 (NF1)—musculoskeletal manifestations.

Features

- Café-au-lait spots, neurofibromas, Lisch nodules
- *Orthopedic*:
  - Scoliosis (dystrophic)
  - Tibial pseudarthrosis
  - Limb overgrowth/undergrowth
  - Cervical kyphosis

Management

- Bracing for early scoliosis
- Surgical fusion for progressive curves
- *Tibial pseudarthrosis*: Excision, intramedullary fixation, BMP, cross-union
- Monitor for malignancy transformation (MPNST)

CHAPTER 11

Trauma and Fracture Management

11.1 General Principles of Trauma

Mozam Hamid Wani, Vineet Aggarwal, Asim Maqbool

Q1. Define trauma. Classify trauma based on severity and mechanism.

(AIIMS JPR 2014)

Definition

Trauma is defined as an injury or damage to tissues caused by the transfer of energy (mechanical, thermal, electrical, chemical) from the environment to the body.

- *Epidemiology*:
  - Leading cause of death under age 45
  - *Common causes*: Road traffic accidents, falls, violence
  - Significant public health burden globally

Classification based on severity

Type	*Description*
Minor trauma	Single system injury, stable vitals (e.g., isolated fracture)
Major trauma	Life-threatening or involving multiple organ systems (e.g., polytrauma)
Polytrauma	Injury to ≥2 body regions with one being life-threatening

Classification Based on Mechanism

Mechanism	*Example*
Blunt trauma	Road traffic accidents, falls
Penetrating trauma	Stab wounds, gunshots
Crush injury	Earthquake victims, industrial accidents
Blast injury	War zones, explosions
Deceleration/Shear	Motor vehicle accidents (e.g., aortic rupture)

Other Classifications

Type	*Example*
Open versus closed	Open fracture versus closed fracture
Primary versus secondary	Primary: direct result of trauma; Secondary: complications like shock, sepsis

Q2. Define polytrauma. Etiopathogenesis, classification, and immune response. Role of DCO.

- *Polytrauma:* A condition where a patient has multiple traumatic injuries, at least one of which is life-threatening.
- Trauma to ≥2 organ systems or body regions with **ISS ≥16**, and one injury potentially life-threatening.

Etiopathogenesis

- *First hit:* Initial trauma → tissue damage → systemic inflammation (SIRS)
- *Second hit:* Surgical intervention or sepsis → overwhelms immune system → MODS
- *Classification:*
  - *By anatomical region*: Head, chest, abdomen, limbs
  - *By severity*: Based on Injury Severity Score (ISS)
  - *By physiological response*: Hemodynamic stability, presence of shock or SIRS

Immune Response

- SIRS → Cytokine storm (IL-6, TNF-α)
- Counter-regulatory **CARS** (compensatory anti-inflammatory response syndrome)
- Balance between SIRS and CARS determines survival

Q3. Priorities in management of polytrauma.

ABCDE of ATLS

1. *A*irway with C-spine control
2. *B*reathing
3. *C*irculation—control bleeding, resuscitate
4. *D*isability—neurological status (GCS)
5. *E*xposure—prevent hypothermia

Orthopedic priorities

- Pelvic binder in pelvic fracture
- External fixation of long bones (DCO)
- Fasciotomy if compartment syndrome
- Avoid early total care in unstable patients

Q4. Define triage. What are its categories and principles?

(AIIMS Patna 2013)

Definition

Triage is the medical process of prioritizing patients based on the **severity of injury and urgency of intervention** required, particularly in mass casualty incidents (MCIs) where resources are limited.

Triage Categories (e.g., START System—Simple Triage and Rapid Treatment)

Category	*Color code*	*Description*	*Example*
Immediate	Red	Life-threatening but treatable injuries	Open pneumothorax, active bleeding
Delayed	Yellow	Serious but not immediately life-threatening	Fracture shaft femur without bleeding
Minimal	Green	Minor injuries, ambulatory patients	Soft tissue injury, minor lacerations
Expectant	Black	Unsalvageable or deceased patients	Massive head injury, cardiac arrest

Principles of Triage

- Aim to **maximize survival** with limited resources
- Prioritize **treatable patients** who can benefit most
- Reassessment is essential as conditions evolve
- Utilized in **natural disasters, mass accidents, war zones**

Q5. What is disaster management? Outline the orthopedic surgeon's role.

Definition

Disaster management is the **organized and coordinated effort** to handle disaster situations to minimize impact on human health and infrastructure.

Phases of Disaster Management

1. *Mitigation*: Reducing risks (e.g., building safety codes)
2. *Preparedness*: Planning, training, mock drills
3. *Response*: Emergency services, triage, stabilization
4. *Recovery*: Rehabilitation, long-term care, policy revision

Orthopedic Surgeon's Role

- Lead triage of orthopedic injuries
- Perform emergency procedures: fracture stabilization, fasciotomy, debridement
- Provide **damage control orthopedics** in unstable patients
- Assist in **rehabilitation planning**
- Work in **coordination with public health** and disaster response teams

Q6. Describe orthopedic management protocols in mass casualty scenarios.

Key Principles

- *Triage:* Prioritize based on life-saving potential and available resources
- *Damage control orthopedics (DCO):*
  - Focus on **temporary stabilization**, often using **external fixators or splints**
  - Avoid prolonged procedures in physiologically unstable patients
- *Definitive treatment:* Once systemic stability is achieved (usually after 48–72 hours)

Initial Measures

- IV fluids, antibiotics (for open wounds)
- Tetanus prophylaxis
- Radiographs for injury assessment
- Application of traction, splints, or external fixators
- Fasciotomy in compartment syndrome

Documentation and Communication

Patient tagging, injury mapping, operative records are crucial for tracking

Q7. Flowchart—disaster planning at state level and concept of triage.

(GMERS Medical College 2015)

FLOWCHART: Disaster management (state level)

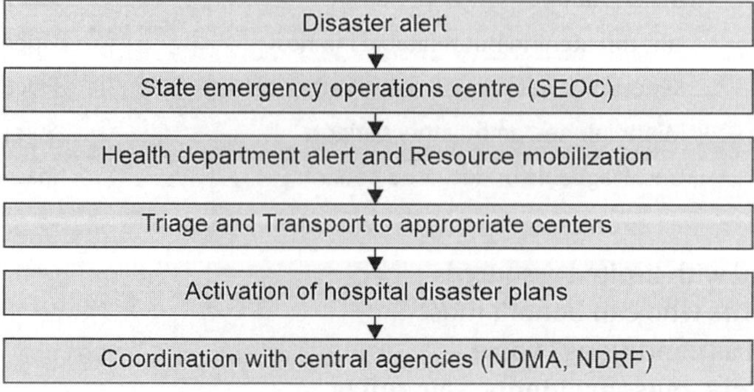

Q8. Describe basic trauma life support (BTLS). What are its key components?

Definition

Basic trauma life support (BTLS) is a standardized **pre-hospital protocol** for early trauma management focused on **assessment, stabilization, and safe transport** of trauma victims.

Key Components (ABCDE Format)

- *A—Airway and C-spine protection:* Jaw thrust, airway adjuncts, cervical collar
- *B—Breathing:* Look, listen, feel; manage open pneumothorax, flail chest
- *C—Circulation:* Control bleeding, IV access (two large bore), fluid resuscitation
- *D—Disability:* Neurological status using GCS, pupil size/reactivity
- *E—Exposure:* Undress patient completely to assess injuries; prevent hypothermia

Other Essentials

- Rapid trauma survey
- Oxygen supplementation
- Splinting of fractures for pain relief and hemorrhage control
- Communication with trauma center for early intervention

Q9. What is ATLS? Describe its primary and secondary surveys.

Definition

Advanced trauma life support (ATLS) is a **systematic and prioritized approach** developed by the American College of Surgeons for managing acutely injured patients.

Primary Survey (ABCDE)

- *A:* Ensure airway patency while maintaining cervical spine stability
- *B:* Assess and support breathing (inspect, palpate, auscultate)
- *C:* Check for pulse, BP, hemorrhage; initiate IV fluids
- *D:* Assess neurological status using AVPU and GCS
- *E:* Expose patient fully but prevent hypothermia

Secondary Survey

- Head-to-toe examination
- Focused history (AMPLE: allergies, medications, past illness, last meal, events)
- *Radiological investigations*: X-ray (CXR, pelvis), FAST, CT scan as required
- Plan definitive care

Q10. What is the MIST protocol in trauma handover?

MIST is a communication format for **structured patient handover** in trauma settings:

- *M—Mechanism of injury:* For example, RTA, fall from height
- *I—Injuries sustained:* For example, open tibial fracture, head trauma
- *S—Signs and vitals:* HR, BP, SpO_2, GCS
- *T—Treatment given:* Fluids, splints, antibiotics, airway management

This ensures **clear, consistent handovers** between EMS, emergency room, and surgical teams.

Q11. What is the 'Golden Hour' and 'Platinum 10 minutes' in trauma care?

(Rajasthan University of Health Sciences 2017)

- *Golden hour:*
    - Refers to the **first 60 minutes** after traumatic injury
    - Most crucial time for intervention to **reduce mortality**
    - Early stabilization and definitive care → improved outcomes

- *Platinum 10 minutes:*
    - The **first 10 minutes on scene** by first responders
    - Target time for **rapid assessment, hemorrhage control, and initiation of transport**

Q12. Write a short note on the "Trimodal Distribution of Death" in trauma.

- *Three peaks:*
    - *Immediate*: Seconds to minutes (brain/spinal cord, major vessels)
    - *Early*: Minutes to hours ("golden hour"; treatable causes like hemothorax, splenic rupture)
    - *Late*: Days to weeks (sepsis, multi-organ failure)

Q13. Discuss the indications for resuscitative thoracotomy in trauma patients.

- *Indications:*
    - Penetrating thoracic injury with cardiac arrest
    - Blunt trauma with signs of life within 10 minutes
- *Goals:*
    - Control cardiac tamponade
    - Cross-clamp aorta
    - Direct cardiac massage

Q14. Explain the role of focused assessment with sonography for trauma (FAST) in trauma evaluation.

(RIMS 2008)

- Non-invasive bedside ultrasound
- *Checks for free fluid:*
    - Peritoneal cavity (hemoperitoneum)
    - Pericardium (tamponade)
    - Pleura (hemothorax)
- Quick and repeatable; integral in hemodynamically unstable trauma patients
    - Damage control resuscitation and surgery

Q15. Principles of trauma scoring systems (ISS, GCS).

Purpose of Trauma Scores

- Quantify injury severity
- Predict prognosis
- Guide triage and resource allocation
- Facilitate communication and research

A. Injury Severity Score (ISS)

Q16. Injury severity score (ISS) in trauma assessment.

What is ISS?

- Anatomical trauma scoring system
- Based on abbreviated injury scale (AIS)

How is ISS Calculated?

- Pick **three most severely injured body regions**

- *Square each AIS score and sum:* ISS = $A^2 + B^2 + C^2$
- *Range:* 0–75
- **ISS >15** → Major trauma
- **ISS = 75** → Unsurvivable (AIS 6 in any one region)

Clinical Utility
- Predicts mortality and morbidity
- Guides triage and referral to trauma centers
- Benchmark for trauma registry data

B. Glasgow Coma Scale (GCS)

Used to assess **level of consciousness** in head injury.

Component	Score
Eye opening (E)	1–4
Verbal response (V)	1–5
Motor response (M)	1–6

Total Score = E + V + M (maximum: 15, minimum: 3)
- *GCS 13–15:* Mild head injury
- *GCS 9–12:* Moderate
- *GCS ≤8:* Severe (requires airway protection)

Q17. Discuss the revised trauma score (RTS) and its clinical significance.

(AIIMS Jodhpur 2008)

- *RTS*: A physiological scoring system
- *Components*:
  - **GCS**, **SBP**, and **RR**
  - Each scored 0–4
- *Used for*: **Triage**, outcome prediction, and trauma system performance

Q18. Write a short note on the abbreviated injury scale (AIS).

- *AIS:* An anatomic scoring system for each injury, ranging from **1 (minor)** to **6 (unsurvivable)**
- *Used in*:
  - Calculating **ISS**
  - Injury classification
  - Research and trauma audits

Q19. MESS—mangled extremity severity score (short note).

Purpose
Helps predict the need for **amputation** in severe limb trauma.

Components (4)

Parameter	Score
Skeletal/Soft tissue injury	1–4
Limb ischemia	1–3 (×2 if >6 hours)
Shock	0–2
Age	0–2

Total score ≥7 → strong predictor of amputation

Q20. Revised trauma score (RTS).

Physiological Trauma Scoring Based On

1. Glasgow coma scale (GCS)
2. Systolic BP
3. Respiratory rate

Formula

RTS = 0.9368 (GCS) + 0.7326 (SBP) + 0.2908 (RR) Range: 0 (worst) to 7.84 (best)

Clinical Significance

- Used in **triage protocols** (e.g., START)
- Early prognostication
- Combined with ISS to calculate **TRISS** (trauma score + injury severity score) → survival prediction

Q21. Explain the pathophysiology of the systemic inflammatory response syndrome (SIRS) in polytrauma.

(PGI Chandigarh 2012)

- *Triggered by:*
  - Massive tissue injury → cytokine release
  - Activation of immune cells
- *Results in:*
  - Widespread **vasodilation, increased capillary permeability, organ dysfunction**
  - May progress to **MODS**

Q22. Discuss the concept of multiple organ dysfunction syndrome (MODS) in trauma.

- *MODS:* Progressive dysfunction of ≥2 organ systems due to trauma and shock
- *Occurs due to*: Persistent SIRS, sepsis, ischemia-reperfusion injury
- *Commonly affected organs*: Lungs, kidneys, liver, heart

Q23. Write a short note on the "second hit phenomenon" in polytrauma.

- *First hit:* Initial trauma insult
- *Second hit:* Subsequent surgery or intervention triggering **exaggerated immune response**
- Leads to worsening of SIRS and potential MODS
- Emphasizes careful **timing of surgery**

Q24. Define damage control orthopedics (DCO). State its indications.

Definition

Damage control orthopedics (DCO) is a **staged surgical approach** where temporary fracture stabilization is prioritized over definitive fixation in severely injured patients to avoid systemic inflammatory overload.

Indications

- **Polytrauma** with ongoing resuscitation needs
- **Chest, abdominal, cranial injuries** with unstable vitals
- High Injury Severity Score (ISS > 25)
- **Coagulopathy, acidosis, hypothermia** ("lethal triad")

Steps

1. External fixation or temporary traction

2. ICU resuscitation (correct pH, temperature, coagulation)
3. Definitive surgery once stabilized

Q25. Discuss fractures in polytrauma patients—damage control orthopedics versus early total care.

(Seth Gordhandas Sunderdas Medical College and KEM Hospital 2013)

Early Total Care (ETC)
- Definitive fracture fixation **within first 24–48 hours**
- Suitable for **hemodynamically stable patients**

Damage Control Orthopedics (DCO)
- Initial **temporary stabilization** (e.g., external fixator)
- Definitive surgery delayed until patient is physiologically optimized

Indications for DCO
- Hemodynamic instability
- Ongoing resuscitation
- Coagulopathy
- Chest/abdominal injuries
- ISS > 18 or "borderline" trauma patient

Advantages
- Reduces risk of **SIRS, ARDS, MOF**
- Improves survival in unstable patients

Definitive Fixation Timing
After 48–72 hours when patient is stable (often in ICU setting)

Q26. Indications and timing of definitive fixation in polytrauma patients.

Key Considerations
- Physiologic status (acid-base balance, lactate)
- Chest/head injury
- Coagulopathy
- Soft tissue status

Timing Strategy

Approach	*Indication*
Early total care (ETC)	Stable patient, ISS <15
Damage control orthopedics (DCO)	Unstable, coagulopathy, chest injury
Safe definitive surgery window	5–10 days after trauma (post-resuscitation)

Indications for Early Definitive Fixation
- Isolated long bone fractures
- Young, stable polytrauma patients
- No major head/chest/abdominal injuries

Q27. Discuss the role of whole-body CT (pan-scan) in polytrauma evaluation.

(Madras Medical College 2012)

- *Used to rapidly identify life-threatening injuries in:* Head, neck, chest, abdomen, pelvis
- *Advantages:*
  - High sensitivity

- Reduced missed injuries
- Improves outcomes in major trauma
- Should be performed **only in stable or borderline patients**

Q28. Explain the clinical significance of the "Lethal Triad" in trauma.

- *Components:*
  - Hypothermia
  - Acidosis
  - Coagulopathy
- *Self-perpetuating cycle leading to:*
  - Poor outcomes
  - High mortality
- *Management includes:*
  - Active warming
  - Buffering acidosis

Q29. Explain the concept of damage control resuscitation (DCR).

[Assam Medical College (affiliated to Srimanta Sankaradeva University of Health Sciences) 2021]

- Aims to prevent **lethal triad** (acidosis, hypothermia, coagulopathy)
- *Components:*
  - Permissive hypotension
  - Hemostatic resuscitation
  - Damage control surgery (minimal, lifesaving)

Q30. Define shock and classify its types in trauma patients.

- *Shock:* Inadequate tissue perfusion leading to cellular hypoxia.
- *Types in trauma:*
  - **Hypovolemic (hemorrhagic)**—most common
  - **Obstructive**—e.g., tension pneumothorax, cardiac tamponade
  - **Cardiogenic**
  - **Distributive**—e.g., neurogenic, septic

Q31. Explain the pathophysiology of hemorrhagic shock.

(CMC Vellore 2013)

- Blood loss → ↓ preload → ↓ stroke volume → ↓ cardiac output
- *Compensatory mechanisms:*
  - Tachycardia
  - Vasoconstriction
  - Increased respiratory rate
- Prolonged hypoperfusion → anaerobic metabolism → lactic acidosis → organ failure

Q32. Discuss the management principles of hemorrhagic shock in trauma.

- **ABC (airway, breathing, circulation) approach**
- *Immediate hemorrhage control:* Direct pressure, tourniquets, surgery, embolization

- *Fluid resuscitation:*
    - Crystalloids (limited use)
    - Blood products
- Early use of **massive transfusion protocol (MTP)**
- Monitor lactate, base deficit

Q33. Management of hypovolemic shock in polytrauma.

(CMC Vellore, PGI Chandigarh)

- *Initial resuscitation:* ABCs, two large bore IV lines
- *Fluids:* 1–2 L warm crystalloids → blood products (1:1:1 PRBC:FFP:Platelets)

Control Bleeding
- *Monitor:* Urine output, lactate, base deficit
- **Definitive fixation** only after stabilization

Q34. Neurogenic shock.

- *Cause:* Spinal cord injury (usually cervical/thoracic)
- *Pathophys:* Loss of sympathetic tone → vasodilation → hypotension, bradycardia
- *Treatment:* Vasopressors (noradrenaline), fluid resuscitation, spinal precautions

Q35. Write a short note on permissive hypotension in trauma resuscitation.

- *Definition:* Maintaining SBP ~80–90 mm Hg until bleeding is controlled
- Goal: Avoid dislodging clots, reduce dilutional coagulopathy
- Contraindicated in **TBI** (requires higher perfusion)

Q36. Discuss the role of massive transfusion protocol (MTP) in trauma patients.

- Initiated when >**10 units of PRBCs in 24 hours** expected
- *Uses balanced resuscitation*:
    - **1:1:1 ratio** of PRBCs:FFP:Platelets
- Incorporates lab-guided therapy (e.g., INR, fibrinogen)
- Reduces mortality from coagulopathy and exsanguination

Q37. Explain the complications of blood transfusion in trauma resuscitation.

(WBUHS 2012)

- Transfusion reactions
- Transfusion-related acute lung injury (TRALI)
- Hypocalcemia (from citrate)
- Hypothermia
- Hyperkalemia
- Dilutional coagulopathy
- Immunosuppression

Q38. Write a short note on tranexamic acid (TXA) and its role in trauma management.

- *Antifibrinolytic:* Inhibits plasminogen activation

- Early TXA (within 3 hours) reduces mortality in bleeding trauma patients (CRASH-2 trial)
- *Dose*: 1g IV bolus + 1g infusion over 8 hours

Q39. Discuss the role of thromboelastography (TEG) in trauma-induced coagulopathy.

(AIIMS BBSR 2015)

- TEG provides **real-time coagulation profile**
- *Assesses*:
  - Clot strength
  - Fibrinolysis
  - Platelet function
- Guides targeted transfusion (e.g., fibrinogen, platelets, cryoprecipitate)

Q40. Biomechanics of trauma and injury patterns.

Mechanisms of Force

Type	*Example*	*Injury pattern*
Compression	Fall from height	Vertebral burst fractures
Tension	Hyperextension	Avulsion injuries
Shear	MVC with twisting	ACL tear, pelvic fractures
Torsion	Skiing	Spiral long bone fractures
Bending	Blow to mid-shaft	Transverse fractures

Injury Patterns

- *Axial load*: Compression fractures (e.g., spine)
- *High-velocity trauma*: Comminution, polytrauma
- *Deceleration injuries*: Ligamentous avulsion, visceral rupture
- Force transmission affects injury type:
  - *Axial loading*: Vertebral compression fractures
  - *Shearing*: Ligamentous injuries
  - *Rotational forces*: Spiral fractures
- *High-energy trauma*: Polytrauma and multi-system injuries
- Patterns vary with age, bone quality, and mechanism

Q41. Role of external fixation in polytrauma patients.

Indications

- Unstable long bone fractures
- Open fractures with soft tissue injury
- Severe polytrauma (ISS > 16)
- Part of **damage control orthopedics (DCO)**
- When immediate definitive fixation is unsafe (e.g., chest/brain injury, coagulopathy)

Advantages

- Quick application (≤30 min)
- Minimally invasive (less blood loss)
- Preserves soft tissues
- Temporary stabilization to allow systemic recovery

Examples

- Spanning knee external fixator in distal femur fracture
- Tibial shaft fracture with severe soft tissue injury

Q42. Fat embolism syndrome (FES) in trauma.

Pathophysiology

- *Mechanical theory:* Fat globules from marrow enter venous circulation → lodge in lungs/brain
- *Biochemical theory:* Free fatty acids cause endothelial damage → ARDS-like picture

Clinical Features (Usually 24–72 hours post-trauma)

- *Respiratory:* Tachypnea, hypoxia, ARDS
- *CNS:* Confusion, agitation, seizures
- *Skin:* Petechial rash (axilla, chest)
- **Retinal hemorrhages**

Gurd's Criteria

- ≥1 major + ≥4 minor criteria
- *Major*: Hypoxia, CNS depression, rash
- *Minor*: Tachycardia, fever, fat in urine/sputum, thrombocytopenia

Prevention

- **Early immobilization/fixation** of long bone fractures
- Gentle reaming during nailing
- High-flow oxygen
- Prophylactic corticosteroids (controversial)

Q43. Acute respiratory distress syndrome (ARDS).

- *Definition:* Non-cardiogenic pulmonary edema due to increased alveolar-capillary permeability.
- *Causes:* Trauma, fat embolism, sepsis.
- *Berlin criteria:*
  - *Onset*: within 1 week of insult
  - Bilateral opacities
  - PaO_2/FiO_2 <300
- *Treatment:* Low tidal volume ventilation, PEEP, prone positioning, treat underlying cause.

Q44. Flail chest.

- *Definition:* Fracture of ≥3 consecutive ribs in ≥2 places → segment moves paradoxically.
- *Clinical:* Paradoxical chest movement, respiratory distress.
- *Management:*
  - Oxygen, pain relief (epidural)
  - Chest physiotherapy
  - Ventilation if severe

Q45. Tension pneumothorax.

- *Definition:* Accumulation of air under pressure in pleural space → mediastinal shift.
- *Signs:* Hypotension, distended neck veins, tracheal deviation, absent breath sounds.
- *Emergency treatment:* Needle decompression (2nd ICS MCL) → chest tube (5th ICS AAL)

Q46. Crush syndrome.

- *Definition:* Systemic effects of muscle crush injury → rhabdomyolysis
- *Triad:* Myoglobinuria, hyperkalemia, renal failure

- *Management:*
    - Aggressive fluids
    - Mannitol, bicarbonate (alkalinize urine)
    - Dialysis if renal failure

Q47. Transportation of polytrauma patient.

- **Golden hour** concept
- *Spinal precautions:* Cervical collar, log roll
- **ATLS protocol** en route
- *Pre-hospital care:* Oxygen, IV access, bleeding control
- Rapid transfer to trauma center

Q48. Urethral injuries.

- Associated with pelvic fractures
- *Signs:* Blood at meatus, high-riding prostate, inability to void
- *Diagnosis:* Retrograde urethrogram (RUG)
- *Treatment:* Suprapubic catheter initially → delayed repair

Q49. Tracheostomy.

- *Indications:*
    - Prolonged ventilation (>10 days)
    - Upper airway obstruction
    - Severe facial trauma
- *Types:* Surgical versus Percutaneous
- *Complications:* Bleeding, infection, tracheal stenosis

Q50. Morel–Lavallée Lesion.

- *Definition:* Closed degloving injury due to shearing forces separating skin/subcutaneous tissue from fascia
- *Sites:* Greater trochanter, pelvis
- *Presents:* Fluctuant swelling, skin necrosis
- *Management:*
    - Compression
    - Drainage (aspiration/surgical)
    - Debridement if infected

Head, Chest, and Abdominal Trauma in Polytrauma Patients

Q51. Write a short note on primary and secondary brain injury.

(RMLIMS 2016)

- *Primary injury*: Direct mechanical damage at time of trauma (e.g., contusion, laceration).
- *Secondary injury*: Cascade of cellular, metabolic, and vascular changes → ischemia, edema, increased ICP.
    - *Prevention*: Oxygenation, perfusion, ICP control.

Q52. Explain the role of intracranial pressure (ICP) monitoring in traumatic brain injury (TBI).

- *Indications:* GCS <8 with abnormal CT or clinical risk factors.
- Maintains **cerebral perfusion pressure (CPP = MAP - ICP)**
- *Normal ICP:* <20 mm Hg
- *Management decisions:* Mannitol, hypertonic saline, decompressive craniectomy.

Q53. Discuss the principles of management of chest trauma in polytrauma patient.

- **ABCDE** (airway, breathing, circulation...) approach
- *Immediate threats:* Tension pneumothorax, open pneumothorax, massive hemothorax, flail chest, cardiac tamponade.
- Chest tube insertion, oxygenation, imaging (CXR, CT), and surgical interventions as needed.

Q54. Write a short note on tension pneumothorax and its management.

(AIIMS Delhi 2013)

- *Definition:* Air enters pleural space and cannot escape → mediastinal shift → compression of heart/lungs.
- *Signs:* Hypotension, JVD, tracheal shift, absent breath sounds.
- *Management:* Immediate needle decompression (2nd ICS MCL) → chest tube placement.

Q55. Explain the management of massive hemothorax in trauma patients.

- **>1,500 mL** blood on initial chest tube or **>200 mL/h** for 3 hours.
- Resuscitation (fluids, blood products), chest tube drainage.
- Surgical intervention (thoracotomy) if ongoing bleeding or hemodynamic instability.

Q56. Discuss the indications for emergency thoracotomy in blunt and penetrating chest trauma.

- *Penetrating trauma:*
  - Cardiac arrest <15 minutes
  - Tamponade, massive hemorrhage
- *Blunt trauma:*
  - Arrest witnessed in trauma bay with signs of life
  - Massive hemothorax or cardiac tamponade

Q57. Explain the role of damage control laparotomy (DCL) in abdominal trauma.

(KGMU 2007)

- Indicated when full repair is unsafe due to physiological derangement.
- *Three phases:*
  1. Initial laparotomy—control hemorrhage/contamination
  2. Resuscitation in ICU
  3. Definitive surgery (re-look)

Q58. Discuss the management of retroperitoneal hematoma in blunt trauma.

- Often associated with pelvic fractures or aortic injuries.
- *Zones:*
  - *Zone I (central)*: Usually operative

  - *Zone II (flank)*: Non-operative unless expanding
  - *Zone III (pelvic)*: Typically non-operative; angiographic embolization if bleeding
- *Imaging:* CT with contrast

Q59. Write a short note on the prophylaxis and management of venous thromboembolism (VTE) in trauma.

- *Prophylaxis:*
  - LMWH, intermittent pneumatic compression devices
  - Initiated once bleeding risk is controlled
- *Management:*
  - Therapeutic anticoagulation (LMWH or unfractionated heparin)
  - Monitor for pulmonary embolism

Q60. Explain the pathophysiology of acute respiratory distress syndrome (ARDS) in trauma patients.

(Bihar University 2015)

- *Cause:* Direct or indirect lung injury → inflammation → alveolar damage.
- *Hallmark:* Non-cardiogenic pulmonary edema.
- *Clinical signs:*
  - Refractory hypoxemia
  - Bilateral infiltrates on chest X-ray
- *Management:*
  - Lung-protective ventilation (low tidal volume)
  - Positive end-expiratory pressure (PEEP)
  - Prone positioning in severe cases

Q61. Write a short note on ventilator-associated pneumonia (VAP) in trauma patients.

- *Definition:* Pneumonia developing ≥48 hours after intubation.
- *Clinical features:* Fever, purulent secretions, new infiltrate on CXR
- *Management:*
  - Empirical antibiotics, de-escalation based on cultures
  - Elevate head of bed, oral care, suctioning to prevent

Q62. Discuss the causes and management of post-traumatic sepsis.

- *Causes:*
  - Open wounds, invasive lines, organ injury
  - Immunosuppression from trauma/surgery
- *Management:*
  - Early recognition and antibiotics
  - Source control (drain abscess, debride wound)
  - Supportive care: fluids, vasopressors, organ support

Q63. Explain the role of early enteral nutrition in trauma patients.

- *Benefits:*
  - Maintains gut mucosal integrity
  - Reduces bacterial translocation
  - Improves immune response

- *Timing:* Initiate within 24–48 hours if no contraindications
- *Preferred route:* Enteral over parenteral when feasible

Q64. Classification and management of open fractures.

Gustilo–Anderson Classification

Type	Description	Contamination	Soft tissue
I	Clean, <1 cm	Minimal	Simple
II	>1 cm, no extensive damage	Moderate	Moderate
IIIA	Extensive soft tissue, still coverable	Severe	Adequate coverage
IIIB	Exposed bone, periosteal stripping	Severe	Requires flap
IIIC	Vascular injury	Severe	Needs vascular repair

Management Principles

- Early debridement (<6 hours)
- Broad-spectrum antibiotics
- Tetanus prophylaxis
- Fracture stabilization (external fixation)
- Soft tissue cover (flaps if needed)
- Definitive fixation once clean

Q65. Principles of initial wound management in trauma.

- ATLS principles first
- Protect wound with sterile dressing
- Photograph wound before debridement
- Early and aggressive irrigation and debridement
- Avoid primary closure in contaminated wounds
- Plan for delayed closure or flap

Q66. Systemic complications of polytrauma.

System	Complication
Respiratory	ARDS, FES
Cardiovascular	Shock, coagulopathy
Renal	AKI (especially in crush syndrome)
CNS	TBI, seizures
GI	Stress ulcers, pancreatitis
Hematological	DIC
Immune	SIRS, sepsis, MODS

Q67. Approach to pelvic fracture with hemodynamic instability.

(GMCJ 2016)

- ABC resuscitation
- Pelvic binder application
- FAST/e-FAST → check for abdominal bleed
- CT angiography
- Angioembolization or surgical packing
- External fixator or C-clamp as needed

Q68. Principles of tourniquet use in trauma surgery.

- *Indications:* Bloodless field for limb surgery
- *Pressures:* 100 mm Hg above SBP (UE), 150 mm Hg above SBP (LE)
- *Duration:* <2 hours preferred
- *Complications:* Nerve palsy, ischemia, rhabdomyolysis
- *Cuff size:* Wide cuffs better

Q69. Primary, secondary, and tertiary survey.

Survey	*Timing*	*Focus*
Primary	Immediate	ABCDE (life-threatening)
Secondary	After stabilization	Head-to-toe assessment
Tertiary	24–48 hours	Missed injuries review

Q70. Role of radiological imaging in acute trauma.

Imaging	*Purpose*
X-ray	FAST skeletal survey
CT scan	Head, chest, abdomen, spine
e-FAST	Peritoneal fluid, hemothorax, pneumothorax
MRI	Cord injury, occult fractures
Angiography	Vascular injury/pelvic trauma

Q71. Principles of splintage and immobilization.

(Kashmir University 2015)

- Reduce pain and bleeding
- Prevent further damage
- Allow transport
- Reduce swelling
- *Types:* Thomas splint, Cramer wire, plaster slab, traction

Q72. Management of crush injuries.

- Early fluids (prevent AKI)
- Mannitol + bicarbonate for myoglobinuria
- Monitor electrolytes (especially K^+)
- Dialysis if needed
- Fasciotomy if compartment syndrome
- Debridement + fracture stabilization

Q73. Define fracture and classify fractures based on etiology, morphology, and biomechanics.

(IMS-BHU 2015)

Definition

A **fracture** is a break in the continuity of bone, usually due to trauma or pathology.

Classification of Fractures

1. *Based on etiology*:
    - Traumatic (e.g., RTA, fall)
    - Pathological (e.g., due to tumor, osteoporosis)
    - Stress (fatigue versus insufficiency)
2. *Based on morphology*:
    - Transverse
    - Oblique
    - Spiral
    - Comminuted
    - Segmental
    - Greenstick, Torus (in children)
3. *Based on biomechanics*:
    - *Tension*: Transverse fracture
    - *Compression*: Oblique fracture
    - *Torsion*: Spiral fracture
    - *Bending*: Butterfly fragment
    - *Shear*: Intra-articular fractures

Q74. Discuss the AO/OTA classification of fractures.

- Developed by **Arbeitsgemeinschaft für Osteosynthesefragen (AO)**
- Universally accepted; used for long bone fractures

Format: [Bone number].[Segment].[Fracture type]

Bone	*Segment*	*Type*
1: Humerus	1: Proximal	A: Simple
2: Radius/Ulna	2: Diaphyseal	B: Wedge
3: Femur	3: Distal	C: Complex

- *Fracture type*:
    - *A*: Extra-articular
    - *B*: Partial articular
    - *C*: Complete articular

Diaphyseal Fractures (Type 2)

- *A:* Simple
- *B:* Wedge
- *C:* Complex

Example: 33.C3 = Distal femur, complete articular, multifragmentary

Q75. Explain the biomechanics of fracture fixation.

Biomechanical Forces in Fractures

- Tension
- Compression
- Bending
- Torsion
- Shear

Fixation Principles

1. *Load sharing versus load bearing:*
   - *IM nails*: Load sharing
   - *Plates*: Load bearing
2. *Stability types*:
   - *Absolute (rigid):* Primary healing (e.g., lag screw, compression plate)
   - *Relative:* Secondary healing (e.g., IM nail, external fixator)
3. *Fixation devices and their mechanics*:
   - *Plates:* Resist bending and torsion
   - *Nails:* Resist axial and torsional loads
   - *External fixators:* Provide adjustable stability
4. *Mechanical properties of implants*:
   - *Stiffness*: Resistance to deformation
   - *Strength*: Maximum load before failure
   - *Elastic modulus*: Slope of stress-strain curve

Q76. Explain the role of periosteum, endosteum, and vascular supply in fracture healing.

(KGMU 2014)

Periosteum

- Highly vascular outer layer of bone
- Source of **osteoprogenitor cells**
- Responsible for **external callus formation**
- Thicker and more active in children

Endosteum

- Lines the medullary cavity
- Contributes to **internal callus** and remodeling
- Source of osteoblasts and osteoclasts

Vascular Supply

- Essential for nutrient and oxygen delivery
- *Vessels involved*:
  - Nutrient artery (diaphyseal region)
  - Periosteal vessels
  - Metaphyseal and epiphyseal arteries
- Damage to blood supply leads to **delayed union or non-union**

Q77. Discuss the concept of stress protection and Wolff's Law.

Wolff's Law

- Bone remodels in response to **mechanical stress** placed upon it.
- *Increased stress*: Bone hypertrophy
- *Decreased stress*: Bone atrophy

Stress Protection:

- Seen when **implants (especially rigid plates)** bear all the load, reducing physiological stress on the bone
- Leads to **bone resorption** beneath the implant → weakening of bone
- More common in load-bearing implants (e.g., femoral plates)

Clinical Implication

- Favor **load-sharing devices** (e.g., IM nails) to prevent stress shielding
- Early **weight-bearing** promotes better remodeling and healing

Q78. Explain the effect of NSAIDs, smoking, and diabetes on fracture healing.

Factor	*Effect on fracture healing*
NSAIDs	Inhibit COX enzymes → ↓ prostaglandin synthesis → interfere with inflammation and callus formation
Smoking	Nicotine causes vasoconstriction, impairs oxygen delivery and angiogenesis, reduces osteoblast activity
Diabetes	Causes microangiopathy, impairs immune response, delays callus formation and increases infection risk

Conclusion

These factors lead to **delayed union, non-union, or poor bone quality**.
Management includes **modification of risk factors** preoperatively and during fracture healing.

Q79. Discuss the principles of fracture reduction—closed versus open reduction.

(AMRU 2013)

Closed Reduction

- Non-invasive method to align fracture fragments manually or via traction
- Aims to restore **length, alignment, rotation**
- Followed by cast/splint/traction
- Used in **minimally displaced fractures**, pediatric cases

Open Reduction

- Surgical exposure of fracture site
- Indicated in **displaced**, **intra-articular**, or **unstable fractures**
- Allows direct visualization and anatomical reduction
- Followed by **internal fixation**

Comparison

Feature	*Closed reduction*	*Open reduction*
Invasiveness	Non-invasive	Surgical exposure
Indication	Simple, stable fractures	Complex, displaced fractures
Risk	Less infection	Higher infection risk
Fixation	Cast/Splint	ORIF with implants

Q80. Explain the concepts of absolute stability versus relative stability.

Stability type	*Description*	*Healing type*	*Examples*
Absolute stability	No motion at fracture site	Primary healing	Compression plating, lag screws
Relative stability	Controlled micromotion allowed	Secondary healing	IM nailing, external fixators, cast

- **Absolute stability** is ideal for **intra-articular fractures**
- **Relative stability** promotes **callus formation** and is suitable for **diaphyseal fractures**

Q81. AO Principles of fracture management.

AO Principles (Four Basic Goals)

1. Anatomical reduction—especially in articular fractures
2. Stable fixation—absolute or relative stability
3. Preservation of blood supply—minimal soft tissue stripping
4. Early and safe mobilization—to prevent joint stiffness and promote healing

Q82. Biological versus mechanical approach to fracture healing.

Feature	*Biological approach*	*Mechanical approach*
Focus	Preserving biology (blood supply)	Achieving mechanical stability
Stability	Relative (bridge plating, nails)	Absolute (lag screws, compression plates)
Healing	Secondary (callus)	Primary (no callus)
Indication	Comminuted, high-energy injuries	Simple fractures needing exact reduction

Q83. Types of fracture stability and their influence on healing.

Stability	*Type of healing*	*Example*
Absolute	Primary (direct osteonal healing)	Compression plating
Relative	Secondary (callus formation)	IM nailing, external fixator
Dynamic	Micromotion to stimulate healing	Functional braces
Rigid	Load-sharing implants	Lag screw fixation

Q84. Primary versus secondary bone healing.

Feature	*Primary healing*	*Secondary healing*
Stability	Absolute	Relative
Callus	Absent	Present
Mechanism	Cutting cones via osteoclasts	Inflammatory → soft callus → hard callus
Seen in	Compression plating	IM nailing, cast, bridge plating

Q85. Modes of internal fixation and biomechanics.

Mode	*Biomechanics*	*Examples*
Compression	Axial stability, absolute stability	Lag screws, compression plates
Neutralization	Protects lag screw	Plate + lag screw
Buttress	Prevents shear in metaphyseal areas	T-plate in distal radius
Bridge	Spans comminuted zone	LCP in segmental fracture
Tension band	Converts tensile force → compression	Patella, olecranon fracture fixation

Q86. Describe the indications for conservative versus surgical management of fractures.

(BFUHS 2013)

Conservative Management
- Undisplaced or minimally displaced fractures
- Fractures in children (due to remodeling potential)
- Medically unfit patients
- *Examples*: Clavicle, humerus, stable distal radius

Surgical Management (ORIF, IMN, External fixator)
- Open fractures
- Displaced intra-articular fractures
- Failed closed reduction
- Pathological fractures
- Fractures with vascular or nerve injury
- Polytrauma patients for early mobilization

Q87. Discuss the role of casts, splints, and functional bracing in fracture treatment.

Device	*Use*
Cast	Circumferential immobilization (e.g., POP cast for Colles' fracture)
Splint	Temporary or partial immobilization (e.g., volar slab, U-slab)
Functional Brace	Allows controlled movement while maintaining alignment (e.g., Sarmiento brace for tibia)

Indications

- Stable fractures
- Early phase post-reduction (splint)
- Definitive treatment in certain diaphyseal fractures

Advantages

- Avoids surgical risk
- Cost-effective
- Encourages early movement (in bracing)

Q88. Principles of initial debridement.

- Timely surgery (preferably <6 hours)
- Wide surgical exposure
- *Excise*:
  - *Skin*: Nonviable, devitalized
  - *Muscle*: 5 Cs: *c*olor, *c*onsistency, *c*ontractility, *c*apillary refill, *c*irculation
  - *Bone*: Floating, devascularized
- *Copious irrigation*: 6–12L saline or with antiseptic
- Mark retained fragments for imaging
- Leave wound open or with temporary VAC

Q89. Role of negative pressure wound therapy (NPWT) in open fractures.

- Reduces edema
- Promotes granulation
- Decreases bacterial colonization
- Temporizes wound for definitive closure or flap
- Often used between **debridements** or before flap

Q90. Current antibiotic prophylaxis guidelines.

Gustilo type	*Antibiotic regimen*	*Duration*
I/II	1st generation cephalosporin (e.g., cefazolin)	24–72 hours
III	Add aminoglycoside (e.g., gentamicin)	3–5 days
Gross contamination (e.g., farm injuries)	Add penicillin/metronidazole	As required

Q91. Management of bone defects in open fractures.

Technique	*Indication*
Masquelet technique	Large segmental loss with soft tissue cover
Bone transport (Ilizarov)	Long-segment loss, infected cases

Continued

Continued

Technique	*Indication*
Autograft (iliac crest, fibula)	Small defects
Allografts	Supplement for large gaps
Induced membrane + graft	Masquelet phase 2

Q92. Masquelet technique.

Two-stage Reconstruction

1. *Stage 1*: Thorough debridement + insertion of cement spacer → induces membrane
2. *Stage 2 (4–8 weeks)*: Remove cement → fill membrane with bone graft (autograft ± BMPs)

Indications

- Segmental bone loss >2–5 cm
- Infected nonunions after sepsis control

Q93. Indications for primary amputation in open fractures.

- Irreparable vascular injury (>6 hours ischemia + crush)
- Extensive soft tissue loss not reconstructible
- Severe contamination (farm injuries, explosions)
- Multiple failed attempts at salvage
- Mangled Extremity Severity Score (MESS) ≥7

Q94. Peri-implant fractures—classification and management.

Definition

Fracture occurring **adjacent to or involving an implant**

Classification

- **Vancouver classification** for periprosthetic hip fractures (e.g., type B1, B2, C)
- Rorabeck for TKR fractures

Management

- Assess fracture type and implant stability
- Fixation (e.g., locking plates, DCS) or revision surgery if implant loose
- Bone grafting if non-union

Q95. Explain the concepts of primary, secondary, and tertiary trauma prevention.

(AIIMS BBSR 2013)

- *Primary prevention:* Prevent injury occurrence (e.g., seat belts, helmets)
- *Secondary prevention:* Early diagnosis and immediate management to reduce impact (e.g., first aid, early imaging)
- *Tertiary prevention:* Rehabilitation and reintegration to reduce long-term consequences (e.g., physiotherapy, prosthetics)

Q96. Explain the pathophysiology and management of burn injuries in trauma patients.

- *Pathophysiology:*
  - *Local injury*: Coagulation, stasis, hyperemia zones (Jackson's burn model).
  - *Systemic response*: ↑ capillary permeability, fluid loss, SIRS.

- *Management (First 24–48 hours):*
  - *Airway*: Suspect inhalation injury.
  - *Breathing*: Monitor for CO poisoning.
  - *Circulation*: Parkland formula for fluid resuscitation (4 mL/kg/%TBSA).
  - Pain control, wound care, tetanus prophylaxis, nutritional support.

Q97. Indications for non-operative management.

- Undisplaced or minimally displaced fractures
- Stable fractures (e.g., clavicle, toe)
- Children with remodeling potential
- Medically unfit patients
- Low-demand elderly
- Closed, low-energy injuries (distal radius, metacarpals)

Q98. Types of bone grafts and their role.

(WBUHS 2018)

Type	*Source*	*Function*
Autograft	Iliac crest, fibula	Osteogenic, osteoinductive, osteoconductive
Allograft	Cadaver bone	Osteoconductive, may be osteoinductive
Xenograft	Animal (rare)	Poor acceptance
Synthetic	Calcium phosphate, BMPs	Scaffold (osteoconductive), sometimes inductive

Roles

- Fill bone defects
- Enhance union (especially in delayed/non-union)
- Structural support (e.g., fibular strut grafts)

Q99. Stress shielding and implant longevity.

- *Definition:* Reduction in physiological stress on bone due to rigid implant taking full load
- *Mechanism:* Bone responds to Wolff's Law → less load → bone resorption
- *Seen in:* Rigid plates, prosthetic stems
- *Effects:*
  - Bone weakening, implant loosening
  - Periprosthetic fractures

Q100. Principles of intra-articular fracture management.

1. *Anatomical reduction*:
   - **Most critical goal** in intra-articular fractures
   - *Aim*: Restore smooth articular surface to prevent **post-traumatic osteoarthritis**
   - Requires **direct visualization** or **fluoroscopic/CT-guided reduction**
   - Cartilage has **poor healing**, so exact apposition is crucial
2. *Stable internal fixation*:
   - Use **rigid fixation** to maintain reduction and allow early motion
   - **Lag screws**, **buttress plates**, or **headless compression screws** often used
   - In cases with severe comminution, consider **fragment-specific fixation**
3. *Preservation of blood supply*:
   - Use **minimally invasive techniques** where feasible

- Avoid stripping periosteum excessively, especially in epiphyseal/metaphyseal areas
- Prefer **biological fixation** methods when soft tissue is compromised

4. *Early mobilization of joint*:
   - Essential to prevent **joint stiffness, adhesions, and cartilage degeneration**
   - Starts as early as **within 3–5 days** post-operative if fixation is stable
   - Use **continuous passive motion (CPM)** in joints like knee, elbow
5. *Management of associated soft tissue injury*:
   - In high-energy trauma, soft tissues are often damaged
   - *Use staged protocol*:
     - *Stage 1*: External fixator to span joint
     - *Stage 2*: Definitive ORIF after soft tissue recovers (swelling ↓, wrinkle sign appears)
6. *Use of CT scan in preoperative planning*:
   - **CT (3D reconstruction)** is often mandatory
   - *Helps visualize*:
     - Articular comminution
     - Depression fragments
     - Involvement of subchondral bone
7. *Assessment of joint congruity post-fixation*:
   - Use **fluoroscopy or arthroscopy** intraoperatively
   - A **step-off >2 mm** in weight-bearing joints (e.g., knee, hip) is unacceptable
   - Ensure **restoration of mechanical axis** in lower limb intra-articular fractures
8. *Rehabilitation and physiotherapy*:
   - *Customized per joint:*
     - *Knee*: Quadriceps strengthening
     - *Elbow*: Flexion-extension arc restoration
   - Protect with partial weight bearing initially (e.g., 6–12 weeks)

Q101. Distraction Osteogenesis (SN).

(GMCJ 2017)

- Concept by **ilizarov**
- **Gradual mechanical distraction** stimulates new bone formation in osteotomy gap
- Bone forms in tension-stress zone
- *Phases:*
  1. Latency
  2. Distraction (1 mm/day)
  3. Consolidation

Q102. Neo-osteogenesis (SN).

- *Refers to new bone formation during*:
  - Distraction osteogenesis
  - Callotasis
- Occurs due to **mechanical tension**, stimulating osteoblast proliferation
- *Ilizarov principle*: Tension-stress leads to regeneration of bone and soft tissues

Q103. Ilizarov technique and applications.

- Based on **distraction osteogenesis**
- Uses **circular external fixator** to stimulate new bone formation

Applications

- Limb lengthening
- Nonunion, especially infected
- Bone defects
- Correction of deformities
- Congenital deficiencies (e.g., PFFD)
- Contracture release (arthrogryposis)

Q104. Bone transport (SN).

- Variant of distraction osteogenesis
- **Segment of bone is moved** across defect
- *Indications*: Bone loss after trauma/infection/tumor
- Performed using **Ilizarov or LRS**
- Generates both **bone and soft tissue**

Q105. Biology of fracture healing AND effect of im nails and plates + osteogenesis modalities.

(NEIGRIHMS 2018)

Intramedullary Nail

- Allows **relative stability**
- Promotes **secondary healing with callus**
- Preserves periosteal blood supply

Plates (Compression)

- Provide **absolute stability**
- Allow **primary bone healing**
- Rigid fixation may reduce callus

Stimulation of Osteogenesis

Modality	***Mechanism***
Ultrasound (LIPUS)	Enhances callus via micro-strain
Electrical stimulation	↑ Osteoblast activity
Bone morphogenetic proteins (BMPs)	Induce mesenchymal cell differentiation
PEMF	Cellular-level bone stimulation

Q106. JESS—Joshi external stabilization system (SN).

- **Mini external fixator**
- *Used in*:
    - Pediatric fractures (especially hand, forearm)
    - Clubfoot correction
    - Facial bone injuries
- *Advantages*: Low cost, customizable, less bulky

Q107. Tension band principle (SN).

- Converts **tensile forces into compressive forces** at fracture site
- Used in fractures under muscle pull (e.g., **olecranon, patella**)

- *Components*:
  - K-wires for alignment
  - **Figure-of-eight cerclage wire** anteriorly
- Promotes **primary healing under compression**

Q108. LCP—locking compression plate (SN).

- Combines benefits of **locking screw fixation** with conventional compression
- **Fixed-angle construct**—plate and screw form a stable unit
- *Useful in*:
  - Osteoporotic bone
  - Periarticular or metaphyseal fractures
- No need for plate-to-bone compression
- Preserves periosteal blood supply

Q109. Merits and demerits of compression locking plate (SN).

Merits
- Fixed-angle stability
- Less reliance on bone quality
- Less periosteal stripping
- Useful in comminuted and osteoporotic fractures

Demerits
- Costly
- Difficult hardware removal
- Over-rigidity can delay union ("stress shielding")

Q110. Locked plating versus conventional plating.

Feature	*Locked plate*	*Conventional plate*
Screw-plate interface	Fixed angle (angular stability)	Compression-based
Use in osteoporotic bone	Excellent	Limited
Bone-plate contact	Less needed (preserves periosteum)	Requires compression
Principle	Internal fixator	Load-sharing/compression

Applications
Periarticular fractures, osteoporotic bones, metaphyseal fractures

Q111. Minimally invasive percutaneous plate osteosynthesis (MIPPO) technique.

(RGUHS 2017)

- Fracture fixation using **indirect reduction** and **small incisions**
- Plate slid submuscularly to bridge fracture
- Preserves **fracture biology and soft tissues**
- *Indications:* Distal tibia, humerus, proximal femur

Advantages
- Less infection
- Preserves periosteum
- Faster healing

Q112. Less invasive stabilization system (LISS).

- Combines locking plate principles + minimally invasive approach
- Ideal for metaphyseal fractures (distal femur, proximal tibia)

Q113. Biological plating (SN).

- Emphasizes **preservation of biology** over rigid mechanical fixation
- Minimizes periosteal stripping
- Uses long plates bridging the fracture zone
- Encourages **callus-based secondary healing**
- Works best in **comminuted, diaphyseal fractures**

Q114. Explain the role of locking plates versus conventional plates in fracture fixation.

(GGMC 2107)

Feature	*Conventional plate*	*Locking plate*
Plate-screw interface	Friction-based compression	Threaded interface—angular stability
Stability	Requires good bone purchase	Better in osteoporotic bone
Use in comminution	Not ideal	Acts as internal fixator (bridge plating)
Periosteal blood supply	Compromised	Preserved (no compression on bone)

Indications for Locking Plates
- Osteoporotic bone
- Periarticular fractures
- Multifragmentary or bridge plating
- Minimally invasive fixation (MIPO)

Q115. Antiglide plate (SN)

- Used in **lateral malleolus (fibula)** and other **oblique fractures**
- Plate resists posterior and inferior displacement (glide)
- Provides **buttress effect**—holds fragment from shearing
- Acts as a tension band on posterolateral fibula

Q116. Screw anatomy and lag screw principle (SN).

Screw Anatomy
- Head
- Shaft
- Threads
- Core diameter versus outer diameter
- Thread pitch

Lag Screw Principle
- Creates **interfragmentary compression**
- Near cortex drilled larger (gliding hole)
- Far cortex drilled smaller (threaded)
- As screw is tightened, fragments are pulled together

Q117. Short Notes

A. *Elastic stable intramedullary nailing (ESIN):*
   - Used in pediatric long bone fractures (femur/tibia)
   - Flexible titanium nails inserted retrograde/antegrade
   - Minimally invasive, preserves physis

B. *Titanium elastic nailing system (TENS):*
   - Pediatric version of ESIN
   - Allows dynamic axial loading and promotes early union
   - Used in femur, tibia, humerus fractures in children (6–14 years)

Q118. Explain the concept of load-sharing versus load-bearing fixation.

(DYPU Pune 2017)

Concept	*Load sharing*	*Load bearing*
Definition	Load is shared between implant and bone	Implant takes full load
Healing	Stimulates callus formation (relative stability)	Less biological stimulation
Implants	IM nail, bridge plating	Plates in segmental fractures
Advantage	Promotes early weight bearing	Useful when bone continuity is compromised

Clinical Relevance

Prefer load-sharing fixation (e.g., IM nails) where bone integrity is sufficient and promotes better healing.

Q119. Discuss the indications for external fixation and its biomechanical principles.

Indications

- Open fractures (especially Gustilo Type IIIB/IIIC)
- Fractures with soft tissue compromise
- Damage control orthopedics in polytrauma
- Infected non-unions
- Limb lengthening (Ilizarov)
- Temporary stabilization (e.g., pelvic fractures)

Biomechanical Principles

- Provides **relative stability**
- Works on **principles of tensioned wires, pins, and rings/bars**
- Stability depends on **pin diameter, spread, and number**
- Frame configuration affects load transfer (unilateral, ring fixator, hybrid)

11.2 Upper Limb Trauma

Sakib Arfee, Abhai Singh Bhadwal, Shyam Singh

Q1. Write a short note on sternoclavicular joint dislocations.

(PGI Chandigarh 2013)

Types
- *Anterior dislocation*: Most common, usually benign.
- *Posterior dislocation*: Rare but serious due to risk to mediastinal structures.

Mechanism
Direct or indirect trauma (e.g., lateral shoulder impact).

Management
- *Anterior*: Closed reduction or observation.
- *Posterior*: Urgent reduction due to risk to trachea, vessels, esophagus—often under general anesthesia or surgically.

Q2. Discuss the mechanism and management of medial clavicle fractures.

Mechanism
High-energy trauma (e.g., motor vehicle accidents, falls).

Diagnosis
Often missed on standard X-rays—CT scan useful.

Management
- Most managed non-operatively.
- Surgical fixation if—displaced, symptomatic non-union, or with posterior dislocation.

Q3. Describe the classification and management of clavicle fractures.

(Asked in: AIIMS Delhi 2022, MUHS Maharashtra 2022)

Introduction
- Clavicle fractures are **common injuries** accounting for **2.6–5% of all fractures.**
- *Mechanism*: Typically due to **direct blow** to the shoulder or fall on an outstretched hand.

Classification
Allman classification (simplified)

Type	Location	Incidence
I	Middle third (midshaft)	~80% (most common)
II	Distal third (lateral end)	~15%
III	Proximal third (medial end)	~5%

Neer's Classification (for Distal Third Fractures)
- *Type I*: Minimal displacement (CC ligaments intact).
- *Type II*: Displaced fracture (CC ligaments torn).
- *Type III*: Intra-articular extension into AC joint.

Management
General principles:
- Most clavicle fractures, especially **non-displaced**, heal well with **conservative treatment**.
- **Surgical fixation** indicated in specific cases.

Non-operative Treatment

- *Indications*:
  - Minimally displaced fractures.
  - No skin tenting or neurovascular compromise.
- *Method*:
  - Arm sling or figure-of-eight bandage for 3–6 weeks.
  - Early gentle mobilization to prevent stiffness.

Operative Treatment

- *Indications*:
  - Open fractures.
  - Skin tenting/impending skin compromise.
  - Neurovascular injury.
  - Displacement >2 cm.
  - Comminuted fractures with >2 fragments.
  - Floating shoulder (clavicle + scapular neck fracture).
- *Methods*:
  - Plate osteosynthesis (superior plating preferred).
  - Intramedullary fixation (elastic nails, threaded pins in selected cases).

Advantages of Surgery

- Better functional outcomes.
- Lower rates of non-union/malunion.
- Faster return to activity.

Q4. Management of non-union of clavicle fractures.

(Asked in: PGI Chandigarh 2021)

Definition

Non-union of clavicle fracture is defined as **failure of union** at **>6 months** post-injury, with clinical symptoms (pain, instability).

Risk Factors

- Significant initial displacement.
- Comminution.
- Smoking, diabetes, open fractures.
- Inadequate immobilization.

Clinical Features

- Persistent pain at fracture site.
- Visible deformity or palpable movement.
- Functional limitation in shoulder movement.

Management

Non-surgical: Considered in **asymptomatic** patients with good shoulder function despite radiological non-union.

Surgical:

- *Indications*:
  - Symptomatic non-union (pain, instability).
  - Functional impairment.
- Procedures:
  1. *Open reduction and internal fixation (ORIF)*: Anatomical reduction with plate fixation (preferably superior plate).

2. *Bone grafting*:
   - Autologous iliac crest bone graft (ICBG) for biological augmentation.
   - Useful in atrophic non-unions.

Outcome
- With proper surgical technique, union rates approach >**90%**.
- Important to optimize biological (graft) and mechanical (stable fixation) environment.

Q5. Indications for conservative versus operative management in clavicular fractures.

(DNB 2024)

Introduction

Clavicle fractures are common injuries, accounting for approximately 2.6–5% of all adult fractures and 35–45% of injuries to the shoulder girdle. The majority involve the middle third of the clavicle. Management can be **conservative** or **operative**, depending on fracture location, displacement, comminution, associated injuries, and patient factors.

A. Conservative Management

Indications:
1. *Undisplaced or minimally displaced fractures*:
   - <2 cm displacement
   - No shortening or malrotation
2. *Middle third clavicle fractures (most common):* Without significant displacement or comminution
3. *Pediatric clavicle fractures*:
   - Excellent remodeling potential
   - Even displaced fractures usually treated non-operatively
4. *Medial end fractures*:
   - Usually stable due to ligamentous support
   - Treated with sling and analgesia
5. *Low-demand elderly patients*: Poor surgical candidates due to comorbidities
6. *Compliant patients*: Willing to accept prolonged immobilization and cosmetic deformity

Method
- Arm sling or figure-of-eight bandage
- Immobilization for 3–4 weeks, followed by physiotherapy
- *Union rates*: 90–95% in non-displaced fractures

B. Operative Management

Absolute indications:
1. Open fractures
2. Neurovascular injury
3. Impending skin perforation
4. *Floating shoulder*: Ipsilateral clavicle and scapular neck fracture
5. Symptomatic non-union or malunion

Relative Indications:
1. *Displaced midshaft fractures*:
   - 2 cm shortening or displacement
   - Comminution with loss of contact
   - Associated with poor functional outcomes if managed conservatively
2. *Bilateral clavicle fractures*: Risk of respiratory compromise
3. *Polytrauma patients*: Need for early mobilization

4. *Athletes or high-demand individuals*: Better functional outcome, faster return to activity
5. *Lateral end fractures with*:
   - Displacement and ligamentous injury (Neer Type II)
   - High risk of non-union

Surgical options:
- *Open reduction and internal fixation (ORIF) using*:
  - Pre-contoured locking plate
  - Intramedullary nailing (in selected cases)

Recent Evidence
- *Canadian Orthopedic Trauma Society (COTS) study (2007)*: Showed better functional outcomes, lower non-union and symptomatic malunion rates with ORIF in displaced midshaft fractures.
- *Meta-analyses*: Favor surgery for displaced midshaft fractures in young active individuals.

Conclusion
Management of clavicular fractures must be **individualized.** Conservative treatment is effective for most non-displaced fractures, especially in children and the elderly. However, **operative treatment** offers superior outcomes in **displaced, comminuted, or high-demand cases**. Thorough clinical evaluation and shared decision-making are key.

Q6. Write a short note on operative fixation of clavicle fracture.

Introduction
Clavicle fractures, particularly those involving the midshaft, are common injuries. While many can be managed conservatively, certain fracture types require surgical intervention to ensure optimal functional outcomes and to prevent complications like non-union or malunion.

Indications for Operative Fixation
1. Displaced midshaft fractures with >2 cm shortening or comminution
2. Open fractures
3. Neurovascular compromise
4. Impending skin perforation
5. Symptomatic non-union or malunion
6. Floating shoulder (ipsilateral scapular neck fracture)
7. Polytrauma patients (early mobilization needed)
8. Bilateral clavicle fractures
9. Athletes and high-demand individuals
10. Displaced lateral end fractures (Neer type II, III)

Surgical Techniques
1. *Open reduction and internal fixation (ORIF):*
   - *Plate fixation (preferred method):*
     - Pre-contoured locking compression plate (LCP) on superior or anterior surface
     - Better mechanical stability and union rates
   - Lag screw fixation in simple oblique fractures
2. *Intramedullary fixation:*
   - Elastic nails, Kirschner wires, or titanium elastic nails (TEN)
   - Minimally invasive
   - Less soft tissue stripping
   - Not suitable for comminuted or lateral-end fractures

Advantages of Operative Fixation
- Faster return to function

- Lower non-union and malunion rates
- Improved cosmetic and functional outcomes
- Early pain relief and shoulder mobilization

Complications
- Infection
- Hardware irritation or prominence
- Neurovascular injury
- Non-union or delayed union
- Plate breakage or loosening

Recent Evidence
Canadian Orthopedic Trauma Society (COTS) study: ORIF in displaced midshaft clavicle fractures resulted in superior union rates and functional outcomes compared to non-operative care.

Conclusion
Operative fixation is the treatment of choice in selected clavicle fractures with clear indications. It promotes early mobilization, restores shoulder function, and prevents complications in high-risk fractures.

Q7. Explain the role of plate fixation versus intramedullary fixation in clavicle fractures.

(GGMC 2011)

Plate Fixation
- *Pros*: Rigid fixation, anatomical reduction, suitable for comminuted fractures.
- *Cons*: Larger scar, risk of plate prominence, infection.

Intramedullary Fixation
- *Pros*: Minimally invasive, smaller incision, less hardware irritation.
- *Cons*: Limited use in comminuted fractures, risk of migration, requires more precise technique.

Choice depends on: Fracture type, location, surgeon expertise, and patient preference.
What are the common mechanisms and treatment options for clavicle fractures?

Q8. Write a note on complications of clavicle fracture.

Early Complications
1. *Neurovascular injury*:
   - Brachial plexus injury
   - Subclavian vessels (artery/vein)
2. Skin tenting or impending perforation
3. Pneumothorax or hemothorax (especially medial fractures)
4. *Associated injuries*:
   - Rib fractures
   - Scapular fractures
   - Pulmonary contusion

Late Complications
1. Non-union (5–15% in displaced midshaft fractures)
2. *Malunion*:
   - Shoulder droop
   - Cosmetic deformity
   - Strength and endurance reduction

3. Chronic pain or thoracic outlet syndrome
4. *Post-traumatic arthritis*: AC or SC joint involvement
5. *Hardware-related issues (if operated)*:
   - Implant prominence
   - Plate breakage or loosening

Q9. Surgical approaches for clavicle fractures.

(MS 2012)

Approach Depends on Fracture Site

1. *Middle third (most common)*:
   - *Superior approach*:
     - Incision over superior clavicle
     - Avoid supraclavicular nerves
     - Better plate contouring
   - *Anterior approach*:
     - Cosmetically better
     - Less hardware prominence
     - Risk to cephalic vein and deltoid detachment
2. *Lateral end*:
   - Extension of deltopectoral approach
   - May require detachment of deltoid and trapezius insertions
3. *Medial end*:
   - Anterior approach to sternoclavicular joint
   - Difficult exposure due to proximity to mediastinal structures

Q10. Neurovascular structures at risk in clavicle fracture.

(DNB 2002)

- Subclavian vein (anterior and inferior to clavicle)
- Subclavian artery
- *Brachial plexus*: Trunks lie posterior to subclavian artery
- Suprascapular nerve
- Thoracic duct (on left side, rare)
- Apex of lung → Risk of pneumothorax

Q11. Floating shoulder injury and its management.

(MS 2016)

Definition

Fracture of **clavicle** + fracture of **scapular neck**, disrupting the **superior shoulder suspensory complex (SSSC)**

Diagnosis

- Suspect in high-velocity trauma
- X-ray (AP, scapular Y)
- CT scan with 3D reconstruction for scapular neck

Management

Non-operative:

- If fractures are minimally displaced
- Shoulder immobilization followed by rehabilitation

Operative:
- Clavicle ORIF → stabilizes SSSC
- Scapular neck ORIF → if significantly displaced (>1 cm or angulated)
- *Indicated if*:
  - 1 cm medialization or angular deformity of scapula
  - Associated with neurovascular injury or open fractures

Q12. Surgical anatomy of AC joint along with classification of AC joint injuries. Briefly discuss the management.

I. Surgical Anatomy of the AC Joint
- *Type*: Planar synovial joint
- *Articulating surfaces*:
  - Lateral end of clavicle
  - Medial margin of acromion
- *Joint capsule*: Weak but reinforced by **AC ligaments** (superior, inferior, anterior, posterior)

Ligamentous Support
1. *Acromioclavicular (AC) ligaments*: Provide **horizontal stability**
2. *Coracoclavicular (CC) ligaments:*
   - Conoid ligament (medial, vertical stability)
   - Trapezoid ligament (lateral, resists axial compression)

Muscular Support
- Deltoid (anteriorly)
- Trapezius (posteriorly)

II. Classification of AC Joint Injuries
Most widely used: Rockwood classification (Types I–VI)

Type	Description	Ligament status	Radiographic findings
I	Sprain of AC ligament	AC sprained, CC intact	Normal X-ray
II	AC ligament tear, CC sprain	AC torn, CC intact/strained	Slight clavicle elevation
III	Both AC and CC ligaments torn	Complete tear	Clavicle elevated with 25–100% displacement
IV	Posterior displacement of clavicle into trapezius	AC and CC torn	Clavicle displaced posteriorly
V	Severe superior displacement (>100%)	AC and CC torn, delto-trapezial fascia stripped	Severe clavicle elevation
VI	Inferior displacement of clavicle under coracoid or acromion	Very rare	Clavicle below acromion or coracoid

III. Management
Non-operative (Types I and II)
- Sling for 1–2 weeks
- Ice, NSAIDs
- Early physiotherapy
- Excellent outcomes in most patients

Controversial (Type III)
- Non-operative for most patients
- *Surgical in*:
  - Athletes
  - Heavy laborers
  - Cosmetic concerns
  - Persistent instability or pain

Operative (Types IV, V, VI or failed Type III)

Surgical Techniques

1. *AC joint stabilization with*:
   - Hook plate
   - Screws
   - TightRope or suture button
   - Endobutton fixation
2. CC ligament reconstruction
3. Distal clavicle excision (Mumford procedure - chronic cases)

Recent Advances

- Arthroscopic-assisted techniques gaining popularity
- Biological grafts (e.g., autograft, allograft) for CC ligament reconstruction
- Suspensory fixation devices (e.g., TightRope, Dog Bone)

Conclusion

Understanding the surgical anatomy and classification of AC joint injuries guides appropriate management. While types I and II are treated conservatively, higher-grade injuries often require surgical intervention for optimal outcomes, especially in active individuals.

Q13. Indications for surgery in AC joint injuries and various surgical techniques.

(DNB 2019)

I. Indications for Surgery in AC Joint Injuries

Rockwood classification of AC joint injuries

Type	Description	Management
I	Sprain of AC ligaments; no displacement	Conservative
II	Ruptured AC ligaments, sprained CC ligaments; slight displacement	Conservative
III	Complete tear of AC and CC ligaments; marked clavicle elevation	Initially conservative; surgical in athletes/manual workers
IV	Posterior displacement of clavicle into/through trapezius	Surgical
V	Severe superior displacement with muscle detachment	Surgical
VI	Inferior displacement (under coracoid/acromion)—rare	Surgical

Surgical treatment is indicated in:

- *Type IV, V, VI*: Always surgical
- *Type III*: Surgical in—
  - Overhead athletes
  - Manual laborers
  - Chronic symptomatic cases
- Failure of conservative treatment

Surgical options:

- Hook plate fixation
- Coracoclavicular ligament reconstruction
- Tightrope/suture button fixation
- Weaver–Dunn procedure (modified or anatomical)

Other surgical indications:

- Chronic pain or dysfunction despite conservative treatment
- Cosmetic deformity causing distress
- High-grade instability on dynamic imaging
- Failed conservative therapy

II. Surgical Techniques for AC Joint Injuries

Technique	Principle	Advantages	Disadvantages
Hook plate fixation	Provides rigid fixation between acromion and clavicle	• Simple technique • Immediate stability	• Subacromial impingement • Need for plate removal • Can cause osteolysis
CC screw fixation	Fixes clavicle to coracoid	• Strong fixation • Widely used	• Risk of screw breakage • Requires removal
Suture loop/Tight Rope (endobutton)	Suspensory fixation between coracoid and clavicle	• Minimally invasive • No hardware removal • Allows micro-motion for healing	• Technically demanding • May loosen over time
Bosworth screw	Large screw between clavicle and coracoid	• Simple • Strong fixation	• Hardware irritation • Requires second surgery for removal
Ligament reconstruction (autograft/allograft)	Anatomic reconstruction of CC ligaments	• Durable fixation • Restores normal biomechanics	• Technically demanding • Longer recovery time
Weaver–Dunn procedure	Transfers coracoacromial ligament to distal clavicle	• Useful in chronic cases • Combines with other methods	• Inferior to anatomic reconstructions • Can stretch out over time
Arthroscopic techniques	Endobutton or graft passed arthroscopically	• Minimally invasive • Cosmetic • Early rehabilitation	• Requires training and setup • Higher cost

Conclusion

Surgical treatment of AC joint injuries is indicated in high-grade injuries (Rockwood IV–VI), chronic symptomatic type III injuries, and failed conservative management. A variety of techniques exist, and the choice should be based on injury chronicity, surgeon expertise, and patient needs. Modern trends favor minimally invasive anatomic reconstruction with strong functional outcomes.

Q14. Fracture scapula.

Type: Long Type

Introduction

Fractures of the scapula are **relatively uncommon**, accounting for about **1% of all fractures** and **3–5% of shoulder girdle injuries**. Due to its **protected anatomical location**, high-energy trauma such as road traffic accidents, falls from height, or crush injuries are typically required to fracture the scapula.

Scapular fractures are often **associated with other injuries**, particularly in the chest wall, upper limb, spine, or head, making their evaluation critical in polytrauma settings.

Anatomy of the Scapula

The scapula is a **flat triangular bone** that forms the **posterior part of the shoulder girdle**. It articulates with:

- Clavicle at the AC joint
- Humerus at the glenohumeral joint

Anatomical Divisions

- Body
- Spine
- Acromion
- Coracoid
- Glenoid cavity
- Scapular neck
- Scapular borders and angles

The scapula is covered by muscles (e.g., trapezius, deltoid, infraspinatus) that protect it and influence fracture displacement.

Mechanism of Injury

- High-energy blunt trauma (e.g., RTA, fall from height)
- Direct trauma to posterior thorax
- Indirect trauma via axial loading through the arm

Classification of Scapular Fractures

Several systems exist, but commonly classified based on anatomical location:

1. *Anatomical classification*:
   - Scapular body fractures (50–60%)
   - Scapular neck fractures
   - Glenoid fractures (articular)
   - Acromion fractures
   - Coracoid fractures
   - Scapular spine fractures
2. *Ideberg classification for intra-articular glenoid fractures*
   (Important for surgical decision-making)
   - *Type I*: Anterior rim fracture
   - *Type II*: Transverse fracture extending medially
   - *Type III*: Inferior fracture
   - *Type IV*: Extends superiorly
   - *Type V*: Combination of II + IV
   - *Type VI*: Comminuted intra-articular

Clinical Features

History:

- High-velocity trauma
- Chest pain, shoulder pain
- History of polytrauma or fall

Examination:

- Local tenderness, swelling, ecchymosis over posterior shoulder
- Limited shoulder range of motion
- Crepitus on scapular movement
- *Check for associated injuries*:
  - Rib fractures
  - Pneumothorax
  - Spine or brachial plexus injury

Investigations

1. *Radiographs*:
   - AP view
   - Lateral scapular (Y) view
   - Axillary view (if tolerated)
2. *CT scan with 3D reconstruction:*
   - *Essential for*:
     - Glenoid fractures
     - Intra-articular involvement
     - Planning surgical approach
3. *Associated investigations*:
   - *Chest X-ray*: Rule out pneumothorax
   - CT thorax for rib, lung injuries
   - Neurovascular assessment

Management

General principles:

- Most scapular fractures are **treated conservatively** due to surrounding musculature providing support and stability.
- Surgical treatment is reserved for displaced fractures, intra-articular involvement, or floating shoulder.

Non-operative Management

Indications:

- *Minimally displaced fractures*:
  - <1 cm displacement in body or spine
  - <5 mm articular step-off in glenoid
- No functional impairment
- No associated shoulder instability

Treatment

- Immobilization in a sling for 2–3 weeks
- Early passive ROM → active ROM from 3–4 weeks
- Strengthening exercises by 6–8 weeks

Operative Management

Indications:

- *Intra-articular glenoid fractures*:
  - 5 mm displacement
  - 20% articular surface involvement
- *Scapular neck fractures*: 40° angulation or >1 cm translation
- *Double disruption of the superior shoulder suspensory complex (SSSC):* "Floating shoulder"
- Unstable acromion/spine fractures causing impingement
- Symptomatic non-unions or malunions
- Open scapular fractures
- Associated neurovascular compromise

Surgical Approaches

- *Judet approach (posterior)*: For body, spine, glenoid neck
- *Modified Judet or lateral approach*: For glenoid rim fractures
- *Anterior approach*: For coracoid or anterior glenoid

Fixation Methods

- Reconstruction plates (3.5 mm)
- Cannulated screws for glenoid fractures
- Locking plates for spine and body fractures

Postoperative Rehabilitation

- Early mobilization with pendulum exercises
- Passive and active-assisted ROM exercises
- Strengthening phase by 6–8 weeks
- Return to full function by 3–6 months

Complications

- Non-union or malunion
- Stiffness and frozen shoulder
- Glenohumeral arthritis (if articular involvement)
- Chronic pain or impingement
- Hardware irritation
- Thoracic outlet syndrome
- Neurovascular injury (brachial plexus, axillary artery)

Prognosis
- Generally good with conservative management
- Intra-articular and displaced fractures may have poorer outcomes if untreated
- Early diagnosis and proper rehabilitation are key for functional recovery

Conclusion
Scapular fractures, though rare, are **clinically significant** due to the potential for **associated injuries and functional impairment**. Most fractures heal well conservatively, but **precise assessment using CT and classification systems** helps in identifying fractures that may benefit from surgery. The emphasis remains on **early mobilization and rehabilitation** for optimal outcomes.

Q15. Describe anterior shoulder dislocation—mechanism, clinical signs, and management.

(Asked in: RGUHS Karnataka 2022, MUHS Maharashtra 2023)

Introduction
- Shoulder is the **most commonly dislocated joint.**
- **Anterior dislocation** accounts for >**95%** of all shoulder dislocations.

Mechanism
- Typically caused by **abduction**, **external rotation**, and **extension** forces.
- *Common scenarios*:
  - Fall onto an outstretched hand (FOOSH).
  - Direct blow to the posterior shoulder.

Clinical Signs
Inspection:
- Arm held in **abduction and slight external rotation.**
- Loss of normal shoulder contour ("**squared-off**" appearance).
- Prominent acromion.

Palpation:
- Empty glenoid fossa.
- Head of humerus palpable under coracoid process.

Neurological: Check **axillary nerve** function (sensory loss over "regimental badge" area).

Management
Emergency management: Immediate reduction under analgesia/sedation (if no contraindications).

Reduction Techniques
- Kocher's method (external rotation method).
- Stimson technique (gravity-assisted).
- Milch technique (abduction and external rotation).

Post-reduction Care
- Confirm reduction by X-ray.
- Sling immobilization for 2–3 weeks (younger patients = shorter immobilization).
- *Early rehabilitation*: Start pendulum exercises once pain decreases.

Surgical Indications
- Recurrent dislocations.
- Associated fractures (Bankart, greater tuberosity).
- Large Hill–Sachs lesions.

Q16. Explain the mechanism and management of anterior shoulder dislocations.

Mechanism
- Forced abduction, extension, and external rotation
- Most common direction of dislocation

Clinical Features
- Arm held in abduction and external rotation
- Flattened deltoid contour

Management
- Immediate closed reduction (e.g., Hippocratic, Kocher's method)
- Post-reduction X-ray to confirm
- Immobilization in sling (1–3 weeks)
- Physiotherapy for rehabilitation
- Recurrent dislocations may need surgical stabilization

Q17. Explain the clinical features and treatment of posterior shoulder dislocations.

Clinical Features
- Arm held in adduction and internal rotation
- Prominent posterior shoulder
- Limited external rotation
- "Lightbulb sign" on X-ray (AP view)

Treatment
- Acute: Closed reduction under anesthesia
- Chronic/Locked: May require open reduction or osteotomy
- Address underlying causes (e.g., seizures, electrocution)

Q18. Management of proximal humerus fracture-dislocation.

(Asked in: PGI Chandigarh 2022)

Introduction
- Often seen in elderly (osteoporotic bone) or young (high-energy trauma).
- Combination of **fracture** of the proximal humerus and **anterior dislocation**.

Classification

Neer classification: Based on number of displaced parts (anatomical neck, surgical neck, greater tuberosity, lesser tuberosity).

Management

Non-operative:
- *Indications*:
  - Minimally displaced fractures.
  - Good reduction achieved after closed manipulation.
- *Method*:
  - Closed reduction under sedation.
  - Immobilization with sling for 3–4 weeks.
  - Early mobilization to prevent stiffness.

Operative

- *Indications*:
  - Failed closed reduction.
  - 3- or 4-part fractures (especially in young patients).
  - Associated vascular injury.
- *Surgical options*:
  - ORIF (locking plates/screws)—preferred for displaced fractures in young.
  - Hemiarthroplasty—in complex fractures in elderly with poor bone stock.
  - Reverse shoulder arthroplasty—in elderly with rotator cuff dysfunction.

Postoperative Care

- Early passive and active-assisted range of motion.
- Avoid prolonged immobilization to prevent frozen shoulder.

Q19. Discuss the indications for open reduction and internal fixation (ORIF) versus shoulder hemiarthroplasty in proximal humerus fractures.

ORIF Indications

- Young patients
- Good bone quality
- 2- or 3-part fractures

Hemiarthroplasty Indications

- Elderly patients
- Comminuted 4-part fractures
- Fracture-dislocations
- AVN risk or failed ORIF

Reverse shoulder arthroplasty may be preferred in elderly with rotator cuff insufficiency.

Q20. Classification of proximal humerus fractures in the elderly and blood supply relevance.

Neer Classification (Most Common)

Based on anatomical parts:

- Greater tuberosity
- Lesser tuberosity
- Articular head
- Shaft

A fragment is defined as "separate" if it is displaced >1 cm or angulated >45°.

Type	*Description*
One-part	No fragment significantly displaced
Two-part	Displacement of one fragment (e.g., surgical neck or tuberosity)
Three-part	Displaced surgical neck + one tuberosity
Four-part	Both tuberosities + surgical neck displaced

Relevance of Blood Supply

- *Main supply*: **Anterior humeral circumflex artery (AHCA)** via **arcuate artery**
- **Posterior humeral circumflex artery (PHCA)** contributes significantly
- Four-part fractures risk **avascular necrosis (AVN)** due to disruption of both AHCA and PHCA
- Management planning requires assessing **vascular viability** of the humeral head

Q21. Treatment of four-part fracture.

Goals

Restore alignment, preserve function, prevent AVN

Elderly (Low Demand/Osteoporotic)

- **Reverse shoulder arthroplasty** (RSA) is preferred
- Avoids dependence on rotator cuff

Younger Patients

- ORIF with locking plate if head is viable
- Hemiarthroplasty if comminution or AVN risk is high

Q22. AVN risk in proximal humerus fractures.

(DNB 2020)

Risk Factors

- 3- or 4-part fractures
- Head-splitting fractures
- Dislocation
- Delay in reduction (>12 hours)
- Disrupted medial calcar
- Open fractures

Impact on Management

- **High AVN risk** leads to considering **arthroplasty (RSA or hemi)**
- **Locking plate fixation** should aim to preserve medial hinge
- AVN may develop late → monitor radiologically
- May require conversion to arthroplasty if symptomatic

Q23. Indications of reverse shoulder arthroplasty in proximal humerus fractures.

(MS 2011)

Indications

- *Elderly patients with*:
    - Comminuted 3- or 4-part fractures
    - Fracture-dislocations
    - Osteoporotic bone precluding fixation
    - Disrupted rotator cuff
    - High AVN risk
- Failed ORIF or hemiarthroplasty
- Chronic non-union or post-traumatic arthritis

Q24. Management of displaced proximal humerus fractures in elderly.

(Asked in: MUHS Maharashtra 2023, PGI Chandigarh 2022)

Challenges in Elderly

- Osteoporotic bone.
- Higher risk of fixation failure.
- Limited functional demand but greater need for pain-free range.

Management Approach

A. *Minimally displaced fractures*:

- Non-operative.
- Sling immobilization for comfort → Early passive mobilization.

B. *Displaced two-part/three-part/ four-part fractures*:

Options:

- *Reverse total shoulder arthroplasty (RTSA)*:
  - Gold standard for complex fractures in elderly.
  - Especially in 3- or 4-part fractures with head-split components.
  - *Advantages*: Reliable function, less dependence on rotator cuff healing.
- *Hemiarthroplasty*:
  - Traditional option.
  - Outcomes less predictable unless tuberosities heal properly.
- *Locking plate fixation*:
  - Younger elderly patients with good bone quality.
  - Anatomical reduction needed to prevent avascular necrosis (AVN).

Key Points in Elderly

- Aim for **early mobilization**.
- Prioritize **pain-free functional range** over perfect radiological union.

Post-operative Care

- Initial sling support.
- Early passive ROM exercises.
- Gradual progression to active and strengthening exercises.

Q25. Discuss the indications for open reduction and internal fixation (ORIF) versus shoulder hemiarthroplasty in proximal humerus fractures.

Introduction

Proximal humerus fractures account for ~4–6% of all fractures and are common in the elderly due to osteoporosis. Treatment is determined by:

- Number of parts involved (Neer classification)
- Bone quality
- Patient age and activity level
- Risk of avascular necrosis (AVN)

The two major surgical options are **ORIF** and **hemiarthroplasty**.

I. Open Reduction and Internal Fixation (ORIF)

Indications

- *2- or 3-part fractures:* Especially surgical neck with/without tuberosity involvement
- *Younger patients (<65 years):* Good bone quality
- Fractures with viable head fragment
- Preserved medial hinge
- Minimal comminution
- High-demand patients (e.g., manual workers, athletes)

Advantages

- Retains native joint
- Better proprioception and strength (if healed well)
- Potential for better range of motion in young patients

Limitations
- Technically demanding
- Failure in osteoporotic bone (screw pullout, non-union)
- Risk of AVN if blood supply compromised

II. Shoulder Hemiarthroplasty

Indications
- Head-splitting fractures
- Anatomically irreducible or severely comminuted 3- or 4-part fractures
- Fracture dislocations
- Osteoporotic bone precluding fixation
- Elderly low-demand patients
- High AVN risk
- Failed ORIF or chronic non-union

Advantages
- Avoids complications of fixation failure
- Reliable pain relief
- Predictable outcomes in low-demand patients

Limitations
- *Functional results depend on*:
  - Tuberosity healing
  - Proper implant positioning
- Loss of overhead motion in some cases

Comparative Table

Feature	*ORIF*	*Hemiarthroplasty*
Ideal age group	< 65 years	> 65 years
Bone quality	Good	Osteoporotic
Fracture type	2- or 3-part, reducible 4-part	Head-splitting, severely comminuted fractures
AVN risk	Lower	Used when risk is high
Outcome dependence	Reduction quality	Tuberosity healing and prosthesis alignment
Rehabilitation	Earlier ROM with stable fixation	Slower if tuberosity repair is done

Conclusion

ORIF is ideal for young, active patients with good bone quality and reconstructible fractures. Hemiarthroplasty is reserved for complex, irreparable fractures in elderly or when the humeral head viability is lost. **Patient selection, fracture pattern, and surgeon experience** determine the success of either approach.

Q26. Intramedullary nailing versus locking plates for proximal humerus fractures.

(MS 2017)

Intramedullary Nailing
- Minimally invasive, smaller incision.
- Preferred in 2-part surgical neck fractures.
- Preserves periosteal blood supply.
- *Cons*: Poor control of tuberosities, rotator cuff violation.

Locking Plates
- Anatomical reduction with good control of fragments.
- Better for 3- and 4-part fractures.

- Enhanced fixation in osteoporotic bone with angular stability.
- *Cons*: Higher soft tissue dissection, risk of AVN if medial hinge lost.

Q27. Management of 3-part proximal humerus fracture with rotator cuff tear.

(DNB 2015)

- Perform ORIF using locking compression plate for fracture fixation.
- Repair torn rotator cuff using suture anchors or transosseous sutures.
- Post-operative rehabilitation includes immobilization in abduction brace followed by passive and active ROM.
- In the elderly with extensive cuff tear and poor bone

Q28. Indications of reverse shoulder arthroplasty in proximal humerus fractures.

(MS 2011)

Reverse shoulder arthroplasty (RSA) is a preferred option in elderly patients with complex proximal humerus fractures where traditional methods such as ORIF or hemiarthroplasty are not feasible or yield poor outcomes.

- Indications include:
- Comminuted 3- or 4-part fractures in elderly.
- Fracture dislocations with rotator cuff tear.
- Head-splitting fractures with poor bone stock.
- Failed ORIF or hemiarthroplasty.
- Chronic non-union or post-traumatic arthritis with rotator cuff deficiency.
- High risk of AVN or poor tuberosity healing potential.

Q29. Management of proximal humerus fractures with splitting of the head.

(DNB 2009)

Head-splitting fractures involve a vertical or horizontal split of the humeral head, often due to axial loading of the abducted arm. These are rare but severe injuries.

Management depends on fracture morphology and viability of the head fragment.

Treatment Options

- *Young patients with large viable fragment*: Attempt ORIF using screws or locking plates.
- *Elderly or in cases with small comminuted fragments*: Proceed with hemiarthroplasty.
- *If associated with rotator cuff tear or poor bone*: Consider reverse shoulder arthroplasty.
- Ensure meticulous surgical planning and restoration of tuberosity and cuff function.

Q30. Treatment of a valgus-impacted proximal humerus fracture.

(MS 2006)

Valgus-impacted fractures of the proximal humerus are a subtype of 3-part fractures characterized by valgus angulation of the humeral head with impaction and preservation of the medial calcar. They are usually stable due to bony buttressing.

Treatment depends on displacement, head viability, and patient factors.

Conservative Management

- Indicated for minimally displaced fractures (<1 cm).
- Sling immobilization for 2–3 weeks followed by ROM exercises.

Operative Management

- ORIF using locking plate for significant displacement or instability.
- Restore neck-shaft angle and maintain medial calcar support.

- Bone grafting or cement augmentation may be used in osteoporotic bone.
- Rarely, RSA in elderly with cuff dysfunction and poor bone quality.

Q31. Cement augmentation in osteoporotic proximal humerus fractures.

(DNB 2003)

Cement augmentation is used as an adjunct to enhance fixation in osteoporotic proximal humerus fractures, especially when using locking plates or screws.

Indications
- Elderly patients with severe osteoporosis.
- Poor purchase of screws in cancellous bone.
- Revision surgeries with compromised bone stock.

Types of cement used
- Polymethylmethacrylate (PMMA).
- Calcium phosphate cement (CPC)—bioresorbable.

Advantages
- Increases construct stability.
- Reduces screw pullout and failure.
- Facilitates early mobilization.

Disadvantages
- Risk of cement leakage and thermal necrosis.
- Non-resorbable nature of PMMA.

Q32. Treatment options in a 4-part proximal humerus fracture in osteoporotic elderly.

(DNB 2024)

Introduction

Proximal humerus fractures are common in the elderly due to:
- Low-energy falls
- Osteoporotic bone

A **four-part fracture**, as per **Neer classification**, involves:
- Displacement of both tuberosities
- Surgical neck fracture
- Articular segment

In the **osteoporotic elderly**, the goal is **pain relief, functional mobility**, and **minimizing complications**, not necessarily anatomical perfection.

Treatment Modalities

1. **Conservative Management**

Indications:
- Non-displaced or minimally displaced fractures
- Medically unfit for surgery
- Very low functional demand

Method:
- Sling immobilization for 2–3 weeks
- Passive-assisted ROM → active ROM by 3–6 weeks

Limitations:
- High risk of malunion, non-union, stiffness
- Poor outcomes in 4-part fractures

2. Operative Management

a. Open reduction and internal fixation (ORIF)
Indications:
- Young or physiologically fit elderly with adequate bone quality
- Preserved humeral head vascularity
- Reconstruction technically feasible

Implants used:
- locking compression plates (LCP)
- Screws with bone graft/cement augmentation

Limitations in elderly:
- Osteoporotic bone → screw cut-out, failure
- High AVN risk
- Poor tuberosity healing → compromised outcome

b. Hemiarthroplasty
Indications:
- Head-splitting fractures
- Unreconstructible head
- Preserved rotator cuff function

Key to success:
- Accurate **tuberosity reconstruction**
- Proper **height and version** of prosthesis

Limitations:
- Pain relief good, but functional outcome depends on tuberosity healing
- High revision rate compared to RSA

c. Reverse shoulder arthroplasty (RSA) preferred option
Indications:
- *Elderly patients with*:
  - Osteoporotic bone
  - Comminuted 3- or 4-part fractures
  - Tuberosity fragmentation
  - Rotator cuff deficiency
- Fracture-dislocation or failed ORIF

Advantages:
- Semi-constrained design → shoulder stability even without cuff
- Early mobilization
- Better functional results than hemiarthroplasty

Considerations:
- Reattachment of tuberosities aids rotation
- Requires post-operative rehabilitation and functional deltoid

3. Cement Augmentation (Adjunct to ORIF)
- Used to improve fixation in osteoporotic metaphyseal bone
- Enhances screw purchase
- Used selectively in combination with plate fixation

Algorithm Summary

Patient factors	*Preferred option*
Very elderly, low demand	Conservative
Elderly with functional goals and poor bone	RSA
Young elderly, good bone and reducible fracture	ORIF
Non-reconstructible head, intact cuff	Hemiarthroplasty

Conclusion

In the osteoporotic elderly with 4-part proximal humerus fracture, **reverse shoulder arthroplasty** is often the **treatment of choice**, providing better pain relief and functional outcomes than fixation or hemiarthroplasty. Careful patient selection and early rehabilitation are vital to optimize recovery.

Q33. Write a detailed long answer on fracture greater tuberosity fracture including its management.

Introduction

The **greater tuberosity** of the humerus is the site of insertion of three rotator cuff tendons:

1. Supraspinatus
2. Infraspinatus
3. Teres minor

Fractures of the greater tuberosity are clinically significant because they can cause:

- Shoulder dysfunction
- Rotator cuff weakness
- Impingement
- Chronic pain

They account for approximately **20% of proximal humerus fractures**, and often occur in:

- Younger patients due to high-energy trauma
- Elderly due to low-energy falls on the outstretched arm

Mechanism of Injury

- Direct trauma to lateral shoulder
- Fall on outstretched arm with abduction and external rotation
- Avulsion injury due to contraction of rotator cuff during dislocation

Frequently associated with:

- Anterior shoulder dislocation
- Rotator cuff injuries

Anatomy and Biomechanics

- The greater tuberosity is located laterally and posteriorly on the humeral head.
- Serves as the insertion site for the supraspinatus (superior facet), infraspinatus (middle facet), and teres minor (inferior facet).
- Its anatomical position and muscle attachments mean even small displacements can significantly affect shoulder mechanics.

Classification

1. Isolated fracture (no dislocation)
2. Associated with anterior shoulder dislocation
3. Comminuted versus non-comminuted
4. *Displacement-based classification*:
    - *Minimally displaced*: <5 mm (≤3 mm in overhead athletes)
    - *Moderately displaced*: 5–10 mm
    - *Severely displaced*: >10 mm

Clinical Features

- Pain, swelling, and tenderness over the lateral shoulder
- Limited active abduction and external rotation
- Associated dislocation signs
- Pain on resisted cuff testing (if tolerated)
- **Check axillary nerve and deltoid function**

Investigations

Radiographs:

- AP, scapular Y, and axillary views
- Look for displacement and comminution

CT scan: Helpful for surgical planning in comminuted or intra-articular fractures

MRI: To assess associated **rotator cuff tears** or **labral injuries** in select cases

Management

A. Non-operative management

Indications:

- Displacement <5 mm (3 mm in overhead athletes)
- No impingement or rotator cuff dysfunction
- Intact rotator cuff

Treatment:

- Arm sling for 1–2 weeks
- Early pendulum and passive ROM exercises
- Active ROM after 3–4 weeks
- Strengthening after 6 weeks

Outcomes: Excellent in minimally displaced fractures with proper rehabilitation

B. Operative Management

Indications:

- Displacement >5 mm
- Impingement on abduction
- Associated shoulder dislocation with a non-reducible fragment
- Overhead athletes with 3 mm+ displacement
- Communution or large displaced fragment
- Rotator cuff involvement

Surgical options:

1. *Open reduction and internal fixation (ORIF)*:
    - *Small fragment*: Cannulated screws, suture anchors
    - *Large fragment*: Screws with or without locking plates
2. *Arthroscopic fixation:* Suture anchors for minimally comminuted avulsion-type injuries
3. *Arthroplasty*: Rare; only if associated with complex proximal humerus or cuff-tear arthropathy in elderly

Rehabilitation

- Immobilization for 2–3 weeks
- Passive and assisted ROM from 2nd to 3rd week
- Full active ROM by 6–8 weeks
- Strengthening from 8–12 weeks

Complications

- Non-union or malunion
- Subacromial impingement

- Stiffness or adhesive capsulitis
- Rotator cuff dysfunction
- Chronic pain
- AVN (rare in isolated greater tuberosity fractures)

Prognosis
- Generally good with proper diagnosis and timely treatment
- Overhead athletes need precise anatomical restoration
- Delayed diagnosis can lead to chronic shoulder dysfunction

Conclusion
Fractures of the greater tuberosity, though often small, are **biomechanically and functionally significant**. Even minor displacement may compromise rotator cuff function and lead to impingement. Early recognition and appropriate treatment, whether conservative or surgical, lead to excellent outcomes in most patients.

Q34. Describe management of humeral shaft fractures. Indications for operative management.

(Asked in: AIIMS Delhi 2022, RGUHS Karnataka 2022)

Introduction
- Humeral shaft fractures account for **3–5% of all fractures**.
- *Mechanism*: Direct trauma, fall on outstretched hand, road traffic accidents.

Management
Non-operative treatment (first-line for most cases):
- *Indications*:
  - Closed fractures.
  - *Acceptable alignment*:
    - <20° anterior angulation,
    - <30° varus/valgus,
    - <3 cm shortening.
- *Methods*:
  - Functional brace (Sarmiento brace).
  - U-slab or hanging cast initially for immobilization.
  - Early mobilization encouraged.

Advantages
- High union rates (85–95%).
- Functional alignment tolerated well due to shoulder and elbow motion adaptability.

Operative Treatment
- *Indications*:
  - Open fractures.
  - Polytrauma patients (early mobilization needed).
  - Segmental fractures.
  - Bilateral humeral fractures.
  - Associated vascular injury (brachial artery).
  - Failure of conservative treatment (non-union/malunion).
  - Radial nerve palsy after manipulation (rare).
  - Floating elbow (ipsilateral humerus + forearm fractures).

Surgical Options
- Open reduction and internal fixation (ORIF) with plating (preferred for most).
- Intramedullary nailing—for segmental fractures or pathological fractures.
- External fixation—temporary for open or infected fractures.

Q35. Radial nerve palsy associated with humeral shaft fracture—management algorithm.

(Asked in: PGI Chandigarh 2022)

Introduction

- Radial nerve is vulnerable due to its course through the spiral groove.
- *Incidence*: ~12% in humeral shaft fractures.

Initial Assessment

- Primary palsy: Present at time of injury.
- Secondary palsy: Occurs after manipulation or during healing.

Management Algorithm

Primary (initial) radial nerve palsy:

- *In closed fractures*: Conservative observation.
    - 70–90% recover spontaneously within 3–6 months.
- Serial clinical and EMG (electromyography) monitoring after 3 weeks.

Immediate Exploration Indications

- Open fracture with nerve palsy.
- Vascular injury requiring repair.
- High-energy trauma with bone fragments likely entrapping the nerve.

Delayed Exploration

- No signs of recovery by 3–4 months.
- EMG shows denervation without reinnervation.

Surgical Options on Exploration

- Nerve repair (primary suture, graft if required).
- Tendon transfers for irreparable injuries (if late presentation).

Summary Flow

Condition	*Management*
Closed fracture + primary palsy	Conservative, observe
Open fracture + palsy	Immediate exploration
No recovery by 3–4 months	Surgical exploration
Intraoperative findings	Repair, graft, or tendon transfer

Q36. Holstein–Lewis fracture and radial nerve injury.

(DNB 2021)

Definition

A **Holstein–Lewis fracture** refers to a **spiral fracture of the distal third of the humeral shaft**. It is classically associated with a **high risk of radial nerve palsy**.

Historical Note

First described by **Holstein and Lewis in 1963**, they observed a notable association between this fracture pattern and radial nerve injury.

Anatomical Basis

- The **radial nerve** spirals around the **posterior aspect of the humerus** in the **radial groove**.
- As it descends into the **distal third**, it **pierces the lateral intermuscular septum** to come **anteriorly**, lying in close proximity to the **periosteum of the humerus**.

- At this level, the nerve is **fixed and tethered**, making it **particularly vulnerable** to injury during:
  - Fracture
  - Manipulation
  - Surgical exposure

Q37. Why is radial nerve injury common in Holstein–Lewis fracture?

1. *Anatomical fixation*: The nerve is tightly bound within the **lateral intermuscular septum**, and this fixed location means that a displaced fracture may stretch or entrap the nerve.
2. *Proximity to fracture site*: The distal third of the humeral shaft is where the radial nerve **transitions from posterior to anterior**, increasing the risk of traction or laceration.
3. *Spiral nature of fracture*: The spiral fracture may cause **rotational displacement**, further increasing the likelihood of nerve entrapment in fracture fragments.
4. *Iatrogenic causes*: During **reduction or nailing**, traction on the limb or manipulation may injure the already vulnerable nerve.

Clinical Features of Radial Nerve Palsy
- **Wrist drop**
- Weakness in finger extension
- Sensory loss over the dorsum of the hand and lateral 3½ fingers (posterior cutaneous branch)

Management
Fracture
- *Most Holstein–Lewis fractures can be managed by*:
  - **Functional bracing, or**
  - **Surgical fixation** (plating preferred in displaced/comminuted fractures)

Radial nerve palsy
- **Most are neuropraxia (90%)** → expectant management
- **Observation for 8–12 weeks** with serial clinical and EMG monitoring
- *Surgical exploration if*:
  - No recovery after 3–4 months
  - Immediate palsy following closed reduction or operative fixation
  - Clinical suspicion of nerve entrapment

Prognosis
- Radial nerve recovery is good in most cases
- Complete functional recovery expected in 70–90% with conservative approach

Conclusion
The Holstein–Lewis fracture is a classic example of **fracture-nerve anatomical correlation.** Due to the unique **location of the radial nerve**, injuries to this region must be carefully monitored for radial nerve palsy. Early recognition and appropriate management of both fracture and nerve are critical for good outcomes.

Q38. Surgical options for pathological humeral shaft fractures.

(DNB 2007)

Introduction
Pathological fractures of the humeral shaft occur due to weakened bone secondary to:
- Metastatic lesions
- Multiple myeloma
- Primary bone tumors

- Benign lesions (e.g., bone cysts, fibrous dysplasia)
- Osteoporosis (rarely causes isolated shaft fractures)

These fractures require **individualized management** focusing on:
- Pain relief
- Immediate stabilization
- Early mobilization
- Preservation of function
- Management of the underlying pathology

Goals of Surgical Treatment
- Immediate mechanical stability
- Pain relief
- Facilitate chemotherapy/radiotherapy
- Restore limb function
- Avoid recurrence and complications

Preoperative Considerations
- Evaluate systemic disease burden
- Assess prognosis and life expectancy
- *Imaging*: X-ray, CT, MRI, and bone scan
- Biopsy if diagnosis uncertain
- Serum studies (e.g., calcium, ALP, tumor markers)

Surgical Options
1. Intramedullary Nailing (IMN)
Most commonly used technique, especially for metastatic lesions
Advantages:
- Load-sharing device
- Minimally invasive
- Protects the entire shaft
- Allows early mobilization

Considerations:
- Use **cephalomedullary nail** if proximal humerus involvement
- Augment with **bone cement (PMMA)** if lytic lesions present

Contraindications:
- Distal humerus extension of lesion
- Severe canal obliteration

2. Plate Osteosynthesis (ORIF)
Indications:
- Fractures involving distal third of shaft
- Lesions not amenable to nailing
- Need for **segmental excision or curettage**

Implants:
- Locking compression plates (LCP)
- Dynamic compression plates (DCP)

Often combined with:
- Curettage of tumor + cement filling or bone graft substitute
- Augmentation with polymethylmethacrylate (PMMA)

Limitations:
- More invasive
- Potential risk of soft tissue and radial nerve injury

3. Endoprosthetic Replacement
Indications:
- Extensive proximal or distal involvement
- Destruction of humeral head or articular surfaces
- Poor bone stock unsuitable for fixation

Types:
- Modular tumor prosthesis
- Total humeral replacement (in selected cases)

Advantages:
- Immediate stability
- Eliminates tumor burden

Disadvantages:
- Higher cost
- Complex procedure
- Functional compromise, especially shoulder/elbow movement

4. Segmental Resection with Cement Spacer
Indications:
- Non-reconstructable segmental bone loss
- Palliative intent
- Short life expectancy

Features:
- PMMA spacer fashioned as temporary or permanent implant
- May be reinforced with intramedullary nail or K-wires

5. Cement-Augmented Fixation (PMMA)
Used in combination with IMN or plating:
- Improves mechanical strength
- Fills voids from lytic lesions
- Immediate pain relief
- Allows chemotherapy and radiotherapy

6. Radiotherapy-assisted Fixation (Adjuvant)
Post-operative external beam radiotherapy:
- Controls tumor progression
- Prevents hardware failure
- Especially useful in myeloma, metastasis

Postoperative care
- Early physiotherapy and ROM
- Continue systemic therapy (chemo/hormonal)
- Monitor for local recurrence
- Radiotherapy if indicated

Conclusion
Surgical management of pathological humeral shaft fractures aims to offer **stability, pain relief, and early mobility**, especially in the **oncological and palliative context**. The choice between intramedullary nailing, plating, or endoprosthesis depends on **fracture location, extent of disease, bone quality**, and **patient prognosis**.

Q39. Hanging cast technique—indications and limitations.

Definition

The **hanging cast technique** is a conservative method for treating **humeral shaft fractures**, particularly those in the **middle and distal third**. It relies on the **gravity-assisted alignment** of the fracture fragments by suspending the arm in a cast, allowing traction and muscle tone to realign the bone.

Technique Description

- A **cylindrical cast** is applied from just below the axilla to just above the wrist.
- The arm is **left to hang vertically** with the **elbow extended**, using the weight of the cast and limb to exert longitudinal traction.
- The shoulder may be supported with a **sling looped around the neck**, but the weight must remain hanging for the reduction to be effective.

Mechanism

- Utilizes the **gravitational pull** of the arm's own weight to **reduce angulation and overlap** at the fracture site.
- **Deltoid and biceps tension** assist in aligning the fragments.
- Works best when **medial and lateral cortices are in contact**

Indications

1. *Middle third or distal third humeral shaft fractures*: Transverse, short oblique, or mildly comminuted patterns
2. *Closed fractures*: With acceptable alignment after initial traction
3. *Patients unfit for surgery*: Medically frail or with comorbidities
4. Temporary management in polytrauma
5. **As a second stage** after initial traction or splinting

Limitations/Contraindications

Absolute contraindications:

- Open fractures
- Vascular injury
- Compartment syndrome

Relative contraindications:

- proximal third shaft fractures (ineffective)
- Radial nerve palsy needing surgical exploration
- Grossly unstable or segmental fractures
- Pathological fractures
- Non-compliant patients
- Obese patients or those with heavy limbs
- Shoulder dislocation associated with fracture

Complications

- Shoulder stiffness or frozen shoulder
- Malunion (varus angulation)
- Skin maceration or cast sores
- Brachial plexus traction neuropathy
- Poor patient tolerance (especially elderly)

Outcome

- Union rates of >90% have been reported with proper technique
- Requires careful monitoring and transition to functional brace as healing progresses

Conclusion

The hanging cast is a **simple, cost-effective**, and time-tested technique for selected humeral shaft fractures. However, careful patient selection, monitoring, and follow-up are critical to ensure optimal results and avoid complications.

Q40. Discuss the pros and cons of plating versus nailing for humeral shaft fracture and which modality to use in laborers.

(MS 2023)

Introduction

Both **plating** and **intramedullary nailing (IMN)** are widely accepted surgical techniques for **humeral shaft fractures**. The choice depends on fracture pattern, patient activity level, soft tissue conditions, and surgeon expertise.

In laborers or heavy manual workers, functional outcome, rotator cuff integrity, and union rate are critical.

I. Plating (Open Reduction and Internal Fixation – ORIF)

Pros

- **Anatomical reduction** and rigid fixation
- **Lower incidence of shoulder problems** (no rotator cuff violation)
- **Better control in comminuted and segmental fractures**
- Preferred in **proximal and distal third shaft fractures**
- Avoids implant impingement around the shoulder

Cons

- **More soft tissue dissection**
- Risk of **radial nerve injury**
- Longer operative time
- Cosmetic scar
- Stress shielding in osteoporotic bone

II. Intramedullary Nailing (IMN)

Pros

- **Minimally invasive**—Smaller incision
- **Preservation of fracture hematoma**
- Early mobilization possible
- Less risk of infection
- Better biomechanical load-sharing device

Cons

- *Shoulder pain and dysfunction due to*: Entry point through rotator cuff (especially with antegrade nailing)
- Higher risk of **malalignment** (especially rotational)
- Difficult fixation in proximal or distal third fractures
- Nail migration or implant prominence
- Delayed union in some studies

Evidence-based Comparison

Factor	*Plating*	*Nailing*
Union rate	Slightly better	Comparable
Shoulder function	Better	Often compromised
Infection risk	Slightly higher	Lower
Blood loss	More	Less
Rotator cuff damage	None	Common (antegrade entry)
Return to activity	Good with proper rehabilitation	May be delayed by shoulder dysfunction

Which Modality for Laborers?

Recommendation: ORIF with Plating

Justification:

- Laborers rely on **full shoulder strength and mobility**.
- IMN may compromise shoulder function due to **rotator cuff violation**.

- Plating offers **rigid fixation** with **better functional outcomes** in high-demand patients.
- **Less risk of shoulder pain**, especially in overhead workers.

Conclusion

Both plating and nailing are acceptable for humeral shaft fractures. However, for **laborers and high-demand individuals**, **plating** is preferred due to **better shoulder outcomes** and **less functional compromise**. Individual patient assessment, fracture characteristics, and surgeon proficiency should guide the final decision.

Q41. Functional bracing and surgical indications in humerus shaft fractures.

(MS 2018)

I. Functional Bracing of Humeral Shaft Fractures

Definition

Functional bracing involves **application of a cylindrical brace** around the arm that allows **early shoulder and elbow motion** while providing **circumferential soft tissue compression** to align and stabilize the fracture.

Principle

- Introduced by **Augusto Sarmiento**
- Uses **hydrostatic pressure** and **muscle action** to maintain alignment
- Enhances **callus formation** by allowing controlled micromotion at the fracture site

Indications

- Most **closed humeral shaft fractures**
- Minimally displaced or short oblique fractures
- **Mid-shaft or distal-third fractures**
- Early mobilization desired
- Patients unfit for surgery

Application Protocol

- Applied after 1–2 weeks of initial splinting or hanging cast
- Brace from **axilla to elbow**, with **padding** and **Velcro straps**
- Shoulder and elbow ROM exercises encouraged

Advantages

- Non-invasive and cost-effective
- Avoids surgical risks (infection, nerve injury)
- Allows early joint motion
- Preserves fracture hematoma and biology

Limitations

- May not control rotation in spiral fractures
- Less effective for proximal third fractures
- Cosmetic deformity (angulation) may occur
- Patient compliance critical
- Skin maceration or pressure sores

Q42. Surgical indications in humerus shaft fractures.

Absolute Indications

1. Open fractures
2. Vascular injury requiring repair
3. Floating shoulder (associated scapular neck fracture)
4. Bilateral humeral fractures

5. Polytrauma requiring early mobilization
6. Failure of conservative treatment (non-union, malunion)

Relative Indications
1. Segmental fractures
2. Fractures with significant shortening (>3 cm)
3. Radial nerve palsy after closed manipulation
4. Pathological fractures
5. Comminuted or spiral fractures not suitable for bracing
6. Proximal or distal third fractures

Surgical Options
- *ORIF with plate fixation*: Gold standard
- *Intramedullary nailing*: For selected cases, less invasive
- *External fixation*: Rarely used, in open or infected fractures

Conclusion
Functional bracing remains a **first-line option** for most closed humeral shaft fractures. However, **surgical intervention is warranted** in unstable patterns, open injuries, polytrauma, or failed conservative care. **Careful patient selection** ensures optimal outcomes with either approach.

Q43. Causes and treatment of humeral shaft non-union.

(DNB 2013)

Definition
Non-union of the humeral shaft refers to **failure of fracture healing** beyond **6–9 months**, with **no radiological progression** and **clinical signs** of persistent mobility or pain at the fracture site.

Types of Non-union
1. *Hypertrophic (vascular)*:
   - Adequate biology, poor mechanical stability
   - "Elephant foot" or "horse hoof" appearance
2. *Atrophic (avascular)*:
   - Poor biology
   - No callus formation; may be associated with bone resorption
3. *Oligotrophic*: Intermediate type, minimal callus formation

Causes of Non-union
- *Biological factors*:
  - Poor blood supply
  - Severe soft tissue damage
  - Infection (especially post-operative)
  - Use of rigid implants suppressing micromotion
  - Radiation or prior surgery
  - *Systemic conditions*: Diabetes, smoking, NSAID overuse
- *Mechanical factors*:
  - Inadequate fracture stability
  - Poor implant selection or technique (e.g., loose IM nail, single cortex plating)
  - Excessive distraction or malalignment
  - Early aggressive mobilization or weight-bearing
- *Patient factors*:
  - Non-compliance with immobilization
  - Malnutrition

- Alcoholism
- Osteoporosis

Clinical Features

- Pain and tenderness at fracture site
- Abnormal mobility or crepitus
- No progression of union on serial X-rays

Radiological Evaluation

- *X-rays*: Assess gap, callus, implant status
- *CT scan*: Helpful for evaluating non-union site
- Blood investigations to rule out infection (CRP, ESR, WBC count)

Treatment Options

I. Non-surgical

- Rarely effective alone
- Bone stimulators (electromagnetic or ultrasound) in early/partial union
- Cast brace with weight loading (selected cases)

II. Surgical Treatment

1. *For hypertrophic non-union (mechanical problem)*:
   - *Rigid fixation with*:
     - Compression plating (e.g., dynamic compression plate - DCP)
     - Exchange nailing (if previously nailed)
   - Preservation of biological environment
   - Optional bone grafting (rarely needed)
2. *For atrophic non-union (biological problem)*:
   - Decortication and debridement of necrotic tissue
   - Rigid internal fixation with locking compression plate (LCP)
   - Autologous iliac crest bone graft or fibular strut graft
   - Consider bone morphogenetic proteins (BMPs) in selected cases
3. *Infected non-union*:
   - *Staged surgery*:
     - *First stage*: Debridement + antibiotic cement spacer
     - *Second stage*: Definitive fixation with bone grafting
   - Consider external fixation (e.g., Ilizarov) in chronic osteomyelitis

Special Considerations

- External fixators (monolateral or ring fixators) for severe soft tissue loss
- **Papineau technique**, Masquelet technique, or vascularized grafts for large bone loss

Conclusion

Non-union of humeral shaft fractures arises from **mechanical or biological failure**, often due to inadequate fixation or poor vascularity. **Tailored surgical intervention** with compression plating, bone grafting, and biomechanical optimization yields high union rates and functional recovery.

Q44. Complications of humeral shaft fractures (including radial nerve palsy).

A. Early Complications

1. *Radial nerve palsy:*
   - Most common nerve injury associated with humeral shaft fractures
   - *Incidence*: ~10–18%, especially in **Holstein–Lewis fractures** (distal third spiral fractures)
   - Usually **neuropraxia**; resolves in 8–12 weeks

Management:
- Observe if initial injury is closed and palsy is present
- EMG/NCS after 3–4 weeks
- *Surgical exploration if*:
    - Open fracture
    - Nerve deficit after manipulation or ORIF
    - No recovery by 3–4 months

2. *Vascular injury*:
    - Rare; more likely in proximal or open fractures
    - Subclavian or brachial artery at risk
3. *Compartment syndrome*: Very rare but possible in high-energy trauma
4. *Skin compromise*: Pressure necrosis in open injuries or due to cast/bracing

B. Late Complications

1. *Non-union*:
    - Incidence ~2–10%
    - *Risk factors*: Inadequate immobilization, infection, distraction, smoking, diabetes
    - Requires surgical fixation with or without bone grafting
2. *Malunion*:
    - Especially varus angulation or shortening
    - May cause functional deficit, cosmetic deformity
3. *Shoulder and elbow stiffness*:
    - Due to prolonged immobilization
    - Early ROM exercises crucial
4. *Infection*:
    - More common in open fractures or post-ORIF
    - Managed with debridement, antibiotics, and possibly implant removal
5. *Implant complications*:
    - Plate loosening or nail migration
    - Stress shielding

Q45. Classification and management of distal humerus fractures.

A. Classification

Classification (based on anatomical location and articular involvement):
- Supracondylar fractures
- Transcondylar fractures
- Intercondylar (T- or Y-type) fractures
- Lateral condyle or medial condyle fractures

AO/OTA Classification

The AO/OTA system classifies fractures based on anatomical location and complexity.

Region Code for Distal Humerus: 13

Types:

Type	*Description*
13-A Extra-articular fractures	Above the condyles
13-B Partial articular fractures	One condyle remains in continuity with shaft
13-C Complete articular fractures	Articular surface separated from shaft and fractured

Subtypes:

- *Type A (extra-articular):*
  - *A1*: Supracondylar, simple
  - *A2*: Metaphyseal wedge
  - *A3*: Multifragmentary
- *Type B (partial articular)*:
  - *B1*: Lateral condyle (capitulum)
  - *B2*: Medial condyle (trochlea)
  - *B3*: Sagittal splits, partial joint involvement
- *Type C (complete articular)*:
  - *C1*: Simple articular + simple metaphyseal
  - *C2*: Simple articular + multifragmentary metaphyseal
  - *C3*: Comminuted articular + comminuted metaphyseal
- *Jupiter Classification (based on columns)*:
  - Unicolumnar (medial/lateral)
  - Bicolumnar (T or Y-shaped)
  - Important for preoperative planning

B. Management

Non-operative

- *Only for*:
  - Non-displaced fractures
  - Medically unfit patients
  - Low-demand elderly with minimal displacement
- *Methods*: Above elbow slab, U-slab, collar and cuff
- *Risk*: Stiffness, non-union, poor elbow function

Operative Treatment (Preferred in Most Cases)

Goals:

- Anatomical reduction
- Stable fixation
- Early mobilization

Surgical approaches: Posterior approach (triceps-splitting, triceps-reflecting or olecranon osteotomy)

Fixation principles:

- *Dual plating (orthogonal or parallel)*: Medial and lateral column fixation
- Locking plates in osteoporotic bone
- Headless compression screws for intercondylar fragments
- Bone grafts for comminution

Post-operative:

- Early passive → active ROM
- Delayed strengthening

Complications

- Stiffness
- Non-union
- Ulnar nerve neuropathy
- Heterotopic ossification
- Implant failure
- Post-traumatic arthritis

Q46. Indications and surgical approaches for ORIF in distal humerus fractures.

Indications for ORIF
- Displaced intra-articular fractures
- Failure of conservative treatment
- Bilateral injuries or polytrauma
- Young patients requiring early mobility
- Open fractures (after initial debridement)
- Non-unions or malunions
- Comminuted or bicolumn fractures

Surgical Approaches
Posterior approach (most common)
1. *Triceps-splitting*: Vertical split in triceps
2. *Triceps-reflecting (Bryan–Morrey)*: Lift triceps off olecranon
3. *Olecranon osteotomy*: Best exposure of joint
    - Preferred for C-type fractures
    - Osteotomy fixed with tension band or screw

Medial and Lateral Approaches
- For unicolumnar fractures (Type B1/B2)
- Minimal exposure needed

Paratricipital Approach
- Triceps preserved
- Suitable for elderly or partial articular fractures

Fixation Principles
- **Orthogonal (90-90)** or **parallel bicolumnar plating**
- Locking plates preferred in osteoporotic bone
- Interfragmentary compression screws for articular reduction

Post-operative
- Early ROM from 2–5 days post-operative
- Elbow brace or hinged splint for protection

Q47. Describe capitulum fractures.

Definition
Fracture involving the **lateral distal articular surface** of the humerus (capitulum), often seen in young adults from falls on an outstretched hand with elbow flexion.

Classification (Modified Bryan and Morrey)
- *Type I (Hahn–Steinthal)*: Large osseous fragment
- *Type II (Kocher–Lorenz)*: Cartilage-dominant fragment
- *Type III*: Comminuted fracture
- *Type IV*: Fracture extends medially into trochlea (Dubberley)

Diagnosis
- Often missed on AP view
- **Lateral elbow X-ray** shows "double arc" or "saucer sign"
- CT scan is useful for pre-operative planning

Management
Non-displaced: Immobilization in long arm cast for 3–4 weeks

Displaced/Comminuted
- ORIF with headless screws (Herbert/acutrac)
- *Approach*: lateral or posterior (extended Kocher)

Non-reconstructable
- Excision of fragment (type II or III)
- Consider elbow arthroplasty in elderly

Complications
- Elbow stiffness
- Avascular necrosis
- Post-traumatic arthritis
- Instability if lateral ligament complex involved

Q48. Discuss the indications and techniques of open reduction and internal fixation (ORIF) in elbow fractures.

(SRIHER 2011)

Indications
- Intra-articular fractures (e.g., distal humerus, radial head)
- Unstable extra-articular fractures (e.g., olecranon with displacement)
- Comminuted or displaced fractures not amenable to conservative treatment
- Elbow instability due to fracture-dislocation

Techniques
- **Posterior approach** commonly used
- Use of plates, screws, tension band wiring depending on fracture type
- *Goal*: Anatomical reduction, stable fixation, early mobilization

---

Q49. Explain the mechanism, diagnosis, and treatment of elbow dislocations.

Definition
Elbow dislocation refers to the loss of congruity between the distal humerus and the proximal radius and ulna.

Mechanism
- *Most common direction*: Posterior dislocation (~90%)
- *Typical cause*: Fall on an outstretched hand (FOOSH) with elbow slightly flexed and forearm supinated
- *Sequential soft-tissue injury pattern*: Lateral collateral ligament (LCL) → anterior capsule → medial collateral ligament (MCL)
  (Circle of Horii theory)

Classification
- *Simple dislocation*: No associated fractures
- *Complex dislocation*: Associated with fractures (radial head, coronoid, etc.)

Diagnosis
- *Clinical*:
  - Obvious deformity, swelling
  - Loss of range of motion
  - Check distal neurovascular status
- *Radiology*:
  - *X-ray (AP and lateral)*: Confirms dislocation direction and rules out fractures
  - *CT scan*: For complex injuries or pre-operative planning

Treatment

Immediate care:

- **Closed reduction under sedation** or general anesthesia
- Neurovascular examination pre- and post-reduction
- **Post-reduction X-rays** to confirm concentric reduction

Immobilization: Posterior splint at 90° flexion for **5–10 days** for simple dislocation

Mobilization:

- Early **active ROM** to avoid stiffness
- Avoid prolonged immobilization (>2–3 weeks)

Surgical indications:

- Incongruent reduction
- Associated fractures (terrible triad, Monteggia variant)
- Recurrent instability
- Entrapped soft tissue or bony fragment

Complications

- **Stiffness** (most common)
- Chronic instability
- Heterotopic ossification
- Ulnar nerve injury
- Myositis ossificans

Q50. Posterior elbow dislocation—clinical features and management.

(Asked in: PGI Chandigarh 2021, MUHS Maharashtra 2023)

Definition

Displacement of ulna and radius posterior to humerus.

Clinical Features

- Obvious deformity.
- Flexed and shortened elbow.
- Inability to move elbow.
- Neurovascular status must be assessed (brachial artery, median/ulnar nerves).

Management

Acute:

- Closed reduction under sedation/anesthesia → longitudinal traction and elbow flexion.
- Confirm reduction by X-ray.
- Immobilization in posterior slab at 90° flexion for 2–3 weeks.

Post-reduction: Early ROM exercises to prevent stiffness.

Surgical: Indicated if associated fractures (complex dislocations) or unstable reduction.

Q51. Differentiation between simple versus complex elbow dislocations.

Feature	*Simple*	*Complex*
Definition	Pure dislocation without fracture	Associated with fractures (radial head, coronoid, olecranon)
Stability post-reduction	Usually stable	Often unstable
Management	Closed reduction, early rehabilitation	May require surgical fixation
Prognosis	Good with rehabilitation	Depends on extent of injury

Q52. Management of complex elbow dislocations (with fractures).

(Asked in: AIIMS Delhi 2021, JIPMER Puducherry 2022)

Definition
Dislocation associated with fractures (radial head, coronoid, olecranon, or capitellum).

Management
Principles:
- Early stable reduction.
- Fix all associated fractures (ORIF if necessary).
- Repair collateral ligaments if instability persists.

Specific protocol:
- Radial head fractures → Fixation or replacement.
- Coronoid fractures → Fixation.
- Ligamentous repair (LCL/MCL).
- Temporary external fixation if joint grossly unstable.

Q53. Divergent elbow dislocation—short note.

Definition
A rare type of elbow dislocation where radius and ulna are displaced in opposite directions with disruption of proximal radioulnar joint.

Mechanism
High-energy trauma or hyperextension + axial load

Associated injuries
- Radial head fracture
- Coronoid fracture
- Interosseous membrane rupture

Treatment
- Closed or open reduction
- Fixation of associated injuries

Q54. Write a short note on ligament reconstruction in chronic elbow instability.

Definition
Surgical repair or reconstruction of collateral ligaments (e.g., **ulnar collateral ligament** in throwers or **lateral ulnar collateral ligament** in posterolateral rotatory instability).

Indications
- Chronic elbow instability
- Failed conservative management
- Recurrent dislocations or subluxations

Procedure
- Autograft (e.g., palmaris longus) or allograft used
- Tensioned and fixed anatomically to restore stability
- Often combined with bony procedures if needed

Q55. Explain the role of hinged external fixators in elbow injuries.

Purpose
- Maintains **elbow alignment** while allowing **controlled motion**
- Used when internal fixation is insufficient to maintain stability

Indications
- Complex fracture-dislocations
- Gross instability post-ORIF
- Comminuted fractures with soft tissue compromise
- Elbow arthrolysis to prevent re-stiffness

Mechanism
- Fixed to humerus and ulna/radius
- Allows flexion-extension but limits rotation/subluxation

Q56. Management of neglected elbow injury.

Definition
Elbow injury not treated or mismanaged for >3 weeks

Common Issues
- Stiffness
- Malunion/non-union (e.g., lateral condyle)
- Chronic dislocation
- Instability
- Heterotopic ossification

Management Depends On
- *Type of injury*:
  - *Neglected dislocation*: Open reduction with V-Y triceps plasty, capsular release, ligament reconstruction if needed
  - *Neglected lateral condyle fracture*: If painful or unstable → ORIF ± bone grafting
  - *Stiff elbow*:
    - *Non-operative*: Physiotherapy, dynamic splinting
    - *Operative*: Open/arthroscopic capsular release, HO excision
- **Physiotherapy** is critical post-operative

Q57. Posterolateral rotatory instability (PLRI)—diagnosis and treatment.

Definition
Posterolateral rotatory instability (PLRI) is the most common form of chronic elbow instability due to lateral ulnar collateral ligament (LUCL) insufficiency.

Etiology
Usually follows trauma, dislocation, or repetitive varus stress (e.g., in overhead athletes).

Pathomechanics
Radius and ulna rotate externally away from the humerus (supination), resulting in posterolateral subluxation.

Clinical Features
Lateral elbow pain, mechanical symptoms (clicking/locking), and apprehension during supination-extension activities.

Diagnosis
- Pivot-shift test of elbow (positive under anesthesia)
- *Imaging*: MRI may show LUCL tear; dynamic fluoroscopy may help.

Treatment
- *Conservative*: Bracing and physiotherapy in mild, non-symptomatic cases.
- *Surgical*: LUCL reconstruction using autograft (palmaris longus/gracilis).
- Postoperative hinged brace with gradual ROM.

Q58. Describe the mechanism of injury of radial head fracture.

Mechanism of Injury
- Radial head fractures typically occur due to:
  1. **Fall on outstretched hand (FOOSH)** with **elbow in extension and forearm in pronation**, transmitting force axially through the radius.
  2. The radial head is forced against the **capitellum**, leading to compression and fracture.
  3. Direct blow to the lateral elbow (less common).

Associated Injuries
- Capitellar fractures
- Elbow dislocation
- Coronoid process fractures
- Interosseous membrane injuries (Essex-Lopresti)
- Distal radioulnar joint (DRUJ) disruption

Q59. Classification and treatment of radial head fractures.

(Asked in: PGI Chandigarh 2021)

Introduction
Radial head fractures occur from **axial load transmitted through the forearm** during a fall.

Mason Classification

Type	*Description*
I	Non-displaced or minimally displaced
II	Displaced (>2 mm) or angulated fracture
III	Comminuted fracture involving the entire head
IV	Radial head fracture with elbow dislocation

Treatment
Type I:
- Non-operative management.
- Sling or posterior splint for a few days.
- Early range of motion to prevent stiffness.

Type II:
- Open reduction and internal fixation (ORIF) (Open Reduction and Internal Fixation) if mechanical block to movement or >2 mm displacement.
- Otherwise conservative management.

Type III:
- Radial head excision (historical).
- **Radial head replacement (arthroplasty)** is preferred today, especially if elbow instability present.

Type IV:
- Reduction of elbow dislocation first.
- Manage radial head fracture depending on fracture type.

Important Surgical Considerations

- Preserve radial head if possible (important stabilizer against valgus stress and axial load).
- Arthroplasty preferred if fixation not feasible.

Q60. Discuss the indications for radial head excision versus prosthetic replacement.

(AIIMS BBSR 2013)

Introduction

Radial head fractures are common elbow injuries. Complex or comminuted fractures that are not amenable to fixation may need excision or prosthetic replacement. Each method has distinct indications.

Radial Head Excision

Indications:

- Isolated radial head fracture (Mason type III or IV) with:
  - **Intact interosseous membrane**
  - **Stable elbow and DRUJ (distal radioulnar joint)**
  - Elderly, low-demand patients
- Chronic non-union or post-traumatic arthritis of radial head
- After failed internal fixation

Contraindications:

- Associated ligamentous injury (LCL/MCL)
- Essex-Lopresti lesion
- Complex instability
- High-demand patients

Complications:

- Valgus instability
- Proximal migration of radius
- Wrist pain (DRUJ dysfunction)
- Ulnar impingement

Radial Head Prosthetic Replacement

Indications

- Comminuted, non-reconstructable radial head fractures (Mason type III or IV)
- Associated elbow instability (terrible triad, LCL/MCL injury)
- Essex–Lopresti injury
- High-demand young patients
- Failed ORIF or radial head excision causing instability

Types of Prosthesis

- Monoblock versus modular
- Press-fit versus cemented

Advantages

- Maintains joint stability
- Prevents proximal migration
- Allows early mobilization

Complications

- Overstuffing (loss of ROM, pain)
- Loosening
- Capitellar erosion
- Implant failure

Comparison

Parameter	Radial head excision	Radial head replacement
Stability	May cause instability	Maintains elbow stability
Suitable for	Elderly, low-demand	Young, high-demand, unstable elbow
Complications	DRUJ issues, valgus deformity	Overstuffing, loosening
Cost	Low	High

Conclusion

Choice between radial head excision and replacement depends on fracture type, associated injuries, and patient profile. Prosthetic replacement is preferred in unstable elbows, while excision may be considered in select elderly or low-demand patients.

Q61. Write a note on Essex–Lopresti injury and why is it missed.

(DNB 2020)

Definition

- A complex injury consisting of:
    - Radial head fracture
    - Interosseous membrane (IOM) disruption
    - Distal radioulnar joint (DRUJ) dislocation/subluxation

Mechanism

- High-energy axial load through the forearm (e.g., fall on outstretched hand).
- Causes proximal migration of the radius after radial head fracture due to IOM tear and DRUJ disruption.

Why is it missed?

- Focus is often on radial head fracture alone.
- DRUJ instability and IOM rupture may not be clinically evident initially.
- Symptoms at DRUJ appear delayed (chronic pain, decreased grip strength, instability).
- Lack of awareness or inadequate radiographic evaluation.

Diagnosis

- Careful examination of **wrist for DRUJ instability**
- **Forearm shortening** (comparison films)
- **MRI** may be needed to detect IOM injury
- Positive ulnar variance at wrist X-ray

Management

- **Radial head replacement (not excision)** if comminuted
- DRUJ stabilization
- IOM rarely repaired but forearm should be stabilized early

Q62. Sideswipe injuries of elbow.

Definition

High-energy injuries due to collision of extended elbow with a protruding object (e.g., pole or vehicle), usually while protruding from a moving vehicle.

Features

- Severe soft tissue injury with open fractures.
- Neurovascular injury common (especially brachial artery, median/ulnar nerve).
- Often involves distal humerus and/or olecranon fractures.

Management
- Emergency debridement and stabilization.
- Vascular repair if needed.
- Soft tissue coverage (flaps).
- Secondary reconstructions or amputation in extreme cases.

1. Management of neglected elbow injury.
2. Floating elbow management.
3. Coronoid fractures.

Q63. Classification and surgical management of olecranon fractures.

(Asked in: PGI Chandigarh 2021, MUHS Maharashtra 2022)

Classification

Mayo classification:

Type	*Description*
I	Non-displaced
II	Displaced, stable
III	Displaced, unstable

Management

Type I: Conservative (immobilization in above-elbow slab at 30–45° flexion).

Type II and III:
- *Tension band wiring (TBW)*: For simple transverse fractures.
- *Plate fixation*: For comminuted, oblique, or unstable fractures.

Early:
- Wound infection.
- Hardware prominence/irritation.

Late:
- Non-union.
- Loss of extension.
- Post-traumatic arthritis.

Q64. Surgical approach to olecranon fractures.

Posterior Approach
- Skin incision midline posterior, curving around olecranon tip
- Reflect triceps laterally/medially

Fixation Techniques
- Tension band wiring (for transverse fractures)
- Plate fixation (comminuted or oblique fractures)
- Intramedullary screws (select cases)

Q65. Write a short note on the terrible triad injury of the elbow.

Definition

Terrible triad of the elbow is a **complex elbow injury** involving:

1. Posterior elbow dislocation

2. Radial head fracture
3. Coronoid process fracture

Mechanism
- High-energy fall on an outstretched hand with valgus and axial load force.
- *Leads to disruption of*:
  - LCL
  - Radial head
  - Coronoid process
  - Often MCL

Clinical Features
- Pain, swelling, deformity
- Inability to move elbow
- Neurovascular exam critical (check for ulnar or radial nerve injury)

Radiology
- *X-ray*: Dislocation, radial head or coronoid fracture
- *CT scan*: Helpful in surgical planning

Management
Goal: Restore bony anatomy and stability

Surgical management:
1. *Radial head*: ORIF or radial head replacement
2. *Coronoid*: Fixation if >10–15% of height or type II/III (Regan–Morrey)
3. *Lateral collateral ligament (LCL)*: Repair always
4. *Medial collateral ligament (MCL)*: Repair if residual instability after the above

Post-operative:
- Early ROM within protected range
- Hinged elbow brace

Complications
- Stiffness
- Heterotopic ossification
- Instability
- Post-traumatic arthritis

Q66. Complications of olecranon fractures.

1. Non-union
Especially in comminuted fractures, elderly, osteoporotic patients, or due to inadequate fixation.

Management:
- Revision fixation with bone grafting
- Consider tension band wiring or plate fixation depending on fracture type

2. Malunion
Leads to mechanical block, deformity, or loss of range of motion

Management: Corrective osteotomy in symptomatic cases

3. Loss of elbow extension strength
From disruption of triceps mechanism or inadequate reattachment.

Management:
- Physiotherapy for muscle strengthening
- Reattachment procedures if needed

4. Hardware prominence and irritation
- Very common due to subcutaneous location of olecranon
- Seen more with tension band wiring

Management: Implant removal after union

5. Stiffness of the elbow
Due to prolonged immobilization or intra-articular injury

Management:
- Early mobilization
- Manipulation under anesthesia (MUA) or arthrolysis

6. Post-traumatic arthritis
Especially if intra-articular step-off is not addressed

Management: NSAIDs, intra-articular injections, or ultimately total elbow arthroplasty in elderly

7. Infection
Particularly in open fractures or following surgery

Management:
- Antibiotics and debridement
- Possible hardware removal if chronic

8. Ulnar nerve neuropathy
Compression, stretching, or iatrogenic injury

Management: Observation, neurolysis, or anterior transposition

9. Triceps weakness or avulsion
Due to inadequate repair

Management: Surgical reattachment

Conclusion
Complications of olecranon fractures are not uncommon and often predictable. Prevention by proper technique and early rehabilitation is essential. Prompt identification and appropriate management help restore function.

Q67. Floating elbow management.

Definition
Ipsilateral humerus and forearm fractures

Significance
Unstable, high-energy injury often associated with neurovascular trauma

Goals
- Stabilize both humerus and forearm fractures
- Restore alignment, rotation, and length
- Prevent compartment syndrome

Management
- *Initial*:
    - Rule out neurovascular compromise

- Splinting and elevation
- Fasciotomy if required

- *Definitive*:
  - Internal fixation of both humerus and radius/ulna fractures
    - Typically humerus first for better control
  - Rigid fixation allows early mobilization

Q68. Coronoid fractures.

Importance
Key to elbow anterior stability

Mechanism
Varus or valgus stress, often with elbow dislocation

Classification

- *Regan and Morrey*:
  - *Type I*: Tip
  - *Type II*: <50% height
  - *Type III*: >50% height

Associated Injuries

- Posterolateral rotatory instability
- Terrible triad (coronoid + radial head + dislocation)

Management

- *Type I*: Usually conservative
- *Type II–III or unstable elbow*:
  - Open reduction and internal fixation (screws or suture lasso)
  - Address radial head or ligamentous injury
  - May require external fixator or hinged brace for stability

Q69. Explain the pathophysiology and management of Monteggia fractures.

(WBUHS 2011)

Definition
A **Monteggia fracture** is defined as a fracture of the **proximal third of the ulna** with **dislocation of the radial head** at the elbow joint.

Pathophysiology
Mechanism of injury:

- *Direct trauma*: Blow to the ulna with elbow flexed.
- *Indirect trauma*: Fall on an outstretched hand with the forearm in hyperpronation or hyperextension.

Forces Involved

- Axial load
- Pronation/supination
- Varus/valgus stress
- The dislocation of the radial head occurs due to **disruption of the annular ligament** and **interosseous membrane** tension imbalance.

Associated Injuries

- Interosseous membrane injury
- Posterior interosseous nerve palsy (especially in children)
- DRUJ instability (rare)

Management

General principles:

- Restore **length**, **alignment**, and **rotation** of the ulna
- Radial head typically **reduces spontaneously** after ulnar fixation

In Adults

- *Always requires surgical management*:
  - **Open reduction and internal fixation (ORIF)** of the ulna using plating (compression/locking plates)
  - Ensure radial head reduction (confirmed on fluoroscopy)
  - Repair of annular ligament if radial head remains unstable
  - Postoperative immobilization for 2–3 weeks followed by physiotherapy

In Children

- Closed reduction and casting may suffice (if fracture is recent and reducible)
- Indications for surgery:
  - Failed closed reduction
  - Delayed presentation (>2 weeks)
  - Irreducible radial head

Conclusion

Early diagnosis and anatomic reduction of the ulna are critical for successful outcome. Delayed or missed diagnosis can lead to chronic instability and functional deficits.

Q70. Write a short note on Bado's classification of Monteggia fractures.

Bado's Classification (1967)

Based on **direction of radial head dislocation** and **pattern of ulnar fracture**.

Type	*Radial head dislocation*	*Ulnar fracture pattern*	*Common mechanism*
I	Anterior	Diaphyseal fracture with anterior angulation	Hyperpronation injury
II	Posterior/Postero-lateral	Diaphyseal fracture with posterior angulation	Backward fall on extended elbow
III	Lateral	Metaphyseal ulnar fracture	Abduction injury
IV	Anterior (like Type I)	Both radius and ulna fractured at same level	High energy trauma

Relevance

- Guides treatment approach and prognosis
- Type I most common (60% in children)
- Type II more common in adults

Q71. Discuss the management of chronic Monteggia fracture-dislocations.

Definition

A Monteggia fracture-dislocation persisting >**3–4 weeks** after injury, with **non-reduction of radial head** and malunited or healed ulna.

Challenges in Management

- Soft tissue contractures around radial head
- Bony remodeling of radial head or capitellum
- Annular ligament fibrosis or rupture
- Limb deformity and loss of motion

Management Strategy

1. *Preoperative evaluation*:
   - X-rays of the forearm and elbow (AP and lateral)
   - CT scan for 3D planning (especially for radial head morphology)

2. *Surgical options*:
    - *Ulnar osteotomy*:
        - Corrects malalignment, restores length and angulation
        - Usually enough to spontaneously reduce radial head
        - Most important step in chronic cases
    - *Radial head reduction*:
        - Open reduction may be needed if radial head does not reduce
        - Remove interposed tissue or reconstruct annular ligament
    - *Annular ligament reconstruction*:
        - Needed if radial head is unstable after ulnar correction
        - Bell-Tawse technique using strip of triceps or lateral fascia
    - *Radial head resection*: Rarely used; only in adults with unreconstructable radial head and low functional demand
3. *Postoperative care*:
    - Immobilization for 3–4 weeks
    - Gradual mobilization under physiotherapy

Prognosis
- Better in children than adults
- Earlier intervention yields better outcomes
- Late reconstruction may not fully restore function

Q72. Transolecranon fracture-dislocation.

(DNB 2008)

Definition
A transolecranon fracture-dislocation is a *complex posterior elbow injury* characterized by:
- Fracture of the olecranon,
- Disruption of the ulnohumeral articulation,
- Preservation of the proximal radioulnar joint (unlike Monteggia).

Mechanism
High-energy trauma (e.g., fall on outstretched hand with flexed elbow or direct blow).

Clinical Features
- Swollen, deformed elbow,
- Loss of elbow extension,
- Painful limited range of motion.

Imaging
- X-ray (AP and lateral)
- CT scan if comminuted to assess articular involvement.

Management
- *Goal*: Anatomical reconstruction of trochlear notch and stable fixation.
- *Surgical*:
    - ORIF with pre-contoured locking plates is the treatment of choice.
    - Reconstruction of any associated coronoid or radial head injuries.
    - Early ROM exercises to prevent stiffness.
- *Post-operative care*:
    - NSAIDs for pain and HO prevention,
    - Physiotherapy.

Q73. Monteggia fracture variants—short note.

Monteggia Fracture

Proximal ulnar shaft fracture + radial head dislocation

Bado Classification

- *Type I*: Anterior radial head dislocation (most common in children)
- *Type II*: Posterior
- *Type III*: Lateral
- *Type IV*: Both bone fracture with radial head dislocation

Variants

Monteggia-equivalent lesions: Ulna fracture with other forms of proximal radial injury (e.g., radial neck fracture, epiphyseal injury)

Management

Open or closed reduction of ulna + radial head alignment

Q74. Heterotopic ossification after elbow trauma and its prevention.

(DNB 2001)

Definition

Heterotopic ossification (HO) is the abnormal formation of bone in soft tissues following trauma or surgery.

Etiology

- Elbow dislocations, fracture-dislocations
- Burns, head/spinal cord injury
- Post-operative elbow surgeries.

Risk Factors

- Delayed treatment
- Extensive dissection
- Associated neurological injury.

Clinical Features

- Pain and stiffness
- Progressive loss of range of motion
- Hard mass on palpation.

Diagnosis

- *X-ray*: HO appears 3–6 weeks post-injury
- Bone scan or CT for early detection and surgical planning.

Prevention

- *NSAIDs*: Indomethacin 75 mg OD for 6 weeks
- *Radiotherapy*: 700–800 cGy within 72 hours of injury or surgery
- Minimize surgical trauma and early motion.

Management

Conservative: Physiotherapy, analgesia

Surgical Excision

Reserved for mature HO (after 6–12 months), when function is **Forearm fractures**

Q75. Management of both bone forearm fractures in adults.

(Asked in: AIIMS Delhi 2022, PGI Chandigarh 2022)

Introduction

- Fractures of both the **radius and ulna** disrupt the **forearm ring**.
- Restoration of both **length**, **alignment**, and **rotation** is critical for **normal pronation-supination**.

Management

Non-operative treatment:

- Rare in adults.
- *Indications*:
    - Minimally displaced fractures.
    - Low-demand patients with high surgical risk.
- *Method*:
    - Above-elbow plaster cast with forearm in neutral/mild supination.
    - Close monitoring with serial X-rays.

Operative treatment (preferred):

- **Open reduction and internal fixation (ORIF)** with **dynamic compression plates (DCP)** or **limited contact dynamic compression plates (LC-DCP)**.
- Each bone plated separately.
- Absolute stability aimed for (compression principle).

Surgical Principles

- Anatomic reduction mandatory (especially rotational alignment of radius).
- Minimum six cortices purchase per fragment (three screws on each side).
- Early gentle range of motion after surgery.

Complications

- Malunion (especially rotational deformities).
- Nonunion or delayed union.
- Compartment syndrome.
- Synostosis between radius and ulna (radioulnar fusion).

Q76. Classify forearm fractures and discuss their management.

Classification

Forearm fractures are classified based on:

1. *Anatomical location*:
    - Proximal third
    - Middle third
    - Distal third
2. *Bone involved*:
    - Isolated radius or ulna fracture
    - Both-bone fractures
    - Monteggia fracture-dislocation (proximal ulna with radial head dislocation)
    - Galeazzi fracture-dislocation (distal radius with DRUJ dislocation)
    - Nightstick fracture (isolated ulna shaft)

3. *Fracture pattern*:
    - Transverse
    - Oblique
    - Spiral
    - Comminuted
    - Segmental

Management
- *Non-operative*:
    - *Indications*: Isolated, undisplaced or minimally displaced fractures.
    - *Method*: Above-elbow cast immobilization for 6–8 weeks.
- *Operative*:
    - *Indications*: Displaced fractures, both-bone fractures, segmental fractures, open fractures, neurovascular compromise.
    - *Method*:
        - **ORIF** with dynamic compression plates (gold standard).
        - **Intramedullary nailing** for select pediatric or comminuted fractures.
        - Address associated dislocations in Monteggia or Galeazzi variants.

Q77. Explain the biomechanical principles of forearm stabilization.

Forearm Biomechanics
- Radius and ulna form a ring with interosseous membrane and proximal/distal radioulnar joints.
- Stabilization depends on anatomical reduction and restoration of radial bow.

Principles of Stabilization
1. *Anatomical reduction*: Essential to restore forearm rotation (pronation-supination).
2. *Restoration of radial bow*: Critical for functional motion.
3. *Stable internal fixation*:
    - Dynamic compression plating (DCP) restores load-sharing ability.
    - Avoids rotational malalignment and non-union.
4. Maintenance of interosseous membrane tension.
5. Alignment of proximal and distal radioulnar joints.

Implants Used
- 3.5 mm DCP or LCP for both bones.
- Low profile locking plates in osteoporotic bone.
- Compression screws and lag techniques for oblique fractures.

Q78. Discuss the complications of forearm fractures and their prevention.

Early Complications
- *Neurovascular injury*: Particularly posterior interosseous nerve or ulnar nerve.
- *Compartment syndrome*: Surgical emergency.
- *Open fractures*: Risk of infection.

Late Complications
- *Malunion*: Leads to rotational deformity and limited supination/pronation.
- *Non-union*: Especially with segmental or comminuted fractures.
- *Re-fracture*: Particularly after plate removal if not adequately remodeled.
- *Cross-union*: Bone bridging between radius and ulna due to excessive callus.
- *Loss of forearm rotation*: Due to poor reduction or interosseous membrane scarring.

Prevention
- Ensure accurate anatomical reduction and stable fixation.
- Early controlled mobilization after union.
- Timely surgical intervention in high-risk fractures.
- Use of prophylactic fasciotomy in high-risk crush injuries.

Q79. Describe Galeazzi fracture-dislocation and its management.

(Asked in: MUHS Maharashtra 2022)

Definition
- Fracture of the **distal third of radius** associated with **dislocation of the distal radioulnar joint (DRUJ)**.
- Known as "**fracture of necessity**"—requires surgery.

Mechanism

Fall on an outstretched hand with axial load and pronation.

Clinical Features
- Deformity and swelling over distal forearm.
- Painful pronation/supination.
- Palpable dislocation at DRUJ.

Radiological Signs
- Widened DRUJ on AP view.
- Dorsal displacement of ulna on lateral view.
- Disruption of ulnar styloid alignment.

Management

Adults:
- ORIF of radial fracture with a plate.
- After radius fixation, reassess DRUJ stability:
  - Stable DRUJ → above-elbow immobilization in supination for 4–6 weeks.
  - Unstable DRUJ → Temporary fixation with percutaneous K-wire across DRUJ + immobilization.

Children

Closed reduction often successful.

Important
- DRUJ stability is key to successful management.
- Failure to recognize DRUJ injury → chronic instability and poor functional outcomes.

Q80. Write a note on Nightstick fracture and indications for operative management.

(DNB 2009)

Definition
- Isolated fracture of the **ulnar shaft**, typically in the mid-diaphyseal region.
- Occurs when the forearm is raised in defense against a blow — hence the term **"Nightstick fracture"**.

Mechanism
- **Direct blow** to the medial forearm (defensive injury)
- Most often seen in **assault victims** or in sports injuries

Clinical Features
- Localized tenderness, swelling, and pain over ulna
- Usually no neurovascular injury

Imaging

X-ray AP and lateral views of the forearm

Management

Non-operative (conservative):

- *Criteria*:
  - Displacement < 50%
  - Angulation <10°
  - No shortening
  - Closed fracture
- *Method*: Functional bracing or long arm cast

Operative Indications

1. Displacement > 50% or angulation > 10°
2. Comminuted fracture
3. Open fracture
4. Segmental or pathological fracture
5. Failure of conservative treatment
6. Patient demands early return to function (athletes, laborers)

Surgical Options

Open reduction and internal fixation (ORIF) with compression plating

Q81. Classify distal radius fractures and discuss their management and complications.

Classification of Distal Radius Fractures

1. *Frykman classification*:
   - Based on radiocarpal and distal radioulnar joint (DRUJ) involvement and ulnar fracture
   - Types I–VIII, increasing complexity
   - *Limitation:* Does not guide treatment or prognosis.
2. *Fernandez classification*:
   - Mechanism-based classification
   - *Type I*: Bending (Colles, Smith)
   - *Type II*: Shearing (Barton's)
   - *Type III*: Compression (impaction)
   - *Type IV*: Avulsion
   - *Type V*: Combined mechanisms
3. *AO/OTA classification*:
   - *Type A*: Extra-articular
   - *Type B*: Partial articular
   - *Type C*: Complete articular
   - Subtypes indicate fracture complexity

Management of Distal Radius Fractures

1. **Non-operative treatment**
   - *Indications*:
     - Minimally displaced fractures
     - Extra-articular fractures
     - Low-demand elderly patients

- *Method*:
    - Closed reduction under anesthesia
    - Below-elbow cast/splint for 4–6 weeks
- *Follow-up*:
    - Serial radiographs to check for displacement
    - Physiotherapy post-immobilization

2. **Operative treatment**
    - *Indications (instability criteria)*:
        - Dorsal angulation >10°
        - Radial shortening >3 mm
        - Intra-articular step-off >2 mm
        - Open fractures
        - DRUJ instability
    - *Surgical options*:
        - *Percutaneous pinning (K-wires)*: In young with simple fractures
        - *External fixation*: Ligamentotaxis for comminuted fractures
        - *ORIF with volar locking plate (VLP)*: Gold standard for unstable fractures
        - *Fragment-specific fixation*: For complex intra-articular patterns

Complications

- Malunion (most common)
- Stiffness of wrist or fingers
- Tendon irritation/rupture (especially EPL with dorsal plates)
- Median nerve compression (carpal tunnel syndrome)
- Complex regional pain syndrome (CRPS)
- DRUJ instability
- Post-traumatic arthritis

Q82. Discuss the classification and changing trends in the management of fracture distal radius in adults.

(AMC 2015)

Changing Trends in Classification

- Shift from anatomical (Frykman) to **mechanism-based (Fernandez)** and **radiographic/articular-based (AO)** systems
- CT-based classification increasing in relevance due to improved preoperative planning

Changing Trends in Management

- *Volar locking plate fixation (VLP):*
    - Preferred surgical method
    - Offers angular stability in osteoporotic bone
    - Allows early mobilization and improved functional outcomes
- *Fragment-specific fixation:*
    - Used in selected comminuted intra-articular fractures
    - Direct fixation of each articular fragment
- *External fixators*: Used less frequently, but still useful in high-energy comminuted/open injuries
- *Arthroscopic-assisted reduction*: Gaining role in precise intra-articular visualization and reduction
- *Role of 3D printing and preoperative planning*: Patient-specific implants and enhanced surgical planning for complex fractures
- *Evidence-based care*:
    - Focus on early range of motion and functional bracing
    - Patient-reported outcomes increasingly prioritized

Q83. Discuss the fracture patterns of distal radius fractures in adults. Also discuss the management and complications of distal radius fractures in adults.

I. Fracture Patterns of Distal Radius in Adults

Fracture patterns of the distal radius depend on:

- Mechanism of injury
- Bone quality
- Position of the wrist at the time of injury

1. **Based on direction of displacement**

- *Colles' fracture:*
  - Extra-articular fracture
  - Dorsal displacement and angulation
  - Usually results from fall on outstretched hand (FOOSH)
- *Smith's fracture*:
  - Extra-articular fracture
  - Volar displacement
  - Fall on flexed wrist
- *Barton's fracture*:
  - Intra-articular fracture-dislocation
  - Shear-type injury
  - Can be dorsal or volar
- *Chauffeur's fracture (radial styloid)*:
  - Intra-articular fracture of radial styloid
  - Due to compression from the scaphoid (car accident injury)
- *Die-punch fracture*:
  - Impaction of the lunate into the lunate fossa
  - Intra-articular depression fracture

2. **Based on AO/OTA classification**

- *Type A*: Extra-articular
- *Type B*: Partial articular (one fragment remains attached to shaft)
- *Type C*: Complete articular (all articular fragments are displaced)

II. Management of Distal Radius Fractures

A. Non-operative Treatment

- *Indications*:
  - Undisplaced or minimally displaced
  - Extra-articular
  - Elderly with low demands
- *Method*:
  - Closed reduction + below-elbow cast
  - Immobilization for 4–6 weeks
- *Follow-up*:
  - Serial radiographs
  - Begin range-of-motion exercises early after cast removal

B. Operative Treatment

Indications:

- Intra-articular displacement >2 mm
- Dorsal tilt >10°
- Radial shortening >3 mm

- Comminuted fractures
- Associated DRUJ instability
- Open fractures or associated neurovascular injury

Surgical options:
- *Orif with volar locking plate (VLP):*
  - Preferred in most unstable and displaced fractures
  - Allows early mobilization
- *External fixator (ligamentotaxis)*:
  - Useful for comminuted fractures
  - Used with or without K-wires
- *Percutaneous pinning*:
  - For simple extra-articular or minimally displaced fractures
  - Used in younger patients
- *Fragment-specific fixation*:
  - Targets individual fragments with mini-plates or screws
  - For highly comminuted intra-articular fractures
- *Arthroscopic-assisted fixation (select centers)*: Better visualization of intra-articular surface
- 3D planning and patient-specific implants (advanced centers)

III. Complications

Early	***Late***
Median nerve compression	Malunion (commonest)
Compartment syndrome	DRUJ dysfunction
Tendon irritation/rupture (EPL)	Complex regional pain syndrome (CRPS)
Infection (if open or post-operative)	Post-traumatic osteoarthritis
Stiffness	Carpal instability

Q84. Colles' fracture—clinical features, radiology, and management.

(Asked in: RGUHS Karnataka 2022, MUHS Maharashtra 2023)

Introduction
- **Colles' fracture** is a **distal radius fracture** occurring approximately **2.5 cm proximal to the wrist joint** with **dorsal displacement and angulation** of the distal fragment.
- Common in elderly females (osteoporotic bone) after a **fall on outstretched hand**.

Clinical Features
- Pain, swelling, and deformity over the wrist.
- **Classical "dinner fork" deformity**.
- Tenderness at distal radius.
- Check for median nerve symptoms (carpal tunnel syndrome risk).

Radiological Features
- *X-ray (PA and lateral views of wrist) shows*:
  - Dorsal displacement of distal fragment.
  - Dorsal angulation.
  - Radial shortening.
  - Loss of normal volar tilt (normally ~11° volar).
  - Possible radial styloid fracture.

Management

Non-operative:

- *Indications*: Extra-articular, minimally displaced fractures.
- *Method*:
    - Closed reduction under sedation (traction + palmar flexion + ulnar deviation).
    - Immobilization in below-elbow cast for 5–6 weeks.
    - Early physiotherapy after cast removal.

Operative:

- *Indications*:
    - Unstable fractures.
    - Intra-articular involvement.
    - Comminuted fractures.
    - Failure to maintain reduction.
- *Options*:
    - Percutaneous pinning.
    - External fixator (ligamentotaxis).
    - **Open reduction and internal fixation (ORIF)** with volar locking plate (gold standard for unstable fractures).

Complications

- Malunion → persistent deformity.
- Median nerve compression (acute or late).
- Complex Regional Pain Syndrome (CRPS).
- Stiffness of wrist and fingers.

Q85. Management of Colles' fracture with post-reduction carpal tunnel syndrome.

(DNB 2024)

Colles' Fracture

Extra-articular distal radius fracture with dorsal displacement.

Post-reduction carpal tunnel syndrome (CTS) may result from:

- Hematoma
- Swelling
- Volar displacement or over-tight cast.

Management

- Immediate cast splitting or removal to relieve pressure.
- Elevation and ice to reduce edema.
- *If symptoms persist (>12–24 hours)*: Perform **urgent carpal tunnel decompression** (open or mini-open).
- Definitive fracture fixation (CRIF or ORIF) depending on instability.

Q86. Surgical approach for Volar Barton's fracture.

(MS 2019)

Volar Barton's Fracture

Intra-articular fracture of volar rim of distal radius with volar displacement.

Surgical Approach

- *Henry's (Volar) approach*:
    - Incision along radial border of FCR tendon.
    - FCR tendon is retracted ulnarly.

  - Protect radial artery and median nerve.
  - Pronator quadratus is elevated to expose distal radius.
- *Fixation*: Volar locking plate for articular congruity and early mobilization.

Q87. Compare Smith's fracture versus reverse Barton's fracture.

(MS 2007)

Feature	Smith's fracture	Reverse Barton's fracture
Type	Extra-articular	Intra-articular
Mechanism	Fall on flexed wrist	High-energy fall on flexed wrist
Displacement	Volar displacement of distal fragment	Volar displacement of articular fragment
Articular involvement	No	Yes
Stability	More stable	Highly unstable
Treatment	Closed reduction and cast or volar plating	ORIF with volar plate (always surgical)

Q88. Discuss the differences between Colles' and Smith's fractures.

Feature	Colles' fracture	Smith's fracture
Mechanism	Fall on outstretched hand (FOOSH)	Fall on flexed wrist
Displacement	Dorsal	Volar
Common in	Elderly osteoporotic females	Younger individuals
Deformity	"Dinner fork"	"Garden spade"
Treatment	Closed reduction or ORIF	Often ORIF due to instability

Q89. Explain the management of Barton's fracture.

Definition

Intra-articular distal radius fracture with dislocation of the radiocarpal joint (volar/dorsal).

Management

- Unstable → ORIF with volar plate (volar more common)
- Early mobilization to avoid stiffness

Q90. Discuss the surgical options for intra-articular distal radius fractures.

- Volar locking plate fixation (most common)
- External fixation (in high-energy comminution or soft tissue injury)
- Percutaneous pinning
- Fragment-specific fixation (when plates can't control small fragments)

Q91. Compare Volar plating versus external fixation for distal radius fractures.

(DNB 2023)

Feature	Volar plating	External fixation
Approach	Open reduction, internal fixation	Minimally invasive, percutaneous pins
Indication	Intra-articular, comminuted fractures	Severely comminuted, open fractures

Continued

Continued

Feature	*Volar plating*	*External fixation*
Stability	More rigid fixation	Less rigid
Early mobilization	Possible	Limited
Soft tissue handling	Risk of surgical wound complications	Less soft tissue trauma
Malunion risk	Lower	Higher in complex fractures
Infection risk	Lower (if wound care adequate)	Higher (pin tract infections)
Functional outcome	Generally better	Comparable in low-demand patients

Conclusion

Volar plating preferred in most displaced fractures; external fixation used in open, highly comminuted, or polytrauma cases.

Q92. Frykman classification of distal radius fractures.

(DNB 2022)

Frykman classified DRFs based on articular involvement and ulnar styloid fracture:

Type	*Fracture type*
I	Extra-articular, no ulnar styloid
II	Extra-articular + ulnar styloid fracture
III	Intra-articular (radiocarpal)
IV	III + ulnar styloid
V	Intra-articular (radioulnar joint)
VI	V + ulnar styloid
VII	Intra-articular (radiocarpal + DRUJ)
VIII	VII + ulnar styloid

Clinical Utility

Limited practical use now; AO classification preferred. Frykman is helpful in teaching and understanding articular involvement.

Q93. Surgical approach for Volar Barton's fracture.

(MS 2019)

Volar Barton's Fracture

Intra-articular distal radius fracture with volar displacement of volar lip fragment.

Surgical Approach

- *Volar (Henry's) approach*:
  - *Incision*: Between FCR and radial artery.
  - Retract FCR medially and radial artery laterally.
  - Pronator quadratus elevated from radius.
  - Fracture visualized and reduced.
  - Fixed using **volar locking plate**.

Key Points

- Early fixation → early mobilization.
- Precaution to avoid FPL and median nerve injury.
- Check for DRUJ stability post-fixation.

Q94. Describe the management of Die-punch fracture in distal end radius.

(DNB 2016)

Definition

A Die-punch fracture is a depression fracture of the lunate fossa of the distal radius caused by axial loading of the lunate.

Management

- *Initial evaluation*: X-ray (PA and lateral), CT for articular depression.
- *Non-displaced fracture*: Closed reduction and immobilization in a cast.
- *Displaced/intra-articular fracture*:
  - *Surgical management*:
    - ORIF via volar approach using buttress plate.
    - Elevation of depressed fragment and bone grafting if needed.
    - Use of subchondral K-wires or screws for articular support.
  - *Post-operative*: Early physiotherapy to prevent stiffness.

Q95. Describe in detail the surgical fixation technique in Chauffeur's fracture.

(DNB 2010)

Definition

Chauffeur's fracture = radial styloid fracture due to axial load transmission through the scaphoid.

Surgical Technique

- *Indications*: Displaced or intra-articular fractures.
- *Approach*: Volar or dorsal radial approach.
- *Steps*:
  - Anatomical reduction under image guidance.
  - Temporary fixation with K-wires.
  - Definitive fixation with a lag screw or buttress plate.
- *Post-operative*: Immobilization 2–3 weeks, then rehabilitation.

Q96. Compare Smith's fracture versus reverse Barton's fracture.

(MS 2007)

Feature	***Smith's fracture***	***Reverse Barton's fracture***
Type	Extra-articular fracture	Intra-articular fracture
Mechanism	Fall on flexed wrist	Fall on flexed wrist with shear
Displacement	Volar angulation of distal fragment	Volar rim fracture with subluxation
Treatment (displaced)	Closed reduction + cast/volar plating	ORIF with volar plate fixation
Stability	Usually stable post-reduction	Unstable, needs surgical stabilization

Q97. Management of DRUJ instability after distal radius fracture.

(MS 2013)

Distal Radioulnar Joint (DRUJ) instability may occur due to:

- Malreduction of distal radius
- TFCC injury
- Ulnar styloid fracture.

Management

1. Correct reduction of distal radius (check ulnar variance and sigmoid notch alignment).
2. *Ulnar styloid fracture*: Base fracture with instability → fix with tension band/K-wire.
3. *Persistent DRUJ instability*:
    - Acute setting → DRUJ pinning in supination (1.6 mm K-wire for 4 weeks).
    - Chronic setting → TFCC repair or reconstruction (arthroscopic/open).
4. *Immobilization*: In supination for 4–6 weeks.

Q98. TFCC injury—short note.

Introduction

The **triangular fibrocartilage complex (TFCC)** is a critical structure that stabilizes the **distal radioulnar joint (DRUJ)** and supports the ulnar side of the wrist. It acts as a cushion between the **ulna** and **carpal bones**.

Anatomy of TFCC

- Triangular fibrocartilage (articular disc)
- Ulnolunate and ulnotriquetral ligaments
- Dorsal and volar radioulnar ligaments
- Sheath of the extensor carpi ulnaris (ECU)
- Meniscus homologue

Mechanism of Injury

- *Traumatic*: Fall on outstretched hand, forced ulnar deviation or rotation.
- *Degenerative*: Repetitive microtrauma, especially with **ulnar positive variance** (ulna longer than radius).

Clinical Features

- Ulnar-sided wrist pain (especially with grip or ulnar deviation)
- Clicking or catching
- Decreased grip strength
- Tenderness over TFCC (fovea sign)
- Positive **ulnar grind test** or **TFCC stress test**

Diagnosis

- *X-ray*: Rule out DRUJ dislocation, ulnar variance.
- *MRI/Arthrogram*: Best for soft tissue visualization.
- *Wrist arthroscopy*: Gold standard for diagnosis and classification.

Palmer Classification (Simplified)

- *Type I (traumatic)*:
    - *IA*: Central perforation
    - *IB*: Ulnar avulsion with/without DRUJ instability
    - *IC*: Distal avulsion
    - *ID*: Radial avulsion
- *Type II (degenerative)*:
    - *IIA*: TFCC wear
    - *IIB–IIE*: Progressive involvement of lunate, ulna, ligaments, arthritis

Management

Conservative:

- Immobilization (wrist splint or cast) for 4–6 weeks
- NSAIDs, activity modification
- Physiotherapy

Surgical:
- Arthroscopic debridement (Type IA)
- TFCC repair (for IB, IC, ID injuries)
- Ulnar shortening osteotomy (for ulnar impaction in degenerative cases)
- DRUJ stabilization procedures (in chronic instability)

Prognosis
- Good in acute, well-managed cases
- Chronic or degenerative tears may require surgical intervention for relief

Q99. Management in suspected scaphoid fracture with negative X-ray.

Clinical Suspicion
- Tenderness in anatomical snuffbox
- Pain on axial thumb compression
- Swelling and pain over scaphoid

X-ray negative? Follow these steps
1. *Initial management*:
   - Immobilize in a **thumb spica cast or splint**.
   - Treat as a fracture until proven otherwise.
2. *Further imaging after 10–14 days*:
   - Repeat X-rays (may show healing if fracture was present).
   - *If still negative but symptoms persist*:
     - *MRI*: Gold standard for early detection.
     - *CT scan*: For assessing displacement or planning surgery.
3. *If MRI confirms fracture*:
   - *Treat based on fracture location*:
     - *Distal pole*: 4–6 weeks cast.
     - *Waist fracture*: 6–10 weeks cast.
     - *Proximal pole*: May require surgical fixation due to poor vascularity.
4. *If MRI is negative*: Discontinue immobilization and reassess clinically.

Q100. Discuss the management of neglected scaphoid fracture with AVN and non-union.

(MS 2022)

Problems in Neglected Scaphoid
- Non-union
- Avascular necrosis (commonly proximal pole)
- Wrist instability or arthritis

Management
- *Non-operative*: Rarely effective.
- *Surgical options*:
  - *Non-union without AVN*: ORIF with bone grafting (vascularized or non-vascularized)
  - *With AVN (especially proximal pole)*:
    - Vascularized bone graft (e.g., 1,2-ICSRA graft)
    - ORIF with Herbert screw or headless compression screw

- *Salvage Procedures (advanced collapse)*:
  - Proximal row carpectomy
  - Scaphoid excision + 4-corner fusion
  - Total wrist arthrodesis (last resort)

Q101. Write a short note on scaphoid fractures and their complications.

Common Site

Waist of scaphoid

Complications

- Nonunion
- Avascular necrosis (AVN) of proximal pole
- Scaphoid nonunion advanced collapse (SNAC wrist)
- Arthritis

Q102. Discuss the indications for percutaneous fixation in scaphoid fractures.

Indications

- Minimally displaced (<1 mm) waist fractures
- Stable fractures with preserved vascularity
- Early return to function (e.g., athletes)

Implant

Headless compression screw

Q103. Explain the pathophysiology and treatment of scapholunate ligament injuries.

Pathophysiology

- Tear of scapholunate interosseous ligament
- Leads to dissociation and abnormal motion (DISI deformity)

Treatment

- *Acute (<6 weeks)*: Direct repair + pinning
- *Chronic*: Capsulodesis or partial wrist fusion

Q104. Discuss the management of perilunate and lunate dislocations.

Perilunate

Capitate dislocated dorsally, lunate remains aligned with radius

Lunate

Lunate dislocated volarly (spilled teacup sign)

Management

- Emergent closed/open reduction
- ORIF and ligament repair often required
- Median nerve decompression if needed

Q105. Bennett's fracture-dislocation—overview.

Definition
Oblique intra-articular fracture at the base of the 1st metacarpal with dislocation of the carpometacarpal joint.

Mechanism
Axial force on flexed thumb (e.g., punch injury).

Pathoanatomy
- Volar-ulnar fragment remains attached to trapezium via volar ligaments.
- Shaft of metacarpal displaced radially and dorsally by **APL** tendon.

Treatment
- Closed reduction + percutaneous K-wire fixation.
- ORIF with lag screw if unstable or comminuted.
- *Goal*: Restore articular congruity and thumb function.

Q106. Differences between Bennett's and Rolando's fractures.

(DNB 2019)

Feature	*Bennett's fracture*	*Rolando's fracture*
Definition	Intra-articular fracture-dislocation at base of 1st metacarpal involving a single fragment	Comminuted intra-articular fracture at base of 1st metacarpal
Fracture pattern	Oblique or simple	Y or T-shaped, comminuted
Mechanism	Axial load through partially flexed thumb	High energy axial load
Stability	Relatively unstable due to pull of APL	Highly unstable due to comminution
Treatment	Closed reduction + K-wire/ORIF	ORIF or external fixation; sometimes salvage difficult
Prognosis	Good with stable fixation	Guarded due to joint involvement and comminution

Q107. Gamekeeper's thumb (Skier's thumb)—diagnosis and management.

(MS 2011)

Definition
Injury to the **ulnar collateral ligament (UCL)** of the **MCP joint** of the thumb.

Etiology
Sudden forced abduction and extension of thumb (skiing injury, chronic valgus stress).

Diagnosis
- Pain and swelling over ulnar aspect of MCPJ.
- *Stress testing*: >30° valgus laxity or 15° greater than opposite side.
- *Stener lesion*: Adducted aponeurosis interposes between UCL and insertion.

Imaging
- *X-ray*: May show avulsion fragment.
- *MRI/USG*: Confirms UCL tear and Stener lesion.

Management
- *Partial UCL tear*: Thumb spica splint for 4–6 weeks.
- *Complete tear or Stener lesion*: Surgical repair.

Q108. Discuss the treatment of phalangeal neck fractures in children.

(DNB 2008)

Characteristics
- Most common in proximal phalanges
- Risk of angulation and growth disturbance

Management
- *Undisplaced/Minimally displaced*: Closed reduction and immobilization with buddy taping or splint
- *Displaced/Unstable*: Closed or open reduction with K-wire fixation
- Immobilization for 3–4 weeks
- Early mobilization to prevent stiffness
- Regular follow-up to monitor growth

Q109. What are the indications for surgical fixation of metacarpal fractures?

Surgical fixation is considered when the fracture is unstable, displaced, or associated with functional impairment. Specific indications include:

Absolute Indications
- Open fractures
- Multiple metacarpal fractures
- Intra-articular fractures with >1–2 mm step-off
- Rotational deformity on clinical examination
- Unstable oblique or spiral fractures
- *Fractures with significant displacement*:
  - 10–15° angulation (2nd and 3rd metacarpal)
  - 30–40° angulation (4th and 5th metacarpal)
- Shortening >5 mm
- Loss of active extension or flexion

Relative Indications
- Failure of closed reduction
- Malalignment after conservative treatment
- Unacceptable cosmetic or functional outcome

Surgical Techniques
- K-wire fixation (closed or open)
- Open reduction and internal fixation (ORIF) with screws or plates

Early fixation helps in **early mobilization**, preventing stiffness and deformity.

Q110. Boxer's fracture and its management.

Definition
Fracture of the 5th metacarpal neck, typically from punching a hard object.

Clinical Features
Swelling, tenderness, and dorsal angulation of the 5th MCP

Radiology
X-ray shows apex dorsal angulation at the 5th metacarpal neck.

Management
- *Acceptable angulation*: up to 40–50°
- *Non-operative*: Ulnar gutter splint for 3–4 weeks
- *Operative indications*:
  - Unacceptable angulation or rotation
  - Open fracture
  - Intra-articular involvement
- *Surgical options*:
  - Closed reduction and K-wire fixation
  - ORIF in case of severe displacement

Q111. Classification of metacarpal fractures.

Classification (based on location)
- *Head*: Intra-articular or comminuted
- *Neck*: Commonly 5th metacarpal (Boxer's fracture)
- *Shaft*: Transverse, oblique, spiral, or comminuted
- *Base*: May involve CMC joint (e.g., Bennett's, Rolando's)

Q112. Complex dislocation of MCP joint (SN).

Definition
MCP joint dislocation that is **irreducible by closed means**.

Cause
Interposition of volar plate or soft tissue

Common Site
Index finger

Clinical Features
- Hyperextension deformity
- Prominent metacarpal head
- Palmar puckering ("buttonholing")

Management
- **Open reduction** via dorsal approach
- Avoid volar approach due to neurovascular structures

Q113. Mallet finger injury, classification, diagnosis, and treatment.

(Asked in: AIIMS Delhi 2021)

Definition
A mallet finger is caused by disruption of the extensor tendon at the distal interphalangeal joint (DIPJ), resulting in an inability to actively extend the DIP.

Classification (Doyle's Classification)
1. *Type I*: Closed tendon rupture without fracture.
2. *Type II*: Open laceration of the extensor tendon.
3. *Type III*: Deep avulsion with loss of skin and tendon.

4. *Type IV*:
   - *IV-A*: Transphyseal injury (pediatrics).
   - *IV-B*: Intra-articular fracture of 20–50% articular surface.
   - *IV-C*: Fracture involving >50% articular surface or with volar subluxation.

Treatment
- *Non-operative*: **Splinting DIPJ in extension/hyperextension** for 6–8 weeks (type I and most type IV-A/B).
- *Surgical*:
  - *Indications*:
    - Volar subluxation of distal phalanx
    - Bony fragment >50% articular surface (type IV-C)
    - Open injuries (type II, III)
    - Failed conservative treatment.
  - *Techniques*: K-wire fixation, tension band wiring, extension block pinning.

Q114. Write a short note on volar plate injuries of the finger.

- *Mechanism*: Hyperextension injury at the PIP joint
- *Findings*: Swelling, tenderness volarly at PIP, limited flexion
- *Diagnosis*: Clinical, with lateral X-ray to rule out avulsion fractures

Management
- Buddy taping or dorsal block splint (20–30° flexion)
- Surgery if large avulsion or joint instability present

Q115. Management of phalangeal fractures.

Types
- Proximal, middle, or distal phalanx fractures
- Transverse, oblique, spiral, comminuted, intra-articular, open, or closed

Non-operative Management
- *Stable, non-displaced fractures*: buddy taping or splinting (e.g., aluminum splint)
- *Immobilization*: 3–4 weeks depending on location and stability

Operative Indications
- Displaced or unstable fractures
- Rotational deformity
- Intra-articular step-off >1–2 mm
- Open fractures
- Multiple phalangeal fractures

Surgical Options
- Closed reduction with percutaneous K-wires
- Open reduction and internal fixation (ORIF) with mini-plates or screws
- External fixation (rarely, in comminuted or open injuries)

Rehabilitation
- Early motion to prevent stiffness
- Hand therapy in complex injuries

Q116. Jersey finger and its surgical management.

Definition

Avulsion of the flexor digitorum profundus (FDP) tendon from the distal phalanx—commonly the ring finger.

Mechanism

Forceful extension of a flexed DIP joint (e.g., grabbing a jersey during sports).

Classification (Leddy and Packer)

- *Type I*: tendon retracted to palm, no bony fragment
- *Type II*: tendon at PIP level, small bony fragment
- *Type III*: large bony fragment with tendon attached, caught at A4 pulley

Clinical Signs

- Inability to flex DIP joint
- Tenderness over volar aspect of distal phalanx

Surgical Management

- *Early repair (<7–10 days)*: Primary tendon reinsertion with suture anchors, pull-out sutures, or mini-screws
- *Bony fragment*: ORIF if large or displaced
- *Chronic cases*: Tendon grafting, two-stage tendon reconstruction, or DIP joint arthrodesis

Post-operative Rehabilitation

Early passive mobilization (Duran or Kleinert protocols)

Q117. Flexor tendon injuries—zones and management.

(Asked in: MUHS Maharashtra 2023)

Introduction

- Flexor tendon injuries are **serious** and often occur from penetrating trauma.
- Tendon injury classified by **zone** (important for prognosis and surgical planning).

Flexor Tendon Zones

Zone	*Location*	*Clinical importance*
I	Distal to FDS insertion	FDP injury alone
II	A1 pulley to FDS insertion ("no man's land")	Both FDS and FDP at risk; difficult repairs
III	Palm (thenar/hypothenar muscles)	Better prognosis
IV	Carpal tunnel	Median nerve injury may coexist
V	Proximal to carpal tunnel (forearm)	Major neurovascular injuries likely

Management

- *Primary repair (within 24 hours ideally)*:
  - Core suture (4- or 6-strand technique) + epitendinous running suture for strength.
  - *Techniques*: Modified Kessler, Bunnell, and Strickland methods.
- *Delayed primary repair:* Between 24 hours to 2 weeks.
- *Secondary repair:* After 2–3 weeks (scar tissue formation), may need tendon grafting.
- *Postoperative care:* Early passive mobilization protocols (Kleinert or Duran protocols) to prevent adhesions.
- *Key point:* Zone II ("no man's land") repairs have **highest failure risk** — require expert technique and strict rehabilitation.

Q118. Management of extensor tendon injuries of the hand.

- *Zones I–VIII (from fingertip to forearm):*
  - *Zone I (Mallet finger)*: Splint DIP in extension for 6–8 weeks
  - *Zone III (Boutonnière)*: PIP splint in extension
  - *Zone V (MCP joint)*: Requires surgical repair
- *Surgical repair* if laceration >50% or with retraction
- *Rehabilitation*: Controlled early motion to prevent adhesions

Q119. Write a short note on neurovascular assessment in upper limb trauma.

- *Essential components*:
  - *Motor*: Radial (thumb extension), median (thumb opposition), ulnar (finger abduction).
  - *Sensory*: Light touch over dermatomes.
  - *Vascular*: Pulses (radial, ulnar), capillary refill, skin color/temp.
- Crucial before and after interventions (reduction/splinting).

Q120. Discuss the biomechanics of upper limb injuries.

Upper limb injuries are influenced by the complex biomechanics of shoulder, elbow, forearm, and wrist joints.

- *Shoulder*: Ball-and-socket joint allows multidirectional motion but is prone to dislocations due to instability.
- *Elbow*: Hinge joint—commonly suffers from valgus stress injuries and hyperextension trauma.
- *Forearm*: Radius and ulna function as a ring; disruption at one point (e.g., fracture) often leads to injury at another (e.g., dislocation).
- *Wrist*: Transmits loads during falls; high incidence of distal radius and scaphoid fractures.
- *Kinetics*: Force transmission from hand to shoulder means a distal injury may affect proximal function.

Q121. Explain the role of early mobilization in upper limb trauma rehabilitation.

- *Prevents stiffness*: Especially important in elbow and hand injuries prone to contractures.
- Maintains joint nutrition and cartilage health through synovial fluid movement.
- *Promotes tendon gliding*: Reduces adhesions in repaired tendons (e.g., after flexor tendon surgery).
- *Enhances functional recovery*: Promotes muscle memory and neuromuscular coordination.
- *Psychological benefit*: Reduces fear-avoidance and enhances patient morale.

Protocols like **early passive motion (Kleinert, Duran)** are used in tendon repairs; **early active-assisted ROM** is common in post-fracture or dislocation cases.

Q122. Discuss the indications for nerve conduction studies (NCS) and electromyography (EMG) in upper limb trauma.

Indications

- Unexplained weakness or numbness after trauma
- Suspected peripheral nerve injury (e.g., radial nerve palsy post-humeral shaft fracture)
- Compression neuropathies (e.g., carpal tunnel post distal radius fracture)
- Delayed recovery or suspected neurapraxia versus axonotmesis

NCS

Evaluates speed and amplitude of nerve signals

EMG

Detects muscle denervation and reinnervation, assesses chronicity

Used typically **3 weeks post-injury** for accuracy.

Q123. Explain the role of imaging modalities (X-ray, CT, MRI, and ultrasound) in diagnosing upper limb injuries.

- *X-ray*: First-line; detects fractures, dislocations, alignment (e.g., Monteggia, Galeazzi injuries)
- *CT scan*: Excellent for complex fractures (intra-articular, scapula, distal humerus)
- *MRI*: Soft tissue injuries—rotator cuff tear, ligamentous injuries, occult fractures, AVN
- *Ultrasound*: Dynamic evaluation of tendons, effusions, nerve entrapments; bedside use

Q124. Write a short note on compartment syndrome of the upper limb.

Definition

A condition where increased pressure within a closed fascial compartment compromises circulation and tissue function.

Most Common Site in Upper Limb

Forearm (especially volar compartment)

Causes

- Fractures (supracondylar humerus, both bone forearm)
- Crush injuries
- Tight casts or dressings
- Burns, prolonged limb compression

Clinical features (6 P's)

- *P*ain (out of proportion and on passive stretch)
- *P*aresthesia
- *P*allor
- *P*aralysis
- *P*ulselessness (late)
- *P*oikilothermia

Diagnosis

- Clinical suspicion is paramount
- Compartment pressure >30 mm Hg or ΔP (diastolic BP - compartment pressure) <30 mm Hg is indicative

Treatment

- Immediate fasciotomy
- Remove constrictive dressings
- Delay closure or use of skin grafts may be needed post-decompression

Q125. Discuss the pathophysiology and management of Volkmann's ischemic contracture.

(MMC 2017)

Definition

A late sequela of untreated or missed compartment syndrome, leading to ischemic necrosis of forearm muscles (mainly flexor group), resulting in fibrosis and contracture.

Pathophysiology

- Initial ischemia → muscle necrosis → fibrous tissue replacement
- Median and ulnar nerves may also be affected
- Leads to claw-like deformity of hand and wrist flexion

Types (Tsuge Classification)

- *Mild*: Only flexor digitorum profundus (FDP) and flexor pollicis longus (FPL)

- *Moderate*: FDP, FPL, and some nerve involvement
- *Severe*: All flexors with gross deformity and nerve damage

Clinical Features
- Claw hand deformity
- Fixed flexion of wrist and fingers
- Muscle wasting
- Nerve deficits

Management
- *Early*: Observation, physiotherapy, dynamic splinting
- *Late*: Surgical interventions
  - Muscle sliding procedures (Max Page, Seddon)
  - Tendon transfers
  - Contracture release
  - Nerve decompression/neurolysis

Q126. Explain the classification and management of open fractures of the upper limb.

Classification
Gustilo-Anderson Classification
- *Type I*: <1 cm clean wound, minimal soft tissue damage
- *Type II*: 1–10 cm wound, moderate soft tissue damage
- *Type IIIA*: Extensive soft tissue injury, adequate bone coverage
- *Type IIIB*: Extensive soft tissue loss, periosteal stripping, requires flap
- *Type IIIC*: Vascular injury requiring repair

Management
1. *Initial care*:
   - Hemostasis, IV fluids, tetanus prophylaxis
   - Broad-spectrum IV antibiotics (e.g., first generation cephalosporin, aminoglycosides if Type III)
2. Surgical principles (within 6–8 hours ideally):
   - *Debridement*: Remove all devitalized tissue
   - *Stabilization*: External fixation preferred initially in high-grade injuries
   - *Wound management*:
     - Delayed closure or VAC dressing
     - Flap coverage (muscle/local/free) if needed (especially Type IIIB)
3. *Definitive fixation*:
   - ORIF once wound is clean
   - Bone grafting if required
4. *Rehabilitation*: Early ROM to prevent stiffness

Q127. Pulseless hand following supracondylar fracture of humerus (SN).

Definition
Absence of distal pulses following a supracondylar humerus fracture, commonly due to brachial artery injury or spasm.

Types
- *Pink pulseless hand*: Hand is perfused but pulse is absent (arterial spasm or kink)
- *Pale pulseless hand*: No perfusion—suggests arterial occlusion or rupture

Management
- **Urgent closed reduction and pinning**
- If still pulseless → **vascular exploration**
- **Doppler/CT angiography** if unclear
- Monitor for compartment syndrome

Q128. Fracture lateral condyle humerus—short note.

Definition
Fracture involving the lateral condyle and extensor origin of humerus in children.

Classification (Milch)
- *Type I*: Lateral to trochlear groove (rare)
- *Type II*: Through trochlear groove (common)

Management
- *<2 mm displacement*: Long arm cast
- *>2 mm or rotated*: Open reduction and internal fixation (K-wires)

Complications
Nonunion, lateral overgrowth, tardy ulnar palsy

Q129. Neglected fracture lateral condyle humerus—short note.

Presentation
Often presents weeks/months later with deformity, limited movement, or tardy ulnar nerve palsy.

Radiology
Nonunion or pseudoarthrosis visible

Management
- *<6 months*: Open reduction + internal fixation
- *>6 months*: Consider corrective osteotomy, ulnar nerve transposition, or ORIF if symptoms

Q130. Thomson's approach to radius with applied anatomy—short note.

Indication
Surgical exposure of proximal and middle third of radius (commonly for ORIF).

Approach
- *Interval*: Between **extensor carpi radialis brevis (ECRB)** and **extensor digitorum communis (EDC)**
- *Position*: Supine, forearm pronated
- *Key steps*:
    - Incise fascia
    - Retract ECRB laterally and EDC medially
    - Protect **posterior interosseous nerve (PIN)**—runs close to radial neck, enters supinator
    - Access radial shaft anterior to supinator

Applied Anatomy
- Avoid injury to PIN (most vulnerable during supinator dissection)
- Maintain soft tissue envelope for bone healing

Q131. Rehabilitation protocols in flexor tendon injury repairs—short note.

Goal

Restore tendon glide, prevent adhesions, and maintain joint mobility.

Phases

1. *Early phase (0–3 weeks)*:
   - Dorsal splint with wrist in slight flexion
   - Passive mobilization (e.g., Kleinert or Duran protocol)
2. *Intermediate phase (3–6 weeks)*:
   - Controlled active mobilization
   - Continue splinting during non-exercise time
3. *Late phase (6–12 weeks)*:
   - Progressive strengthening
   - Discontinue splint gradually
4. *>12 weeks*:
   - Unrestricted activity
   - Functional rehabilitation and work conditioning

Note: Close collaboration with hand therapist is essential

Q132. Discuss the principles of rehabilitation following upper limb fractures.

(JIPMER 2011)

Key Principles

- *Immobilization phase*: Pain control, edema reduction, joint protection.
- *Mobilization phase*: Early ROM exercises of uninvolved joints, gradual loading of affected limb.
- *Strengthening phase*: Progressive resistance training, coordination exercises.
- *Functional training*: Task-specific rehabilitation (grip strength, writing, lifting).
- *Multidisciplinary care*: Includes physiotherapists, occupational therapists, and orthopedic follow-up.

Q133. Explain the role of physical therapy in shoulder dislocation recovery.

Goals

- *Acute phase*: Pain reduction, immobilization, isometric strengthening.
- *Intermediate phase*: ROM recovery (especially external rotation and abduction), scapular stabilization.
- *Late phase*: Strengthening rotator cuff and deltoid, proprioceptive retraining.
- *Prevent re-dislocation*: Focus on dynamic stability and activity modification (especially in athletes).

Q134. Write a short note on the role of dynamic splints in hand injuries.

Definition

Devices that apply a controlled force to assist or resist motion.

Uses

- Promote **early motion** while protecting healing structures (e.g., tendon repairs).
- Prevent joint contractures (e.g., boutonnière deformity).
- Restore hand function in nerve palsy (e.g., radial nerve palsy).

Types

Extension/flexion assist, radial/ulnar deviation assist.

Q135. Discuss the principles of post-operative rehabilitation in elbow trauma.

Phases
- *Phase 1 (0–2 weeks)*: Pain/edema control, splinting, passive ROM if stable.
- *Phase 2 (2–6 weeks)*: Controlled active-assisted ROM, avoid varus/valgus stress.
- *Phase 3 (6+ weeks)*: Full ROM, strengthening, proprioception, functional training.

Key Consideration
Prevent **elbow stiffness** and **heterotopic ossification**.

Q136. Explain the role of occupational therapy in hand trauma rehabilitation.

Role
- Restores **functional independence** in ADLs (grasp, writing, dressing).
- Custom **splint fabrication** for protection or correction.
- **Sensory re-education** (after nerve injuries).
- *Vocational rehabilitation*: Adapting work tasks or tools.
- **Scar management** and **edema control techniques**.

Mobilization in upper limb trauma rehabilitation
- Prevents stiffness, muscle atrophy, and joint contractures.
- Enhances circulation and reduces edema.
- Improves functional outcomes and promotes early return to ADLs.
- Should be guided by fracture stability and soft tissue healing status.

11.3 Lower Limb Trauma

Vipin Sharma, Sajad Ahmad Wani

General Principles of Lower Limb Trauma

Q1. Discuss the biomechanics of lower limb trauma.

(KMC Manipal 2013)

Mechanism of Injury

- Axial loading (e.g., falls from height)—femoral, tibial plateau, calcaneal fractures.
- Rotational forces—spiral fractures, ligamentous injuries.
- Direct blow/trauma—transverse or comminuted fractures.
- High-velocity trauma (e.g., RTAS)—complex, open, segmental, or floating knee injuries.

Forces Influencing Fracture Patterns

- *Compressive*: Shortening of limb, impaction.
- *Tensile*: Avulsion-type fractures.
- *Shear*: Seen in oblique fractures.
- *Torsional*: Spiral configurations.

Understanding these forces helps predict **fracture configuration**, **soft tissue damage**, and guides **treatment planning**.

Q2. Explain the importance of neurovascular assessment in lower limb injuries.

Vascular Assessment

- *Check pulses*: Femoral, popliteal, dorsalis pedis, posterior tibial.
- *Look for signs of ischemia*: Pallor, pulselessness, pain, paresthesia, paralysis.
- Doppler/CT angiography if vascular injury is suspected.

Neurological Assessment

- *Femoral nerve*: Hip flexion, knee extension.
- *Sciatic nerve*:
  - *Peroneal division*: Foot dorsiflexion, eversion.
  - *Tibial division*: Plantarflexion, toe flexion.
- Document sensory and motor deficits.

Early and repeated assessments are essential for detecting **compartment syndrome**, evolving nerve injuries, or missed vascular compromise.

Q3. Discuss the role of imaging (X-ray, CT, MRI) in evaluating lower limb fractures.

X-rays

- First-line modality.
- Minimum of **two orthogonal views** (AP and lateral).
- Include **joint above and below**.

CT Scan

- Ideal for intra-articular fractures (e.g., tibial plateau, distal femur).
- Provides 3D fracture mapping—helps in preoperative planning.

MRI

- Soft tissue, ligamentous, and occult fractures.
- Used in evaluating **ACL/PCL, meniscus**, and **osteochondral lesions**.

In polytrauma, **whole-body CT (pan-scan)** may be required.

Q4. Write a short note on the management of open fractures of the lower limb.

Initial Management (Golden Hour Principles)

- **ATLS protocol.**
- Broad-spectrum **IV antibiotics** (within 1 hour).
- **Tetanus prophylaxis.**
- Sterile dressing, splinting.

Surgical Management

- **Debridement** within 6–12 hours ("Time is tissue").
- **Fracture stabilization** (external fixator preferred in the initial stage).
- Delayed or staged wound closure (or flap coverage for Grade III injuries).

Gustilo-Anderson Classification

Guides **antibiotics**, **surgical timing**, and **fixation options**.

Pelvic Ring Injuries

Q5. Classification and management of pelvic ring injuries.

(Asked in: PGI Chandigarh 2022, AIIMS Delhi 2021, BHU Varanasi 2022)

Introduction

- Pelvic ring fractures are **high-energy injuries** often associated with **life-threatening hemorrhage**, visceral, and neurovascular injuries.
- **Early stabilization is critical** for survival.

Classification

Mechanism-based (Young and Burgess classification):

Type	*Mechanism*	*Features*
Lateral compression (LC)	Side impact	Iliac wing or pubic rami fractures; sacral compression
Anteroposterior compression (APC)	Frontal impact	Open book pelvis; pubic symphysis disruption
Vertical shear (VS)	Fall from height	Vertical displacement; sacroiliac joint disruption
Combined mechanism	Mixed forces	Complex patterns

Stability-based (Tile Classification)—(Discussed separately below)

Management

Initial management:

- **ATLS protocol**—treat life-threatening conditions first.
- **Pelvic binder** or **sheet wrapping** to compress the pelvis and reduce hemorrhage.
- Early identification and control of bleeding (angioembolization or pelvic packing if needed).

Definitive management:

- *Stable injuries*: Non-operative treatment.
  - Bed rest, analgesia, protected weight-bearing.
- *Unstable injuries*: Operative treatment.
  - External fixation (temporary or definitive).
  - Internal fixation (plating of anterior ring, iliosacral screws for posterior ring).

Goals

- Hemorrhage control.
- Restore pelvic ring stability.
- Enable early mobilization to prevent complications like DVT, pneumonia.

Q6. Describe tile classification and principles of treatment of pelvic fractures.

(Asked in: RGUHS Karnataka 2022, CMC Vellore 2023)

Tile Classification (Based on Stability)

Type	*Description*	*Stability*
A	Stable pelvic ring fractures	Stable
B	Rotationally unstable, vertically stable ("open book" injuries)	Partially stable
C	Rotationally and vertically unstable (complete disruption)	Completely unstable

Principles of Treatment

Type A (stable):
- Non-operative management.
- Bed rest, analgesics, gradual mobilization.

Type B (rotationally unstable):
- Initial stabilization with **pelvic binder**.
- *Definitive fixation*:
    - Anterior ring—plate and screw fixation (ORIF).
    - Posterior ring—often requires iliosacral screw fixation.

Type C (rotationally and vertically unstable):
- Life-threatening emergency.
- Temporary external fixation or C-clamp in emergency settings.
- *Definitive surgery*:
    - ORIF for anterior and posterior ring.
    - Iliosacral screws, plates, or lumbopelvic fixation as needed.

Key Points
- **Hemorrhage control is priority** initially.
- **Early stabilization reduces mortality and improves functional outcomes.**
- Multidisciplinary management often required (ortho, general surgery, vascular, urology teams).

Q7. Pelvic fractures and hemorrhage control in trauma. Classify pelvic fractures and discuss their management.

Classification
- *Stable fractures*: No disruption of pelvic ring integrity (e.g., avulsion fractures).
- *Unstable fractures*: Disruption of the ring in ≥2 places or rotational/vertical instability.

Based on Stability
- Anteroposterior compression (APC)
- Lateral compression (LC)
- Vertical shear (VS)

Management
- *Stable fractures*: Conservative (bed rest, analgesia, physical therapy).
- *Unstable fractures*:
    - Initial resuscitation
    - External fixation
    - Angioembolization or preperitoneal packing (if bleeding)
    - Definitive internal fixation

Q8. Explain the role of pelvic binders in acute pelvic fractures.

- Temporarily stabilizes the pelvic ring and **reduces pelvic volume**.
- Indicated for **hemodynamically unstable** patients with suspected pelvic fractures.
- Applied at the level of the **greater trochanters**, not the iliac crest.
- Helps tamponade venous bleeding and reduce shear forces.

Q9. Explain the role of preperitoneal packing (PPP) in pelvic trauma.

- Indicated in **uncontrolled venous bleeding** with hemodynamic instability.
- Pads placed in the preperitoneal space compress the bleeding pelvic vessels.
- Often combined with external fixation for pelvic stability.
- Quick and effective in emergency settings where angioembolization is delayed/unavailable.

Q10. Discuss the indications for angioembolization in pelvic fractures.

- Ongoing **arterial bleeding** after pelvic stabilization.
- CT scan showing active contrast extravasation ("blush").
- Persistent hypotension despite resuscitation and pelvic binder.
- Used selectively in **hemodynamically stable** or stabilized patients.

Q11. Management of a young woman with APC 3 pelvic injury in shock (SN).

- *APC III*: Complete disruption of symphysis pubis and both sacroiliac joints—pelvis unstable in all directions.
- *Initial management (ATLS protocol)*:
  - *Resuscitation*: IV fluids, blood transfusion.
  - *Pelvic binder*: Apply early to reduce pelvic volume and control bleeding.
- *Definitive management*:
  - *Hemorrhage control*: Angioembolization or preperitoneal packing if ongoing bleeding.
  - *Surgical fixation*:
    - Anterior plating of pubic symphysis.
    - Posterior SI screw or lumbopelvic fixation.
- *Multidisciplinary care*: Ortho + trauma + vascular + ICU.

Acetabular Fractures

Q12. Describe Letournel's classification of acetabular fractures.

Asked in: PGI Chandigarh 2021, KGMU Lucknow 2022

Letournel–Judet classification is the most widely used system to categorize acetabular fractures based on involvement of anterior and posterior columns and walls.

Elementary Fractures (5 types)—Involve Only One Part

Type	*Description*
1. Posterior wall	Most common. Fragment of posterior wall, often with dislocation
2. Posterior column	Fracture extending from greater sciatic notch to obturator foramen
3. Anterior wall	Rare. Involves anterior wall and acetabular roof
4. Anterior column	From iliac wing to pubis. Common in elderly
5. Transverse	Horizontal fracture splitting both columns, separating superior acetabulum

Associated Fractures (5 types)—Combinations of Elementary Fractures

Type	*Description*
1. Posterior column + Posterior wall	Common variant; unstable
2. Transverse + Posterior wall	Seen with dashboard injury and dislocation
3. T-Shaped	Transverse fracture + vertical limb separating anterior and posterior columns
4. Anterior column + Posterior hemi-transverse	Common in elderly; requires column stabilization
5. Both column fracture	Entire acetabulum is detached from the pelvis; "floating acetabulum"

Radiological Clues (Judet Views)
- AP view
- Obturator oblique (anterior column + posterior wall)
- Iliac oblique (posterior column + anterior wall)

Q13. Management of acetabular fractures.

Initial Management
- **Traction (skeletal)** to maintain reduction, reduce soft tissue compromise.
- *Imaging*: **AP pelvis, Judet views, CT scan with 3D recon.**

Indications for Non-operative Treatment
- Minimally displaced (<2 mm)
- Congruent joint
- Elderly or high-risk surgical patients

Operative Indications
- Displacement >2 mm
- Incongruent joint
- Posterior wall fractures with instability
- Presence of intra-articular fragments

Surgical Timing

Preferably within 7–10 days to reduce complications.

Q14. Approaches for surgical fixation of acetabular fractures.

Choice of approach depends on fracture type, location (anterior versus posterior), surgeon expertise, and patient factors.

Posterior Approaches

Approach	*Indication*
Kocher–Langenbeck	Posterior wall and column fractures; transverse fractures
Position: Lateral/Prone	
Risks: Sciatic nerve injury	

Anterior Approaches

Approach	*Indication*
Ilioinguinal	Anterior column, anterior wall, both-column fractures
Spares abdominal contents	
Risks: Femoral neurovascular bundle injury	

Modified stoppa (intrapelvic approach) indiacted in anterior column, transverse, both-column

- Better medial visualization of quadrilateral plate
- Avoids iliac fossa dissection

Extended Approaches

Approach	Description
Extended iliofemoral	Allows access to both columns but with high morbidity
Triradiate (tri-approach)	Combines anterior and posterior incisions

Combined Approaches

- Used in complex and both-column fractures
- Staged or simultaneous anterior-posterior fixation

Q15. Modified Stoppa's approach (SN).

- *Indication*: Commonly used for anterior acetabular fractures and some pelvic fractures.
- *Incision*: Pfannenstiel (transverse suprapubic) incision.
- *Technique*:
  - Dissection through the rectus abdominis and space of Retzius.
  - Offers access to the quadrilateral plate and anterior column.
- *Advantages*:
  - Reduced blood loss compared to ilioinguinal approach.
  - Avoids inguinal neurovascular structures.
- *Complications*: Injury to corona mortis, bladder, or obturator nerve if not carefully dissected.

Q16. Complications of acetabular fractures.

Acetabular fractures, particularly those involving the weight-bearing dome or with displacement, carry a significant risk of complications. These can be **early** or **late**:

1. Early Complications

a. *Neurovascular injury*:
   - **Sciatic nerve** (especially peroneal division) is commonly at risk, particularly in posterior column or dislocation-type injuries.
   - Femoral artery or vein injury is rare but serious.

b. *Vascular injury and hemorrhagic shock*:
   - Especially in high-energy injuries.
   - Pelvic venous plexus or ilio-lumbar vessels may be source of bleeding.

c. *Deep vein thrombosis (DVT) and pulmonary embolism (PE)*: Due to prolonged immobility and trauma-associated hypercoagulability.

d. *Infection*:
   - Higher in open fractures or post-operatively.
   - Requires debridement, antibiotics, and possibly hardware removal.

e. *Associated Injuries*: Fractures of pelvis, femur, spine, or abdominal and urogenital trauma.

2. Late Complications

a. *Post-traumatic osteoarthritis*:
   - Most common late complication.
   - Due to incongruent joint surface, cartilage damage, or AVN.
   - May require total hip replacement.

b. *Avascular necrosis (AVN) of the femoral head*:
   - Especially with associated dislocation or fracture-dislocation.
   - Risk increases with delay in reduction (>6 hours).
c. *Heterotopic ossification*:
   - Formation of bone in soft tissues around the joint.
   - Risk factors: extensive surgical dissection, head injury.
   - May cause stiffness and reduced ROM.
d. *Malunion/Nonunion*:
   - Especially in non-operative or poorly reduced fractures.
   - Leads to joint incongruity and functional impairment.
e. *Chronic pain and limp*: Due to joint incongruity, muscle weakness, or nerve injury.
f. *Hardware complications*: Prominent screws, implant breakage, or loosening.
g. *Sciatic Nerve palsy (Late onset)*: Due to stretching or scar entrapment.

3. Functional Complications
- Gait abnormalities
- Leg length discrepancy
- Reduced hip ROM
- Impaired ability to return to pre-injury activity level

Q17. Direct anterior approach (DAA) to the hip joint (SN).

(AIMS Kochi 2013)

- *Indication*: Total hip arthroplasty, selected femoral neck fractures.
- *Incision*: Anterior, over the tensor fascia lata.
- *Intermuscular plane*: Between sartorius and tensor fascia lata (Smith–Petersen interval).
- *Advantages*:
  - Muscle-sparing (no detachment of hip abductors).
  - Faster recovery and lower dislocation rates.
- *Limitations*:
  - Steep learning curve.
  - Limited exposure in obese or muscular patients.

Proximal Femur and Hip Fractures

Management of Femoral Head Fractures
- *Classification*: Pipkin classification (types I–IV).
- *Initial management*:
  - Urgent reduction if dislocated to prevent AVN.
  - CT scan to assess fracture details.
- *Definitive management*:
  - *Type I/II*: ORIF if large or displaced fragments; excision of small fragments.
  - *Type III*: ORIF; often poor prognosis due to neck fracture.
  - *Type IV*: Treat acetabular and head fracture appropriately.
- *Complications*: AVN, post-traumatic arthritis, heterotopic ossification.
  - Classify fracture-dislocation of hip. Outline the principles of management of each type.
  - Describe the blood supply of head of femur at various ages and how will you manage a case of fracture neck of femur in a 50 years old male.

Q18. Pipkin classification of femoral head fractures.

The **Pipkin classification** is used to categorize **femoral head fractures** typically associated with **posterior hip dislocations**. It is crucial for guiding management and predicting outcomes.

Type	Description	Notes/Management considerations
I	Fracture of the femoral head below (inferior to) the fovea capitis (non-weight-bearing portion)	Often treated conservatively or with fragment excision if small
II	Fracture of the femoral head above (superior to) the fovea capitis (weight-bearing portion)	Requires anatomical reduction, often ORIF (open reduction internal fixation)
III	Type I or II fracture with associated femoral neck fracture	Poor prognosis due to high risk of avascular necrosis; may require arthroplasty in older patients
IV	Type I or II fracture with associated acetabular fracture (usually posterior wall)	Requires treatment of both femoral head and acetabular injuries, often surgical

Clinical Notes

- **Urgent reduction** of any dislocation is critical to reduce the risk of **AVN**.
- CT scan helps define fracture pattern and plan surgery.
- **Surgical approach** varies based on type and associated injuries (anterior versus posterior approach).

Q19. Classify fractures of the femoral neck and discuss their management.

Classification (By Anatomical Location)

1. *Subcapital*: Just below the femoral head.
2. *Transcervical*: Across the mid-neck.
3. *Basicervical*: At the base of the neck.

Management Strategy (Based on Age, Displacement, And Bone Quality)

Patient profile	Management
Young (<60 years), non-displaced	Cannulated screws (preserve native hip)
Young with displaced fractures	Urgent ORIF (risk of AVN); consider THA if failed
Elderly (>60 years), displaced	Hemiarthroplasty or Total Hip Arthroplasty (THA)
Elderly, non-ambulatory	Cemented hemiarthroplasty

Q20. Garden classification and management of femoral neck fractures.

(Asked in: JIPMER Puducherry 2022, AMU Aligarh 2022)

Introduction

- Femoral neck fractures are common, especially in **elderly osteoporotic individuals**.
- High risk of **avascular necrosis (AVN)** and **non-union**.

Garden Classification (Based on Degree of Displacement on AP X-ray)

Type	Description
Garden I	Incomplete, valgus impacted fracture
Garden II	Complete fracture, non-displaced
Garden III	Complete fracture, partially displaced
Garden IV	Complete fracture, completely displaced

Clinical Use

Determines risk of AVN and helps guide treatment choice.

Management

Young patients (<60 years):

- *Aim*: Preserve native femoral head.
- *Garden I and II*: Internal fixation with cannulated cancellous screws (CCS) or dynamic hip screw (DHS).

- *Garden III and IV*:
    - Closed or open reduction + internal fixation with multiple screws.
    - Early surgery (<6–12 hours) improves head survival.

Elderly patients (>60–65 years):
- *Aim*: Early mobilization and weight-bearing.
- *Garden I and II*: Internal fixation if bone quality good.
- *Garden III and IV*:
    - Hemiarthroplasty (cemented or uncemented).
    - Total hip arthroplasty (THA)—if active, independent, and pre-injury good mobility.

Key Points
- Early diagnosis and surgical stabilization are crucial.
- Displacement degree decides between **fixation** versus **replacement**.

Q21. Explain Pauwels' classifications of femoral neck fractures.

Pauwels' Classification (Based on Angle of Fracture Line)
1. *Type I*: <30° to horizontal
2. *Type II*: 30°–50°
3. *Type III*: >50°

Higher angle = more **shear forces** more **greater instability** and risk of **non-union**.

Q22. Describe the vascular supply of proximal femur. Enumerate the possible complications of an intracapsular fracture neck of femur and management options in a 65 years old male.

Vascular Supply of the Proximal Femur
1. *Medial femoral circumflex artery (mfca)—primary supply*:
    - *Branch of*: Profunda femoris (deep femoral artery).
    - *Retinacular branches (posterior-superior)*: Enter femoral head at posterosuperior neck.
    - **Most critical** for femoral head viability.
2. *Lateral femoral circumflex artery (LFCA)*:
    - Contributes minor anterior supply.
    - Less significant in head perfusion.
3. *Artery of ligamentum teres (obturator artery branch)*:
    - Supplies the **fovea capitis**.
    - Important in children; limited role in adults.
4. *Intraosseous and subsynovial vessels*: Supplementary; not sufficient alone.

Complications of Intracapsular Fracture Neck of Femur
- Avascular necrosis (AVN)—due to disrupted blood supply.
- Nonunion—high due to lack of cambium layer, synovial fluid inhibiting healing.
- Malunion—uncommon but possible.
- Shortening and limb length discrepancy
- Deep vein thrombosis (DVT)
- Infection—especially post-surgery.
- Osteoarthritis—late complication.
- Implant failure in internal fixation.

Management in a 65-year-old Male
Factors to Consider
Physiological age, activity level, comorbidities, fracture type (displacement), bone quality.

Displaced Fracture (Garden III/IV)
Preferred treatment: Arthroplasty
- *Hemiarthroplasty (mod active patients with low demands)*: Cemented bipolar prosthesis often used.
- *Total hip arthroplasty (THA)*: For more active, independent patients with good acetabular cartilage.

Undisplaced Fracture (Garden I/II)
- Internal fixation with **cannulated screws** or **dynamic hip screw (DHS)**.
- *Goal*: Preserve native hip.

Q23. Discuss the role of hemiarthroplasty versus total hip arthroplasty in femoral neck fractures.

Hemiarthroplasty
- Replaces **only femoral head.**
- *Indications*:
  - Low-demand elderly
  - Poor cognitive status
  - Comorbidities

Total Hip Arthroplasty (THA)
- Replaces **both femoral head and acetabulum.**
- *Indications*:
  - Active elderly patients
  - Pre-existing arthritis
  - Garden III/IV fractures with good mobility

THA has better functional outcomes but slightly higher dislocation risk.

Q24. Discuss the complications of femoral neck fractures and their prevention.

Early Complications
- Avascular necrosis (AVN) of femoral head (due to retinacular artery disruption)
- Non-union
- DVT/PE
- Infection
- Delirium in elderly

Late Complications
- Osteoarthritis
- Implant failure or cut-out
- Shortening and gait disturbance

Prevention
- Prompt fixation (<6–12 hours ideally)
- Stable and anatomical reduction
- Appropriate implant selection
- Early mobilization
- DVT prophylaxis and multidisciplinary care (especially in elderly)

Q25. Management of intertrochanteric fractures—discuss implants and choice.

(Asked in: MUHS Maharashtra 2023, PGI Chandigarh 2022)

Introduction

- Intertrochanteric fractures occur between **greater and lesser trochanters**.
- Elderly are most commonly affected.

Implants and Choice

Dynamic hip screw (DHS):

- Best for **stable** two-part fractures (AO/OTA 31A1).
- Provides controlled collapse and compression at fracture site.
- Requires intact posteromedial cortex for stability.

Proximal femoral nail (PFN):

- *Preferred for unstable fractures*:
  - Comminuted
  - Reverse oblique
  - Subtrochanteric extension
  - Lateral wall fractures.
- *Advantages*:
  - Intramedullary load-sharing device.
  - Short lever arm → less mechanical failure.
  - Less blood loss, minimally invasive.

Other options

- *Proximal femoral nail antirotation (PFNA)*: Improved design with helical blade.
- Cement-augmented implants for osteoporotic bone.

Surgical Goals

- Achieve anatomical or near-anatomical reduction.
- Restore medial support and neck-shaft angle.
- Promote early mobilization.

Q26. Unstable trochanteric fractures (SN).

- *Definition*: Comminuted, reverse oblique, or fractures with posteromedial support loss.
- *Management*:
  - *Implants*:
    - Proximal femoral nail (PFN)—preferred for unstable patterns.
    - Dynamic hip screw (DHS)—not ideal due to higher failure in unstable cases.
  - *Surgical principles*:
    - Restoration of medial support.
    - Stable fixation to allow early mobilization.
- *Complications*: Implant failure, malunion, nonunion, varus collapse.

Q27. Explain the indications for dynamic hip screw (DHS) versus proximal femoral nailing (PFN).

Factor	*DHS*	*PFN*
Fracture pattern	Stable intertrochanteric fractures	Unstable, reverse oblique, subtrochanteric
Surgical technique	Open reduction, lateral plate	Minimally invasive, intramedullary
Weight-bearing	May be delayed in comminuted cases	Allows early full weight-bearing
Biomechanics	Extramedullary (longer lever arm)	Intramedullary (more biomechanically sound)

Q28. Discuss the classification of trochanteric fractures and how does it influence the management.

Classification of Trochanteric Fractures and Its Influence on Management

Trochanteric fractures (also called **intertrochanteric fractures**) are extra-capsular fractures of the proximal femur between the **greater and lesser trochanters**. Classification helps in predicting **stability, complications, and choosing appropriate treatment.**

AO/OTA Classification (A1–A3)

Most widely used radiological classification:

Type	*Description*	*Stability*	*Management*
31-A1	Simple two-part fracture	Stable	DHS or short PFN
31-A2	Multi-fragmentary with posteromedial comminution	Unstable	PFN (preferably long)
31-A3	Reverse oblique or transverse pattern (extends into subtrochanteric region)	Highly unstable	Long PFN

Evans Classification

Based on stability and postero-medial integrity:

- *Stable*: Intact posteromedial cortex (lesser trochanter).
- *Unstable*: Comminution of posteromedial cortex, reverse oblique fracture, or subtrochanteric extension.

Boyd and Griffin Classification

Older system, less used now:

- *Type I*: Simple, two-part fractures.
- *Type II*: Comminution of medial cortex.
- *Type III*: Comminution with subtrochanteric extension.
- *Type IV*: Intertrochanteric fracture with involvement of the shaft.

Influence on Management

Stable fractures:

- *Devices*:
  - Dynamic hip screw **(DHS)** is often sufficient.
  - **Short PFN** can be used too.
- **Early mobilization** possible.

Unstable fractures:

- *Preferred implant*: **Proximal femoral nail (PFN)**—offers better stability and load sharing.
- *Reverse oblique and subtrochanteric extension*: Require **long PFN**.
- DHS is contraindicated due to risk of medial collapse.

Q29. Periprosthetic fractures around the hip—short note.

Definition

Fractures occurring **around or near hip implants**, especially THA

Classification: Vancouver System

Type	*Location*	*Implant stability*	*Bone stock*
A	Trochanteric	Stable	Good
B1	Around stem	Stable	Good
B2	Around stem	Loose stem	Good
B3	Around stem	Loose	Poor bone
C	Well below the stem	Irrelevant	Variable

Management

- *A*: Conservative or tension band
- *B1*: ORIF
- *B2/B3*: **Revision THA with long-stem + fixation**
- *C*: ORIF as per standard fracture protocol

Always assess implant stability radiographically or intra-operatively.

Q30. Write a short note on subtrochanteric fractures of the femur.

Definition

Subtrochanteric fractures are fractures that occur within **5 cm distal to the lesser trochanter**, in the proximal shaft region of the femur.

Etiology

- High-energy trauma in young adults (e.g., RTAs, falls from height)
- Low-energy trauma in the elderly with osteoporotic bones
- Pathological fractures (e.g., metastasis, bisphosphonate-induced atypical fractures)

Classification

Russell–Taylor classification (based on piriformis fossa involvement):

- *Type I*: Piriformis fossa intact
- *Type II*: Piriformis fossa involved (limits intramedullary entry)

Clinical Features

- Pain, swelling, deformity
- Limb shortening and external rotation
- Inability to bear weight

Management

- *Surgical treatment is standard*:
  - Proximal femoral nailing (PFN)—gold standard
  - Long cephalomedullary nails
  - Bridge plating in select cases or revision
- *Post-operative care*: Early mobilization, DVT prophylaxis, physiotherapy

Q31. Discuss the biomechanical challenges in treating subtrochanteric fractures.

Subtrochanteric region has **unique biomechanical properties** that make treatment complex:

1. *High mechanical stress zone*:
   - Region subjected to **high compressive and tensile forces** during ambulation.
   - Has a **bending moment arm** due to its position below the hip joint.
2. *Cortical bone dominance*:
   - Subtrochanteric region is composed mainly of dense cortical bone.
   - Less vascular → **slower healing**, prone to **non-union**.
3. *Fracture patterns*:
   - Often **comminuted**, **spiral**, or **reverse oblique**—difficult to reduce and stabilize.
   - May extend proximally toward the greater trochanter or distally into the shaft.
4. *Implant challenges*:
   - Requires **load-sharing fixation**.
   - **Intramedullary fixation (PFN)** is biomechanically superior as it:
     - Resists bending and rotational forces.
     - Shares axial load with the bone.
   - **Plate fixation** carries higher risk of stress risers and implant failure.

5. *Malalignment risks*:
    - Malreduction (especially **varus malalignment**) increases failure risk.
    - Entry point for nail must be precise; **piriformis versus trochanteric entry** depends on anatomy and fracture pattern.

Femoral Shaft Fractures

Q32. Classify femoral shaft fractures and discuss their management.

(MUHS 2016)

Classification (AO/OTA System—32 Series)
- *Type 32-A*: Simple fractures (transverse, oblique, spiral)
- *Type 32-B*: Wedge fractures
- *Type 32-C*: Complex (comminuted, segmental)

Management
Adults:
- *Intramedullary nailing (IMN)*: Gold standard (especially for diaphyseal fractures)
- *External fixation*: Temporary stabilization in polytrauma/open fractures
- *Plating*: In select cases (e.g., distal shaft, periprosthetic, open fractures)

Children:
- *<5 years*: Conservative (hip spica)
- *5–10 years*: Elastic nailing (TENS)
- *>10 years*: Rigid IMN or submuscular plating

Q33. Explain the indications for intramedullary nailing in femoral shaft fractures.

Indications
- Closed, isolated mid-shaft fractures
- Polytrauma patients (as part of ETC or DCO)
- Pathological fractures
- Segmental fractures
- Open fractures (type I/II; type III after debridement)

Allows **early mobilization**, load-sharing, minimal soft tissue disruption.

Q34. Write a short note on the use of plating versus nailing in femoral shaft fractures.

Aspect	*Nailing*	*Plating*
Approach	Minimally invasive	Open or submuscular
Biomechanics	Load-sharing	Load-bearing
Indications	Midshaft, segmental, polytrauma	Distal/proximal shaft, periprosthetic
Union rate	Higher	Slightly lower
Complications	Fat embolism, malalignment	Higher infection risk, non-union in comminution

Q35. Discuss the complications of femoral shaft fractures, including fat embolism syndrome.

(GGMC 2013)

Early Complications
- *Fat embolism syndrome (FES)*:
    - *Triad*: Respiratory distress, petechiae, altered mental status

- Occurs 24–72 hours post-injury
- Prevented by early fixation
- Hemorrhagic shock
- Compartment syndrome
- Open fractures → infection risk

Late Complications
- Malunion (especially in rotational deformity)
- Non-union
- Implant failure
- Knee stiffness
- Limb length discrepancy

Q36. Explain the role of reamed versus unreamed nailing in femoral shaft fractures.

Factor	*Reamed nailing*	*Unreamed nailing*
Canal preparation	Enlarged to fit larger diameter nail	Nail passed without reaming
Advantages	Better implant fit, stability, union rate	Less heat, preserves endosteal blood supply
Disadvantages	Risk of fat embolism, thermal necrosis	Reduced stability, higher non-union risk
Preferred in	Most cases (except severe chest trauma)	Open fractures, polytrauma (as damage control)

Q37. Principles and techniques of femoral shaft fracture fixation in adults.

(Asked in: AIIMS Delhi 2022, KGMU Lucknow 2022)

Introduction
- Femoral shaft fractures are typically **high-energy injuries** and are considered **life and limb-threatening**.
- *Goals of treatment*: **Early stabilization, anatomic alignment, early mobilization.**

Principles of Fixation

Initial management:
- ATLS protocol first (address life-threatening injuries).
- Temporary stabilization with skeletal traction (Thomas splint) if definitive surgery delayed.

Definitive fixation principles:
- Restore length, alignment, and rotation.
- Stable fixation to allow early mobilization.
- Preserve biology (minimal periosteal stripping).

Techniques of Fixation

Intramedullary nailing (gold standard):
- **Reamed antegrade intramedullary nail** preferred in most adults.
- *Entry points*:
  - Piriformis fossa (classical).
  - Greater trochanter (preferred now to avoid soft tissue disruption).

Subtypes:
- *Antegrade nailing*: Standard for midshaft fractures.
- *Retrograde nailing*: Indicated for distal third fractures, polytrauma, obese patients, or ipsilateral injuries.

Open reduction and internal fixation (ORIF) with plate:
- *Indications*:
  - When nailing not feasible (very proximal or distal fractures).
  - Peri-implant fractures.
- Less favored compared to nailing due to larger exposure and risk of infection.

External fixation:

- Temporary stabilization in polytrauma or open fractures with contamination.
- Definitive external fixation in some cases of severe open fractures.

Q38. Indications and advantages of intramedullary nailing in femoral fractures.

(Asked in: PGI Chandigarh 2021, MUHS Maharashtra 2023)

Indications for Intramedullary Nailing

Primary indications:

- Closed diaphyseal fractures (simple or comminuted).
- Polytrauma patients (early stabilization to reduce systemic complications).
- Segmental fractures.
- Pathological fractures.
- Some open fractures (Gustilo grade I/II).
- Bilateral femoral fractures.

Special indications: Femoral shaft fractures associated with ipsilateral femoral neck fractures (with modified techniques).

Advantages of Intramedullary Nailing

Biomechanical benefits:

- **Load-sharing device**—aligns with mechanical axis of femur.
- High strength, better resistance to bending and torsional forces.

Biological benefits:

- **Preserves soft tissue envelope and periosteal blood supply**.
- Reduced incidence of infection compared to plating.

Functional outcomes:

- Allows **early mobilization** and **early weight-bearing** (depending on fracture configuration).
- **High union rates** (~95%).

Other benefits:

- Minimal surgical exposure.
- Lower incidence of malunion compared to non-operative treatment

Q39. Write a short note on floating knee injuries and their management.

Definition

Simultaneous **ipsilateral fractures** of the **femur and tibia**, usually from **high-energy trauma**.

Classification (Fraser's)

- *Type I*: Diaphyseal fractures of both bones
- *Type II*: Involves intra-articular extension

Management

- **Damage control** initially (external fixators)
- *Definitive fixation*:
  - **Intramedullary nails** (antegrade femur, retrograde tibia or vice versa)
  - **Plating** if the intra-articular component
- Early **mobilization** and **physiotherapy**
- Address associated **vascular/nerve injury**

Prognosis depends on
- Soft tissue injury
- Articular involvement
- Timing and type of fixation

Distal Femur and Knee Injuries

Q40. Classify distal femur fractures and discuss their management.

Anatomical Classification
- *Supracondylar*: Above the condyles
- *Intercondylar*: Extending into the joint space
- *Comminuted*: Multiple fragments, often with articular involvement

Fracture Pattern
- Transverse
- Oblique
- Comminuted
- Segmental

Management

Type	*Treatment approach*
Extra-articular	Locking compression plate (LCP) or retrograde IM nail
Intra-articular	Anatomical reduction + locking plate (ORIF)
Osteoporotic bones	Locking plate + bone graft or cement augmentation

CT scan with 3D recon is essential for intra-articular planning.

Q41. Explain the AO classification of distal femur fractures (33 series).

- *33-A*: Extra-articular
  - *A1*: Simple
  - *A2*: Metaphyseal wedge
  - *A3*: Complex
- *33-B*: Partial articular (one condyle)
  - *B1*: Lateral condyle
  - *B2*: Medial condyle (e.g., Hoffa)
  - *B3*: Sagittal plane split
- *33-C*: Complete articular (bicondylar)
  - *C1*: Articular simple, metaphyseal simple
  - *C2*: Articular simple, metaphyseal multifragmentary
  - *C3*: Both articular + metaphyseal complex

Q42. Discuss the indications for locking plate fixation in distal femur fractures.

Indications
- Comminuted fractures
- Osteoporotic bone

- Periprosthetic fractures
- Metaphyseal-diaphyseal extension
- Fractures with poor bone stock or open injuries

Advantages
- Angular stability
- Less soft tissue stripping (MIPO technique)
- Suitable for poor bone quality

Q43. Write a short note on Hoffa fractures and their surgical management.

Definition
Coronal plane fracture of the **femoral condyle** (usually lateral)

Classification
- Part of AO 33-B2
- Letenneur classification (based on location and fragment size)

Management
- Always **surgical** (non-union risk with conservative treatment)
- *Approach*:
  - Lateral/medial parapatellar or posterior
  - Fixation with **lag screws** (antero-posterior or postero-anterior) ± plate

Q44. Classification and treatment of patellar fractures.

Classification
- Transverse (most common)
- Vertical
- Stellate/Comminuted
- Osteochondral
- Pole fractures (superior/inferior)

Management

Type	*Treatment*
Non-displaced	Cylinder cast or extension brace
Displaced with extensor lag	Tension band wiring (TBW)
Comminuted pole fracture	Partial patellectomy with repair
Osteochondral fragments	ORIF or excision

Q45. Management of knee dislocations and vascular injuries.

Types (Kennedy Classification)
- Anterior (most common)
- Posterior
- Medial, lateral
- Rotatory (rare)

Associated Injuries
- Popliteal artery (~40%)—limb-threatening
- Peroneal nerve (~25%)

Management Steps

1. Reduce immediately
2. Check pulses, Doppler/CTA
3. If vascular compromise → Emergency exploration
4. External fixator if grossly unstable or open
5. Definitive ligament reconstruction later

Q46. Indications and techniques for external fixation in knee injuries.

(*Source: Orthodnb.com*)

Indications

- Open fractures
- Polytrauma (damage control)
- Gross instability (e.g., fracture-dislocation)
- Compartment syndrome
- Soft tissue compromise

Technique (For Spanning Knee Fixator)

- Pins in **distal femur** and **proximal tibia**
- Avoid joint capsule
- Maintain ~10° knee flexion
- Convert to internal fixation once stable

Q47. Explain the management of multi-ligament knee injuries.

Definition

Injury to ≥2 major knee ligaments (ACL, PCL, MCL, LCL)

Initial Care

- Knee reduction and immobilization
- Vascular assessment critical (compartment pressure, pulses)

Definitive Care

- *Staged reconstruction preferred*:
  - Address extra-articular ligaments first (MCL, LCL)
  - ACL/PCL in second stage (4–6 weeks later)
- **Bracing and physiotherapy** critical in both stages

One-stage repair used in some centers with experienced teams.

Tibial Plateau and Shaft Fractures

Q48. Schatzker classification and management of tibial plateau fractures.

(Asked in: RGUHS Karnataka 2022, AIIMS Delhi 2021)

Introduction

- Tibial plateau fractures involve the **proximal tibial articular surface**.
- Caused by **axial loading** with **varus/valgus stress**.
- Important due to risk of **joint incongruity**, **instability**, and **post-traumatic arthritis**.

Schatzker Classification

Type	*Description*
I	Lateral plateau split fracture
II	Lateral plateau split + depression fracture
III	Lateral plateau pure depression fracture
IV	Medial plateau fracture
V	Bicondylar fracture (both medial and lateral plateaus)
VI	Plateau fracture with metaphyseal-diaphyseal dissociation

Management

Non-operative:

- *Indications*:
  - Undisplaced fractures (<2 mm step-off).
  - Stable knee joint.
- *Method*:
  - Long leg cast or hinged knee brace.
  - Non-weight bearing for 6–8 weeks.
  - Early passive ROM exercises.

Operative:

- *Indications*:
  - Displacement >2 mm
  - Depression >5 mm
  - Instability
  - Open fractures
  - Associated compartment syndrome.
- *Surgical options*:
  - ORIF with buttress plating (lateral/medial plating depending on fracture type).
  - Percutaneous cannulated screws (for simple split fractures).
  - Dual plating for bicondylar fractures.
  - Bone grafting/substitutes for depressed fractures.

Key Surgical Principles

- Restore joint congruity.
- Maintain mechanical axis.
- Allow early mobilization without compromising fixation.

Q49. Discuss the role of dual plate fixation in tibial plateau fractures.

Indications

- **Bicondylar fractures** (Schatzker V, VI)
- Posteromedial/lateral fragments
- Comminuted plateau with metaphyseal-diaphyseal extension

Advantages

- Provides **stable fixation** for both columns
- Allows early **mobilization** and weight-bearing
- Reduces malunion in **valgus/varus** injuries

Techniques

- Medial and lateral plates via dual incisions or MIPO approach
- Restoration of articular surface with elevation and bone grafting as needed

Key Points to Remember

- *Distal femur*: CT is essential for articular involvement; locking plates are preferred for osteoporotic bones.
- *Knee dislocation*: Always check for **popliteal artery** injury (Doppler/CT angiogram).
- *Tibial plateau*: Schatzker types V and VI require **dual plate** fixation.

Tibial Shaft Fractures

Q50. Management of open tibial shaft fractures.

(Asked in: JIPMER Puducherry 2022, CMC Vellore 2023)

Introduction

- Open tibial fractures are common due to **subcutaneous location** of the tibia.
- High risk of **infection, nonunion, and soft tissue complications**.

Classification

Gustilo–Anderson Classification:

Type	Description
I	Clean wound <1 cm
II	Wound >1 cm without extensive soft-tissue damage
IIIA	Extensive soft-tissue damage, adequate bone coverage
IIIB	Extensive periosteal stripping, requires soft-tissue flap
IIIC	Associated with vascular injury requiring repair

Management Steps

Emergency phase:

- ATLS protocol first.
- Broad-spectrum IV antibiotics ASAP (within 3 hours).
- Tetanus prophylaxis.
- **Irrigation and debridement**—remove all devitalized tissue.

Stabilization:

- External fixator as **temporary or definitive fixation** initially.
- Internal fixation (IM nailing or plating) once infection controlled (preferably within the "safe window" of 5–7 days).

Soft tissue coverage:

- Early soft tissue closure preferred (within 72 hours if possible).
- Local rotational flaps or free flaps for large defects (IIIB).

Definitive Fixation Options

Fracture type	Preferred fixation
Gustilo I/II	Early IM nailing
Gustilo IIIA	Debridement + early IM nailing if feasible
Gustilo IIIB	External fixator initially, delayed internal fixation after soft tissue coverage
Gustilo IIIC	Limb salvage versus amputation decision depending on vascular repair success

Key Points

- Early antibiotic + meticulous debridement are **cornerstones**.
- External fixation often used temporarily in contaminated wounds.
- Aim for union **without infection**.

Q51. Role of negative pressure wound therapy (NPWT) in open fractures.

(Asked in: BHU Varanasi 2022)

Definition

Negative pressure wound therapy (NPWT): Application of **sub-atmospheric pressure** (–75 to –125 mm Hg) to a wound via a sealed dressing connected to a vacuum pump.

Mechanism of Action

- Removes exudate and edema.
- Increases blood flow and granulation tissue formation.
- Reduces bacterial load.

Indications in Open Fractures

- After initial debridement, when immediate soft tissue coverage not possible.
- Temporary wound management before definitive closure or flap.
- Complex wounds with large soft tissue defects.

Advantages

- Decreases infection rates.
- Reduces need for repeated debridements.
- Helps bridge to flap coverage.
- Shortens hospital stay in some cases.

Limitations

- Should not delay definitive wound coverage beyond 5–7 days.
- Not a substitute for proper surgical debridement.

Q52. Classify tibial shaft fractures and discuss their management.

AO/OTA Classification (42 series)

- *Type A*: Simple (transverse, oblique, spiral)
- *Type B*: Wedge fractures
- *Type C*: Complex/comminuted or segmental fractures

Management Strategy

Patient/Fracture profile	*Preferred treatment*
Stable, closed, low-energy	Functional bracing or casting (rare today)
Unstable or displaced	Intramedullary nailing (IMN) (gold standard)
Comminuted, segmental	IMN or bridge plating
Polytrauma or open fracture	External fixation as temporary or definitive
Children	Elastic nailing (TENS) or casting

Q53. Explain the indications for intramedullary nailing in tibial fractures.

Indications

- Displaced diaphyseal fractures
- Segmental or comminuted fractures
- Pathological fractures
- Polytrauma requiring early mobilization
- Certain open fractures (after debridement)

Contraindications

- Skeletal immaturity
- Proximal or distal metaphyseal fractures with poor IMN control
- Active infection (relative)

Nail can be **reamed or unreamed** depending on soft tissue condition.

Q54. Write a short note on the complications of tibial shaft fractures.

Early Complications

- Compartment syndrome
- Open fractures → infection
- Neurovascular injury
- Fat embolism

Late Complications

- Non-union or delayed union (more common than femur due to subcutaneous bone)
- Malunion (varus/valgus deformities)
- Infection (especially in open or plated cases)
- Knee stiffness or anterior knee pain (post IM nailing)

Q55. Discuss the role of external fixation in tibial fractures.

Indications

- **Open fractures** (especially Gustilo type IIIB/C)
- **Severe soft tissue injury** (precluding internal fixation)
- **Polytrauma patients** (damage control orthopedics)
- **Temporary stabilization** in unstable patients

Types

- Uniplanar external fixator (bridging knee/ankle if needed)
- Circular fixators (ilizarov) for complex non-union or bone loss

Important for **soft tissue care**, **wound access**, and temporary stability.

Q56. Early and definitive management of open tibia fractures.

(Asked in: MUHS Maharashtra 2022, CMC Vellore 2023)

Early Management

Emergency room:

- Splint limb.
- IV antibiotics.
- Tetanus prophylaxis.
- Cover wound with sterile dressing.

Surgical debridement:

- Within 6 hours ideally ("golden period").
- Remove all devitalized tissue.

Temporary stabilization: External fixator if severe contamination or soft tissue compromise.

Definitive Management

Type I/II: Early **intramedullary nailing** after thorough debridement.

Type IIIA: Intramedullary nailing + soft tissue management (may require split skin graft).

Type IIIB:
- *Staged protocol*:
  - Initial external fixation.
  - Early flap coverage (muscle or free flap)—ideally within 72 hours.
  - Later conversion to internal fixation if needed.

Type IIIC:
- Immediate vascular repair.
- Decision between **limb salvage versus primary amputation** based on severity (mangled extremity severity score—MESS).

Important Points
- Early debridement and early soft tissue coverage decrease infection rates dramatically.
- Reamed nails preferred in adult open tibia fractures after wound control.

Q57. Explain the concept of tibial nonunion and its management.

(RUHS 2011)

Definition

Failure of fracture healing after **9 months** with no signs of progression over **3 months**.

Types
- *Hypertrophic (vascular)*: Mechanical instability
- *Atrophic (avascular)*: Biological deficit

Management

Type	*Treatment*
Hypertrophic	Exchange nailing, compression plating
Atrophic	Bone grafting + stable fixation
Septic	Debridement, antibiotics, staged reconstruction

Bone stimulators or BMPs may be used adjunctively.

Distal Tibia and Ankle Fractures

Q58. Classify distal tibia fractures and discuss their management.

AO Classification (43 Series)
- *Type A*: Extra-articular
- *Type B*: Partial articular (one part of the joint involved)
- *Type C*: Complete articular (joint surface and metaphysis)

Management

Fracture type	*Treatment modality*
Stable extra-articular	Cast immobilization (rare)
Unstable extra-articular	MIPO or ORIF
Intra-articular/pilon	Staged protocol—spanning external fixator → delayed ORIF
Open or high-energy	Initial external fixation, followed by definitive fixation

Q59. Explain the concept of pilon fractures and their treatment principles.

Definition

Comminuted intra-articular distal tibial fractures involving the plafond, often from axial loading (e.g., fall from height).

Treatment Principles

1. **Initial spanning external fixator** (to allow soft tissue recovery)
2. CT imaging for pre-operative planning
3. **Delayed ORIF** (7–14 days post-injury)
4. MIPO techniques to reduce soft tissue trauma
5. Bone grafting in metaphyseal voids (if required)

Avoid early ORIF to prevent wound complications.

Q60. Management of pilon fractures.

Definition

Fracture of distal tibia involving the articular surface, often with fibular fracture.

Management

- *Initial*:
  - Temporary spanning external fixator for soft tissue recovery.
  - Elevation, ice, and monitoring for compartment syndrome.
- *Definitive*:
  - ORIF once swelling subsides.
  - MIPO (minimally invasive) technique if soft tissues are fragile.
  - External fixation in highly comminuted cases or poor soft tissue.

Q61. Indications for ankle arthrodesis following trauma.

- Severe post-traumatic arthritis with pain and deformity.
- Failed ORIF or nonunion.
- Infection or avascular necrosis.
- Gross instability or deformity uncorrectable by soft tissue procedures.
- Charcot joint in selected cases.

Q62. Write a short note on the use of spanning external fixators in pilon fractures.

Purpose

Temporize fracture while soft tissues recover before ORIF

Advantages

- Reduces swelling
- Maintains length and alignment
- Protects joint reduction (ankle/spanning across ankle)
- Allows soft tissue monitoring and wound care

Timing

Typically used **for 7–14 days** before definitive surgery

Q63. Weber classification of ankle fractures—management principles.

(Asked in: PGI Chandigarh 2021, MUHS Maharashtra 2022)

Introduction

- Ankle fractures are among the **most common lower limb fractures**.
- Stability of the ankle depends mainly on the **relationship between the fibula, tibia, and syndesmosis**.

Weber (Danis–Weber) Classification: (Based on the Level of Fibular Fracture Relative to the Syndesmosis)

Type	*Description*
Weber A	Fracture below the syndesmosis
Weber B	Fracture at the level of syndesmosis
Weber C	Fracture above the syndesmosis

Management Principles

Weber A:

- Usually stable as syndesmosis is intact.
- *Non-operative treatment*:
  - Below-knee cast immobilization for 4–6 weeks.
  - Early weight-bearing as tolerated.

Weber B:

- May be stable or unstable.
- Stress radiographs or clinical judgment to assess syndesmotic stability.
- *Stable*: Conservative management (cast).
- *Unstable*: ORIF with plates and screws.

Weber C:

- Syndesmosis disrupted—always unstable.
- Requires ORIF for fibula + Syndesmotic screw fixation.
- Non-weight bearing until healing.

Important

Always assess for associated medial malleolus fracture or deltoid ligament injury—affects stability and decision-making.

Q64. Discuss the management of syndesmotic injuries of the ankle.

Diagnosis

- Positive squeeze test, external rotation test
- Widened tibiofibular clear space on imaging
- Confirmed with stress X-rays or weight-bearing CT

Management

Stability	*Treatment*
Stable	Conservative, cast immobilization
Unstable	Syndesmotic screw or suture-button fixation (TightRope)
Associated fracture	Fix the fracture and stabilize syndesmosis

Syndesmotic screws usually removed at 3–4 months post-operative.

Q65. Write a short note on the management of posterior malleolar fractures.

(AIIMS JPR 2011)

Indications for Fixation

- Fragment >25–30% of articular surface
- Posterior instability (posterior talar subluxation)
- Associated syndesmotic injury

Fixation Techniques

- **Posterolateral approach** preferred
- Direct reduction and **posterior-to-anterior screw** fixation
- Alternative: anterior indirect reduction with AP screws (less ideal)

Q66. Discuss the role of weight-bearing CT in evaluating ankle fractures.

Why Use It?
- Assesses **functional stability** of the syndesmosis and joint congruity
- Detects subtle malreductions not seen on non-weight-bearing imaging

Advantages
- Improved accuracy in evaluating **rotational malalignment**
- Superior to fluoroscopy and static X-rays in planning surgery
- Helpful in **post-operative assessment** of reduction and screw placement

Q67. Calcaneal fractures—mechanism, classification, radiology, management.

Mechanism of Injury
- High-energy axial load (e.g., fall from height).
- May be associated with spine or lower limb fractures.

Classification
- *Sanders classification (based on coronal CT through posterior facet)*:
  - *Type I*: Non-displaced
  - *Type II*: Two-part
  - *Type III*: Three-part
  - *Type IV*: Comminuted
- *Essex-Lopresti (based on X-ray)*: Tongue-type or joint-depression type.

Radiological Evaluation
- *X-rays*: Lateral, axial (Harris), and AP views of foot.
- *CT scan*: Gold standard for intra-articular assessment.

Management
- *Non-displaced*: Conservative with cast, elevation, and NWB.
- *Displaced intra-articular*: ORIF or minimally invasive fixation.
- *Comminuted/unfit patients*: Primary subtalar arthrodesis.

Q68. Classification and treatment of displaced intra-articular calcaneal fractures.

Classification
- *Sanders CT-based*:
  - *Type I*: Non-displaced
  - *Type II–IV*: Displaced (increasing severity/comminution)

Treatment
- *Acute*:
  - *Sanders I–II*: ORIF preferred.
  - *Type III–IV*: ORIF or primary fusion in low-demand patients.
- *Malunited*:
  - Corrective osteotomy
  - Subtalar arthrodesis if painful arthritis develops.
  - Bone grafting if necessary.

Q69. Write a short note on the role of open reduction and internal fixation (ORIF) in calcaneal fractures.

(KMC Manipal 2018)

Indications for ORIF
- Displaced intra-articular fractures with >2 mm step-off.

- Restoration of Bohler's angle (<20° suggests collapse).
- Open fractures or those with skin compromise.

Benefits
- Anatomical reduction of the subtalar joint.
- Restoration of heel height and alignment.
- Improved functional outcomes in selected patients.

Q70. Principles of fixation for calcaneal fractures.

- *Restore anatomy*: Length, height, width, and **Böhler's angle**.
- Reduce subtalar joint surface anatomically.
- *Stable fixation*: Plate and screws or minimally invasive methods.
- *Soft tissue care*: Wait for wrinkle sign before ORIF.
- *Rehabilitation*: Early ROM, delayed weight bearing (~10–12 weeks).

Q71. Talar fractures.

Introduction
- Talar fractures are **relatively rare** but **clinically significant** due to the talus's key role in ankle and hindfoot motion and its **delicate blood supply**.
- These fractures are often the result of **high-energy trauma** and carry a high risk of **complications** such as **avascular necrosis** (AVN) and post-traumatic arthritis.

Anatomy of the Talus
- *Divided into*: Head, neck, body, lateral process, and posterior process.
- *Articulations*:
  - Ankle joint (tibia and fibula with talar body)
  - Subtalar joint (talus and calcaneus)
  - Talonavicular joint (head of talus and navicular)
- *Blood supply*:
  - Posterior tibial artery → **artery of tarsal canal** (supplies body)
  - Dorsalis pedis → **artery of sinus tarsi**
  - Delicate intraosseous anastomosis—fractures can compromise perfusion, especially of the body.

Mechanism of Injury
- *Typically high-energy trauma*: RTA, fall from height.
- Forced **dorsiflexion** of the ankle often implicated in **talar neck fractures**.
- Snowboarders commonly sustain **lateral process fractures**.

Classification Systems

1. *Hawkins classification (for Talar neck fractures)*:

Type	Description	AVN Risk
I	Non-displaced	~0–15%
II	Subtalar dislocation	~40–50%
III	Subtalar + ankle dislocation	~90%
IV	Subtalar + ankle + talonavicular dislocation	~100%

2. *AO/OTA classification*:
- For body, neck, and process fractures.
- More comprehensive but less commonly used in clinical practice.

Clinical Features
- **Pain**, swelling, deformity of the ankle/hindfoot.
- **Inability to bear weight**.

- May present with **open wounds** or **associated dislocations.**
- Examine for **neurovascular compromise** and **compartment syndrome**.

Radiological Evaluation
- *X-rays*: AP, lateral, oblique ankle views. Can miss subtle fractures.
- *CT scan*: Gold standard—defines fracture pattern, displacement, comminution.
- *MRI*: For detecting **AVN** or subtle osteochondral injuries.

Management

A. *Non-displaced fractures (e.g., Hawkins type I)*
- *Conservative management*:
    - Short leg cast
    - Non-weight bearing for 6–8 weeks
    - Close radiological follow-up

B. *Displaced fractures (Hawkins II–IV, body fractures)*
- *Surgical management*:
    - **Urgent reduction** of dislocations to prevent AVN.
    - **Open reduction and internal fixation (ORIF)** with screws/plates.
    - *Approach*: anteromedial, anterolateral, or dual incision as needed.

C. *Lateral or posterior process fractures*
- *Small fragments*: Excision
- *Large or intra-articular*: ORIF

Post-operative Care
- Immobilization in a cast or boot.
- **Non-weight bearing for 8–12 weeks.**
- Regular monitoring with X-rays and/or MRI for signs of AVN.
- Gradual return to weight bearing once healing confirmed.

Complications
- *Avascular necrosis (AVN)*: Especially in displaced neck/body fractures.
- *Post-traumatic arthritis*: Subtalar and ankle joints.
- Malunion/Nonunion
- Infection, especially in open fractures.
- Osteonecrosis with collapse of talar dome
- Stiffness and chronic pain.

Prognosis
- Dependent on fracture type and quality of reduction.
- Non-displaced fractures have good outcomes.
- Displaced fractures with AVN may require salvage procedures like **arthrodesis** or **total ankle replacement** in the long term.

Q72. Discuss the surgical options for talus fractures.

Types of Talus Fractures
- *Neck fractures*: Most common; classified by Hawkins classification.
- *Body fractures*: Less common; often associated with high-energy trauma.

Surgical Options
- *ORIF*: Standard treatment for displaced fractures to restore joint congruity.
- *Arthrodesis*: Considered in cases with avascular necrosis or post-traumatic arthritis.
- *Delayed reconstruction*: For neglected or malunited fractures.

1. Management and Complications of Talar Neck Fractures

Management

- *Initial*: Immobilization, non-weight-bearing, urgent reduction if dislocated.
- *Definitive*:
  - *Non-displaced*: Cast and non-weight bearing.
  - *Displaced (Hawkins II–IV)*: Open reduction and internal fixation (ORIF) with screws or plates.
  - **CT scan** to assess comminution and alignment.

Complications

- Avascular necrosis (AVN)—most feared complication, especially Hawkins III–IV.
- Post-traumatic arthritis—subtalar and ankle joint.
- Malunion or nonunion
- Talar collapse
- Infection (in open fractures or post-surgery).

Dislocation of Talus

- Often due to high-energy trauma.
- May be total or subtalar dislocation.
- **Urgent reduction** is critical to preserve vascularity.
- Often requires ORIF.
- High risk of **AVN**, arthritis, and stiffness.

Lisfranc and Midfoot Injuries

Q73. Explain the management of navicular stress fractures.

Management

- *Conservative*: Non-weight-bearing cast immobilization for 6–8 weeks; effective in many cases.
- *Surgical*: Indicated for high-level athletes, nonunion, or when conservative treatment fails; involves internal fixation.

Q74. Lisfranc injury—diagnosis, classification and management.

(Asked in: AIIMS Delhi 2022, JIPMER Puducherry 2023)

Introduction

- *Lisfranc injury*: **Disruption of the tarsometatarsal joints.**
- *Mechanism*: Indirect trauma—axial load on plantarflexed foot (e.g., fall from height, sports injuries).
- **Critical to diagnose early** to prevent chronic instability and arthritis.

Diagnosis

Clinical:

- Midfoot swelling and bruising (especially plantar ecchymosis—classic sign).
- Pain on midfoot palpation and torsion stress.
- Inability to bear weight.

Radiology:

- X-rays (AP, oblique, lateral views).
  - *Key signs*:
    - Diastasis >2 mm between 1st and 2nd metatarsal bases.
    - Malalignment of medial cuneiform and base of 2nd metatarsal ("Fleck sign"—avulsion at Lisfranc ligament site).
- **Weight-bearing X-rays** if doubt persists.
- CT scan to assess fracture-dislocation details.

Classification

Hardcastle classification:

Type	*Description*
A	Total incongruity (homolateral displacement)
B	Partial incongruity (isolated medial or lateral displacement)
C	Divergent displacement (medial + lateral shift)

Myerson modified Hardcastle Classification—more detailed, currently favoured.

Management

Non-operative:

- *Indications*: Non-displaced injuries (<2 mm displacement).
- *Method*:
  - Below-knee cast.
  - Strict non-weight-bearing for 6–8 weeks.

Operative:

- *Indications*:
  - Any displacement >2 mm.
  - Instability under stress imaging.
- *Procedure*:
  - Open reduction and internal fixation (ORIF) with screws/plates.
  - Primary arthrodesis in severe ligamentous injuries (controversial but increasingly favoured).

Key Points

- **Early recognition** and **anatomic reduction** are crucial to avoid late arthritis.
- **Missed Lisfranc injuries** → poor outcomes.

Q75. Describe midfoot injuries and principles of treatment.

(Asked in: PGI Chandigarh 2022, KGMU Lucknow 2022)

Introduction

- Midfoot includes **tarsometatarsal joints (Lisfranc)**, **naviculocuneiform**, and **calcaneocuboid joints**.
- Injuries result from **high-energy trauma** (RTAs, falls).

Types of Midfoot Injuries

- Lisfranc injuries (TMT joint disruptions).
- Fracture-dislocations involving navicular or cuboid.
- Crush injuries.

Principles of Treatment

Diagnosis:

- High suspicion clinically.
- *Early imaging*: Weight-bearing X-rays, CT scan if necessary.

Non-operative treatment:

- *Indications*:
  - Non-displaced fractures.
  - Stable joints on stress testing.
- *Method*:
  - Below-knee cast immobilization.
  - Non-weight-bearing for 6–8 weeks.

Operative treatment:
- *Indications*:
  - Displaced fractures.
  - Midfoot instability.
- *Surgical options*:
  - ORIF with screws and/or plates to restore joint congruity.
  - Primary arthrodesis for purely ligamentous injuries or severe crush injuries (especially at Lisfranc joint).

Rehabilitation:
- Early ROM exercises after immobilization.
- Delayed weight-bearing until radiological union.

Key Points
- **Anatomic reduction** is critical in midfoot to restore normal foot arch and avoid arthritis.
- Untreated displacement → **chronic pain, flatfoot deformity, and arthrosis**.

Q76. Explain the classification and treatment of metatarsal fractures.

Classification
- *By location*: Base, shaft, neck, or head.
- *By displacement*: Nondisplaced or displaced.
- *Specific types*:
  - *Avulsion fractures*: Common at the base of the 5th metatarsal.
  - *Jones fractures*: Transverse fracture at the metaphyseal-diaphyseal junction of the 5th metatarsal.
  - *Stress fractures*: Often in the 2nd and 3rd metatarsals.

Treatment
- *Nondisplaced fractures*: Conservative management with immobilization and gradual weight-bearing.
- *Displaced fractures or multiple metatarsal fractures*: May require surgical fixation.

Q77. Write a short note on stress fractures of the foot and their management.

Common Sites
- Metatarsals (especially 2nd and 3rd).
- Navicular bone.
- Calcaneus.

Management
- *Low-risk fractures*: Rest, activity modification, and gradual return to activity over 6–8 weeks.
- *High-risk fractures*: May require non-weight-bearing immobilization or surgical intervention if conservative treatment fails.

Quick Mindmap: Lower Limb Trauma Revision
- *Lower limb trauma*:
  - *Pelvic ring injuries*: Tile Classification
  - *Acetabular fractures*:
    - Letournel classification
    - Surgical approaches
  - *Neck of femur and intertrochanteric*:
    - Garden Classification
    - DHS versus PFN
  - *Femoral shaft fractures*: Nailing principles
  - *Tibial plateau and shaft*:
    - Schatzker types
    - Gustilo classification (open fractures)

- *Ankle and calcaneum*:
  - Weber classification
  - Sanders classification
- *Midfoot injuries*:
  - *Lisfranc injuries*: Fleck sign

Soft Tissue Injuries and Ligamentous Injuries in the Lower Limb

Q78. Discuss the pathophysiology and treatment of quadriceps tendon rupture.

(AIMS Kochi 2011)

Pathophysiology

- Often occurs in patients >40 years, especially with chronic comorbidities (e.g., diabetes, renal failure).
- Rupture usually occurs 1–2 cm above the patella.
- *Mechanism*: Sudden eccentric contraction of quadriceps (e.g., trying to prevent a fall).

Clinical Features

- Inability to extend the knee actively.
- Palpable gap above the patella.
- Patella baja on X-ray.

Treatment

- *Acute rupture (<3 weeks)*: Surgical repair (end-to-end suture or suture anchors).
- *Chronic rupture*: Tendon reconstruction using autograft or allograft.

Q79. Explain the management of patellar tendon rupture.

Clinical Features

- Sudden pain and inability to extend the knee.
- Palpable gap below the patella.
- Patella alta on lateral radiograph.

Management

- *Surgical repair*:
  - Primary repair using non-absorbable sutures through transosseous tunnels in the patella.
  - Augmentation with wire or cerclage if needed.
- *Rehabilitation*: Immobilization followed by gradual physiotherapy focusing on ROM and quadriceps strength.

Q80. Write a short note on medial and lateral collateral ligament injuries of the knee.

MCL Injuries

- *Mechanism*: Valgus stress.
- *Grades*: I (mild sprain) to III (complete tear).
- *Treatment*:
  - *Grade I–II*: Conservative with bracing, rest, and physiotherapy.
  - *Grade III*: Often non-operative but may require repair if associated with multi-ligament injury.

LCL Injuries

- *Mechanism*: Varus stress.
- Often associated with posterolateral corner injuries.
- Grade III often needs surgical reconstruction.

Q81. Discuss the surgical and conservative management of Achilles tendon ruptures.

Conservative
- Indicated in sedentary individuals or those with comorbidities.
- Functional brace or cast in plantarflexion, followed by early mobilization protocols.

Surgical
- *Open repair*: Traditional method, higher risk of wound complications.
- *Percutaneous or minimally invasive repair*: Lower risk of wound issues, faster recovery.

Rehabilitation
- Early ROM exercises.
- Gradual weight-bearing.
- Return to sports in 4–6 months depending on strength and recovery.

Nerve and Vascular Injuries in Lower Limb Trauma

Q82. Write a short note on vascular injuries associated with lower limb fractures.

Common Scenarios
- *Femur fractures*: Profunda femoris artery injury.
- *Knee dislocations/tibial plateau fractures*: Popliteal artery.
- *Distal tibia fractures*: Anterior tibial artery.
- *Pelvic trauma*: Iliac vessels.

Signs
- Absent distal pulses
- Expanding hematoma
- Bruit/Thrill
- Cold, pulseless limb

Investigations
- Doppler ultrasound
- CT angiography (gold standard in trauma)

Management
- *Temporary*: Tourniquet or direct pressure
- *Definitive*: Vascular repair, bypass graft, or stenting + fracture stabilization

Q83. Discuss the indications for vascular repair in lower limb trauma.

(Kashmir University 2013)

Indications
- *Hard signs of vascular injury*:
    - Active bleeding
    - Pulsatile hematoma
    - Absent distal pulses
    - Limb ischemia
- Confirmed vessel disruption on CTA
- Associated open fractures with exposed vessels

Options
- Primary repair
- Vein graft (saphenous)

- Bypass grafting
- Temporary shunting (in DCO scenario)

Timing

Ischemia time >6 hours leads to high risk of limb loss (critical golden period).

Q84. Explain the role of fasciotomy in lower limb compartment syndrome.

Causes

- Tibial shaft fractures
- Crush injuries
- Reperfusion after prolonged ischemia

Clinical Features (6 P's)

- *P*ain out of proportion (earliest sign)
- *P*aresthesia
- *P*allor
- *P*ulselessness (late)
- *P*aralysis
- *P*oikilothermia

Diagnosis

Clinical + Compartment pressure measurement (>30 mm Hg or ΔP <30 mm Hg)

Surgical Fasciotomy

- *Two-incision, four-compartment fasciotomy for leg*:
    - *Lateral*: Anterior + lateral compartments.
    - *Medial*: Superficial and deep posterior compartments.

Post-operative

Wound left open or skin grafted later.

Summary Flowchart: Approach to Suspected Neurovascular Injury in Lower Limb Trauma

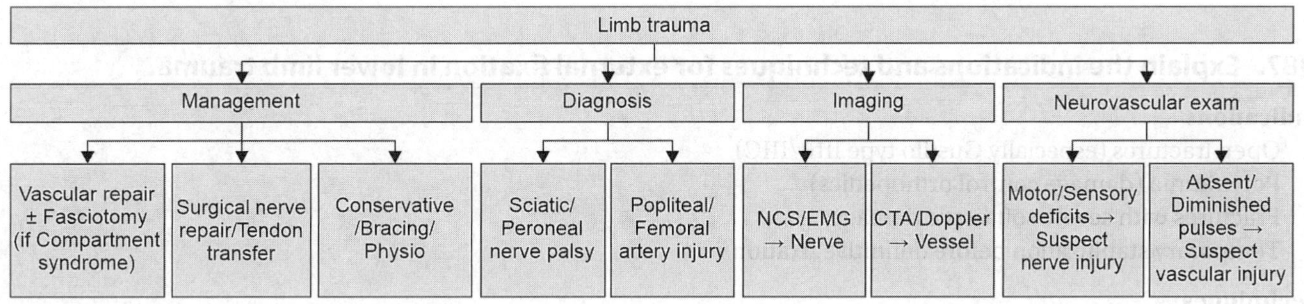

Q85. Discuss the complications of lower limb fractures and their prevention.

Early Complications

- Vascular injury
- Compartment syndrome
- Open fractures with infection risk
- DVT/PE

Late Complications

- Non-union/delayed union
- Malunion
- Joint stiffness
- Post-traumatic arthritis
- Chronic pain syndromes

Prevention Strategies
- Early fracture stabilization
- Prompt soft tissue care
- DVT prophylaxis
- Physiotherapy initiation
- Nutritional support

Q86. Write a short note on compartment syndrome of the lower limb.

(PGI Chandigarh)

Definition

A limb-threatening condition caused by **increased pressure within a closed osteofascial compartment**, impairing circulation and nerve function.

Classic Signs (6 P's)
1. *P*ain (disproportionate, on passive stretch)
2. *P*allor
3. *P*ulselessness (late)
4. *P*aresthesia
5. *P*aralysis
6. *P*oikilothermia

Diagnosis
- Clinical
- Compartment pressure >30 mm Hg or ΔP (diastolic—compartment pressure) <30 mm Hg

Management
- **Emergency fasciotomy**
- Avoid elevation
- Monitor renal function (rhabdomyolysis risk)

Q87. Explain the indications and techniques for external fixation in lower limb trauma.

Indications
- Open fractures (especially Gustilo type IIIB/IIIC)
- Polytrauma (damage control orthopedics)
- Fractures with severe soft tissue damage
- Temporary stabilization before definitive fixation

Techniques
- **Uniplanar or biplanar fixators**
- Pin insertion avoiding neurovascular bundles
- **Pin care** is vital to prevent pin-tract infections

Often used as a **bridge** to internal fixation or for definitive treatment in **severe soft tissue injury**.

Rehabilitation and Post-Trauma Recovery (Lower Limb)

Q88. Discuss the principles of rehabilitation following lower limb fractures.

Key Principles
- *Pain management*: NSAIDs, ice, elevation, nerve blocks.
- *Edema control*: Compression, elevation, lymphatic massage.

- *Joint mobility*: Early range of motion (ROM) to prevent stiffness.
- *Muscle strengthening*: Isometric initially, then isotonic exercises.
- *Functional training*: ADL retraining (e.g., standing, stair climbing).
- *Gait re-education*: With assistive devices (crutches, walker).
- *Psychological support*: For motivation and adherence.

Multidisciplinary Involvement
- Ortho surgeon
- Physiotherapist
- Occupational therapist
- Pain specialist

Q89. Explain the role of early weight-bearing in lower limb trauma recovery.

Benefits of Early Weight-bearing
- Stimulates **osteogenesis** and bone healing via Wolff's law.
- Prevents disuse atrophy and osteoporosis.
- Improves **circulation** and reduces DVT risk.
- Enhances **joint proprioception** and balance.

Indications
- Stable fracture fixation (e.g., IM nailing, locking plates)
- Post-operative hip arthroplasty

Caution

Avoid in cases of **non-union risk**, complex fractures, or poor fixation.

Q90. Write a short note on the importance of gait training after lower limb surgery.

Gait Training Goals
- Re-establish **normal walking pattern**
- Promote **symmetry and weight shift**
- Prevent abnormal compensations (e.g., hip hiking, circumduction)
- Improve **confidence** and reduce fall risk

Tools Used
- Parallel bars
- Crutches, walkers
- Weight-shifting exercises
- Mirror feedback or video-assisted correction

Stages
1. Non-weight bearing (NWB)
2. Partial weight bearing (PWB)
3. Full weight bearing (FWB)

Q91. Discuss the role of functional braces in tibial and femoral fractures.

Definition

Functional braces are orthoses that allow controlled motion at the fracture site while maintaining stability.

Common Uses
- Tibial shaft fractures (especially post-casting)
- Femoral shaft fractures during late healing phases

Advantages
- Encourages early mobility
- Enhances bone healing by micro-motion
- Reduces muscle atrophy and joint stiffness
- Cost-effective alternative to surgery in select cases

Types
- Patellar tendon-bearing (PTB) brace for tibia
- Sarmiento brace for femoral fractures

Q92. Explain the use of orthotics in lower limb fracture rehabilitation.

(NEIGRIHMS 2013)

Purpose of Orthotics
- Support weak joints
- Prevent deformities
- Aid in ambulation
- Improve alignment during healing

Common Orthoses
- *Ankle-foot orthosis (AFO)*: For foot drop due to peroneal nerve injury
- *Knee-ankle-foot orthosis (KAFO)*: For femur/tibia fractures in polio/post-trauma
- *Shoe lifts*: For limb length discrepancies post-fracture
- *Customized insoles*: Redistribute pressure, aid shock absorption

When to Use
- During **late healing phase** or in **neuromuscular deficits**
- Post-operative or post-casting recovery

FLOWCHART: Rehabilitation phases after lower limb fracture

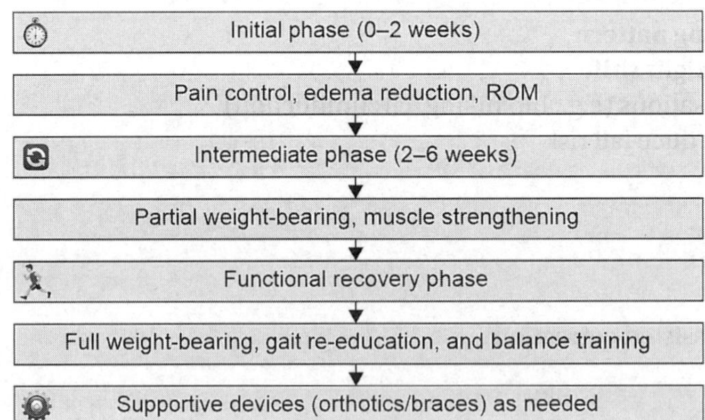

11.4 Spinal Trauma

Tahir Afzal, Pankaj Vir Singh

Basic Concepts and Biomechanics

Q1. Biomechanics of spinal injuries.

(RGUHS 2011)

Forces Acting on Spine
- Axial loading (compression)
- Flexion/Extension
- Shear
- Rotation/Torsion
- Distraction

Injury Mechanisms

Mechanism	*Common injury*
Flexion	Wedge fractures, anterior compression
Flexion-distraction	Chance fractures
Axial compression	Burst fractures
Rotation	Fracture-dislocation
Shear	Translational injuries
Hyperextension	Posterior element injury (elderly, ankylosed spine)

Injury pattern depends on force vector, energy, and spine segment involved.

Q2. Three-column theory by Denis (spinal trauma).

Denis' Three Columns (Thoracolumbar Spine)

Column	*Structures included*	*Role*
Anterior	Anterior half vertebral body, disc, ALL	Resists compression
Middle	Posterior half body, posterior annulus, PLL	Key stabilizer
Posterior	Pedicles, facets, lamina, spinous process,PLC	Resists tension, distraction

Clinical Relevance
- *Stable injury*: 1-column involved
- *Unstable injury*: ≥2 columns disrupted
- Middle column integrity is critical for surgical decision-making

Q3. Tension band principle—short note.

Definition
Posterior spinal elements resist flexion forces like a tension band.

Principle
- In flexion, anterior column compresses; posterior column distracts
- Posterior ligamentous complex (PLC) and bony arches act as a tension band to prevent excessive flexion or failure
- Helps maintain **kyphotic alignment and stability**

Surgical Application
- Posterior spinal instrumentation (e.g., rods, hooks) uses this principle
- Especially important in kyphosis correction, trauma fixation

Q4. Posterior ligamentous complex (PLC) in spine stability.

PLC Components
- Supraspinous ligament
- Interspinous ligament
- Ligamentum flavum
- Facet joint capsules

Importance
- Key tension band resisting flexion/distraction forces
- Damage leads to spinal instability (even if bones appear intact)
- Evaluated on MRI (best to assess disruption)

Clinical Implications
- PLC injury = **unstable injury**
- Often mandates surgical stabilization
- Present in **Chance fractures**, flexion-distraction injuries

Spinal Cord Injury and Stability Mechanisms

Q5. Role of the posterior ligamentous complex (PLC) in spine stability.

PLC Components
- Supraspinous ligament
- Interspinous ligament
- Ligamentum flavum
- Facet joint capsules

Function
- Acts as a **tension band** resisting flexion and distraction forces
- Maintains alignment and kyphotic control
- Key contributor to **posterior column** in Denis' three-column theory

Clinical Significance
- *PLC disruption*: **Unstable spine**
- Detected by MRI (discontinuity, edema)
- Critical in **Thoracolumbar Injury Classification and Severity Score (TLICS)**

TLICS factor	*PLC disruption*
0	Intact
2	Indeterminate
3	Definite disruption (requires surgery)

Q6. Concept of spinal cord injury without radiographic abnormality (SCIWORA).

Definition
Clinical evidence of spinal cord injury without evidence of fracture or dislocation on plain X-ray or CT.

Seen in
- **Pediatric patients** (especially <8 years)

- More elastic spine → transient subluxation causes cord damage
- Commonly cervical spine

Clinical Types
- Complete
- Incomplete (Brown-Sequard, anterior cord, central cord)

Investigations
MRI is gold standard (cord edema, hemorrhage, ligamentous injury)

Management
- Immobilization (rigid cervical collar)
- High-dose steroids (controversial)
- Early physiotherapy and rehabilitation

Q7. Mechanisms of spinal cord injury.

Mechanism	*Description*	*Common injuries*
Hyperflexion	Anterior compression, posterior tension	Wedge fracture, flexion teardrop, Chance fracture
Hyperextension	Posterior compression, anterior tension	Central cord syndrome (especially in elderly with spondylosis)
Axial loading	Vertical force causing burst of vertebral body	Burst fracture
Rotation	Twisting with shear	Fracture-dislocation
Distraction	Pulling forces, seen in seatbelt injuries	Chance fracture
Shearing	Translational forces	Dislocations, high-grade instability

These mechanisms often overlap in high-energy trauma.

Q8. Role of compensatory mechanisms in preventing spinal cord injury.

(DYPU Pune 2016)

Compensatory Mechanisms
- Mobility of vertebral column absorbs force
- Elasticity of spinal cord (especially in children)
- Dural slack accommodates minor vertebral displacement
- Wider spinal canal (e.g., in cervical spine) allows transient deformation
- *CSF cushioning*: Distributes compressive force
- *Ligamentous stretch*: Delays disruption

Relevance
- These mechanisms explain **SCIWORA** in children and **delayed onset** cord injury
- Loss of these compensations (e.g., in ankylosing spondylitis) leads to **higher injury risk**

Spinal Fracture Classifications

Q9. Denis classification of spinal fractures.

Based on the Three-column Theory (Thoracolumbar Spine)

Column	*Structures included*
Anterior	Anterior half vertebral body, disc, anterior longitudinal ligament (ALL)
Middle	Posterior half vertebral body, posterior annulus, posterior longitudinal ligament (PLL)
Posterior	Pedicles, laminae, spinous process, facet joints, posterior ligamentous complex (PLC)

Fracture Types

Type	Column involved	Description
Compression	Anterior	Wedge fracture
Burst	Anterior + Middle	Comminution, canal compromise
Seat-belt (Chance)	All three	Flexion-distraction
Fracture-dislocation	All three	Instability, translation

Unstable if ≥2 columns are involved (especially middle)

Q10. AO spine classification system for spinal trauma (thoracolumbar).

Modern, comprehensive system combining morphology, neurological status, and PLC integrity.

A. Morphological Types

Type	Description
A (Compression)	*A1*: Wedge *A2*: Split *A3*: Incomplete burst *A4*: Complete burst
B (Distraction)	*B1*: Posterior ligamentous injury *B2*: Anterior tension band (e.g., hyperextension) *B3*: Translational
C (Translation)	Translational/rotational displacement

Neurologic Status (N)

- *N0*: Intact
- *N1*: Transient deficit
- *N2*: Radicular
- *N3*: Incomplete spinal cord
- *N4*: Complete cord injury

Posterior Ligamentous Complex (PLC) Integrity (M)

- *M0*: Intact
- *M1*: Indeterminate
- *M2*: Disrupted

AO classification guides surgical decision-making more comprehensively than Denis.

Q11. Magerl classification of thoracolumbar fractures (short note).

Precursor to AO classification—based purely on **mechanism of injury**.

Types

Type	Mechanism	Subtypes
A	Compression	A1 (wedge), A2 (split), A3 (burst)
B	Distraction	B1 (posterior tension), B2 (anterior tension)
C	Rotation/Translation	C1–C3 depending on displacement

Later modified into **AO classification** by adding neurological and soft-tissue criteria.

Q12. Role of MRI in evaluation of spinal trauma.

(TNMGR Chennai 2022)

Introduction

MRI is essential for evaluating soft tissue and spinal cord injuries following trauma, which X-rays and CT often miss.

Indications for MRI in Spinal Trauma

- Neurological deficit not explained by X-ray/CT (e.g., SCIWORA)
- Suspected ligamentous injury
- Pre-reduction MRI in suspected disc herniation (before manipulating subluxations)
- Evaluation of spinal cord contusion/edema/hemorrhage

What MRI Detects

- Cord edema (T2 hyperintensity)
- Cord hemorrhage (poor prognosis)
- Disc herniations compressing cord
- Ligamentous injuries (anterior/posterior longitudinal ligament, ligamentum flavum, etc.)
- Epidural hematoma

MRI Sequences Useful

- T1/T2 weighted images
- STIR (for soft tissue injuries)
- Gradient Echo (for hemorrhage)

Quick Exam-oriented Table

MRI role	*Details*
Cord status	Edema, hemorrhage
Ligaments	PLC injuries
SCIWORA detection	MRI diagnosis essential
Pre-reduction planning	Disc herniation before reduction

Crisp Flowchart

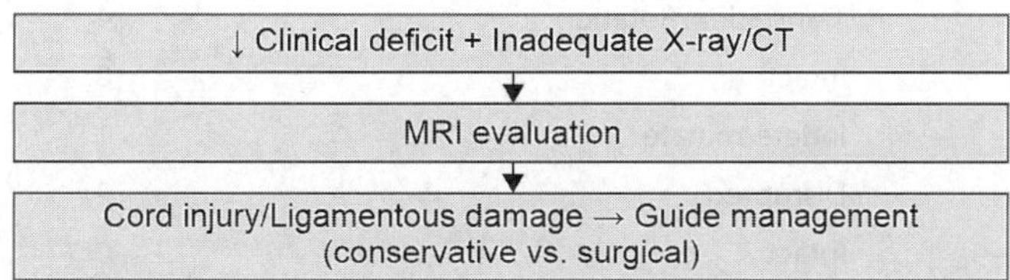

Spinal Classification Systems for Injury and Instability

Q13. Thoracolumbar injury classification and severity score (TLICS).

Purpose

Guides decision-making (conservative versus surgical) in thoracolumbar spine trauma.

Components

Category	*Description*	*Score*
Injury morphology	Compression	1
	Burst	2
	Translation/Rotation	3
	Distraction	4

Continued

Continued

Category	Description	Score
PLC integrity	Intact	0
	Suspected	2
	Definite injury	3
Neurologic status	Intact	0
	Nerve root injury	2
	Complete cord injury	2
	Incomplete cord injury	3
	Cauda equina	3

Total Score Interpretation

Total score	Treatment
≤ 3	Non-operative
4	Surgeon discretion
≥ 5	Surgical stabilization indicated

MRI is essential to evaluate PLC integrity.

Q14. Subaxial cervical spine injury classification system (SLIC).

Purpose

Management of subaxial (C3–C7) cervical spine injuries.

Components

Category	Description	Score
Injury morphology	Compression	1
	Distraction	3
	Translation/Rotation	4
Discoligamentous complex (DLC)	Intact	0
	Indeterminate	1
	Disrupted	2
Neurological status	Intact	0
	Root injury	1
	Complete cord injury	2
	Incomplete cord injury	3
	Ongoing cord compression	+1

Total Score Interpretation

Total score	Recommendation
< 4	Conservative
= 4	Surgeon discretion
> 4	Surgical fixation

Q15. White and Panjabi's classification of spinal instability.

Purpose

First biomechanical classification of spinal instability.

Parameters Evaluated

Factor	*Instability threshold*
Translation	>4.5 mm
Sagittal rotation	>11°
Kyphotic angulation	>20°
Vertebral body collapse	>50%
Disc space loss	>50%
Neurological status	Presence of deficit
Pain and deformity	Functional limitation

The system classifies **clinical and radiographic instability** and is used to assess surgical need.

Cervical Spine Trauma—Atlanto-occipital and Axial Injuries

Q16. Management of odontoid fractures in adults.

(Asked in: RGUHS 2023, MUHS 2023)

Classification (Anderson and D'Alonzo)
- *Type I*: Avulsion of the tip of dens (stable)
- *Type II*: Fracture at the base of the odontoid (most common, unstable)
- *Type III*: Fracture through body of C2 involving dens (better healing potential)

Mechanism
- High-velocity trauma (e.g., RTA)
- Falls in elderly (osteoporotic fractures)

Clinical Features
- Neck pain, limited range of motion
- Neurological symptoms (if associated cord injury)

Investigations
- X-ray cervical spine (AP, lateral, open-mouth odontoid view)
- CT scan for bony detail
- MRI for ligamentous injury or cord compromise

Management

Type I: Cervical collar immobilization

Type II:
- Difficult to heal; high nonunion risk
- *Young patients*: Anterior odontoid screw fixation (preserves rotation)
- *Elderly or poor bone quality*: Posterior C1–C2 fusion (Gallie/Brooks/Harms technique)
- *Non-surgical (for non-displaced fractures in high-risk surgical candidates):* Halo vest immobilization

Type III: Generally heals well with external immobilization (halo/cervical collar).

Complications
- Nonunion
- Pseudarthrosis
- Neurological deterioration if untreated

Q17. Describe SCIWORA—diagnosis and management principles.

(Asked in: JIPMER Puducherry 2022, MUHS Maharashtra 2023)

Definition

Spinal cord injury without radiographic abnormality (SCIWORA): Clinical evidence of spinal cord injury without abnormalities seen on plain X-rays or CT scans.

Epidemiology

- *More common in children due to*:
  - Ligamentous laxity,
  - Elastic spinal column,
  - Relatively large head size.

Mechanism

- Stretching of the spinal cord without bony injury during trauma.
- Hyperflexion, hyperextension, or axial loading forces.

Diagnosis

Clinical:
- Neurological deficits appearing immediately or delayed after trauma (within 48 hours).
- Symptoms range from mild sensory loss to complete paralysis.

Imaging:
- *X-ray/CT*: Normal.
- *MRI*: Investigation of choice.
  - Shows cord edema, hemorrhage, or ligamentous injury.

Management Principles

Acute management:
- Immobilization with rigid cervical collar or brace.
- Steroid use (high-dose methylprednisolone) remains controversial and institution-dependent.

Definitive management:
- *Conservative in most cases*:
  - Prolonged immobilization (6–12 weeks).
  - Gradual mobilization once healing confirmed.
- *Surgery only if*:
  - MRI shows cord compression due to herniated disc or instability.
  - Progressive neurological deterioration.

Rehabilitation:
- Early physiotherapy and occupational therapy essential.
- Long-term neurorehabilitation if persistent deficits.

Prognosis

- Better if MRI shows cord edema alone.
- Poorer outcome if hemorrhagic changes present.

Q18. Canadian C-spine rule.

- *Purpose*: Clinical decision tool to determine need for imaging after trauma.
- *High-risk criteria*: Age ≥65, dangerous mechanism, extremity paresthesias.
- *Low-risk criteria*: Simple rear-end collision, sitting position, ambulatory, delayed onset pain.
- *Neck rotation <45°*: Imaging required.

Q19. Halo traction in cervical spine injuries.

- *Used for*: Odontoid, Hangman's, facet dislocations.
- *Benefits*: Rigid immobilization, non-operative option.
- *Complications*: Pin loosening, infection, dysphagia.
- *Duration*: Usually 8–12 weeks.

Q20. Central cord syndrome.

- Common in elderly with spondylosis and hyperextension injury.
- *Findings*:
  - Upper limb weakness > lower limb.
  - Variable sensory loss.
  - Bladder dysfunction may occur.
- *Management*: Conservative initially; decompression surgery if needed.

Q21. Anterior cord syndrome.

- Due to anterior spinal artery infarction or flexion/compression trauma.
- *Loss of*:
  - Motor function.
  - Pain and temperature below the lesion.
- *Preserved*: Proprioception and vibration.
- Poor prognosis.

Q22. Brown–Séquard syndrome.

- Hemisection of the spinal cord, often from penetrating trauma.
- *Ipsilateral*: Motor loss, proprioception, vibration.
- *Contralateral*: Pain and temperature loss.

Prognosis
Best among incomplete cord injuries; many regain function with rehabilitation.

Q23. Management of atlanto-occipital dislocation (AOD).

Definition
Disruption of occiput-C1 articulation → highly unstable and often fatal.

Types
- Anterior (most common)
- Posterior
- Vertical (worst prognosis)

Diagnosis
- *CT scan*: Measure **basion-dens interval (BDI)** >12 mm
- *MRI*: Evaluate tectorial membrane, alar ligament
- *Radiographs*: Harris criteria, Powers ratio (>1 = AOD)

Management

Step	***Description***
Emergency immobilization	Hard collar or halo (initial)
Surgical stabilization	Occipitocervical fusion (O-C2 or O-C3)

Continued

Continued

Step	Description
Avoid traction	May worsen injury
Neurological monitoring	High spinal cord injury risk

Most patients require **early surgical fixation**.

Q24. Classification and treatment of atlantoaxial fractures.

Fractures at C1-C2 junction include:
- Jefferson fracture (C1 burst)
- Odontoid fracture (C2 peg)
- Hangman's fracture (C2 pedicle)

Classification Summary

Injury	Type	Management
Jefferson	C1 ring fracture (usually 4-part)	Halo for stable, fusion if unstable
Odontoid	Anderson and D'Alonzo (Type I–III)	See Q25
Hangman's	Levine-Edwards	See Q26
C1-C2 dislocation	Ligamentous disruption	Posterior C1–C2 fusion

Key to management: **Assess transverse ligament** for instability.

Q25. Odontoid fractures—Anderson and D'Alonzo classification and management.

Type	Description	Treatment
I	Avulsion of tip (alar ligament)	Hard collar
II	Base of dens (most common, unstable)	*Controversial*: Surgery (lag screw or posterior C1–C2 fusion) preferred in elderly/nonunion
III	Extends into C2 body	Better healing → halo or rigid collar

Type II has highest risk of nonunion due to poor blood supply.

Q26. Hangman's fracture—pathophysiology and treatment.

(Asked in: RGUHS 2023)

Definition

Traumatic bilateral fracture of C2 pars interarticularis.

Mechanism

- Hyperextension + distraction
- Seen in MVAs, suicidal hanging

Classification (Levine–Edwards)

Type	Features	Treatment
I	<3 mm translation, no angulation	Rigid collar or halo
II	>3 mm displacement or angulation	Halo or posterior fusion
IIA	Angulation >11° with minimal displacement (flexion-distraction)	Posterior C2–C3 fusion
III	Facet dislocation at C2–C3	Surgical fixation (anterior/posterior)

Avoid traction in Type IIA. Most unstable fractures need posterior stabilization.

Lower Cervical and Evaluation Tools

Q27. Facet dislocations of the cervical spine—short note.

Definition

Dislocation of facet joints usually due to flexion-distraction and/or rotation trauma.

Types

Type	*Description*
Unilateral	<25% translation, stable
Bilateral	>50% anterior translation, unstable, often cord injury

Clinical Features

- Neck pain, deformity
- Neurologic deficits (often severe in bilateral)

Radiology

- *X-ray*: Perched/locked facets, step-off
- *CT*: Precise fracture detail
- *MRI*: Disc herniation, ligament injury

Management

Injury	*Treatment*
Unilateral	Traction + reduction; posterior fusion if unstable
Bilateral	Early reduction (closed/open), followed by fixation (anterior/posterior)

Avoid closed reduction if MRI shows large disc herniation.

Q28. Jefferson fracture—management.

Definition

Burst fracture of C1 (atlas) involving anterior and posterior arches, usually due to axial loading.

Diagnosis

- **CT scan** is gold standard
- Open ring on odontoid view (lateral mass displacement)

Stability Check

- Transverse ligament integrity = key to stability
- **Lateral mass displacement >7 mm** → ligament rupture

Management

Stability	*Treatment*
Stable	Hard collar or Philadelphia collar (6–12 weeks)
Unstable	Halo vest or C1–C2 posterior fusion

Avoid traction in suspected ligament disruption.

Q29. Canadian C-spine rule—importance in evaluation.

Purpose

Rule out cervical spine injury in alert, stable trauma patients to avoid unnecessary radiographs.

Stepwise Rule

1. *High-risk factors*: Imaging
   - Age ≥65
   - Dangerous mechanism (fall >3 ft, axial load, MVA at high speed)
   - Paresthesia in extremities
2. *Low-risk factors*: Safe ROM check
   - Simple rear-end MVC
   - Sitting position in ED
   - Ambulatory at any time
   - Delayed neck pain
   - Absence of midline tenderness
3. *Active neck rotation >45°*: No imaging

Validated tool with >**99% sensitivity** for cervical spine injury.

Q30. Role of Halo traction in cervical spine fracture management.

Definition

Rigid external fixation system that immobilizes the head and cervical spine.

Indications

- Type II odontoid fractures (young/stable)
- Jefferson fracture (stable or reducible)
- Hangman's fracture (type I, II)
- Distraction reduction (pre-operative in dislocations)
- Non-surgical candidates

Components

- Halo ring (fixed to skull)
- Vest with uprights
- Pins (4–6)

Complications

- Pin site infection
- Loosening, overdistraction
- Dysphagia
- Skull perforation (rare)

Provides **360° cervical immobilization**, especially useful in C1–C2 injuries.

Thoracic and Thoracolumbar Spine Trauma

Q31. Classify thoracolumbar fractures and discuss their management.

(Himachal Pradesh University Shimla 2016)

Most used classification: **AO Spine Classification**

AO Thoracolumbar Classification

Type	*Description*	*Examples*
A	Compression	*A1*: Wedge: *A3/A4*: Burst
B	Distraction	*B1*: Flexion-distraction (Chance)
C	Translation/rotation	Unstable dislocations

Management Based on TLICS

TLICS score	*Approach*
≤3	Conservative (brace, rest)
=4	Surgeon discretion
≥5	Surgical fixation (posterior/anterior)

MRI is essential for PLC status; neurological status dictates urgency.

Q32. Concept of burst fractures and treatment principles.

Burst Fracture

Compression injury causing vertebral body fragmentation and canal compromise.

Features

- Axial load + flexion
- Retropulsion of fragments into spinal canal
- Common at T12–L1

Key Assessment

- Vertebral height loss
- Canal compromise on CT/MRI
- PLC integrity
- Neurologic status

Treatment

Stability	*Management*
Stable, no deficit	Brace or TLSO
Unstable or neuro deficit	Posterior pedicle screw fixation ± decompression
Severe comminution or kyphosis	Anterior + posterior fusion may be needed

Q33. Chance fracture—short note.

Definition

Flexion-distraction injury involving all 3 columns (bony or ligamentous).

Mechanism

- Seat-belt injury (lap belt), especially in MVC
- Flexion around a fulcrum

Imaging

- Horizontal fracture through posterior elements (CT)
- *MRI*: PLC and disc status

Management

Type	*Treatment*
Bony Chance fracture	Brace (TLSO) 8–12 weeks
Ligamentous or unstable	Posterior instrumentation and fusion
With abdominal injury	Multidisciplinary care (often associated with bowel trauma)

Unstable if PLC or disc disrupted → surgery needed.

Q34. Role of vertebroplasty and kyphoplasty in thoracic spine fractures.

Indications

Osteoporotic vertebral compression fractures (VCFs) causing pain/disability.

Vertebroplasty

- Injection of cement (PMMA) into collapsed vertebra
- Stabilizes microfractures
- Pain relief in 1–2 days

Kyphoplasty

- Balloon insertion → height restoration → cement injection
- Preferred if height loss or kyphotic deformity present

Indications

- Painful osteoporotic VCF unresponsive to conservative treatment
- Vertebral hemangioma
- Myeloma or metastasis with collapse

Complications

- *Cement leakage*: Neural compression, pulmonary embolism
- Adjacent segment fracture

Not used for unstable burst fractures or posterior wall compromise.

Advanced Spine Trauma Management

Q35. Role of vertebroplasty and kyphoplasty in thoracic spine fractures.

Used in **stable, osteoporotic vertebral compression fractures (VCFs)**—See previous detailed answer.

Q36. Role of minimally invasive spine surgery (MISS) in spinal trauma.

Minimally invasive spine surgery (MISS) refers to using percutaneous, muscle-sparing techniques with image-guided navigation for fracture fixation or decompression.

Applications in Trauma

Indication	*Procedure*
Unstable burst fractures	Percutaneous pedicle screw fixation
Fractures with canal compromise	MISS decompression (e.g., tubular laminectomy)
Pathological fractures	Kyphoplasty/vertebroplasty
Polytrauma	Early stabilization with minimal morbidity

Advantages

- Reduced blood loss, shorter hospital stay
- Less postoperative pain and infection risk
- Early mobilization
- Ideal in elderly or high-risk patients

Limitations

- Steep learning curve

- Radiation exposure
- Limited by severe deformity or multi-column injury

Q37. Indications for short-segment versus long-segment fixation in thoracolumbar fractures.

- *Short-segment fixation*: One level above and below fracture
- *Long-segment fixation*: ≥2 levels above and below

Comparison Table

Criteria	*Short-segment*	*Long-segment*
Indications	Isolated burst fracture, intact PLC, good bone	Severe comminution, multilevel injury, osteoporosis
Stability	Less stable in severe burst	More rigid and kyphosis-preventing
Motion preservation	Better	Less (more segments fused)
Implant strain	Higher risk of implant failure	Less risk
Common additions	Intermediate screws at fracture level	Often not needed

Current Trend

- **Short-segment with intermediate screws** at fracture level improves biomechanics
- Used commonly in **AO type A3/A4 fractures** with minimal posterior ligament disruption

Thoracolumbar Burst and Flexion-sistraction Injuries

Q38. Clinical and radiological evaluation of unstable burst fractures.

[Dr Ram Manohar Lohia Institute of Medical Sciences (RMLIMS) Lucknow 2011]

Burst Fracture

Axial compression injury with posterior wall involvement and possible retropulsion into spinal canal.

Clinical Evaluation

- History of fall from height or axial load
- Midline back pain, tenderness
- Step deformity or gibbus
- Neurological deficits (paraparesis/paraplegia) → important prognostic marker
- Associated polytrauma (calcaneal, pelvic fractures)

Radiological Evaluation

Modality	*Key Findings*
X-ray (AP/lateral)	Loss of vertebral height, kyphosis, increased interpedicular distance
CT scan	Fragment comminution, retropulsion into canal, canal compromise
MRI	PLC integrity (critical for stability), spinal cord compression, disc injury

Unstable Features

- Involvement of >50% vertebral body height
- >30° kyphosis
- >50% canal compromise
- PLC disruption on MRI
- Neurological deficit
- TLICS ≥5

Q39. Management of burst fractures of the spine.

Management depends on **stability, neurology, and TLICS score.**

Conservative Management

- **Stable fracture**, intact PLC, neurologically normal
- **Brace** (TLSO) for 8–12 weeks
- Serial imaging and neuro monitoring

Surgical Management

Indication	*Procedure*
Unstable burst fracture	Posterior pedicle screw fixation
Neurological deficit	Decompression ± stabilization
Severe kyphosis (>30°)	Posterior fusion with or without osteotomy
Retropulsed fragments with deficit	Anterior decompression ± corpectomy + cage + posterior stabilization

Preferred construct: **Short-segment fixation with intermediate screws** at fracture level for added stability.

Q40. Management of flexion-distraction injuries (e.g., Chance fracture).

These are **posterior column injuries** due to flexion around a fulcrum (e.g., seatbelt injuries).

Classification

- *Bony chance fracture*: Horizontal fracture of vertebra including posterior elements
- *Ligamentous chance fracture*: Involves PLC and disc without bony continuity

Diagnosis

- *X-ray*: Horizontal fracture line, widened interspinous space
- *CT*: Bony integrity
- *MRI*: Assess **PLC and disc status**

Treatment

Type	*Treatment*
Bony injury (intact PLC)	Brace (TLSO) 10–12 weeks
Ligamentous or disc injury	Posterior pedicle screw fixation (2 above and 2 below if unstable)
Neurological deficit	Decompression + stabilization
Associated intra-abdominal injury	Delay surgery, multidisciplinary care

Surgery is Indicated If

- Kyphosis >20°
- Disruption of PLC
- Neurological deficit
- Multi-level injury

Lumbar Spine Trauma

Q41. Biomechanics of lumbar spine injuries.

(West Bengal University of Health Sciences Kolkata 2016)

The lumbar spine is designed to provide **stability and flexibility** to the trunk while transmitting axial loads.

Key Biomechanical Concepts

- *Motion segments*: Each lumbar motion segment includes two vertebrae and the intervening disc.

- *Weight bearing*: Primarily through vertebral bodies and intervertebral discs
- *Facet joints*: Resist shear and rotation
- *Posterior ligamentous complex (PLC)*: Acts as a tension band in flexion

Mechanisms of Injury

Force type	*Resulting injury*
Axial compression	Burst fractures
Flexion-distraction	Chance fractures
Shear and rotation	Fracture-dislocations
Hyperextension	Pars injuries, spondylolysis

Biomechanical failure depends on the **magnitude and direction** of force, bone quality, and ligament integrity.

Q42. Lumbar flexion-distraction injuries—short note.

Often referred to as **Chance fractures** at the thoracolumbar junction (T12–L2).

Mechanism
- Hyperflexion around a fixed fulcrum (e.g., seatbelt injury)
- Common in MVAs with lap belts

Features
- Horizontal fracture through posterior elements
- Can be **bony**, **ligamentous**, or **mixed**
- May be associated with **abdominal organ injury**

Management

Type	*Treatment*
Bony fracture (stable)	Brace (TLSO) for 10–12 weeks
Ligamentous/Posterior column disruption	Posterior pedicle screw fixation
Associated neurological deficit	Decompression + fixation
Abdominal trauma	Surgical delay ± coordination with general surgery

MRI is critical for evaluating soft tissue and ligamentous integrity.

Q43. Classification and management of lumbar burst fractures.

Burst Fracture
Vertebral body fracture due to axial load with retropulsion of fragments.

Classification (AO Spine)

Type	*Description*
A3	Incomplete burst (one endplate)
A4	Complete burst (both endplates)

Evaluation
- *CT scan*: Assess canal compromise, bony fragments
- *MRI*: PLC disruption, spinal cord involvement

Instability Factors
- Loss of vertebral height >50%
- Kyphosis >30°

- Canal compromise >50%
- Neurological deficit
- PLC injury (confirmed on MRI)

Management

Criteria	*Treatment*
Stable, neurologically intact	Brace or TLSO
Unstable (PLC rupture, kyphosis, deficit)	Posterior instrumentation ± decompression
Severe canal compromise with deficit	Anterior corpectomy + cage + posterior stabilization

Advanced Lumbar Spine Trauma Management

Q44. Conservative versus Surgical management of lumbar fractures.

(Assam Medical College Dibrugarh 2012)

Conservative Management

Indications:
- Stable fractures (no PLC disruption)
- Minimal kyphosis (<20°)
- Intact neurology
- TLICS score ≤3

Modalities:
- TLSO brace for 8–12 weeks
- Activity modification
- Serial imaging + neuro monitoring

Advantages:
- Non-invasive
- Preserves spinal mobility

Limitations:
- Poor compliance
- Progressive deformity risk
- Delayed neurological deterioration (rare)

Surgical Management

Indications:
- Neurological deficit
- Instability (PLC rupture, kyphosis >30°)
- Retropulsed fragment compressing canal
- TLICS ≥5

Goals:
- Decompression
- Stabilization
- Early mobilization

Approaches:
- Posterior pedicle screw fixation
- Anterior corpectomy + cage (for severe canal compromise)
- Minimally invasive fixation (in selected cases)

Role in Decision-making
- Helps differentiate **burst fracture from stable compression**
- Identifies **ligamentous Chance injuries**
- Contraindication for closed reduction if significant disc herniation seen in facet dislocations

Q45. Principles of lumbar spine fusion in unstable fractures.

Fusion aims to **restore spinal stability** in the face of instability or neurological compromise.

Indications for Fusion
- PLC disruption
- Recurrent/Progressive instability
- Multi-column injuries
- Failed conservative treatment
- Revision surgery

Principles

Principle	*Description*
Restore alignment	Correction of kyphosis/lordosis
Rigid fixation	Pedicle screws and rods
Neural decompression	If neurological deficit present
Fusion bed preparation	Endplate decortication, use of graft
Graft material	Autograft (iliac crest) or allograft or cages
Avoid excessive motion segments	Minimize loss of mobility

Types of Fusion
- Posterolateral fusion (most common)
- *Interbody fusion (TLIF/PLIF)*: Restores anterior column
- *Combined anterior + posterior*: For severe cases (e.g., corpectomy)

Spinal Cord Injury (SCI) and Neurological Deficits

Q46. Pathophysiology of acute spinal cord injury.

SCI involves **primary** and **secondary** injury phases.

Primary Injury
- Occurs at time of trauma
- Mechanical damage: compression, contusion, shear, laceration
- Disruption of axons, blood vessels, membranes

Secondary Injury
Begins within minutes, continues for days–weeks

Process	*Effect*
Ischemia and hypoxia	↓ Perfusion leads to further neural injury
Excitotoxicity	Excess glutamate → Ca^{2+} influx → neuronal apoptosis
Inflammation	Cytokines, neutrophils, macrophages → edema
Lipid peroxidation	Cell membrane degradation
Demyelination	Conduction failure

Target of most interventions: Limit secondary injury

Q47. American Spinal Injury Association (ASIA) impairment scale.

[Institute of Medical Sciences Banaras Hindu University (BHU) Varanasi 2019]

Standardized system to classify severity of SCI.

ASIA Impairment Scale (AIS)

Grade	*Description*
A	*Complete*: No sensory or motor function in S4–S5
B	*Incomplete*: Sensory preserved below level including S4–S5, no motor
C	*Incomplete*: Motor preserved below level; >50% muscles < grade 3
D	*Incomplete*: Motor preserved; ≥50% muscles ≥ grade 3
E	Normal sensory and motor function

Neurological Level
Most caudal segment with **normal motor and sensory** function on both sides

ASIA is used for prognosis and monitoring recovery.

Q48. Role of steroids in acute spinal cord injury.

Methylprednisolone was historically used to reduce secondary injury.

NASCIS-2 Protocol
- 30 mg/kg IV bolus over 15 minutes
- Then 5.4 mg/kg/h infusion for 23 hours
- Initiate within **8 hours of injury**

Current Evidence
- *Controversial due to risk of*:
  - Sepsis
  - GI bleeding
  - Delayed wound healing

Current Recommendations
- **Not routinely recommended**
- May be considered in **select cases** after risk-benefit assessment (per AANS guidelines)

Focus now on early surgery, hemodynamic support, and neuroprotective trials.

Q49. Spinal shock versus neurogenic shock—short note.

Feature	*Spinal shock*	*Neurogenic shock*
Definition	Temporary loss of spinal cord reflexes below injury	Distributive shock due to loss of sympathetic tone
Cause	SCI (especially complete)	Cervical or upper thoracic SCI (T6 and above)
Duration	Hours to weeks	Acute—minutes to days
Signs	Flaccid paralysis, areflexia, loss of autonomic function	Hypotension, bradycardia, warm dry skin
End of shock	Return of bulbocavernosus reflex	Stabilization of vitals
Management	Supportive	Fluids, vasopressors (norepinephrine), atropine

Both can coexist in cervical spine trauma.

Advanced Spinal Cord Injury Management

Q50. Management of autonomic dysreflexia in SCI patients.

(Narayana Medical College Nellore Andhra Pradesh 2017)

Autonomic dysreflexia (AD) is a life-threatening sympathetic overactivity in patients with SCI at or above T6.

Triggers
- Bladder distension (most common)
- Bowel impaction
- Pressure sores
- Ingrown toenails, tight clothing

Symptoms
- Severe hypertension
- Bradycardia
- Pounding headache
- Flushing, sweating above lesion level
- Blurred vision, anxiety

Management (Acute)
1. *Sit patient upright*: ↓ BP
2. *Remove noxious stimuli*:
   - Check Foley catheter (kinks, obstruction)
   - Rectal exam for impaction
3. *Pharmacologic*:
   - Nifedipine (sublingual)
   - Nitroglycerin paste
   - Avoid beta-blockers (risk of unopposed α-adrenergic activity)

Prevention
- Regular bowel/bladder regimen
- Avoid tight clothing
- Educate patient/caregivers

Q51. Long-term complications of spinal cord injury.

System	*Complications*
Neurological	Chronic pain, spasticity, neuropathic pain
Urological	Neurogenic bladder, UTI, stones, renal failure
Gastrointestinal	Constipation, autonomic dysreflexia
Musculoskeletal	Contractures, heterotopic ossification, osteoporosis
Cardiovascular	DVT, PE, orthostatic hypotension
Skin	Pressure ulcers
Psychological	Depression, anxiety, loss of self-esteem
Sexual	Erectile dysfunction, fertility issues

Multidisciplinary long-term care is essential.

Q52. Role of neuroprotective agents in spinal cord injury—short note.

Neuroprotective agents aim to **limit secondary injury** and preserve neural tissue.

Current Investigational Agents

Agent	*Mechanism*
Methylprednisolone	Anti-inflammatory, antioxidant (controversial)
Riluzole	Sodium channel blocker—reduces glutamate toxicity
Minocycline	Inhibits microglial activation
GM1 ganglioside	Enhances neuroplasticity
Hypothermia	Reduces metabolic demand, limits inflammation
Stem cell therapy	Experimental—axonal regeneration

Most are under clinical trials—not yet standard care.

Q53. Pathophysiology and stages of spinal shock.

Spinal Shock

Temporary areflexia and loss of motor/sensory/autonomic function below injury level.

Pathophysiology

- *Disruption of descending excitatory inputs*—loss of reflex arcs
- Neurons become hyperpolarized—unresponsive
- Gradual re-emergence as excitability returns

Stages of Spinal Shock

Stage	*Duration*	*Features*
I: Areflexia	0–1 day	Flaccid paralysis, areflexia
II: Initial reflex return	1–3 days	Some reflexes (bulbocavernosus) reappear
III: Early hyperreflexia	4 days–1 month	Hyperexcitability, polysynaptic reflexes
IV: Spasticity	1–12 months	Monosynaptic reflexes return, spasticity develops

End of spinal shock

Return of **bulbocavernosus reflex**.

Q54. Management principles in traumatic spinal cord injury (TSCI).

Goal

Prevent secondary damage, decompress cord, stabilize spine, rehabilitate patient.

Initial Management (ATLS Protocol)

- Airway with cervical spine protection
- *Breathing*: Monitor respiratory effort (diaphragmatic function, especially in C4 and above)
- *Circulation*: Avoid hypotension, maintain MAP >85 mm Hg

Specific Management

Step	*Principle*
Immobilization	Hard collar/spine board initially
Imaging	X-ray, CT, MRI (for soft tissue and cord)
Steroids	Not routinely recommended (see NASCIS-2)
Surgery	Early decompression + stabilization (<24 hours) improves outcome
Medical	DVT prophylaxis, catheter care, pressure sore prevention
Rehabilitation	Begin as early as medically feasible

Q55. Spinal cord injury without radiographic abnormality (SCIWORA).

Seen in **children**, due to flexible spinal column but vulnerable cord

Diagnosis

Imaging	*Findings*
X-ray/CT	Normal
MRI	Cord edema, hemorrhage, ligament injury
Clinical	Motor/sensory deficit ± delayed onset

Pathophysiology
- Stretching of cord without bony damage
- Often involves **hyperextension**

Management
- Immobilization (cervical collar for 3–6 months)
- Steroids—controversial, not routine
- Activity restriction
- Rehabilitation for deficits
- Serial neurological monitoring

Prognosis
Good in mild cases, guarded if hemorrhage or persistent deficit.

Assessment and Imaging in Spinal Trauma

Q56. Role of X-ray, CT, and MRI in evaluating spinal fractures.

(GMCJ 2013)

Modality	*Role*	*Limitations*
X-ray	First-line for screening; detects gross fractures, alignment	Low sensitivity for subtle injuries
CT	Gold standard for bony injury; 3D recon useful for planning surgery	Poor soft tissue detail
MRI	Best for soft tissues, cord, ligaments, disc, edema	Longer scan time, expensive

When to prefer MRI
- Suspected ligamentous injury
- Neurological deficit without CT/X-ray findings
- Assess spinal cord injury severity
- Evaluate epidural hematoma or disc herniation

Q57. Importance of STIR sequences in spinal trauma MRI—short note.

STIR: Short tau inversion recovery (fat-suppressed T2 sequence).

Advantages in Trauma
- Enhances detection of **bone marrow edema**
- Highlights **soft tissue edema**
- Differentiates acute versus chronic fractures
- Detects ligamentous injuries and paraspinal muscle damage

Crucial for diagnosing occult or non-displaced fractures not seen on CT.

Q58. Concept of dynamic flexion-extension radiographs in cervical spine injuries.

Used to evaluate occult instability in cervical spine, especially in
- Whiplash injuries
- Post-trauma with normal static imaging

Key Points
- Must be done **under supervision** after excluding gross instability
- Dynamic lateral X-rays taken in **active flexion and extension**
- *Helps identify*:
  - **Ligamentous instability**
  - Delayed dislocations
  - Subtle subluxations

Contraindicated in acute phase with pain or neurological deficit.

Q59. Role of diffusion tensor imaging (DTI) in spinal cord injury assessment.

(Amrita Institute of Medical Sciences Kochi Kerala 2011)

Diffusion tensor imaging (DTI) is an advanced MRI technique that maps **white matter tracts.**

Utility in SCI

Parameter	Clinical relevance
Fractional anisotropy (FA)	↓ FA indicates axonal damage
Mean diffusivity (MD)	↑ MD indicates edema or necrosis

Advantages
- **Early prediction of neurological recovery**
- Detects microstructural changes before visible on conventional MRI
- Useful for monitoring spinal cord repair in research

Not yet routine but gaining ground in clinical research settings.

Q60. Role of MRI in evaluation of spinal trauma.

MRI is essential for assessing soft tissues and cord pathology.

Specific MRI Uses in Trauma

Indication	MRI findings
Neurological deficit	Cord edema, hemorrhage, transection
Ligamentous injury	PLC disruption
Disc herniation	Cord/root compression
Epidural hematoma	Signal voids compressing thecal sac
SCIWORA	Cord injury without bone changes
Infection versus neoplasm	Differentiation via marrow and soft tissue signal

MRI is crucial in **surgical planning, prognosis, and guiding conservative versus operative management.**

Surgical and Non-surgical Management in Spinal Trauma

Q61. Indications for surgical versus Conservative management in spinal fractures.

Criteria	Conservative	Surgical
Stability	Stable fractures (e.g., compression, minor wedge)	Unstable (3-column, burst with PLC injury)
Neurology	Intact neuro exam	Progressive or existing neuro deficit
TLICS score	≤3	≥5
Deformity	Minimal kyphosis <20°	Kyphosis >30°, vertebral height loss >50%
Canal compromise	Absent or minimal	Severe retropulsion
Pain	Tolerable, improving	Intractable despite rest

TLICS is a key decision tool.

Q62. Pedicle screw fixation in spine trauma—short note.

(Grant Medical College Mumbai 2009)

Pedicle screws allow 3-column stabilization via posterior approach.

Indications
- Unstable thoracolumbar burst fractures
- Translational injuries
- Fixation for decompression (e.g., laminectomy)
- Correcting kyphosis

Advantages
- Rigid fixation
- Load-sharing construct
- Allows indirect decompression (ligamentotaxis)

Limitations
- Risk of screw malposition
- May require fusion in long term
- Less effective in osteoporotic bone

Q63. Anterior versus posterior spinal fusion—indications and techniques.

Feature	Anterior fusion	Posterior fusion
Indications	Vertebral body collapse, anterior column instability	PLC disruption, deformity correction
Approach	Transthoracic, retroperitoneal	Midline posterior
Technique	Corpectomy + cage + plate	Pedicle screws + rods
Advantage	Direct decompression of canal	Familiar, less morbidity
Drawback	More invasive	Less load-sharing for anterior column

Often combined (360° fusion) in severe trauma.

Q64. Role of spinal orthoses.

Cervical Collars
- Used in stable cervical fractures

- **Philadelphia** or soft collar
- Limits flexion-extension

Thoracolumbosacral Orthosis (TLSO)
- Supports mid/lower thoracic and lumbar injuries
- Used in conservative management

Jewett Brace
- For anterior column compression fractures
- Promotes hyperextension

Limitations
- Compliance dependent
- Skin issues in prolonged use
- Ineffective in high instability or neuro deficits

Q65. Complications of spinal fusion surgery—short note.

Type	*Examples*
Intraoperative	Dural tear, bleeding, neural injury
Immediate post-operative	Infection, wound dehiscence, hematoma
Late	Pseudoarthrosis, implant failure, adjacent segment degeneration
Neurological	New/worsened deficits, radiculopathy
Systemic	DVT, pulmonary complications, ileus

Long-term monitoring and physiotherapy are key post-fusion.

Complications of Spinal Trauma

Q66. Post-traumatic kyphosis—causes and management.

Causes
- Improper healing of burst/wedge fractures
- PLC injury left untreated
- Inadequate surgical fixation
- Osteoporotic collapse

Management
- *Observation*: Mild deformity (<20°), no pain
- *Bracing*: TLSO or Jewett
- *Surgical Correction*:
    - Indicated for kyphosis >30°, instability, or neurological symptoms
    - **Posterior osteotomy + pedicle screw fixation**
    - ± Anterior reconstruction in severe collapse

Early surgical fixation prevents kyphotic progression.

Q67. Syringomyelia after SCI—short note.

Syringomyelia
Fluid-filled cyst (syrinx) in spinal cord, may occur months to years after SCI.

Pathophysiology
- Disrupted CSF flow
- *Cord ischemia*: Cavitation
- Pressure from scarring or arachnoiditis

Features
- Segmental pain
- Dissociated sensory loss (pain/temp ↓; proprioception preserved)
- Motor weakness, spasticity

Management
- **MRI** for diagnosis
- **Syringotomy/shunt surgery** if progressive
- Treat underlying tethering or arachnoiditis

Q68. Pressure ulcers in SCI—risk factors and management.

Risk factors	*Prevention*	*Management*
Immobility, sensory loss, poor nutrition	2-hour turning, pressure-relief mattresses, skin care	Debridement, dressings, antibiotics, flap surgery
Moisture (incontinence)	Incontinence control	Off-loading

Most common over sacrum, heels, and trochanters.

Q69. Heterotopic ossification in SCI—management.

Abnormal bone formation in soft tissues near joints (usually hips, knees).

Clinical
- Swelling, warmth, ↓ ROM
- Appears 3–12 weeks post-SCI

Diagnosis
X-ray, **alkaline phosphatase** ↑, **triple-phase bone scan** (early)

Management
- NSAIDs (indomethacin)
- Bisphosphonates
- ROM physiotherapy
- Surgical excision (after maturation) in severe cases

Prevent contractures, monitor progression.

Q70. Spinal instability—short note.

Inability of spine to maintain alignment under physiological loads—pain, deformity, neuro risk.

Management Options
- *Conservative*: Bracing (TLSO, collar) in stable fractures
- *Surgical*:
  - Posterior stabilization (pedicle screws)
  - Anterior reconstruction (corpectomy + cage)
  - Combined (360° fusion)

White and Panjabi or **TLICS** help define instability.

Q71. Neuropraxia, axonotmesis and neurotmesis—short notes.

[Maharashtra University of Health Sciences (MUHS) Nashik 2017]

Type	Pathology	Recovery	Example
Neuropraxia	Conduction block, no axonal damage	Complete, days–weeks	Whiplash, transient cord injury
Axonotmesis	Axonal damage with intact sheath	Regeneration at 1–3 mm/day	Crush injury
Neurotmesis	Complete nerve transection	No recovery without surgery	Lacerations, root avulsion

Sunderland classification expands to 5 grades.

Vertebral Artery Injuries (VAI) Associated with Cervical Spine Trauma

Overview:

- The **vertebral arteries** ascend through the **transverse foramina (C6 to C1)** and enter the skull to supply the posterior brain.
- VAI occurs in **0.5–2%** of blunt trauma patients and is **underdiagnosed** due to subtle presentation.

Mechanism of Injury

Mechanism	Description
Hyperextension + rotation	Common cause
Fracture through transverse foramen	Especially C1–C6
Subluxation/dislocation	C1–C2 instability (e.g., Jefferson, Hangman's fracture)
Flexion-distraction	Can stretch or tear the artery
Atlantoaxial injuries	High risk of arterial injury due to mobility

Clinical Features

- Often **asymptomatic** initially
- **Delayed stroke** (posterior circulation)
- Dizziness, vertigo, ataxia, diplopia
- **Horner's syndrome**
- Posterior headache or neck pain

Imaging and Diagnosis

Modality	Role
CT angiography (CTA)	First-line, rapid, sensitive
MRI/MRA	Useful for ischemic changes and dissection
Digital subtraction angiography (DSA)	Gold standard (used selectively)

Management

Category	Intervention
Antithrombotic therapy	Heparin → warfarin or aspirin (for Grade I–II VAI)
Surgical decompression or stabilization	If associated with unstable spine fracture
Endovascular stenting or embolization	In selected cases (pseudoaneurysm or bleeding)

Biffl Grading System (VAI)

Grade	Injury description
I	Luminal irregularity or dissection with <25% narrowing
II	Dissection or thrombus with >25% narrowing

Continued

Continued

Grade	***Injury description***
III	Pseudoaneurysm
IV	Occlusion
V	Transection with extravasation

Summary Box (For Viva or Long Answer)

- VAI is a serious but **often silent complication** of cervical trauma.
- **Transverse foramen fracture or C1–C2 dislocation** → high risk
- Must **screen with CTA** in high-risk injuries.
- **Stroke prevention** via anticoagulation is key in early management.

Q72. Describe vertebral artery injuries associated with cervical spine trauma.

(Source: JIPMER 2023)

Introduction

Vertebral artery injuries (VAI) can complicate cervical spine trauma, leading to posterior circulation strokes if not identified early.

When to Suspect Vertebral Artery Injury

- High cervical spine fractures (C1–C3)
- Fractures involving transverse foramen (especially C6–C1)
- Subluxations/rotational injuries
- Facet dislocations

Clinical Features

- Often asymptomatic initially
- *May present with*:
  - Dizziness
  - Diplopia
  - Nystagmus
  - Posterior circulation stroke (late)

Imaging Modalities

- *CT angiography (CTA)*: First-line investigation
- *MR angiography (MRA)*: Alternative
- *Doppler ultrasound*: Screening tool (less sensitive)

Management

- *Stable injury without symptoms*: Antiplatelet therapy (Aspirin)
- *Symptomatic or severe injury*:
  - Anticoagulation (Heparin → Warfarin)
  - Endovascular stenting in selected cases
- *Associated cervical fracture requiring surgery*: Take extreme care to avoid worsening VAI during fixation

Quick Exam-Oriented Table

Aspect	***Detail***
Suspect VAI	High cervical injuries (C1–C3)
Imaging	CTA preferred
Management	Antiplatelets/Anticoagulation

Crisp Flowchart

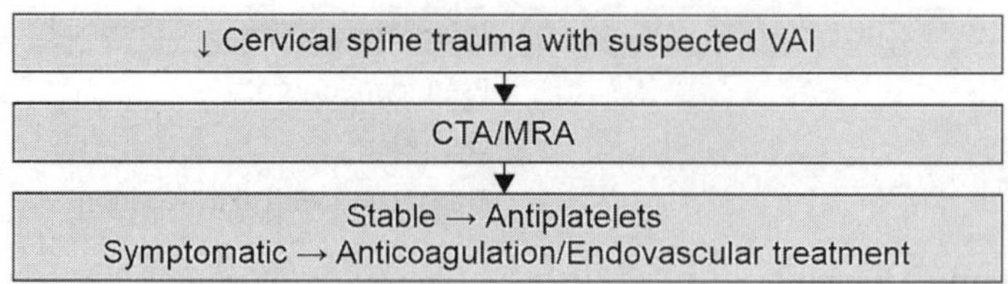

Q73. Short notes: Neuropraxia, axonotmesis, and neurotmesis in spinal trauma.

(Source: TNMGR Chennai 2021)

Based on Seddon's and Sunderland's Classification

Type	*Definition*	*Prognosis*
Neuropraxia	Conduction block without axonal disruption	Excellent (full recovery in days to weeks)
Axonotmesis	Axonal disruption with intact connective tissue (endoneurium, perineurium)	Good (regeneration possible at 1–3 mm/day)
Neurotmesis	Complete nerve transection including connective tissue	Poor (requires surgical repair)

Key Points

Neuropraxia:
- Temporary conduction block
- Seen after mild stretch injuries

Axonotmesis:
- Axon disrupted, but Schwann cell tubes intact
- Recovery possible via axonal regrowth

Neurotmesis:
- Entire nerve severed
- Surgical repair mandatory (nerve grafting)

Spinal Cord Neuropraxia (e.g., After Minor Hyperextension in Cervical Spine Trauma)
- Also called "spinal cord concussion"
- Temporary paralysis, full recovery expected

Quick Exam-oriented Table

Injury type	*Recovery*
Neuropraxia	Days to weeks
Axonotmesis	Weeks to months (axon regrowth)
Neurotmesis	Surgery required

Crisp Flowchart

↓ Nerve injury

Neuropraxia → Conservative management
Axonotmesis → Conservative + monitor recovery
Neurotmesis → Surgical exploration and repair

Spinal Cord Injury Rehabilitation

Q74. Rehabilitation protocols after spinal cord injury.

(Source: MUHS Maharashtra 2023)

Introduction

Rehabilitation after SCI aims to maximize functional independence, prevent complications, and reintegrate the patient into society.

Phases of Rehabilitation

Acute phase (first few days to weeks):
- Spinal immobilization
- Prevention of secondary complications (DVT, pressure sores)
- Chest physiotherapy to prevent pneumonia
- Passive range-of-motion (ROM) exercises

Subacute phase (2–6 weeks):
- Mobilization (bed mobility, wheelchair training)
- Strengthening preserved muscles
- Bladder and bowel training
- Orthotic management if required

Chronic phase (>6 weeks):
- Gait training (for incomplete SCI)
- Advanced wheelchair skills
- Vocational rehabilitation (job retraining, education)

Multidisciplinary Team Involvement
- Physiotherapists
- Occupational therapists
- Rehabilitation medicine specialists
- Psychologists
- Orthotists

Goals
- Independence in activities of daily living (ADLs)
- Maximal community reintegration
- Psychological adaptation

Quick Table

Phase	*Focus*
Acute phase	Prevent complications
Subacute phase	Mobilization, strengthening
Chronic phase	Community reintegration

Crisp Flowchart

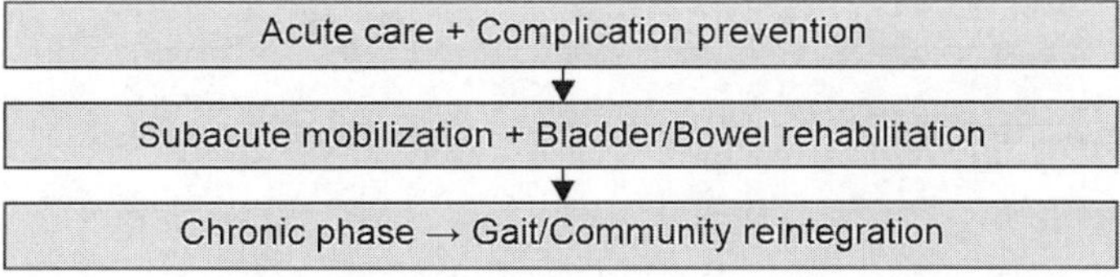

Q75. Role of functional electrical stimulation (FES) in spinal cord injury.

(Source: TNMGR Chennai 2023)

Definition

Functional electrical stimulation (FES) is the application of electrical currents to elicit functional muscle contractions in paralyzed muscles.

Mechanism

- Stimulates peripheral motor nerves below the injury level
- Produces controlled muscle contractions to perform functional tasks

Applications in SCI

- Restoration of hand function (FES hand orthosis)
- Standing and ambulation (FES-assisted walking)
- Improvement of cardiovascular fitness
- Prevention of muscle atrophy and osteoporosis

Advantages

- Improved muscle strength and endurance
- Better cardiovascular health
- Enhanced psychological wellbeing

Limitations

- Requires intact peripheral nerve pathways
- Costly equipment
- Need for regular sessions and compliance

Quick Table

Application	*Example*
Hand function	FES hand glove
Standing/Walking	FES-assisted gait devices

Crisp Flowchart

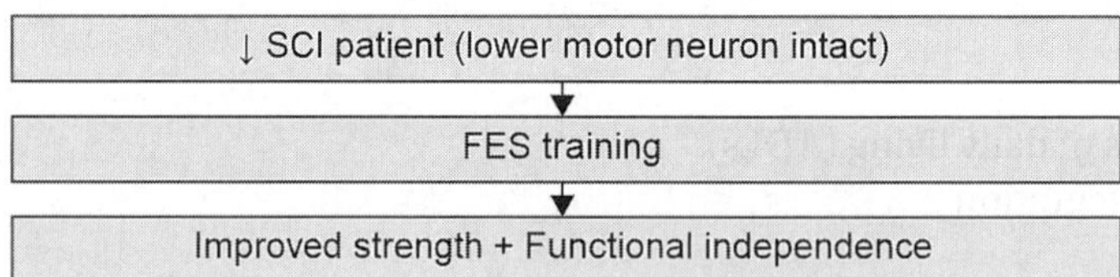

11.5 Pediatric Trauma

Ashish Nehru, Kushagra Pathak, Irfan Ahmed Poswal

General Principles of Pediatric Trauma

Q1. Discuss the anatomical and biomechanical differences between pediatric and adult bone. How do these differences influence fracture patterns, healing, and treatment approaches in children?

Anatomical Differences
- Presence of growth plates (physes)
- Thick periosteum with strong osteogenic potential
- More porous and pliable bones
- Higher cartilage content
- Greater vascular supply

Biomechanical Differences
- Bones can bend more before breaking (leading to greenstick/plastic deformation)
- Energy absorption differs due to increased elasticity

Influence on Fractures
- Fractures often incomplete (torus, greenstick)
- Higher remodeling potential
- Faster healing
- Unique patterns like growth plate fractures (Salter–Harris)

Treatment Implications
- Prefer conservative management (casting)
- Avoid physeal damage to prevent growth disturbances
- Surgical fixation with flexible nails (ESIN) preferred when necessary

Q2. What are the unique considerations in pediatric fracture healing?

- *Growth potential*: Fractures near physes can remodel significantly
- *Remodeling capacity*: High in young children; greater in metaphyseal regions
- *Rapid healing*: Shorter immobilization periods
- *Risk of growth disturbance*: Physeal injuries can lead to angular deformities or limb length discrepancies
- *Thick periosteum*: Aids reduction and healing
- *Compliance*: Challenges with immobilization and rehabilitation

Q3. Explain the importance of periosteal reaction in pediatric fracture healing.

- *Thick and active periosteum*: Enhances callus formation and stabilization
- *Facilitates reduction*: Acts as a tension band aiding realignment
- *Faster healing*: Promotes early bridging of fracture fragments
- *Protective role*: Reduces displacement and aids containment in greenstick fractures

Q4. Explain the concept of bone remodeling and its effect on pediatric fracture management.

- *Definition*: Process of bone reshaping during healing under mechanical stress
- *High in children*: Especially <10 years old
- *Directional correction*: Can correct angulation in the plane of joint movement
- *Clinical impact*: Allows acceptance of more angulation in non-operative treatment

Q5. Remodeling potential in pediatric fractures

- *Age-dependent*: Greater in younger children
- *Plane of motion*: Deformities in the plane of joint movement remodel better
- *Fracture location*: Metaphyseal > Diaphyseal
- *Time factor*: Remodeling occurs over months to years

Q6. How does age, fracture location, and plane of deformity affect remodeling capacity?

- *Age*:
    - *<10 years*: Excellent remodeling potential
    - *Adolescents*: Decreased potential
- *Fracture location*:
    - Near physis > Mid-diaphyseal
    - Upper limb > Lower limb
- *Plane of deformity*:
    - In sagittal/coronal plane of joint motion = better remodeling
    - Rotational deformities = poor remodeling

Q7. Write a short note on plastic deformation and its clinical relevance.

- *Definition*: Permanent bending of bone without a visible fracture line
- *Seen in*: Forearm and fibula of young children
- *Mechanism*: Sub-yield strength repetitive force or sustained pressure
- *Relevance*:
    - May require careful correction
    - Missed diagnosis can lead to functional deformity
    - Radiographs may appear normal—requires clinical suspicion

Q8. Discuss the role of casting versus surgical intervention in pediatric fractures.

Casting

- Preferred in most pediatric fractures
- Benefits from high remodeling potential
- Fewer complications, cost-effective

Surgical Indications

- Open fractures
- Displaced physeal injuries
- Failed closed reduction
- Multiple injuries/polytrauma
- Fractures with high risk of malunion (e.g., displaced femoral shaft, unstable forearm)

Surgical Methods

- ESIN
- Plate fixation
- K-wiring

Conclusion

Conservative management is the mainstay, but surgical intervention is increasing with evolving techniques and need for earlier mobilization.

Greenstick and Buckle (Torus) Fractures—Differences, Radiological Features, and Treatment

Q9. Greenstick fractures.

Definition

An incomplete fracture where one cortex breaks and the other bends, resembling a green twig being bent.

Mechanism

Bending force causes failure on the tension side, while compression side remains intact.

Radiological Features

- Fracture line visible on tension side
- Concavity toward intact cortex
- Periosteal disruption on one side only

Treatment

- Closed reduction may be required to restore alignment
- Immobilization in a cast (above-elbow if forearm involved)
- Frequent follow-up due to potential for re-angulation

Q10. Buckle (torus) fractures.

Definition

Incomplete fracture characterized by buckling of the cortex due to compressive force.

Mechanism

Axial loading compresses the bone leading to bulging of the cortex (usually at the metaphysis)

Radiological Features

- Subtle bulge or buckle on one side
- No clear fracture line
- Intact periosteum

Treatment

- No reduction needed
- Short immobilization (3–4 weeks)
- Removable splints preferred in modern practice

Differences between Greenstick and Torus Fractures

Feature	*Greenstick fracture*	*Torus (buckle) fracture*
Definition	Incomplete fracture with cortical break on one side and bend on other	Compression injury with cortical buckling
Mechanism	Bending force	Axial compressive force
Cortex Involved	One cortex breaks, opposite side bends	Both cortices remain intact (buckled)

Continued

Continued

Feature	Greenstick fracture	Torus (buckle) fracture
Radiology	Fracture line and angulation	Bulge or buckle without fracture line
Periosteum	Disrupted on one side	Intact
Treatment	May need reduction and long cast	No reduction, short-term splint/cast

Q11. Indications and complications of external fixation in pediatric fractures.

(Grant Medical College Mumbai 2014)

Indications

- Open fractures (especially Gustilo type IIIB and IIIC)
- Polytrauma with unstable patient needing damage control orthopedics
- Segmental bone loss
- Fractures with severe soft tissue injury (e.g., degloving)
- Pediatric pelvic fractures
- Temporary stabilization in fracture-dislocation or compartment syndrome
- Infected nonunion (ilizarov fixator)

Complications

- Pin tract infections (most common)
- Pin loosening or breakage
- Refracture after removal
- Neurovascular injury during pin insertion
- Delayed union or nonunion
- Joint stiffness due to prolonged immobilization
- Overgrowth or growth plate disturbance if pins placed near physis

Principles of Amputations in Children

Unique considerations:

- Presence of growth plates—may lead to overgrowth of bone stump
- Preservation of limb length is critical
- Avoidance of disarticulations when possible
- Myodesis and periosteal preservation for better prosthetic fitting
- Consider prosthetic planning at time of surgery

Surgical principles:

- Gentle tissue handling
- Bone cutting proximal to the physis
- Soft tissue balancing (myoplasty/myodesis)
- Early rehabilitation and prosthesis fitting
- Long-term follow-up for bone overgrowth and prosthetic adaptation

Common sites:

- Below-knee amputation is preferred over Syme's
- Above-elbow preferred over disarticulation at shoulder

Compartment Syndrome in Children and Volkmann Ischemic Contracture

Pathophysiology:

- Increased pressure (>30 mm Hg) within a closed osteofascial compartment
- Leads to ischemia of muscles and nerves

Causes:

- Supracondylar humerus fracture (most common)
- Forearm fractures

- Crush injuries
- Tight casts

Clinical features (5 Ps):
- *P*ain out of proportion
- *P*allor
- *P*aresthesia
- *P*aralysis (late)
- *P*ulselessness (very late)

Assessment:
- Passive stretch pain (early sign)
- Compartment pressure measurement (>30 mm Hg or $\Delta P < 30$ mm Hg)

Management:
- Immediate bivalving of cast
- Urgent fasciotomy
- Delay leads to fibrosis and contracture

Volkmann ischemic contracture (VIC):
- Result of missed compartment syndrome
- Fixed flexion deformity of fingers and wrist
- Muscle fibrosis, especially FDS and FDP

Surgical treatment:
- Muscle slide procedures (Max Page)
- Tendon lengthening or transfers
- Contracture release or osteotomy in late cases

Q12. Open fractures in children and management and difference compared to adults.

(PGI Chandigarh 2011)

Classification

Gustilo-Anderson (type I to IIIC)

Initial Assessment
- Assess neurovascular status
- Photograph wounds
- Cover with sterile dressing
- Tetanus prophylaxis

Antibiotic Protocol
- *Type I*: First generation cephalosporin
- *Type II*: Add aminoglycoside
- *Type III*: Add metronidazole or penicillin

Surgical Timing
- Early debridement (within 6–8 hours ideally)
- Delayed primary closure or secondary intention based on contamination

Differences Compared to Adults
- Better healing capacity
- Thicker periosteum—better containment of hematoma
- Less risk of nonunion
- Less aggressive hardware usage

Pediatric Head, Spine, and Polytrauma

Q13. Unique features of pediatric spine injuries compared to adults.

(Asked in: RGUHS Karnataka 2022, AIIMS Delhi 2021)

1. *Anatomical differences*:
   - Large head-to-body ratio increases torque on cervical spine.
   - Ligaments more elastic → higher risk of SCIWORA.
   - Incomplete ossification of vertebrae; growth plates present.
   - Shallow and horizontally oriented facet joints.
   - Underdeveloped neck musculature.
2. *Injury patterns*:
   - More common at upper cervical spine (C1–C3) in young children.
   - Injuries often ligamentous, not bony.
   - SCIWORA more prevalent in children (up to 25–30% of SCIs).
3. *Clinical features*:
   - May present with minimal or no radiological findings.
   - Higher rate of complete neurological deficits with minimal trauma.
4. *Healing and remodeling*:
   - Greater remodeling potential.
   - Risk of growth disturbance and late deformity (kyphosis/scoliosis).

Q14. Assessment and management of pediatric polytrauma.

1. *Primary assessment—ABCDE (as per ATLS)*:
   - *Airway*: Ensure cervical spine protection.
   - *Breathing*: Assess for rib fractures, pneumothorax (uncommon in infants).
   - *Circulation*: Early signs of shock may be subtle; estimate blood volume.
   - *Disability*: AVPU or Pediatric GCS; spinal precautions.
   - *Exposure*: Full body check; avoid hypothermia.
2. *Secondary assessment*:
   - Detailed head-to-toe exam.
   - Imaging: FAST, X-rays, CT, MRI.
3. *Management principles*:
   - Multidisciplinary pediatric trauma team.
   - Prioritize life-threatening injuries.
   - Early fluid resuscitation (20 mL/kg isotonic crystalloids).
   - Monitor for missed injuries; repeat exams are essential.
   - Pain management and psychological support.

Q15. Explain the role of the Glasgow coma scale (GCS) in children.

Modified Pediatric GCS

- Accounts for age-appropriate responses.
- *Eye opening (E)*: Same as adult.
- *Verbal response (V)*: Infant—Coos/babbles → cries → irritable → moans → none.
- *Motor response (M)*: Same as adult.

GCS score	*Severity*
13–15	Mild TBI
9–12	Moderate TBI
≤8	Severe TBI

Uses

- Rapid neurological assessment.
- Guides airway management decisions.
- Determines urgency of neurosurgical referral.

Q16. Short note—management of pediatric spinal trauma.

1. *Initial stabilization*:
    - Immobilization with pediatric-sized cervical collar and spinal board.
    - Avoid flexion during transport.
2. *Diagnosis*:
    - X-ray, CT for bony injury.
    - MRI is essential in suspected SCIWORA.
3. *Treatment*:
    - Most are managed non-operatively.
    - *Surgery indicated for*:
        - Instability
        - Neurological deficit
        - Progressive deformity
    - Brace or halo vest for immobilization.
4. *Long-term follow-up*:
    - Monitor for scoliosis or kyphosis.
    - Growth-related deformities may appear late.

Q17. SCIWORA in children—concept, diagnosis, and management.

(Asked in: PGI Chandigarh 2022, JIPMER Puducherry 2022)

Definition

- **Spinal cord injury without radiographic abnormality** on X-ray/CT.
- Common in age <8 years due to ligamentous elasticity and spinal cord vulnerability.

Diagnosis

- *MRI is the gold standard*: May show edema, hemorrhage, cord contusion.
- High index of suspicion in neurologically abnormal child with normal X-rays/CT.

Management

- *Immobilization*: Cervical collar for 6–12 weeks.
- *Steroids*: Controversial in pediatric age group.
- *Rehabilitation*: Essential—physical therapy, occupational therapy.

Prognosis

Variable. Better outcomes in patients with incomplete deficits.

Q18. Biomechanics of pediatric cervical spine injuries.

1. *Anatomical contributors*:
   - *Larger head:mass ratio*: Greater flexion-extension torque.
   - *Horizontally oriented facets*: Less mechanical resistance.
   - *Elastic ligaments*: Increased translational movement.
   - *Shallow vertebral bodies*: Increased shear forces.
2. *Injury pattern by age*:
   - *<8 years*: More injuries at C1–C3.
   - *8 years*: Shift toward adult pattern (C5–C7).
3. *Mechanisms*:
   - Flexion-extension injuries most common.
   - Distraction and shear forces more significant than compression.

Q19. Management of atlantoaxial instability in children.

Etiologies
- *Congenital*: Down syndrome, os odontoideum.
- *Inflammatory*: Juvenile rheumatoid arthritis.
- Trauma.

Diagnosis
- Lateral cervical spine X-ray in flexion/extension.
- CT for bony anatomy.
- MRI for spinal cord compression.

Management
- *Conservative*: Cervical collar if no instability or symptoms.
- *Surgical*:
  - Posterior C1–C2 fusion (e.g., Brooks or Harms technique).
  - *Indications*: >5 mm atlantodental interval, neurological symptoms, progressive instability.
- *Post-operative immobilization*: Halo vest or rigid collar.

Pediatric Upper Limb Fractures and Injuries

Q20. Injuries due to fall on outstretched hand (FOOSH).

(BFUHS 2011)

Mechanism
Axial load transmission from hand → wrist → forearm → elbow → shoulder.

Common Injuries by Age Group
- *Children*:
  - Supracondylar humerus fracture
  - Lateral condyle fracture
  - Greenstick/torus fractures
  - Clavicle fracture
- *Adolescents*:
  - Distal radius Salter–Harris fracture
  - Radial head/neck fracture

- *Adults*:
    - Colles' fracture
    - Scaphoid fracture
    - Radial head fracture
- *Elderly*:
    - Proximal humerus fracture
    - Olecranon fracture
    - Wrist fracture-dislocations

Complications
- Neurovascular injury (especially brachial artery, median nerve)
- Compartment syndrome
- Malunion, stiffness

Q21. Conservative versus operative management in pediatric clavicle fractures.

Conservative Management (Mainstay)
- *Indications*:
    - Midshaft fractures with minimal displacement
    - Greenstick/Incomplete fractures
    - No neurovascular compromise
- *Methods*:
    - Arm sling or figure-of-eight bandage
    - Rest, analgesia
    - Healing in 3–6 weeks

Operative Management
- *Indications*:
    - Open fractures
    - Neurovascular injury
    - Skin tenting or threatened skin
    - Severely displaced or comminuted fractures
    - Nonunion (rare in children)
- *Surgical approaches*:
    - Anterior approach
    - Plate fixation (preferably precontoured locking plate)
    - Intramedullary fixation (in select cases)

Evidence
Most pediatric clavicle fractures heal well conservatively. Surgery is reserved for complications or high-demand athletes in select cases.

Q22. Supracondylar fractures of humerus in children

Classification: Gartland Classification
- *Type I*: Undisplaced
- *Type II*: Displaced with intact posterior cortex
- *Type III*: Completely displaced
- *Type IV*: Multidirectionally unstable (posterior and anterior)

Clinical Presentation
- Pain, swelling around elbow
- S-shaped deformity (extension type)

- Loss of elbow function
- *Neurovascular signs*: Check radial pulse, cap refill, median/radial nerve exam

Radiological Evaluation

- AP and lateral elbow X-rays
- Anterior humeral line (should intersect middle third of capitellum)
- Fat pad sign (occult fracture)
- Baumann's angle (normal 70–75°)
- Assess for posterior displacement and rotation

Emergency Management

- Neurovascular assessment → monitor for compartment syndrome
- Immobilize limb (above-elbow slab with elbow flexed ~30–40°)
- Admit if pulseless or displaced

Operative Indications

- Gartland type II (controversial)
- Type III and IV
- Vascular compromise or compartment syndrome
- Open fractures
- Irreducible fractures or failed closed reduction

Q23. Management of supracondylar humerus fractures.

Type I (Undisplaced)

- Immobilization with above-elbow cast in 90–100° flexion
- *Duration*: 3 weeks
- Monitor neurovascular status

Type II (Displaced, Posterior Cortex Intact)

- Closed reduction + casting in flexion
- K-wire fixation if unstable or neurovascular risk

Type III/IV (Completely Displaced/Multidirectional)

- *Closed reduction and percutaneous pinning (CRPP)*:
  - Crossed K-wires (greater stability but ulnar nerve risk)
  - Lateral entry wires (less ulnar nerve risk)
- Open reduction (anterior approach) if irreducible or vascular injury

Complications

- Vascular injury (brachial artery)
- Nerve injury (median > radial > ulnar)
- Cubitus varus deformity (malunion)
- Stiffness, compartment syndrome

Follow-up

- Weekly X-rays to monitor reduction
- Wire removal after 3–4 weeks

Q24. Management of pink pulseless and white pulseless hand in supracondylar fractures.

(Asked in: RGUHS Karnataka 2022)

Definitions

- *Pink pulseless hand*: Hand is warm, pink, well-perfused but radial pulse is absent.
- *White pulseless hand*: Hand is pale, cold, pulseless—indicating critical ischemia.

Management Algorithm

Condition	*Action*
Pink pulseless hand	Close monitoring after closed reduction and percutaneous pinning (CRPP). No exploration if hand remains pink. Vascular spasm may be the cause.
White pulseless hand	Emergency reduction. If no improvement—immediate surgical exploration for arterial injury (usually brachial artery).

Surgical Steps for Exploration
- Open reduction
- Arterial inspection (contusion/thrombosis/laceration)
- Fogarty catheter for clot removal
- Interposition graft if needed (e.g., saphenous vein)

Q25. Management of vascular injury in supracondylar fracture.

(Asked in: RGUHS Karnataka 2022)

Classification: Gartland System
- *Type I*: Undisplaced
- *Type II*: Displaced with intact posterior cortex
- *Type III*: Completely displaced
- *Type IV*: Multidirectional instability (recently added)

Vascular Injury Management
- Prompt neurovascular exam
- Pulse examination (radial/brachial), capillary refill
- Immediate reduction (closed) if vascular compromise
- If pulse doesn't return—surgical exploration
- Duplex Doppler or CTA if equivocal

Q26. Complications of supracondylar fractures.

(Asked in: RGUHS Karnataka 2022, JIPMER Puducherry 2022)

Early Complications
- *Neurovascular injury*: Median > Radial > Ulnar nerve
- *Compartment syndrome*: Volkmann's ischemic contracture
- Malreduction

Late Complications
- Cubitus varus (most common)
- Myositis ossificans
- Elbow stiffness
- Growth arrest or limb length discrepancy

Q27. Management of neglected supracondylar fractures.

(Asked in: CMC Vellore 2023)

Definition

Presentation >2–3 weeks after injury with malunion or stiffness.

Management Depends on
- Degree of malunion (especially varus deformity)

- Elbow stiffness
- Functional deficit
- Neurovascular symptoms

Options
- No treatment if function is preserved
- Corrective osteotomy (e.g., lateral closing wedge for cubitus varus)
- Rehabilitation for stiffness
- Avoid aggressive physiotherapy to prevent myositis

Q28. Lateral condyle fractures of the humerus in children.

Classification
- **Milch I and II** (as above)
- *Jakob's classification*:
  - *Type I*: <2 mm displacement
  - *Type II*: 2–4 mm, with intact cartilage hinge
  - *Type III*: >4 mm, complete displacement and rotation

Clinical Features
- Pain, swelling over lateral elbow
- Lateral prominence
- Limited range of motion
- Ecchymosis

Radiology
- AP, lateral, and internal oblique views
- MRI/arthrogram in doubtful displacement

Management
- *Non-operative*: Type I (<2mm) with intact hinge → cast
- *Operative*: Type II/III → Open reduction and internal fixation (ORIF) with K-wires

Complications
- Lateral condyle non-union (most feared)
- Tardy ulnar nerve palsy
- Growth arrest/physeal bar

Q29. Milch classification of lateral condyle fractures.

Standard Classification
- *Milch Type I*: Fracture line **lateral to trochlear groove, through the capitulotrochlear sulcus**.
  - Salter–Harris IV
  - Rare
- *Milch Type II*: Fracture line **passes through the trochlear groove**
  - Salter–Harris II
  - Most common
  - More unstable

Q30. Short note on Monteggia fractures in children.

Definition
Fracture of the proximal ulna with dislocation of the radial head.

Common Features in Children
- *More plasticity*: Greenstick ulnar fracture common
- Radial head dislocation often missed
- May be associated with nerve palsies (posterior interosseous)

Q31. Importance of early diagnosis and treatment in monteggia fractures.

- Early recognition (within 2–3 weeks) allows for **closed reduction.**
- *Delayed diagnosis may lead to*:
  - Irreducible radial head
  - Chronic dislocation
  - Loss of pronation/supination
- Late cases often require **osteotomy, annular ligament reconstruction**, and open reduction.
- **Missed Monteggia** is one of the most common malpractice scenarios in pediatric elbow trauma.

Q32. Monteggia equivalents and management principles in children.

Monteggia Equivalents
- Radial neck fracture with ulnar fracture
- Radial head dislocation with greenstick ulna bowing
- Isolated radial head dislocation (controversial)
- Ulna fracture with radial epiphyseal separation

Management Principles
- *Prompt diagnosis*: Careful X-ray of elbow and forearm
- *Type I injuries*: Closed reduction, long arm cast in supination
- *Type II-IV or displaced fractures*: ORIF of ulna, radial head reduction

Q33. Etiology, Bado classification, management, and challenges of Monteggia fractures in children.

Etiology
- Fall on outstretched hand with forced pronation
- Direct trauma to forearm

Bado Classification

Type	*Direction of radial head dislocation*	*Ulna fracture type*
I	Anterior	Anterior angulated diaphyseal
II	Posterior	Posterior angulated metaphyseal
III	Lateral	Metaphyseal fracture
IV	Anterior (both bones fractured)	Radius + ulna fractured

Management
- *Acute*: Reduce ulnar fracture → radial head usually reduces spontaneously
  - Closed reduction + cast
  - Unstable or irreducible → ORIF
- *Neglected (>3 weeks)*:
  - Ulnar osteotomy
  - Open reduction of radial head
  - Annular ligament reconstruction if needed

Diagnostic Challenges

- Missed radial head dislocation
- Incomplete ulna fracture may hide injury
- Always X-ray elbow with forearm trauma

Q34. Management of radial neck fractures in children.

Classification (Judet)

- *Type I*: <30° angulation
- *Type II*: 30–60° angulation
- *Type III*: >60° angulation or >3 mm displacement

Treatment

Type	*Management*
I	Conservative (immobilization)
II	Closed reduction → casting
III	Attempt closed reduction → percutaneous K-wire leverage or Metaizeau technique
Failed closed reduction	Open reduction and internal fixation (rarely needed)

Q35. Short note on pulled elbow (Nursemaid's Elbow).

Definition

Subluxation of radial head from under annular ligament due to longitudinal traction (e.g., child lifted by hand).

Age Group

1–4 years.

Presentation

- Child refuses to use arm
- Elbow slightly flexed, forearm pronated
- No swelling or bruising

Diagnosis

Clinical; X-rays usually normal.

Treatment

- *Reduction maneuver*:
  - Supination + flexion (classic), or
  - Hyperpronation (more effective)
- Instant relief with click

No immobilization required; recurrence is possible.

Q36. Classification and management of unreduced posterior elbow dislocation in a 10-year-old.

(AIIMS Delhi 2019)

Classification of Elbow Dislocation

- *By direction*:
  - Posterior (most common)
  - Posterolateral (most frequent subtype)
  - Posteromedial
  - Anterior
  - Medial/Lateral

- *By complexity*:
  - *Simple dislocation*: No associated fracture
  - *Complex dislocation*: Associated with fracture (e.g., coronoid, radial head)

Management of Unreduced Posterior Dislocation in a 10-year-old
- *History*: Pain, deformity, inability to move elbow, swelling
- *Examination*: Look for neurovascular compromise
- *Imaging*: X-rays (AP/lateral), CT if needed to assess chronicity and bone injury

Management
- *If <3 weeks*:
  - Attempt **closed reduction under GA**
  - If fails—**open reduction**
- *If >3 weeks (neglected)*:
  - Soft tissue contractures likely—**open reduction**
  - *May need*:
    - Triceps lengthening
    - Collateral ligament repair
    - Temporary stabilization with K-wires or external fixator
- *Post-operative rehabilitation*:
  - Physiotherapy to regain motion
  - Watch for stiffness and myositis ossificans

Q37. The radiographic appearance seemed harmless (TRASH) injuries.

The radiographic appearance seemed harmless (TRASH) injuries are **pediatric elbow injuries with subtle or misleading X-ray findings** but serious consequences if missed.

Common TRASH Injuries
- Monteggia fracture-dislocation
- Lateral condyle fractures
- Medial epicondyle fracture with incarceration
- Radial neck fracture
- Transphyseal separation of distal humerus (especially <2 years)

Key Points
- Always correlate **clinical findings with X-ray**.
- Obtain comparison views or MRI if needed.
- Missed injuries lead to malunion or deformity.

Q38. Short note on Essex–Lopresti injury.

Definition
A rare **forearm injury** involving:
- Radial head fracture
- Disruption of interosseous membrane
- Distal radioulnar joint (DRUJ) dislocation

Mechanism
Axial load transmitted through forearm (e.g., fall on outstretched hand).

Diagnosis
- Tender radial head
- DRUJ instability
- Pain on forearm compression

Treatment
- Radial head repair/fixation
- Interosseous membrane restoration (experimental)
- DRUJ stabilization (K-wires or cast)

Q39. Floating elbow in children.

Definition
Ipsilateral **fracture of humerus and forearm bones**—a severe injury pattern indicating high-energy trauma.

Mechanism
Fall from height or high-velocity trauma

Imaging
- Full limb X-ray (elbow to wrist + shoulder)
- CT if intra-articular

Associated Risks
- Compartment syndrome
- Neurovascular injury
- Open fractures
- Growth plate injuries

Surgical Principles
- Fix both humerus and forearm (usually ESIN or plating)
- *Sequence*: Usually forearm first (to restore length), then humerus
- *Immobilization*: Often needed post-operative with regular NV checks

Complications
- Stiffness
- Malunion
- Compartment syndrome

Q40. Monteggia versus Galeazzi fractures in children.

Feature	*Monteggia*	*Galeazzi*
Definition	Proximal ulna fracture + radial head dislocation	Distal radial shaft fracture + DRUJ dislocation
Mechanism	Fall on outstretched hand + forced pronation	Fall with axial load on outstretched hand
Management	Reduce ulna—radial head reduces spontaneously; ORIF if unstable	Reduce radius and DRUJ; cast or ORIF in older children
Complications	Missed diagnosis, posterior interosseous nerve injury	DRUJ instability, growth disturbance

Q41. Cubitus varus—causes, clinical features, and management.

Causes
- Malunion of supracondylar humerus fracture (most common)
- Growth disturbance
- Surgical malreduction

Clinical
- Medial deviation of extended forearm (gunstock deformity)
- No functional impairment
- Cosmetic concern

Management
- *Cosmetic correction*: Lateral closing wedge osteotomy
- *Techniques*: French osteotomy, dome osteotomy

Q42. Cubitus valgus—causes, clinical features, management.

Causes
- Nonunion of lateral condyle humerus fracture
- Congenital deformities
- Malunion

Clinical
- Lateral deviation of forearm
- Stretch on ulnar nerve → tardy ulnar nerve palsy

Management
- *Mild*: Observation
- *Symptomatic*:
  - Corrective osteotomy
  - Ulnar nerve transposition if palsy present

Q43. Distal radius fractures in pediatric population—classification, clinical features, radiological signs, treatment, complications.

(IMS-BHU 2017)

Classification
- *Based on displacement*:
  - Undisplaced
  - Displaced
- *Based on fracture type*:
  - Greenstick
  - Buckle (torus)
  - Complete transverse
  - *Physeal injuries (Salter-Harris classification)*:
    - Type I—physeal separation
    - Type II—through physis + metaphysis
    - Type III—through physis + epiphysis
    - Type IV—through all 3 (epiphysis, physis, metaphysis)
    - Type V—crush injury

Clinical features
- Pain, swelling at wrist
- Deformity (dorsal angulation—"dinner fork" deformity)
- Decreased range of motion
- Possible associated ulnar fracture or DRUJ injury

Radiological signs
- *X-ray (AP and lateral views)*:
  - *Location*: Metaphyseal/physeal
  - Displacement, angulation, comminution
  - Physeal widening or disruption
  - Compare with opposite side if needed

Treatment

Fracture type	*Management*
Buckle/Greenstick	Below elbow cast for 3–4 weeks
Undisplaced physeal/metaphyseal	Cast immobilization
Displaced metaphyseal	Closed reduction + cast
Unstable fractures	CRIF with K-wires
Salter-Harris IV/V	Often require open reduction and fixation

Follow-up

Weekly X-rays to monitor displacement, especially in physeal injuries.

Complications

- *Growth arrest (Salter-Harris V or after physeal injury)*: Leads to angular deformity, shortening
- *Malunion*: Acceptable angulation varies with age; remodeling potential is high in young children
- Compartment syndrome (rare)
- Distal radioulnar joint (DRUJ) instability
- Refracture
- Physeal bar formation

Q44. Draw a labeled diagram of brachial plexus and discuss Erb's palsy in a 3-year-old.

Brachial Plexus Formation

- *Roots*: C5–T1
- *Trunks*: Upper, middle, lower
- *Divisions*: Anterior, posterior
- *Cords*: Lateral, posterior, medial
- *Branches*: 5 terminal (musculocutaneous, axillary, radial, median, ulnar)

Erb's Palsy (C5–C6 Injury)

Etiology:

- *Birth trauma*: Excessive traction on shoulder
- Shoulder dystocia during delivery

Clinical features:

- Arm hangs by side, internally rotated
- Forearm extended and pronated
- "Waiter's tip" posture
- Absent Moro reflex on affected side
- *Muscle weakness*: Deltoid, biceps, brachialis, supraspinatus

Investigations:

- MRI (brachial plexus)
- Nerve conduction studies (NCS), EMG after 3 weeks

Management

Time	*Strategy*
Birth to 3 months	Observation + physiotherapy
3–6 months	EMG/NCV evaluation
If no improvement by 3–6 months	Surgical exploration, nerve grafting, or neurolysis
Older children (>2 years)	Tendon transfers (e.g., latissimus to biceps)

Pediatric Hip Trauma and Disorders

Q45. Management of pediatric pelvic fractures.

Key Differences from Adults

- Pediatric pelvis is more elastic—more stable
- Greater remodeling capacity
- High association with **polytrauma and internal injuries**

Classification

- *Torode and Zieg*:
  - *Type I*: Avulsion fractures
  - *Type II*: Iliac wing
  - *Type III*: Simple ring injuries
  - *Type IV*: Ring disruption + acetabular or unstable fractures

Imaging

- *X-ray*: AP pelvis
- *CT*: For complex patterns, intra-articular extension
- *MRI*: Soft tissue and cartilage

Management

Type	*Treatment*
I and II	Non-operative, bed rest, analgesia
III	Conservative with close monitoring
IV	Often require surgical stabilization

Associated Injuries

Abdominal, urogenital, and vascular

Q46. 4-year-old boy with groin pain after fall—approach.

Differential Diagnoses

- Transient synovitis (most common)
- Septic arthritis
- Occult fracture (neck of femur)
- DDH
- Perthes disease

Approach

1. *History and Clinical Exam*: Fever, limp, pain
2. *Imaging*:
   - X-ray pelvis (AP)
   - Ultrasound hip (effusion?)
   - MRI if X-ray normal but high suspicion
3. *Lab Tests*: CBC, CRP, ESR (to rule out infection)

Initial Management

- Bed rest, analgesia
- Further treatment based on diagnosis

Q47. Neck of femur fracture in 10-year-old—classification and management.

Delbet Classification

- *Type I*: Transphyseal (worst prognosis)
- *Type II*: Transcervical
- *Type III*: Cervicotrochanteric
- *Type IV*: Intertrochanteric

Management

- Early reduction and internal fixation (within 6–12 hours)
- Use cannulated screws or pediatric hip plates
- Immobilization in hip spica may follow
- Avoid closed reduction in transphyseal (Type I)—high AVN risk

Complications

- Avascular necrosis (most serious)
- Coxa vara
- Limb length discrepancy
- Premature physeal closure

Q48. Management of DDH in trauma.

Special Considerations

In a child with known or suspected DDH, trauma can cause dislocation or complicate management.

Approach

1. *Imaging*:
   - X-ray pelvis (Shenton's line, Hilgenreiner's line)
   - Ultrasound if <6 months
2. *Acute trauma in DDH*:
   - If traumatic dislocation—urgent reduction
   - MRI post-reduction to check congruency
3. *Chronic cases*:
   - Pavlik harness if <6 months
   - Closed or open reduction with pelvic/femoral osteotomy if older

Q49. Short note on post-traumatic AVN of femoral head in children.

Etiology

Mostly seen after femoral neck fractures or hip dislocation

Mechanism

Damage to **retinacular arteries**—compromised epiphyseal blood flow

Clinical

- Pain, limp
- Stiff hip
- May appear weeks after trauma

Diagnosis

- *MRI*: most sensitive for early AVN
- *X-ray*: Sclerosis, fragmentation, collapse

Management

- *Conservative in early stages*: NWB, observation

- *Surgical*: Core decompression, varus osteotomy, joint preservation
- Prognosis worse in transphyseal or delayed cases

Q50. Management of pediatric hip dislocations.

(AIIMS BBSR 2017)

Mechanism
- Low-energy trauma in young children due to ligamentous laxity
- Posterior dislocation most common

Diagnosis
- *Clinical*: Flexed, adducted, internally rotated hip
- *X-ray*: AP + lateral view

Management
1. Urgent closed reduction under GA (within 6 hours)
2. *Post-reduction imaging*: Confirm concentric reduction (MRI or CT)
3. *Immobilization*: Hip spica or bed rest
4. *Rehabilitation*: Gradual weight bearing

Complications
- AVN (10–15%)
- Growth disturbance
- Recurrent dislocation (in DDH)

Q51. Complications of untreated traumatic hip dislocation in children.

1. *Avascular necrosis (AVN)*:
    - Most common and serious complication
    - Occurs due to prolonged disruption of blood supply to femoral head (especially medial femoral circumflex artery)
    - Risk increases significantly if reduction is delayed beyond 6–12 hours
2. *Chondrolysis*:
    - Damage to articular cartilage from prolonged dislocation
    - Leads to joint stiffness and degeneration
3. *Growth disturbance*:
    - *Involvement of physis leads to*:
        - Premature physeal closure
        - Coxa vara/valga
        - Limb length discrepancy
4. *Joint stiffness*: Due to fibrosis, capsular tightness, or intra-articular adhesions
5. *Recurrent dislocations*: Ligamentous injury, capsule laxity, or unrecognized developmental dysplasia
6. *Degenerative arthritis*: Late consequence due to AVN, incongruent reduction, or chondral damage
7. *Sciatic nerve injury*: Can occur during dislocation or closed reduction attempts

Q52. Short note—transient synovitis versus septic arthritis of the hip in children.

Feature	*Transient synovitis*	*Septic arthritis*
Etiology	Post-viral inflammation	Bacterial infection (e.g., *Staphylococcus aureus*)
Onset	Gradual	Sudden
Age group	3–8 years	Any age, especially <3 years

Continued

Continued

Feature	***Transient synovitis***	***Septic arthritis***
Fever	Mild or absent	High-grade
Pain	Mild to moderate	Severe, constant
Systemic features	Absent or mild	Prominent (irritability, toxic)
Weight bearing	Usually able (limp)	Refusal to bear weight
Hip position	Mild flexion and abduction	Flexion, abduction, external rotation (FABER)
Investigations	ESR/CRP mildly elevated	ESR/CRP, WBC markedly raised; positive blood culture
Ultrasound	Effusion present	Effusion + synovial thickening
Joint aspiration	Clear or straw-colored fluid	Purulent fluid, high WBC count, positive Gram stain/culture
Treatment	*Conservative*: rest, NSAIDs	Urgent joint drainage + IV antibiotics

Pediatric Lower Limb Fractures and Injuries

Q53. Classification of femoral shaft fractures in children.

1. *Based on pattern*:
   - Transverse
   - Oblique
   - Spiral
   - Comminuted
   - Segmental
2. *Based on location*:
   - Proximal third
   - Middle third (most common)
   - Distal third
3. *Based on displacement*:
   - Undisplaced
   - Displaced (angulated, rotated, shortened)
4. *By age group—treatment guidelines*:

Age group	***Preferred treatment***
<6 months	Pavlik harness
6 months to 5 years	Traction followed by hip spica
5–10 years	Elastic intramedullary nailing (TENS)
>10 years or heavier children	TENS/ORIF/plating depending on weight and fracture type

Q54. Role of hip spica casting in pediatric femoral fractures.

(NEIGRIHMS 2011)

Indications
- *Age*: 6 months to 5 years
- Isolated closed fracture
- *Acceptable shortening*: <2 cm
- Transverse/Short oblique patterns

Technique
- Initial skin/skeletal traction—followed by hip spica
- *Position*: 90° hip flexion, 45° abduction, 30° knee flexion

Advantages
- Excellent remodeling in young children
- Avoids surgery
- Cost-effective

Disadvantages
- Difficult hygiene
- Parent burden
- Limb length discrepancy if malaligned

Q55. Management of pediatric tibial fractures.

Types
- Diaphyseal fractures (common)
- Physeal injuries
- Toddler's fracture (undisplaced spiral fracture of tibia)
- Tibial spine avulsions

Treatment

Type	*Management*
Undisplaced	Cast (long leg)
Displaced	Closed reduction + casting
Unstable or open fractures	Elastic nails (TENS) or plating
Physeal injuries	Salter-Harris type–specific; surgical if displaced
Toddler's fracture	Long leg cast for 3–4 weeks

Complications
- Malunion (valgus or procurvatum)
- Compartment syndrome (especially with proximal fractures)

Q56. Short note on management of pediatric ankle fractures.

Types
- Malleolar fractures
- Triplane fracture
- Tillaux fracture (SH III)
- Salter–Harris types (physeal injuries)

Investigations
- X-ray (AP, lateral, mortise)
- CT for triplane/Tillaux

Management
- *Non-displaced*: Long leg cast
- *Displaced physeal*: Closed/open reduction + K-wires or screws
- *Triplane/Tillaux*: ORIF often required for anatomical joint restoration

Complications
- Physeal bar
- Growth disturbance
- Premature closure—angular deformities

Q57. Implications of physeal injuries in lower limb fractures.

(WBUHS 2013)

Concerns

Lower limb physis contribute significantly to growth (e.g., distal femur 40%, proximal tibia 25%)

Complications

- Physeal arrest—angular deformity
- Limb length discrepancy
- Bar formation—asymmetric growth

Management Strategies

- Early detection (MRI, CT)
- Physeal-sparing techniques
- Monitoring with growth charts
- Epiphysiodesis or corrective osteotomy if needed

Q58. Ankle fractures in adolescents—classification and management.

Common Types

- *Tillaux fracture*: SH III fracture of anterolateral distal tibia
- *Triplane fracture*: Involves metaphysis, physis, and epiphysis in three planes

Mechanism

External rotation on a partially fused physis

Imaging

- AP, lateral, and mortise X-rays
- CT for 3D assessment

Management

Type	*Treatment*
Non-displaced	Long leg cast
Displaced (>2 mm)	ORIF (often with cannulated screws)

- Close monitoring for **growth disturbances and post-traumatic arthritis**

Physeal and Growth Plate Injuries

Q59. Short note on the growth plate and its significance in pediatric fractures.

Growth Plate (Physis)

- Cartilaginous layer near the ends of long bones
- Responsible for longitudinal bone growth

Significance in Pediatric Fractures

1. *Weakest zone in pediatric bone*: Most fractures in children occur at or near the physis
2. High **remodeling potential** in young bones due to physeal activity
3. *Injuries can lead to*:
    - Growth arrest
    - Angular deformity
    - Limb length discrepancy
4. Importance in **classification and treatment planning** (e.g., Salter–Harris)

Q60. Structure and function of the growth plate (Physis).

Zonal Anatomy (from epiphysis to metaphysis)

1. *Reserve (resting) zone*:
   - Storage of cells
   - Poor vascularity
2. *Proliferative zone*:
   - Rapid mitotic division of chondrocytes
   - Linear growth
3. *Hypertrophic zone*:
   - Cell enlargement and matrix calcification
   - Most common site for fractures
4. *Zone of calcification*: Cartilage turns to bone
5. *Metaphyseal bone*: Primary spongiosa formation

Functions

- **Longitudinal growth** of bone
- **Shock absorption** due to cartilage elasticity
- Acts as **barrier** to infection and tumor spread

Physeal Injuries and Salter–Harris Classification

Salter–Harris Classification

Type	*Description*	*Prognosis*	*Examples*
I	Through physis only	Excellent	Slipped capital femoral epiphysis (SCFE)
II	Physis + metaphysis	Good	Distal radius
III	Physis + epiphysis	Variable	Distal tibia
IV	Through epiphysis, physis, metaphysis	Poorer	Lateral condyle humerus
V	Physeal compression/crush	Worst	Distal femur

Mnemonic: SALTR
(S → I, A → II, L → III, T → IV, R → V)

Clinical Significance of Salter–Harris Classification

- *Helps predict risk of growth disturbance*:
  - *Type I and II*: Usually minimal risk
  - *Type III–V*: High risk of **physeal bar**, deformity, limb length discrepancy
- *Guides treatment*:
  - *Type I/II*: Closed reduction and immobilization
  - *Type III–V*: Often need ORIF to restore joint congruity

Prognostic Implications and Principles of Management

Prognosis Factors

- Age (younger = higher remodeling potential)
- Location of physis (distal femur, proximal tibia → more growth contribution)
- Type of Salter–Harris injury
- Timing and quality of reduction

Management Principles

- Anatomic reduction in intra-articular (type III/IV)
- Gentle manipulation to avoid physeal damage
- Fixation (K-wire or screw) across physis only if essential
- *Long-term follow-up*: X-rays every 6 months to detect growth disturbances early

Q61. Long-term consequences of physeal injuries.

1. *Complications of premature physeal closure*:
   - *Limb length discrepancy (LLD)*:
     - Most pronounced when injury occurs in physes contributing significant longitudinal growth (e.g., distal femur, proximal tibia)
     - More severe if injury occurs at a younger age
   - *Angular deformity*:
     - Occurs if part of the physis closes (partial growth arrest)
     - E.g., genu varum or valgum due to asymmetric closure
   - *Joint incongruity*:
     - Especially in intra-articular physeal fractures (Salter–Harris III/IV)
     - Leads to early osteoarthritis
   - *Recurrent fractures*: Due to altered mechanics or weakened metaphyseal bone
2. *Impact on long-term bone development*:
   - Growth plate is critical for longitudinal bone growth.
   - *Injury can*:
     - Halt growth (in type V injuries)
     - Cause premature asymmetrical closure (leading to deformity)
     - Result in **physeal bar formation**, replacing cartilage with bone bridge

Pathophysiology of Physeal Arrest

- Injury disrupts the germinal and proliferative zones
- **Bar (bony bridge)** forms between metaphysis and epiphysis
- Prevents uniform longitudinal growth

Diagnosis of Physeal Arrest

- *X-rays*: Suspect when deformity or shortening is noted
- *MRI*: Best for early diagnosis, shows cartilage disruption
- *CT scan*: Accurately defines bar location and size
- *Bone age assessment*: To predict future growth potential

Q62. Management of growth plate injuries in children.

Clinical Approach

1. Accurate classification (Salter–Harris)
2. Anatomic reduction if intra-articular
3. Gentle manipulation—avoid additional physeal injury
4. Stabilization (with K-wires/screws avoiding physis when possible)
5. Regular follow-up to monitor for deformity or growth arrest

Treatment of Physeal Arrest

Options based on bar size and location:

Bar size	*Treatment*
<30% of physis	Physeal bar resection ± interposition (fat, silastic)
>50% of physis	Epiphysiodesis (of contralateral limb) or corrective osteotomy
Angular deformity + bar	Osteotomy to correct alignment
Limb length discrepancy >2 cm expected	Consider contralateral epiphysiodesis or limb lengthening

Prognostic Factors

- Younger children are at higher risk due to greater remaining growth
- Early detection improves outcomes
- *Location matters*: Distal femur and proximal tibia have major contributions to limb growth

Summary

- Growth plate injuries may seem benign initially but have **major long-term consequences** like deformity and shortening.
- Premature closure, if asymmetrical, causes **angular deformity**; if complete, causes **limb shortening**.
- Timely diagnosis, anatomic reduction, and surveillance are essential.
- Physeal bar resection may help if identified early and in small bars.

Non-accidental Injuries (Child Abuse) and Special Conditions

Q63. Orthopedic manifestations of child abuse.

Child abuse often presents first to orthopedic services.

Common Orthopedic Findings

- Fractures in various healing stages
- Classic metaphyseal lesions (CMLs)
- Posterior rib fractures
- Spiral fractures in non ambulant children
- Multiple fractures without adequate history
- Fractures inconsistent with developmental stage

Red Flags

- Delay in seeking care
- Vague or changing history
- Inconsistent injury mechanism
- Injuries in non-mobile infants

Q64. Classic metaphyseal lesion (CML).

(AMC 2014)

Definition

A highly specific radiological sign of non-accidental trauma seen in infants.

Location

Metaphyses of long bones: distal femur, proximal/distal tibia, proximal humerus

Mechanism

- Shear forces during violent shaking or pulling
- Affects the metaphyseal corner, resulting in:
  - **"Bucket-handle"** appearance on lateral view
  - **"Corner fracture"** on AP view

Significance

- Virtually pathognomonic for child abuse in infants
- Must differentiate from normal variants and metabolic bone disease

Q65. Role of skeletal survey in suspected child abuse.

Indication

Suspected NAI, especially in children <2 years old

Protocol (as per ACR/AAP)

21 images covering skull, spine, chest, abdomen, pelvis, upper/lower limbs, hands/feet

Purpose
- Detect occult fractures
- Determine fracture age/stage of healing
- Document previous injuries
- Guide further investigations (e.g., bone scan or follow-up skeletal survey in 2 weeks)

Q66. Differences between accidental and non-accidental fractures.

Feature	Accidental	Non-accidental
History	Consistent, timely	Vague, delayed, changing
Developmental appropriateness	Matches injury	Does not match (e.g., fracture in non-walking infant)
Injury site	Bony prominences	Ribs, metaphyses, scapula, sternum
Fracture pattern	Isolated	Multiple, various healing stages
Accompanying signs	Absent	Bruises, burns, retinal hemorrhages

Q67. Osteogenesis imperfecta (OI) and its mimicry of child abuse.

Definition
A congenital connective tissue disorder characterized by brittle bones.

Key Features
- Multiple fractures (often mistaken for abuse)
- Blue sclera
- Dentinogenesis imperfecta
- Hearing loss
- Family history

Differentiating from Abuse
- Genetic testing
- Collagen type I analysis
- Clinical features (OI fractures occur with minimal trauma but have consistent pattern)

Q68. Importance of multidisciplinary management in child abuse.

Team Members
- Pediatrician
- Orthopedic surgeon
- Radiologist
- Social worker
- Child protection services
- Psychologist

Objectives
- Ensure child safety
- Document injuries legally and accurately
- Rule out mimics (e.g., OI)
- Provide rehabilitation
- Prevent future episodes
- Provide counseling and support

Q69. Short note on child abuse–related fractures (non-accidental injuries).

Common Fracture Types
- Classic metaphyseal lesions (CMLs)
- Posterior rib fractures
- Scapular, spinous process, or sternum fractures
- Long bone fractures in infants (especially spiral fractures)
- Multiple fractures in various healing stages

Age of Concern
Most cases occur in children <3 years, especially <1 year

Diagnosis
- History inconsistent with injury
- Full skeletal survey
- Rule out metabolic bone disease
- Multidisciplinary evaluation

Pediatric Fracture Complications and Late Sequelae

Q70. Complications and management of pediatric fractures.

(KMC Manipal 2016)

1. *Early complications*:
   - Neurovascular injury (e.g., brachial artery in supracondylar fracture)
   - Compartment syndrome
   - Infection (in open fractures)
   - Loss of reduction in cast
2. *Late complications*:
   - Malunion (e.g., cubitus varus)
   - Non-union (rare in children)
   - Growth arrest/physeal bar formation
   - Limb length discrepancy
   - Avascular necrosis (e.g., femoral neck, scaphoid)
   - Joint stiffness/myositis ossificans

Management Principles
- Early identification through regular follow-up
- Radiographic monitoring
- Address complications based on type:
- *Malunion*: Osteotomy
- *Growth arrest*: Bar resection or corrective surgery
- *AVN*: Non-weight-bearing, surgical decompression, osteotomy

Q71. Causes and management of malunion in children.

Causes
- Inadequate reduction
- Failure of immobilization
- Growth modulation following fracture
- Physeal injury
- Natural remodeling insufficient (especially in older children or near joint)

Common Examples

- Cubitus varus after supracondylar fracture
- Genu valgum/varum after tibial fracture
- Rotational deformities after femoral or forearm fractures

Management

- *Deformity*: Treatment
- *Mild (<10°)*: Observation
- *Moderate*: Growth modulation (e.g., hemiepiphysiodesis)
- *Severe*: Corrective osteotomy (e.g., lateral closing wedge for cubitus varus)

Q72. Short note on limb length discrepancy (LLD) following pediatric fractures.

Causes

- Overgrowth post-fracture (especially femur)
- Growth arrest due to physeal injury (Salter–Harris V)
- Malunion with angular deformity
- Infection or osteomyelitis affecting the physis

Diagnosis

- Serial limb length measurements
- Scanogram or EOS imaging for accurate assessment
- Bone age and growth potential estimation

Management

- *Predicted*: LLD strategy
- *<2 cm*: Observation or shoe lift
- *2–5 cm*: Epiphysiodesis of contralateral limb
- *>5 cm*: Limb lengthening (Ilizarov/Precice nail) or shortening

Q73. Pathophysiology and treatment of avascular necrosis (AVN) in pediatric fractures.

Common Sites

- Femoral head (neck fractures)
- Proximal humerus
- Talus
- Scaphoid

Pathophysiology

- *Fracture*: Disruption of blood supply (e.g., retinacular arteries in femoral neck)
- *Ischemia*: Osteocyte death → Bone collapse
- Especially critical in intracapsular fractures and fractures with high displacement

Clinical Features

- Persistent pain, limp, stiffness
- Radiographic sclerosis, flattening, fragmentation

Diagnosis

- *MRI*: Most sensitive for early detection
- *X-ray*: Shows late changes (crescent sign, collapse)

Treatment

- Non-weight bearing in early stages
- Bisphosphonates (experimental)

Surgical:
- Core decompression
- Varus/valgus osteotomy
- Epiphyseal-sparing fixation
- Hip containment procedures (e.g., shelf acetabuloplasty in hip AVN)

Q74. Write a note on heterotopic ossification (HO) after elbow trauma and ways to prevent it.

(DNB 2001)

Definition

Heterotopic ossification (HO) is the abnormal formation of mature lamellar bone in non-osseous soft tissues, often following trauma or surgery.

Pathophysiology

- Triggered by local tissue trauma, hypoxia, and inflammatory cytokines.
- Mesenchymal stem cells differentiate into osteoblasts under inappropriate stimuli.
- Bone forms in periarticular soft tissues like muscles, tendons, and ligaments.

Common Sites Post-elbow Trauma

- Brachialis muscle
- Collateral ligaments
- Posterior capsule
- Intermuscular planes around the elbow

Clinical Features

- Painful, stiff elbow
- Decreased range of motion (especially flexion and extension)
- Palpable mass (in mature HO)
- Neuropathy (especially ulnar nerve) if extensive

Imaging

- *X-ray*: Early calcification (2–6 weeks post-injury)
- *CT scan*: More sensitive for early bone formation
- *Bone scan (3-phase)*: Shows increased uptake in early HO
- *MRI*: Soft tissue edema and differentiation from infection/tumor

Risk Factors

- High-energy elbow trauma (e.g., fracture-dislocations)
- Delayed or prolonged surgery
- Multiple surgeries
- Neurological injuries (e.g., head injury, spinal cord injury)
- Severe burns
- Prolonged immobilization

Prevention Strategies

1. *Pharmacological*:
    - *NSAIDs (e.g., indomethacin 75 mg/day for 6 weeks)*:
        - Inhibits prostaglandin synthesis and osteogenesis
        - Effective in early prophylaxis
    - *Bisphosphonates*: Controversial, less commonly used
    - *Selective COX-2 inhibitors (e.g., Celecoxib)*: Similar efficacy with fewer gastrointestinal side effects

2. *Radiation therapy*:
    - Low-dose external beam radiation (700–800 cGy) within 72 hours post-injury/surgery
    - Prevents mesenchymal cell differentiation
3. *Early mobilization*: Gentle ROM exercises started early post-injury or surgery to reduce HO risk
4. *Surgical technique*:
    - Minimize soft tissue trauma
    - Meticulous hemostasis
    - Limit duration of surgery

Treatment of Established HO

- *Observation*: In asymptomatic or mildly symptomatic cases
- *Physical therapy*: Maintain joint motion
- *Surgical excision*:
    - Indicated for functional limitation
    - Delayed until bone matures (~6–12 months)
    - Often combined with post-operative prophylaxis (NSAIDs/radiation)

11.6 Trauma in Special Populations

Sumeet Singh Charak, Sajad Ahmad Wani

Geriatric Fractures

Q1. Geriatric fractures (osteoporotic fractures).

(Asked in: AIIMS Delhi 2022, PGI Chandigarh 2022, MUHS Maharashtra 2022)

Introduction

- **Osteoporotic fractures** result from low-energy trauma (e.g., fall from standing height).
- Reflect **underlying bone fragility** due to decreased bone mineral density (BMD).
- *Common fracture sites*:
  - Hip (Femoral neck, Intertrochanteric)
  - Vertebrae (compression fractures)
  - Distal radius (colles fracture)
  - Proximal humerus

Key Principle

"Fix the fracture + Treat the bone"

Q2. Types of hip fractures in the elderly.

(Asked in: JIPMER Puducherry 2022, CMC Vellore 2023)

Types of Hip Fractures

1. *Femoral neck fracture (intracapsular)*:
   - *Subtypes*: Undisplaced, displaced (Garden classification)
   - Risk of avascular necrosis (AVN) and nonunion
   - *Treatment*: Hemiarthroplasty or total hip arthroplasty (THA) in elderly
2. *Intertrochanteric fracture (extracapsular)*:
   - Stable versus Unstable types (Evans classification)
   - Usually treated with internal fixation (DHS or PFN)
3. Subtrochanteric Fracture (less common, complex fixation)

Clinical Importance

- Early surgery (within 48 hours) improves outcomes
- Consider comorbidities, bone quality, and mobility status in planning treatment

Q3. Definition of fragility fracture.

(Asked in: RGUHS Karnataka 2023)

Definition

- **Fragility fractures** are defined as fractures that occur due to **a fall from standing height or less**, or without significant trauma.
- Indicative of **osteoporosis** and low bone strength.
- Most common in elderly, especially postmenopausal women.

Common Fragility Fracture Sites
- Vertebral compression fractures
- Proximal femur (hip fractures)
- Distal radius
- Proximal humerus

Pathophysiology
- Decreased BMD → Increased bone fragility
- Trabecular bone (rich in vertebrae and femoral neck) more susceptible

Q4. Why is a multidisciplinary approach required in fragility fracture patients?

(Asked in: AIIMS Delhi 2021, RGUHS Karnataka 2022)

Rationale for Multidisciplinary Management
- *Elderly patients with fragility fractures often have*:
  - *Multiple comorbidities*: Diabetes, cardiac diseases, COPD
  - Polypharmacy, malnutrition, frailty
  - Cognitive impairment, fall risk, and functional decline

Multidisciplinary Team Includes
- Orthopedic surgeon
- Geriatrician or physician
- Physiotherapist
- Dietician
- Occupational therapist
- Social worker

Benefits
- Preoperative risk optimization
- Better pain management
- Early mobilization
- Fall prevention strategies
- Improved bone health (osteoporosis treatment)
- Reduced length of stay, complications, and mortality

Conclusion
A team-based, patient-centered model significantly improves functional recovery and long-term outcomes in elderly fracture care.

Q5. Define secondary prevention of fragility fractures.

(Asked in: JIPMER Puducherry 2022)

Definition
Secondary prevention involves measures taken **after the first fragility fracture** to **prevent future fractures**.

Key Components
- *Osteoporosis treatment*: Bisphosphonates, denosumab, teriparatide
- **Calcium + Vitamin D supplementation**
- *Fall prevention*: Home safety, strength training, balance exercises
- *Fracture liaison services (FLS)*: Coordinated care pathway to ensure follow-up and prevention

Focus is on **preventing the second fracture**, which has higher morbidity and mortality risk.

Q6. Management of fragility fractures.

(General Question; Also Referenced in: PGI Chandigarh 2022, MUHS Maharashtra 2023)

Definition Recap

- Fractures due to **low-energy trauma** (fall from standing height or less)
- Indicative of **osteoporotic bone**

Management Includes

A. *Fracture management ("fix the fracture")*:
  - *Hip fractures*: Surgery within 48 hours → THA/Hemiarthroplasty/PFN/DHS
  - *Vertebral fractures*: Conservative or Vertebroplasty/Kyphoplasty (selected cases)
  - *Distal radius, humerus*: ORIF or conservative based on displacement and function

B. *Bone health management ("treat the bone")*:
  - DEXA scan to assess BMD
  - Start anti-osteoporotic therapy (e.g., bisphosphonates, denosumab, teriparatide)
  - Address nutritional deficiencies

C. *Fall prevention*: Environmental modifications, balance training, footwear, medication review

D. *Multidisciplinary care*: As outlined above in Q4.

Q7. Explain the challenges of managing polytrauma in elderly patients.

Challenges

- *Reduced physiological reserves*:
  - *Cardiac*: ↓ Cardiac output
  - *Renal*: Impaired filtration → fluid/electrolyte imbalances
  - *Pulmonary*: ↓ Lung compliance, vital capacity
- *Multiple comorbidities*:
  - Diabetes, hypertension, COPD, CKD
  - *Polypharmacy*: ↑ Drug interactions
  - *Anticoagulants*: ↑ Bleeding risk
- *Atypical presentations*:
  - No tachycardia despite hemorrhage
  - Minimal pain expression due to neuropathy or dementia
  - Delayed signs of infection or sepsis
- *Increased complications*:
  - Delirium
  - Pressure ulcers
  - Nosocomial infections
  - Prolonged hospital stay and mortality

Management Principles

- Early comprehensive geriatric assessment (CGA)
- Multidisciplinary care approach
- Conservative fluid resuscitation (avoid overload)
- Early definitive fixation and **early mobilization**
- Monitor for complications (delirium, AKI, infection)

Q8. Discuss the assessment and management of intertrochanteric fracture in an elderly patient.

Assessment

- *History*: Fall from standing height, pain in groin/thigh, inability to bear weight
- *Examination*: Shortened, externally rotated limb
- *Imaging*: AP/lateral hip X-ray; CT if fracture pattern unclear

Management

- *Preoperative optimization*:
  - Cardiac, pulmonary, electrolyte review
  - Evaluate antiplatelet/anticoagulant status
  - *Pain control*: Fascia iliaca block, paracetamol
- *Surgical fixation (within 48 hours)*:
  - *Stable fractures*: Dynamic hip screw (DHS)
  - *Unstable/comminuted*: Proximal femoral nail (PFN)
  - *Severely osteoporotic or non-ambulatory*: Consider hemiarthroplasty
- *Post-operative care*:
  - Early mobilization with physiotherapy
  - DVT prophylaxis
  - Osteoporosis management and fall prevention

Q9. Discuss fragility fractures and their management in osteoporosis.

Definition

Fractures resulting from **low-energy trauma** (e.g., fall from standing height) due to **osteoporotic bone** weakness.

Common Sites

- Vertebral compression fractures
- Proximal femur
- Distal radius
- Proximal humerus

Management Overview

A. *Fracture management*:
  - Based on site and stability
    - *Hip*: DHS, PFN, hemiarthroplasty
    - *Vertebra*: Conservative or vertebroplasty
    - *Radius/Humerus*: ORIF or conservative

B. *Osteoporosis treatment*:
  - Calcium (1,000–1,200 mg/day) and vitamin D (800–1,000 IU/day)
  - Bisphosphonates (e.g., Alendronate, Risedronate)
  - Teriparatide for high-risk, non-union, severe osteoporosis
  - Denosumab in patients intolerant to bisphosphonates

C. *Fall prevention*:
  - Home modifications
  - Balance training, strength exercises
  - Vision correction, medication review

D. *Fracture liaison services (FLS)*: Coordinated care to prevent secondary fractures and ensure compliance with osteoporosis treatment

Q10. Explain the role of teriparatide in fracture healing.

What is Teriparatide?

- **Teriparatide** is a recombinant form of **parathyroid hormone (PTH 1–34)**
- It is an **anabolic (bone-building)** agent that **stimulates osteoblast activity**, thereby promoting **new bone formation**

Mechanism of Action

- *Intermittent administration leads to*:
  - Activation of osteoblasts
  - Enhanced **bone matrix synthesis**

- Improved **callus formation and remodeling**
- Increased **biomechanical strength** of healing bone

Indications in Fracture Healing
- Osteoporotic fractures (especially hip, vertebra, wrist)
- Delayed union and nonunion
- Stress fractures (e.g., navicular, tibia)
- Spinal compression fractures
- Periprosthetic fractures in osteoporotic bone

Dosage
- 20 mcg subcutaneously once daily
- *Recommended duration*: 6 to 24 months

Benefits
- Accelerates **fracture union**
- Increases **callus volume and density**
- Improves outcomes in patients with **poor bone stock**
- May reduce the need for revision surgeries in high-risk cases

Contraindications
- Paget's disease of bone
- Bone metastases or skeletal malignancies
- Hypercalcemia
- Prior radiation therapy to bone
- Children or young adults with open growth plates

Conclusion
Teriparatide is a valuable adjunct in managing **challenging fracture cases**, particularly in **osteoporotic or metabolically compromised bone**, with well-documented benefits in **fracture healing acceleration** and **functional recovery**.

Q11. Atypical femoral fractures (AFF).

Definition
Low-energy transverse fracture in subtrochanteric or femoral shaft region, often associated with **long-term bisphosphonate use**

Etiopathogenesis
- Suppressed bone turnover → microdamage accumulation
- Typically occurs **without trauma or with minimal trauma**

Radiographic Features
- Transverse fracture line
- Cortical thickening (lateral cortex)
- Beaking of cortex
- Bilateral symmetry (often prodromal pain)

Management
- *Acute fractures*:
  - Cephalomedullary nailing (e.g., PFN)
  - Delay weight-bearing if incomplete fracture
- *Incomplete fractures*:
  - Discontinue bisphosphonates
  - Conservative treatment if asymptomatic or prophylactic nailing if symptomatic

- *Adjunct therapy*:
  - Teriparatide (anabolic therapy)
  - Calcium and vitamin D supplementation

Q12. Explain the management principles of pathological fractures.

Definition

Fractures occurring in bone **weakened by disease**—metabolic, neoplastic, or infectious.

Common Causes

- *Benign tumors*: Bone cysts, fibrous dysplasia
- *Malignant tumors*:
  - Metastasis (breast, prostate, lung)
  - Multiple myeloma
- *Infections*: Chronic osteomyelitis
- *Metabolic bone disease*: Osteoporosis, Paget's disease, osteomalacia

Management Principles

1. *Stabilize the fracture*:
   - Load-bearing implant preferred (e.g., **cemented intramedullary nail**, **prosthetic reconstruction**)
   - Avoid standard internal fixation without reinforcement in metastatic lesions
2. *Treat the underlying pathology*:
   - Biopsy if diagnosis uncertain
   - Radiotherapy for metastatic lesions
   - Chemotherapy for myeloma, metastasis
   - Bisphosphonates or denosumab for bone protection
3. *Goals*:
   - Pain relief
   - Restore mobility
   - Prevent further pathological fractures

Q13. Explain periprosthetic fractures—classification and management.

Definition

Fractures occurring **around or adjacent to orthopedic implants** [e.g., total hip replacement (THR), total knee replacement (TKR)]

Common Sites

- Femur (around THR)
- Tibia/Patella (after TKR)
- Humerus (around shoulder prosthesis)

Classification (Vancouver for THR)

Type	*Location*	*Implant stability*
A	Trochanteric (greater/lesser)	Stem is stable
B1	Around stem	Stem stable
B2	Around stem	Stem loose
B3	Around stem	Stem loose + poor bone stock
C	Distal to the stem/prosthesis	Irrelevant to prosthesis

Management

- *Type A*: Conservative or tension band wiring
- *B1*: **ORIF** with locking plate ± cable system
- *B2/B3*: **Revision arthroplasty** with long-stem prosthesis ± bone grafting
- *C*: Treat like independent femoral shaft fracture (standard fixation)

Key Principle

Always assess **implant stability** and **bone quality** on imaging and intraoperatively.

Q14. Discuss the management of pathological fractures due to bone metastasis.

(Asked in: MUHS Maharashtra 2023, KGMU Lucknow 2022)

Common Sites

- Spine
- Proximal femur
- Pelvis
- Humerus

Goals of Management

1. Pain relief (primary patient concern)
2. Mechanical stabilization to prevent/improve mobility
3. Allow early mobilization to avoid complications (DVT, pneumonia)
4. Improve quality of life and reduce caregiver dependency

Management Strategy

- *Stabilize fracture*: Cemented IM nails, plates, or endoprostheses
- *Adjuvant therapy*: Radiotherapy for local control, bisphosphonates/denosumab for bone resorption
- *Multidisciplinary care*: Oncology + orthopedics + palliative team
- *Consider prognosis*: Use scoring systems (e.g., Tokuhashi score for spine)

Q15. Explain the purpose of Mirels' scoring system

(Asked in: RGUHS Karnataka 2022)

Purpose

- **Predicts fracture risk** in long bones affected by metastatic lesions
- **Guides decisions** on **prophylactic fixation** to prevent complete fracture

Mirels' Criteria (each scored 1–3)

Parameter	*1 point*	*2 points*	*3 points*
Site	Upper limb	Lower limb	Peritrochanteric
Pain	Mild	Moderate	Functional pain
Lesion type	Blastic	Mixed	Lytic
Size	<1/3 cortex	1/3–2/3	>2/3 cortex

- *Score* ≥9: Strong indication for prophylactic fixation

Prevent fracture rather than repair one in metastatic bone disease.

Q16. Discuss the considerations in managing pediatric polytrauma.

Physiological Differences

- *Larger body surface area*: ↑ fluid and heat loss
- *Smaller blood volume*: Rapid decompensation

- Immature immune and organ systems
- Higher basal metabolic rate

Key Considerations
- Children may **compensate well initially** but deteriorate rapidly
- *Pediatric trauma scores*: PTS, AIS, ISS adapted for children
- Follow **pediatric-specific resuscitation protocols** (e.g., weight-based dosing, Broselow tape)
- **Emotional support** and **family-centered care** crucial
- *Avoid hypothermia*: Use warming blankets, warm fluids
- Suspect **non-accidental trauma** when history is unclear

Management Strategy
- ATLS-like approach adapted to pediatrics
- Early airway management (small-sized tubes)
- Low threshold for imaging but avoid excessive radiation
- Multidisciplinary care (pediatric trauma team, intensivist, surgeon)

Q17. Discuss the impact of obesity on trauma outcomes and management.

Risks and Challenges
- *Airway management difficulty*: Short neck, redundant soft tissue
- Vascular access difficulty
- *Imaging limitations*: Poor quality or weight-restricted tables
- ↑ *Risk of*:
  - Wound infections
  - Deep vein thrombosis (DVT)
  - Pulmonary complications (e.g., ARDS, hypoventilation)
  - Pressure ulcers

Pharmacological Considerations
- *Altered drug kinetics*: Use **ideal body weight** for water-soluble drugs
- Adjust **antibiotic** and **analgesic** dosing accordingly

Management Modifications
- Bariatric-sized **equipment** and **operating tables**
- **Aggressive VTE prophylaxis**
- Optimize patient positioning and oxygenation
- Early mobilization, incentive spirometry to reduce pulmonary complications

Q18. Write a short note on trauma in pregnant patients.

Unique Aspects
- *Two patients are involved*: **Mother and fetus**
- **Physiological adaptations** of pregnancy influence trauma management and response

Key Concerns
- *Supine hypotension syndrome*: Gravid uterus compresses IVC → ↓ venous return and maternal hypotension
- *Altered physiology*:
  - ↑ Heart rate
  - ↓ Blood pressure (especially second trimester)
  - Dilutional anemia

Management Principles
- **Left lateral tilt** (≥15°) or wedge under right hip → relieves IVC compression
- *Stabilize the mother first*: Fetal survival depends on maternal well-being

- **Fetal monitoring** (if fetus is viable, usually >24 weeks)
- **Avoid teratogenic drugs** (e.g., NSAIDs in late pregnancy, certain antibiotics)
- Administer **Rh immunoglobulin** to Rh-negative mothers after trauma

Trauma team should coordinate with obstetricians and anesthetists for optimal outcomes.

Q19. Describe the physiological changes in pregnancy that influence trauma response.

Cardiovascular
- ↑ Blood volume by ~40–50%
- ↓ Systemic vascular resistance → ↓ BP in early pregnancy
- ↑ HR (10–15 bpm)
- Compensation masks early hemorrhage signs

Respiratory
- ↑ Minute ventilation (↑ tidal volume)
- ↓ Functional residual capacity
- ↑ Oxygen demand → hypoxia develops quickly

Hematologic
- **Dilutional anemia**
- ↑ Coagulability → hypercoagulable state

Clinical Relevance
- Early signs of shock may be **subtle or delayed**
- Aggressive monitoring needed

Q20. Mention the risks of aortocaval compression during positioning of pregnant patients.

Definition
Aortocaval compression occurs when the gravid uterus compresses the **inferior vena cava and abdominal aorta**, especially when patient is supine.

Risks
- Maternal **hypotension** and decreased cardiac output
- **Decreased uteroplacental perfusion** → fetal hypoxia or bradycardia
- **Syncope**, nausea, dizziness in mother

Prevention
- **Left lateral tilt** (≥15°)
- Place wedge/pillow under right hip
- Avoid supine position >20 weeks, gestation

Q21. List the anesthetic considerations in orthopedic surgery for pregnant women.

General Considerations
- **Protect the fetus while optimizing maternal status**
- Prefer **regional anesthesia** over general when possible

Key Points
- **Avoid teratogenic agents** (especially in first trimester)
- Ensure **left lateral tilt** to prevent IVC compression
- Maintain **oxygenation, normocapnia, and normotension**
- Use drugs **classified as safe in pregnancy**

- Monitor **fetal heart rate** (if gestation >24 weeks)
- Avoid **NSAIDs late in pregnancy** (risk of premature ductus arteriosus closure)

Anesthesia must be tailored with close coordination between orthopedics, anesthesia, and obstetrics.

Q22. Identify the clinical signs of compartment syndrome in pregnancy and their fetal implications.

Clinical Signs of Compartment Syndrome (Same as General Population)
- **Pain out of proportion** to injury
- Pain on **passive stretch**
- **Paresthesia**, pallor, pulselessness, paralysis (late signs)
- Tense swelling

Special Considerations in Pregnancy
- **Edema may be masked by physiological changes**
- Early diagnosis critical to prevent **maternal and fetal compromise**

Fetal Implications
- **Maternal hypotension and metabolic acidosis** from untreated compartment syndrome can lead to **fetal distress or demise**
- **Emergency fasciotomy** must not be delayed in suspected cases

Prompt recognition and intervention is vital to protect **both maternal limb function and fetal well-being**.

Q23. Explain the thromboembolic risks associated with immobilization in pregnant trauma patients.

Background
Pregnancy is a **hypercoagulable state** due to:
- ↑ Fibrinogen and clotting factors (VII, VIII, X)
- ↓ Fibrinolytic activity

Risks Enhanced by Trauma and Immobilization
- Deep vein thrombosis (DVT)
- Pulmonary embolism (PE)
- Iliac vein compression by gravid uterus

Contributing Factors
- Reduced mobility post-trauma
- Venous stasis (IVC compression)
- Endothelial injury

Prevention
- *Low molecular weight heparin (LMWH)*: Safe in pregnancy
- Graduated compression stockings
- Early mobilization when possible
- Avoid warfarin (teratogenic, especially in first trimester)

Q24. What imaging modalities are considered safe during pregnancy for orthopedic injuries?

Safe Modalities
- *Ultrasound (USG)*: No ionizing radiation, safe in all trimesters
- *MRI*: Preferred for soft tissue and spinal injuries; no radiation

Conditional Use

- *X-ray with shielding*: Acceptable with **abdominal lead shielding**, especially for extremities
- *CT scan*: Avoid unless essential (e.g., pelvic trauma, head injury); use shielding

ALARA principle (As Low As Reasonably Achievable) principle applies to all imaging decisions

Q25. State the indications for cesarean section in pelvic fractures during active labor.

Indications

- *Mechanical obstruction*: Malalignment or narrowing of the birth canal from pelvic fracture
- *Unstable pelvic ring*: Risk of displacement during labour
- Fetal distress
- *Open pelvic fractures*: Risk of infection with vaginal delivery
- Recent internal fixation of pelvic bones

Multidisciplinary decision (orthopedics + obstetrics)

Q26. Outline ethical considerations in balancing maternal and fetal risks during orthopedic surgery.

Ethical Principles

1. *Autonomy*: Inform and involve the mother in decision-making
2. *Beneficence*: Aim to benefit both mother and fetus
3. *Non-maleficence*: Avoid harm (e.g., teratogenic drugs, radiation)
4. *Justice*: Equal care irrespective of fetal viability

Key Considerations

- Prioritize **maternal survival**
- Avoid unnecessary delays in urgent care
- Involve **informed consent** and detailed counseling
- Consider **viability of fetus** in surgical/anesthetic planning

Q27. Describe safe pain management options for pregnant women with fractures.

Safe Options

- *Paracetamol (acetaminophen)*: First-line
- *Opioids (short-term, lowest dose)*: For example, morphine, fentanyl

Use with Caution

- *NSAIDs*: Avoid in third trimester (risk of premature ductus arteriosus closure, oligohydramnios)
- *Regional anesthesia*: Effective and safe for limb surgeries

Avoid

- COX-2 inhibitors
- Tramadol in first trimester (possible fetal anomalies)

Pain control is essential to prevent maternal distress, which can compromise fetal oxygenation.

Q28. List the components of a primary and secondary trauma survey in pregnant polytrauma patients

Primary Survey (ABCDE)

- *A*irway with cervical spine protection
- *B*reathing and ventilation
- *C*irculation (consider uterine compression → supine hypotension)

- *D*isability (neurologic status)
- *E*xposure with environmental control

Modifications
- **Left lateral tilt** or wedge under right hip
- Early fetal heart monitoring (if ≥24 weeks, gestation)

Secondary Survey
- Detailed head-to-toe assessment
- Obstetric evaluation (USG for fetal viability, placental abruption)
- *Labs*: Rh typing, Kleihauer–Betke test (to assess fetal-maternal hemorrhage)
- Tetanus prophylaxis
- Radiology as needed (with shielding)

Q29. Assess a pregnant woman with suspected pelvic fracture following trauma. Discuss maternal-fetal physiological responses, injury implications, and communication strategies with the patient and obstetric team.

(CMC Vellore 2017)

Assessment Strategy
- **ATLS protocol** with left lateral positioning
- Assess vitals, GCS, and **pelvic stability**
- Monitor **fetal heart rate**, uterine tone, and vaginal bleeding
- Perform **focused obstetric USG**

Maternal-fetal Physiological Considerations
- Uterine rupture or placental abruption may occur even without external signs
- Hemorrhagic shock can occur with minimal external bleeding
- Maternal hypotension → fetal hypoxia

Communication Strategy
- *Early involvement of multidisciplinary team*: Ortho + Obstetrics + Anesthesia + Neonatology
- Provide **clear, empathetic explanations** to the patient/family
- *Document counseling and consent regarding*:
  - Imaging needs
  - Surgery/Anesthesia risks
  - Fetal viability and outcomes

Goal
Optimize care for both mother and fetus while ensuring ethical transparency and collaborative decision-making.

Q30. Discuss anatomical and physiological changes in pregnancy that affect orthopedic fracture management. Describe proper surgical positioning to prevent aortocaval compression and outline how to counsel patients about radiation risks.

Anatomical and Physiological Changes in Pregnancy
Cardiovascular:
- ↑ Blood volume (40–50%) → hemodilution
- ↓ Peripheral resistance → lower BP in second trimester
- ↑ Heart rate

Respiratory:
- ↑ Tidal volume and minute ventilation
- ↓ Functional residual capacity
- Diaphragm elevation

Musculoskeletal:
- **Relaxin hormone** → ligamentous laxity → ↑ joint mobility
- Altered gait and posture → ↑ fall risk
- Lumbar lordosis exaggeration

Hematologic:
- *Hypercoagulability*: ↑ risk of thromboembolism

Surgical Positioning to Prevent Aortocaval Compression
- Avoid supine position beyond 20 weeks, gestation
- Use **left lateral tilt (≥15°)** or place wedge under **right hip**
- *Prevents compression of IVC*: Maintains venous return and fetal perfusion

Radiation Risk Counseling
- *Counseling points*:
    - Use imaging only when essential
    - Shield abdomen and pelvis
    - Risks depend on **dose and gestational age**
    - *<50 mGy*: low fetal risk
    - MRI and ultrasound are safe modalities
- Reassure patient about **precautions and benefits outweighing risks**
- Involve obstetric team if advanced imaging is required

Q31. Evaluate the orthopedic management of a pregnant woman with lower limb trauma. Include anesthesia planning, surgical precautions, and empathetic communication with the patient and obstetric team.

Orthopedic Management Overview

Assessment:
- ATLS protocol with **left lateral tilt**
- Stabilize fractures as per urgency
- Minimize immobilization to reduce **DVT risk**

Surgical management:
- Delay surgery only if safe for both mother and fetus
- **Definitive fixation preferred over temporary** in most cases
- Use **low radiation** techniques (fluoroscopy with shielding)

Anesthesia Planning
- Regional anesthesia preferred (e.g., spinal/epidural)
- *If GA is needed*:
    - Ensure left lateral tilt
    - Use non-teratogenic drugs
    - Monitor maternal oxygenation and BP closely

Empathetic Communication
- Explain condition, imaging, anesthesia risks in **clear, reassuring terms**
- Involve **multidisciplinary team** early
- Document **shared decision-making** and informed consent
- *Address maternal concerns about*:
    - Surgery effects on fetus
    - Breastfeeding if postpartum
    - Mobility and recovery post-injury

Q32. Describe how to identify and manage compartment syndrome in a pregnant trauma patient. Include the maternal-fetal risks and how to perform a clinical limb exam while maintaining patient dignity.

(DYPU Pune 2017)

Identification

- *Classic signs*:
  - Pain out of proportion
  - Pain on passive stretch
  - Tense, swollen compartment
  - Paresthesia, pallor, paralysis, pulselessness (late signs)
- May be **masked** in pregnancy due to generalized edema or altered pain perception

Maternal-fetal Risks

- *Untreated compartment syndrome*: Ischemic muscle necrosis, acidosis
- *Systemic complications*: **Hypotension**, fetal hypoxia
- Potential for **multi-organ failure** and fetal compromise

Management

- High index of suspicion
- Immediate **fasciotomy** if clinical diagnosis is evident
- Avoid delay for imaging or pressure measurement if signs are classic

Clinical Limb Examination with Dignity

- *Ensure privacy*: Use screens or cover non-examined areas
- Have a **female assistant or chaperone** present
- Explain every step before and during the examination
- Minimize patient exposure and discomfort
- Encourage questions and reassure the patient of the necessity of the exam

Early diagnosis and intervention are critical for **saving the limb and protecting fetal health.**

Q33. Explain the risk and prevention of thromboembolism in immobilized pregnant trauma patients. Demonstrate the role of mechanical prophylaxis and patient education.

Risk Factors

- *Pregnancy is a hypercoagulable state*:
  - ↑ Clotting factors (VII, VIII, X, fibrinogen)
  - ↓ Protein S and fibrinolysis
- *Trauma and immobilization add*:
  - Venous stasis (IVC compression)
  - Endothelial injury
  - Reduced ambulation

Prevention

1. *Pharmacological prophylaxis*:
   - **LMWH** (e.g., enoxaparin)—safe and preferred
   - Avoid warfarin (teratogenic, especially in first trimester)
2. *Mechanical prophylaxis*:
   - Intermittent pneumatic compression (IPC) devices
   - Graduated compression stockings
   - Use in **high-risk patients** or those contraindicated for anticoagulants

3. *Patient education*:
   - Importance of **early mobilization**
   - Recognizing **DVT signs** (swelling, calf pain, redness)
   - Compliance with stockings or medication
   - **Hydration** and limb elevation

Q34. Interpret imaging in pregnant women with orthopedic trauma. Discuss safe modalities, fetal protection principles, and coordination with radiology to address patient anxiety.

Safe Imaging Modalities
- *Ultrasound*: No radiation; safe for soft tissue/muscle injury
- *MRI*: No ionizing radiation; safe in all trimesters

Limited Use
- *X-ray*:
  - Acceptable for extremity and chest imaging
  - Use **lead shielding** over abdomen
- *CT scan*:
  - Use only if essential (e.g., pelvic fracture, head trauma)
  - Apply ALARA principle (As Low As Reasonably Achievable)

Fetal Protection Principles
- Shielding abdomen/pelvis
- Limit exposure field
- Use fastest, lowest-dose protocols

Addressing Anxiety
- **Involve radiologist** in counseling
- Clearly explain **risk–benefit ratio**
- Reassure with facts (e.g., <50 mGy has negligible fetal risk)
- Offer **written consent** and allow support person presence if possible

Q35. Describe the obstetric and orthopedic considerations in a pregnant woman with a pelvic fracture in active labor. Explain when cesarean section is indicated and how to communicate surgical plans empathetically.

(AIIMS JPR 2011)

Obstetric Considerations
- Evaluate **pelvic dimensions** and stability
- Assess **fetal well-being**
- Monitor for **vaginal bleeding** or uterine rupture

Orthopedic Considerations
- Check stability of the pelvic ring
- Avoid stress on recent **pelvic fixation** or hardware

Indications for Cesarean Section
- Malaligned pelvis obstructing delivery
- Unstable pelvic ring or recent fixation
- Associated soft tissue injury or infection
- Fetal distress

Empathetic Communication

- Involve the **multidisciplinary team** (ortho, OB-GYN, anesthesia)
- Explain risks, delivery options, and recovery implications
- Respect patient's preferences; provide **psychological support**
- Use **visual aids** or diagrams if helpful

Q36. Outline the surgical planning for a femur fracture in a pregnant woman. Discuss safe patient positioning, maternal-fetal risk considerations, and ethical communication.

Surgical Planning

- Perform **early definitive fixation** to prevent complications (e.g., DVT, pneumonia)
- Prefer **closed intramedullary nailing** if feasible

Patient Positioning

- **Left lateral tilt** (≥15°) or wedge under right hip
- Avoid supine hypotension syndrome (IVC compression)

Maternal-fetal Considerations

- Minimize blood loss
- Use non-teratogenic drugs and anesthesia
- Fetal monitoring (if viable gestation)

Ethical Communication

- Explain urgency and surgical options
- Discuss imaging and anesthesia safety
- Obtain **informed consent**, balancing **maternal life versus fetal safety**
- Reassure about team coordination and fetal monitoring

Q37. Discuss pain management strategies in orthopedic trauma during pregnancy. Explain safe use of regional anesthesia and considerations in drug selection.

Pain Management Options

Safe drugs:

- *Paracetamol (acetaminophen)*: First line
- *Opioids (short-term)*: Morphine, fentanyl—safe in moderation

Avoid or use with caution:

- *NSAIDs*: Avoid in third trimester (ductus arteriosus closure risk)
- *Tramadol*: Use cautiously (possible teratogenicity)
- Avoid **COX-2 inhibitors**

Regional Anesthesia

- Preferred for **lower limb surgeries**
- **Spinal or epidural blocks** safe and effective
- Reduces need for systemic opioids
- Avoids airway challenges in pregnant patients

Additional Considerations

- Adjust doses based on **physiological changes**
- Multimodal pain strategies
- Discuss **breastfeeding safety** post-operatively

Q38. Describe a multidisciplinary approach to managing polytrauma in a pregnant woman. Include trauma survey protocols and empathetic communication with the patient and her family.

Key Principles

- Pregnancy involves **two patients**: mother and fetus.
- Prioritize **maternal stabilization** to optimize fetal outcome.
- Requires coordinated **multidisciplinary care**.

Multidisciplinary Team Includes

- Trauma surgeon
- Orthopedic surgeon
- Obstetrician
- Anesthesiologist
- Radiologist
- Neonatologist (if >24 weeks gestation)
- Social worker/psychologist

Trauma Survey Protocols (Modified ATLS)

Primary survey (ABCDE):

- *Airway*: Secure with cervical spine protection
- *Breathing*: High-flow oxygen; avoid hypoxia
- *Circulation*: Left lateral tilt (≥15°) to relieve IVC compression
- *Disability*: Assess GCS; consider eclampsia/seizures
- *Exposure*: Avoid hypothermia; check for hidden injuries

Note: Apply **fetal heart rate monitoring** (>24 weeks)

Secondary survey:

- Detailed head-to-toe exam
- Focused Obstetric USG (rule out placental abruption)
- *Labs*: CBC, blood group, Rh typing, Kleihauer-Betke test
- Imaging with shielding (as needed)

Empathetic Communication

- Use **simple, supportive language**
- Explain risks and procedures to both patient and family
- Address **fetal concerns compassionately**
- Involve family in shared decision-making
- Provide psychological support and continuous updates

Goals of Management

- Prevent maternal death → ensures fetal survival
- Timely orthopedic and obstetric interventions
- Optimize fetal health while minimizing maternal complications

Q39. Discuss the treatment of stress fractures in athletes.

Definition

Microscopic bone injuries due to repetitive submaximal loading without sufficient rest

Common Sites

- Tibia (most common)
- Metatarsals (especially second)

- Femoral neck
- Navicular bone
- Pelvis

Risk Factors
- Sudden increase in training intensity
- Poor footwear or running surface
- Vitamin D or calcium deficiency
- *Female athlete triad*: Disordered eating, amenorrhea, osteopenia

Diagnosis
- *X-ray*: Often normal initially (changes may appear after 2–3 weeks)
- *MRI*: Most sensitive and specific
- *Bone scan*: Shows early uptake (less specific)

Management
Conservative:
- Rest, activity modification (4–8 weeks)
- Protected weight bearing (boot or cast)
- *Nutritional support*: Calcium, vtamin D
- Address biomechanical issues (orthotics)

Surgical:
- *Indicated for high-risk sites*:
  - Femoral neck (risk of displacement/AVN)
  - Navicular bone
- Fixation with **screws or intramedullary devices**

Key Concept
- Prevention through **training balance**, **nutrition**, and **early detection**
- Emphasize **gradual progression** in training programs

CHAPTER 12

Sports Injuries and Soft Tissue Disorders

Sanjeev Gupta, Mozam Hamid Wani, Deepali Gupta

I. Fundamentals and Classification

Q1. Classify sports injuries. Differentiate between acute and chronic injuries.

Classification

A. *Based on onset*:
- *Acute injuries*: Sudden onset due to a specific trauma
  Examples: Fracture, ligament tear, muscle strain, contusion
- *Chronic injuries*: Gradual onset due to overuse
  Examples: Tendinopathy, stress fracture, bursitis

B. *Based on tissue type*:
- *Soft tissue*: Muscle, tendon, ligament (strain, sprain)
- *Bone*: Fractures, stress fractures
- *Joint*: Dislocations, cartilage injury

C. *Based on severity (grades)*:
- *Grade I*: Mild
- *Grade II*: Moderate
- *Grade III*: Complete rupture

Differences

Feature	*Acute injury*	*Chronic injury*
Onset	Sudden	Gradual
Cause	Trauma	Repetitive stress
Example	ACL tear, fracture	Tendinitis, stress fracture
Management	RICE, surgical if needed	Load modification, rehabilitation

Q2. Classification and pathophysiology of sports injuries.

(RUHS 2011)

A. Classification

(Similar to Q1: Acute/Chronic, Soft/Hard tissue)

B. Pathophysiology

- *Acute Injuries:* Direct trauma → inflammation → tissue disruption → repair phase (fibrosis or regeneration)

- *Chronic (overuse) injuries:*
  - Microtrauma > repair capacity
  - Disrupted collagen (in tendons)
  - Neovascularization, nociceptor sensitization → pain and dysfunction

Tendon example: Collagen disarray + increased ground substance → **tendinopathy**

Q3. Overuse injuries—examples and management.

Definition

Injuries from repetitive submaximal loading without adequate rest

Examples

- Tennis elbow (lateral epicondylitis)
- Patellar tendinopathy (jumper's knee)
- Shin splints
- Swimmer's shoulder
- Stress fractures

Management

1. Rest/Modification of activity
2. *Physiotherapy*: Eccentric loading, stretching
3. NSAIDs/Analgesics
4. *Orthotics*: Shoes/Inserts
5. Gradual return to sport
6. PRP injections or shockwave therapy (select cases)

Q4. Biomechanics of knee ligament injuries in athletes.

Common ligaments

ACL, PCL, MCL, LCL

Mechanism of Injury

Ligament	*Common mechanism*
ACL	Valgus + internal rotation + hyperextension (non-contact pivoting injury)
PCL	Dashboard injury or hyperflexion
MCL	Direct blow to lateral side
LCL	Varus stress

Biomechanical Concepts

- **Q-angle, landing mechanics, hamstring-quadriceps ratio**
- Poor biomechanics → increased ACL risk (e.g., valgus collapse during landing)

Q5. Role of biomechanics in sports injury prevention.

Importance

- Identifies faulty movement patterns → corrects them
- Reduces injury risk

Applications

- ACL prevention programs (neuromuscular training)
- Gait analysis in runners

- Core strengthening to reduce lower back injuries
- Jump landing technique correction (plyometrics)

Preventive Programs
- FIFA 11+ (for soccer)
- Prevent injury and enhance performance (PEP) program

II. Knee Injuries

Q6. What are the common sports-related injuries of the knee?

Soft Tissue Injuries
- *Ligamentous:*
  - Anterior cruciate ligament (ACL) tear—most common in pivoting sports
  - Medial collateral ligament (MCL) sprain
  - Posterior cruciate ligament (PCL) injury
  - Lateral collateral ligament (LCL) injury
  - *Meniscal*: Medial > lateral meniscus tear
- *Tendon:*
  - Patellar tendinitis (jumper's knee)
  - Quadriceps tendon strain
- *Cartilage:*
  - Chondral/Osteochondral injuries
  - Osteochondritis dissecans

Bone and Joint Injuries
- Tibial plateau fractures
- Patellar dislocation
- Stress fractures (e.g., tibial)

Q7. Meniscal injuries—clinical features, imaging, and management.

Clinical Features
- Joint line tenderness (medial/lateral)
- Locking/Catching sensation
- Swelling (delayed effusion)
- Positive McMurray's or Apley's test
- Difficulty squatting or twisting

Imaging
- *MRI*: Gold standard
  - Identifies tear pattern, location (red vs. white zone)
  - Associated injuries (ACL, chondral damage)

Management

Type	*Treatment*
Small, peripheral tear	Conservative (RICE, rehabilitation)
Large, unstable tear	Arthroscopic repair (especially in red zone)
Complex or degenerated tear	Partial meniscectomy

Meniscus preservation preferred in young athletes.

Q8. Principles of rehabilitation following ACL reconstruction.

(IMS-BHU 2017)

Phases of Rehabilitation

Phase	*Goals*
Immediate post-operative (0–2 weeks)	Pain control, ROM (0–90°), quadriceps activation
Early phase (2–6 weeks)	Full ROM, reduce swelling, closed-chain exercises
Strength phase (6–12 weeks)	Improve strength, proprioception
Agility/Running (3–6 months)	Gradual return to jogging/sport-specific drills
Return to sport (6–9 months)	Hop tests, functional assessment, psychological readiness

Key Points

- Emphasis on **quadriceps strength**
- Avoid open-chain exercises early
- **Functional testing** before return to sport
- Graft maturation ~9 months

Q9. Treatment of multiligament knee injuries in athletes.

Definition

Involvement of ≥2 major ligaments (ACL, PCL, MCL, LCL/posterolateral corner)

Assessment

- *Vascular status*: **Check for popliteal artery injury**
- *Neurological*: **Common peroneal nerve**
- Use **KD classification (Kennedy)**

Imaging

- *MRI*: All ligamentous structures
- *CT angiography*: If vascular injury suspected

Treatment Strategy

Injury type	*Treatment*
KD I–II with intact neurovascular	Early/Delayed reconstruction (ACL ± PCL)
KD III/IV or vascular injury	Emergency vascular repair + staged ligament reconstruction
Chronic dislocations	Complex—may need osteotomies or constrained prostheses

Surgical Principles

- **Anatomic repair/reconstruction**
- **Staged or single-stage** depending on soft tissue condition
- **Rehabilitation** crucial—slower than isolated ACL rehabilitation

Q10. What is the unhappy triad of the knee?

Also known as **O'Donoghue's triad**, typically occurs due to **valgus stress with external rotation** in contact sports.

Classical Triad

1. Anterior cruciate ligament (ACL) tear
2. Medial collateral ligament (MCL) tear
3. Medial meniscus injury (historically)

Modern MRI evidence shows **lateral meniscus** involvement is more common.

Mechanism

- Lateral blow to the knee (valgus)
- Twisting or pivoting while foot is planted

Clinical Features

- Pain, swelling, instability
- Positive Lachman's test, valgus stress test, McMurray's test

Management

- *Isolated MCL*: Conservative with bracing
- *ACL ± meniscus*: Surgical reconstruction (especially in athletes)
- Post-operative rehabilitation

Q11. Medial tibial stress syndrome (MTSS)—shin splints.

Definition

Exercise-induced pain along the **posteromedial tibial border**, usually in runners.

Etiology

Repetitive microtrauma → inflammation of **periosteum**, **tibialis posterior**, or **soleus** origin.

Risk Factors

- Overtraining, flat feet, improper footwear
- Tight gastrocnemius-soleus complex

Clinical Features

- Dull, aching pain during or after exercise
- Tenderness along distal one-third of medial tibia

Investigations

- Clinical diagnosis
- Rule out stress fracture (X-ray or MRI)

Management

- Rest, ice, NSAIDs
- Correct biomechanical abnormalities
- Activity modification
- Stretching/Strengthening exercises
- Orthotics if needed

Q12. Hamstring injuries—classification and management.

Classification

Based on **site and severity**:

Grade	*Description*	*Symptoms*
I	Minor strain, no loss of function	Tightness, minimal pain
II	Partial tear	Pain, weakness, bruising
III	Complete rupture	Sudden severe pain, loss of function

Common Sites

Proximal hamstring (biceps femoris most common)

Management

Type	Treatment
Grade I–II	RICE, NSAIDs, physiotherapy
Grade III	May require surgical repair (complete avulsion)
Rehabilitation	Progressive stretching, strengthening, eccentric training

Reinjury risk high if return to play is premature.

Q13. Anterior shoulder instability—surgical treatment options.

(AIIMS BBSR 2013)

Etiology

Recurrent anterior dislocation, often due to trauma (abduction + external rotation)

Associated Lesions

- *Bankart lesion*: Anterior inferior labral tear
- *Hill-Sachs lesion*: Posterosuperior humeral head impaction fracture

Surgical Options

Surgery	Indications	Key points
Arthroscopic Bankart repair	Most common for soft-tissue Bankart lesions	Anchors labrum to glenoid rim
Latarjet procedure	Glenoid bone loss >20–25%	Transfer coracoid to anterior glenoid
Remplissage procedure	Large engaging Hill-Sachs lesions	Fill defect with infraspinatus tendon
Capsular shift	Multidirectional instability	Tightens capsule; rare in modern practice

Postoperative rehabilitation

- Sling immobilization (2–4 weeks)
- ROM → Strength → Sport-specific training
- Return to sports in 4–6 months

Q14. Patellar tendinopathy (Jumper's Knee)—pathogenesis and management.

Definition

Chronic overuse injury of the **patellar tendon**, common in jumping athletes (e.g., basketball, volleyball).

Pathogenesis

- **Microtrauma** → failed healing response
- Degeneration of **tendon fibers** at the **inferior pole of the patella**
- **Neovascularization** and collagen disorganization

Clinical Features

- Anterior knee pain (especially with jumping, squatting)
- Tenderness at inferior patella pole
- Pain on resisted knee extension

Imaging

- *Ultrasound*: Hypoechoic tendon thickening
- *MRI*: Signal intensity at the patellar tendon origin

Management

Stage	*Treatment*
Acute	Activity modification, ice, NSAIDs
Subacute	Eccentric quadriceps training (Alfredson protocol)
Refractory	PRP injections, shockwave therapy, surgical debridement (rare)

Q15. Patellar dislocation and recurrent instability—diagnosis and treatment.

Acute Patellar Dislocation

Usually **lateral**, due to twisting trauma with valgus force on a flexed knee

Clinical Features

- History of sudden knee pain and "popping out"
- Swelling, tenderness on medial patella (MPFL rupture)

Imaging

- *X-ray*: Look for patellar tilt or subluxation
- *MRI*: Evaluate MPFL injury, osteochondral fragments

Management

Type	*Treatment*
First-time dislocation	Closed reduction, immobilization, physiotherapy
Recurrent instability	Surgical—MPFL reconstruction, lateral release, tibial tubercle osteotomy (TTT) if high Q-angle
Rehabilitation	Focus on quadriceps (especially vastus medialis obliquus) strengthening

Surgical Indications

- Two dislocations
- MPFL tear with high-grade trochlear dysplasia or malalignment

Q16. Principles of return-to-sport (RTS) after orthopedic injuries.

Return-to-sport (RTS) is a **staged, individualized decision** to minimize reinjury risk and optimize performance.

Key Principles

1. *Tissue healing timelines:*
    - *Bone*: 6–8 weeks
    - *Tendon/Ligament*: 3–6 months
2. *Functional testing*:
    - Limb symmetry index ≥90%
    - Hop tests, strength, proprioception
3. *Psychological readiness*:
    - Fear of reinjury (assessed by ACL-RSI scale)
    - Confidence and motivation
4. *Sport-specific drills*: Gradual reintroduction to sport intensity
5. *Multidisciplinary team*: Surgeon, physio, trainer, psychologist

Criteria-based Progression (Example: ACL)

- No effusion or pain
- Full ROM and strength
- ≥90% hop test performance
- 6+ months post-operative

III. Ankle and Foot Injuries

Q17. Common sports-related injuries of the ankle.

1. *Lateral ankle sprain (most common):*
   - Involves anterior talofibular ligament (ATFL) > calcaneofibular ligament (CFL)
   - *Mechanism*: Inversion + plantar flexion
2. *High ankle sprain (syndesmotic injury):* Involves anterior inferior tibiofibular ligament (AITFL), interosseous ligament
3. *Achilles tendinopathy or rupture:* Overuse or explosive loading (running, jumping)
4. *Peroneal tendon injuries:* Subluxation or tear in athletes
5. *Stress fractures:* Navicular, 5th metatarsal (Jones), tibia
6. *Plantar fasciitis:* Heel pain in runners

Q18. Syndesmotic ankle injury—diagnosis and management.

Definition
Injury to distal tibiofibular syndesmosis (AITFL, PITFL, interosseous membrane)

Mechanism
External rotation of foot + dorsiflexion (e.g., football tackle)

Clinical Features
- Pain above lateral malleolus
- Positive squeeze test, external rotation test

Imaging
- *X-ray:* Widened tibiofibular clear space
- *MRI:* Gold standard for ligamentous injury

Management

Type	*Treatment*
Stable (Grade I)	RICE, walking boot, early rehabilitation
Unstable (Grade II/III)	Syndesmotic screw or suture button fixation
Return to sport	6–12 weeks depending on healing

Q19. Achilles tendon rupture—pathophysiology and management.

Pathophysiology
- Eccentric overload → tendon degeneration → rupture (typically 2–6 cm above calcaneus)
- Common in 30–50 years old recreational athletes

Clinical Features
- Sudden "pop", pain in calf
- *Thompson test*: Negative (no plantar flexion)
- Palpable gap

Imaging
Ultrasound or MRI if clinical doubt

Management

Option	Indications
Conservative	Non-displaced tears, non-athletes—functional brace in equinus
Surgical	Young, active, or large gaps—open or percutaneous repair

Rehabilitation

- Early weight bearing
- Gradual dorsiflexion stretching, heel raises

Q20. Stress fractures in athletes—management principles.

Common Sites

Tibia, navicular, 2nd metatarsal, 5th metatarsal (jones)

Pathophysiology

Repetitive microtrauma > bone resorption exceeds formation

Risk Factors

- Female athlete triad
- Poor nutrition, overtraining

Diagnosis

- *Clinical*: Local pain, activity-related
- *Imaging*: X-ray may be normal; **MRI is the gold standard**

Management

Type of bone	Treatment
Low risk (tibia shaft, metatarsals)	Rest, offloading, gradual return
High risk (navicular, femoral neck)	Protected weight bearing ± surgical fixation

Q21. Chronic exertional compartment syndrome (CECS).

Definition:

A reversible, exercise-induced increase in intracompartmental pressure that compromises neuromuscular function.

Pathophysiology

- *During exercise:* Increased blood flow → muscle expansion (up to 20%) → rise in intracompartmental pressure
- *Inadequate fascial compliance:* Tight or inelastic fascia prevents expansion → compresses capillaries and nerves
- *Result:* Ischemia → pain, paresthesia → symptom relief on cessation of activity

Most Common Sites

Anterior and lateral compartments of the leg (especially in runners)

Clinical Features

Feature	Description
Pain	Bilateral, predictable, occurs at a specific time into exercise
Tightness	Localized to affected compartment
Paresthesia	Often in dermatome supplied by affected nerves
Weakness	Foot drop if anterior compartment is involved
Recovery	Symptoms subside with rest (15–30 minutes)

Diagnosis

Clinical suspicion: History is key (exercise-induced symptoms with relief at rest)

Compartment pressure testing

- *Gold standard:*
  - *Pre-exercise:* >15 mm Hg
  - *1 minute post-exercise:* >30 mm Hg
  - *5 minute post-exercise:* >20 mm Hg

MRI/Near-infrared spectroscopy (NIRS): Useful adjuncts (less commonly used)

Differential diagnoses:

- Medial tibial stress syndrome (shin splints)
- Stress fracture
- Popliteal artery entrapment
- Nerve entrapment

Management

Conservative:

- Activity modification
- Physical therapy (stretching, gait retraining)
- NSAIDs (limited role)
- Orthotics

Surgical:

- *Fasciotomy: Definitive treatment:*
  - Open or endoscopic
  - High success rate (~70–90%)
  - Recurrence rate 10–15%

Prognosis:

- Good with surgery
- Poor compliance to conservative treatment → persistent symptoms

Shoulder Injuries in Sports

Q22. Common shoulder injuries in sports.

- Dislocations (anterior > posterior)
- Rotator cuff injuries (especially supraspinatus tear in overhead athletes)
- Superior labrum anterior to posterior (SLAP) lesions
- Shoulder impingement syndrome
- Acromioclavicular joint injuries
- Biceps tendonitis

Q23. Common shoulder dislocations in athletes and their treatment.

(NEIGRIHMS 2015)

Type	*Mechanism*	*Features*	*Management*
Anterior (most common)	Abduction + external rotation	Flattened deltoid, arm abducted	Reduction → immobilization → rehabilitation surgery in recurrent cases
Posterior	Seizures, electric shock, trauma	Arm held in adduction + internal rotation	Closed reduction → immobilization; surgery if locked
Inferior (luxatio erecta)	Rare, hyperabduction	Arm held above head	Closed reduction + sling

Q24. Rotator cuff injuries in overhead athletes.

Causes
- Repetitive microtrauma (throwing, swimming)
- Impingement + tendon degeneration

Clinical Features
- Pain on overhead activity
- Night pain
- Weakness of abduction and external rotation

Tests
- Empty can test
- Drop arm test

Imaging
MRI: Best modality

Treatment
- *Conservative:* Rest, physiotherapy, NSAIDs
- *Surgical:* Arthroscopic repair for full-thickness tears or failed conservative treatment

Q25. Superior labrum anterior to posterior (SLAP) lesions.

Definition
Tear of the superior labrum where biceps tendon anchors.

Causes
- Overhead activities (e.g., throwing, swimming)
- Trauma (fall on outstretched hand)

Types
Snyder classification (Type I–IV)

Diagnosis
- O'Brien test, Speed's test
- MRI arthrogram

Treatment
- *Type I–II:* Debridement, tenotomy/tenodesis
- *Type III–IV*: Repair (especially in young active patients)

Q26. Shoulder dislocations in athletes—clinical features and management.

Clinical Features
- History of trauma
- "Dead arm" sensation
- Prominent acromion, flattening of shoulder
- Positive apprehension and relocation tests (for instability)

Management
1. *Acute:* Closed reduction, immobilization
2. *Rehabilitation:*
   - Focus on proprioception, scapular control
   - Rotator cuff strengthening

3. *Surgical:*
    - Indicated in young athletes with recurrent instability
    - Bankart repair (arthroscopic/open)
    - Latarjet procedure for bony defects

V. Elbow, Wrist, and Hand Injuries in Sports

Q27. Traumatic elbow injuries in athletes.

Injury	*Mechanism*	*Presentation*	*Management*
Elbow dislocation	Fall on outstretched hand	Pain, deformity, swelling	Reduction + immobilization, rehabilitation
Radial head fracture	Valgus stress, FOOSH	Lateral elbow pain, limited supination	Mason classification-based treatment
Olecranon fracture	Direct trauma	Swelling, loss of extension	Tension band wiring or plating
Capitellum fracture	Shearing force	Lateral pain, block to motion	ORIF if displaced

Q28. What is Tommy John surgery?

(CMC Vellore 2017)

- *Definition*: Reconstruction of the **ulnar collateral ligament (UCL)** of the elbow.
- *Indication*: Overhead athletes (e.g., baseball pitchers) with **chronic UCL injury**.
- *Graft used*: Palmaris longus tendon (or gracilis).
- *Technique*: Docking technique or figure-8 technique.
- *Rehabilitation*:
    - 6 months to 1 year for return to sports.
    - Progressive throwing program.

Q29. UCL injury in thrower's elbow—pathophysiology and management.

- *Pathophysiology:*
    - Repetitive valgus stress → microtrauma of UCL (especially anterior band)
    - Common in baseball pitchers
- *Clinical features:*
    - Medial elbow pain during acceleration phase of throwing
    - Instability, reduced performance
- *Diagnosis:*
    - Moving valgus stress test (sensitive)
    - MRI with contrast (for UCL tear)
- *Management:*
    - *Non-operative*: Rest, physiotherapy (mild/moderate)
    - *Surgical*: Tommy John surgery (for complete tear/high-demand athletes)

Q30. Wrist and hand injuries in sports—list and management.

Injury	*Sport*	*Management*
Scaphoid fracture	Football, fall sports	Thumb spica cast or ORIF
TFCC tear	Racquet sports, gymnastics	Splinting, arthroscopic repair
Gamekeeper's thumb (UCL of thumb)	Skiing, rugby	Thumb spica, surgery if Stener lesion

Continued

Continued

Injury	*Sport*	*Management*
Boxer's fracture (5th metacarpal)	Punching	Closed reduction and ulnar gutter splint
Mallet finger	Basketball, volleyball	Extension splint for 6–8 weeks
Jersey finger (FDP avulsion)	Rugby, football	Surgical repair
Hook of hamate fracture	Golf, racquet sports	Immobilization or excision

Q31. Management of gamekeeper's (Skier's) thumb.

- *Definition:* Injury to the **ulnar collateral ligament (UCL)** of the thumb MCP joint.
- *Mechanism:* Valgus stress due to sudden abduction (e.g., fall with ski pole).
- *Clinical features:*
    - Pain/swelling at MCP joint
    - Weak pinch grip
    - Tenderness on ulnar side of MCP
- *Diagnosis:*
    - Stress test for valgus instability
    - MRI for complete tear or Stener lesion
- *Management:*
    - *Partial tear:* Thumb spica splint/cast for 4–6 weeks
    - *Complete tear or Stener lesion:* Surgical repair

Q32. Scapholunate ligament injuries—diagnosis and treatment.

- *Definition:* Disruption of the **scapholunate interosseous ligament** (SLIL), the most important carpal stabilizer.
- *Mechanism:* FOOSH injury causing wrist hyperextension.
- *Clinical features:*
    - Dorsal wrist pain
    - Watson's test positive (painful clunk on radial deviation)
- *Diagnosis:*
    - X-ray: Widened scapholunate gap (>3 mm = Terry Thomas sign)
    - MRI or arthroscopy (gold standard)
- *Management:*
    - *Acute, partial tear:* Immobilization
    - *Complete tear:* Direct repair ± dorsal capsulodesis
    - *Chronic:* SLAC wrist → salvage (proximal row carpectomy or partial wrist fusion)

Q33. Clinical relevance of segond fracture in sports injuries.

- *Definition:* Avulsion fracture of the **lateral tibial plateau** (anterior lateral capsule attachment).
- *Mechanism:* Internal rotation and varus stress—commonly seen in sports trauma.
- *Clinical significance:*
    - **Pathognomonic for ACL tear**
    - Often associated with lateral meniscus injury
- *Diagnosis:* Seen on AP knee X-ray (small lateral bony fragment)
- *Management:*
    - Treat as part of ACL reconstruction plan
    - Address associated injuries during arthroscopy

VI. Muscle, Tendon, and Soft Tissue Injuries

Q34. Grading and management of muscle strains.

(KMC Manipal 2013)

Grading

- *Grade I (mild):* Few muscle fibers torn, minimal strength loss or swelling.
- *Grade II (moderate):* Partial muscle tear, more pain/swelling, reduced strength.
- *Grade III (severe):* Complete tear, significant loss of function, palpable defect.

Management

- *Acute (first 48–72 hours):*
  - *RICE*: Rest, Ice, Compression, Elevation
  - NSAIDs cautiously
- *Subacute (after 72 hours):*
  - Physiotherapy: gentle ROM, stretching
  - Ultrasound or TENS if needed
- *Rehabilitation:* Progressive loading, strengthening exercises
- *Grade III:* May require surgical repair

Q35. Rehabilitation protocol for hamstring injuries.

Phases

1. *Acute phase (0–5 days):*
   - RICE
   - Avoid aggressive stretching
   - Protected weight-bearing if severe
2. *Subacute phase (5–14 days):*
   - Gentle ROM, isometrics
   - Begin eccentric strengthening
3. *Rehabilitation phase (2–6 weeks):*
   - Dynamic exercises, balance, proprioception
   - Gradual return to sports-specific drills
4. *Return-to-play criteria:*
   - Pain-free sprinting
   - Normal strength and flexibility
   - Symmetry on functional tests

Q36. Quadriceps strain—grading and rehabilitation principles.

Grading (same as muscle strains)

- *Grade I:* Minor, mild discomfort
- *Grade II:* Partial tear, pain on knee extension
- *Grade III:* Complete rupture, severe loss of strength

Rehabilitation principles

- **Early rest + compression**
- **ROM preservation** (knee and hip)

- *Quadriceps strengthening:* Start isometric, progress to isotonic and eccentric
- *Stretching:* Initiate once pain subsides
- *Functional retraining:* Jumping, sprinting before return to play

Q37. Pathogenesis and management of tendinopathies.

Examples
- Achilles tendinopathy
- Patellar tendinopathy (Jumper's knee)
- Lateral epicondylitis (Tennis elbow)

Pathogenesis
- Overuse → microtrauma → failed healing → collagen disorganization → neovascularization
- Tendinosis, not inflammation (degenerative)

Management
- Rest/Activity modification
- *Physiotherapy:*
  - Eccentric loading exercises (mainstay)
  - Isometric holds for pain relief
- *Modalities:* US therapy, shockwave
- Orthotics/Bracing (especially elbow straps or heel lifts)
- NSAIDs (short-term for pain)
- *PRP injections:* Some evidence for refractory cases
- *Surgery:* Reserved for chronic non-responsive cases

Q38. Management of patellofemoral pain syndrome (PFPS).

(MUHS 2011)

Goals
- Relieve pain
- Improve patellar tracking
- Correct biomechanical abnormalities

Management plan
1. *Conservative (mainstay):*
   - *Activity modification:* Avoid squatting, stairs, prolonged sitting
   - *Physiotherapy:*
     - *Strengthening*: Vastus medialis oblique (VMO), hip abductors
     - *Stretching*: Iliotibial band, hamstrings, quadriceps
     - Patellar mobilization techniques
   - Taping/Bracing (McConnell taping)
   - *Footwear/Orthotics:* Correct overpronation if present
2. *Medical:*
   - NSAIDs short-term
   - Ice application post-activity
3. *Surgical (rare, only if refractory):*
   - Lateral release
   - Tibial tuberosity transfer

Q39. Osgood–Schlatter disease—definition and treatment.

Definition

A self-limiting traction apophysitis of the tibial tubercle due to repetitive strain from quadriceps in active adolescents (typically 10–15 years)

Clinical Features

- Pain/swelling over tibial tubercle
- Aggravated by activity, relieved by rest

Management

- **Rest/Activity modification**
- **Ice application**
- **NSAIDs** for pain
- **Quadriceps and hamstring stretching**
- **Knee strap/bracing**
- Rarely requires surgery (e.g., ossicle excision in persistent cases)

Q40. Phases of rehabilitation in sports injuries.

1. *Acute/Protection phase:*
   - RICE/POLICE
   - Immobilization (if needed)
   - Pain/Swelling control
2. *Subacute/Recovery phase:*
   - Restore ROM
   - Begin gentle strengthening
   - Proprioception training
3. *Strengthening phase:*
   - Progressive resistance training
   - Functional exercises
   - Cardiovascular conditioning
4. *Return to sport phase:*
   - Sport-specific drills
   - Psychological readiness
   - Reinjury prevention strategies

Q41. RICE versus POLICE protocols.

Component	*RICE*	*Police*
R	Rest	Protection
I	Ice	Optimal loading
C	Compression	Loading → promotes healing via mechanotransduction
E	Elevation	Ice, compression, elevation (same)

Key Difference

POLICE emphasizes **"optimal loading"** instead of complete rest, promoting early mobilization under guidance.

Q42. Imaging modalities used in sports injuries and their indications.

Modality	*Indications*	*Strengths*
X-ray	Fractures, avulsions, dislocations	Quick, widely available
Ultrasound	Tendon tears (Achilles, rotator cuff), muscle strains, effusions	Dynamic, bedside, radiation-free
MRI	Soft tissue injuries (ligaments, cartilage, tendons, menisci), occult fractures	Excellent soft tissue contrast
CT scan	Complex fractures (e.g., spine, pelvis), bony architecture	3D reconstruction, bone clarity
Bone scan	Stress fractures, occult injuries, inflammation	Whole-body screening, sensitive
DXA (DEXA)	Bone mineral density (stress fractures risk)	Evaluates osteoporosis/athlete triad

Q43. Role of platelet-rich plasma (PRP) and stem cell therapy in sports injuries.

(RUHS 2018)

Platelet-rich Plasma (PRP)

- Autologous concentrate of platelets with growth factors
- *Mechanism:* Releases PDGF, TGF-β, VEGF to enhance healing
- *Indications:*
    - Lateral epicondylitis (tennis elbow)
    - Patellar tendinopathy
    - Achilles tendinopathy
    - Muscle strains
    - Mild to moderate OA
- *Benefits:* Minimally invasive, accelerates healing

Stem Cell Therapy

- Mesenchymal stem cells (MSCs) used
- *Sources:* Bone marrow aspirate, adipose tissue
- *Indications:*
    - Cartilage defects (knee OA)
    - Tendon injuries
    - Labral/meniscal degeneration
- *Limitations:* Cost, regulatory issues, need more RCTs

Q44. Role of PRP in soft tissue injury management.

Applications

- *Tendinopathies*
    - Chronic lateral epicondylitis
    - Rotator cuff pathology
    - Patellar and Achilles tendinopathy
- *Ligament injuries:* Mild-moderate MCL, ATFL sprains
- *Muscle injuries:* Grade I–II strains

Benefits

- Accelerated healing via growth factors
- Reduced downtime
- Minimally invasive outpatient procedure

Limitations

- Variable results in RCTs
- Lack of standardized preparation and dosing
- More beneficial in chronic than acute injuries

VIII. Prevention and Conditioning

Q45. Principles of sports injury prevention and conditioning programs.

A. Key Principles

Principle	*Explanation*
Pre-participation screening	Detects underlying risks (e.g., cardiac, joint instability)
Warm-up and cool-down	Enhances flexibility and reduces injury risk
Sport-specific conditioning	Tailored exercises improve biomechanical and neuromuscular control
Strength and endurance training	Prevents overuse injuries and enhances performance
Flexibility exercises	Reduces muscle tightness, improves joint mobility
Proprioception and balance training	Prevents ankle/knee sprains, especially post-injury
Technique optimization	Poor form can predispose to overuse and acute trauma
Gradual progression	Avoids overtraining, promotes adaptation
Protective equipment	Bracing, footwear, and gear appropriate for the sport
Education and awareness	Coaches, athletes, and parents must understand injury signs and prevention

Q46. Rehabilitation protocols following ligament reconstruction.

Phases of rehabilitation

Phase	*Timeline*	*Goals*	*Key interventions*
I. Immediate post-operative	0–2 weeks	Pain control, ROM (0–90°), reduce swelling	Cryotherapy, heel slides, quad sets, compression
II. Early rehab	2–6 weeks	Full ROM, restore gait	Closed-chain exercises, stationary bike, proprioception
III. Intermediate	6–12 weeks	Strengthening, dynamic balance	Leg press, squats, resistance band exercises
IV. Advanced strength	3–6 months	Agility, plyometrics, neuromuscular control	Sport-specific drills, running program
V. Return to sport	6–9 months+	Full function, psychological readiness	Functional tests (e.g., hop tests), clearance by physician

Return to Play Criteria

- Symmetrical strength ≥90%
- No effusion or pain
- Psychological readiness (e.g., ACL-RSI scale)
- Functional hop and agility tests passed

IX. Concussion and Neurological Injuries

Q47. Clinical features and management of concussions in sports.

Definition

A **concussion** is a mild traumatic brain injury (mTBI) caused by biomechanical forces resulting in transient neurological dysfunction without structural brain injury.

A. Clinical Features

1. *Symptoms:*
    - *Physical:* Headache, dizziness, nausea, blurred vision, balance problems
    - *Cognitive*: Confusion, feeling "foggy", amnesia, difficulty concentrating
    - *Emotional:* Irritability, depression, mood swings
    - *Sleep:* Drowsiness, insomnia, hypersomnia

2. *Signs:*
    - Loss of consciousness (in <10% cases)
    - Delayed verbal/motor responses
    - Vacant stare, disorientation
    - Poor coordination or balance
    - Slurred speech
3. *Red flags (indicating severe injury):*
    - Repeated vomiting
    - Seizures
    - Focal neurological deficit
    - Worsening headache
    - Decreased level of consciousness

B. Assessment Tools

- Sport Concussion Assessment Tool 6 (SCAT6)—standard sideline tool
- Balance Error Scoring System (BESS)
- Immediate Post-Concussion Assessment and Cognitive Testing (ImPACT)—neurocognitive tool

C. Management Protocol

Phase	*Action*
Immediate (sideline)	Remove from play, assess ABCs, rule out red flags, apply SCAT6
Rest phase (24–48 hours)	Physical and cognitive rest (no screen time, reading, etc.)
Gradual return to play (RTP)	Follows a stepwise protocol (see below)
Medical clearance	Mandatory before RTP

D. Return to Play (RTP) Guidelines (Graduated Protocol)

(Based on latest Consensus Statement on Concussion in Sport, 2022)

Stage	*Activity*	*Goal*
1	Daily activities that do not provoke symptoms	Recovery
2	Light aerobic exercise	Increase heart rate
3	Sport-specific drills	Add movement
4	Non-contact training drills	Coordination and thinking
5	Full contact practice	Restore confidence
6	Return to sport	Normal gameplay

Note: 24 hours minimum between stages; return only if asymptomatic.

E. Prevention:

- Proper protective equipment
- Coaching on safe techniques
- Rule enforcement (e.g., penalties for head contact)
- Education and awareness among athletes and staff

X. Viva/Short Form Question and Answer

Q48. What is the O'Donoghue triad?

[Institute of Medical Sciences Banaras Hindu University (BHU) Varanasi 2019]

Also called the **"unhappy triad"**:

- *Injury to*:
    1. Anterior cruciate ligament (ACL)
    2. Medial collateral ligament (MCL)
    3. Medial meniscus (earlier thought lateral meniscus, but more commonly medial)

Q49. Name clinical tests for ACL injury.

- Lachman test (most sensitive)
- Anterior drawer test
- Pivot shift test

Q50. Which is the most commonly injured rotator cuff tendon?

Supraspinatus tendon (located under the acromion, prone to impingement and tears)

Q51. Best investigation for ligament injuries?

Magnetic resonance imaging (MRI): Gold standard for soft tissue (ligament/tendon) injuries.

Q52. What is Baker's cyst in athletes?

- *A popliteal fluid-filled synovial cyst often arising from:*
  - Knee joint effusion
  - Meniscal tears or intra-articular pathology
- Located between the **medial head of gastrocnemius and semimembranosus tendon**

Q53. What is femoroacetabular impingement (FAI) syndrome?

- A condition where abnormal contact between **femoral head-neck** and **acetabulum** causes hip pain.
- *Types:*
  - **Cam** (bony bump on femoral head-neck)
  - **Pincer** (acetabular overcoverage)
  - **Mixed**
- *Treatment:* Activity modification, physiotherapy, NSAIDs; arthroscopic correction if needed.

Q54. What are the risk factors for patellar instability?

- Shallow trochlear groove
- Patella alta
- Increased Q angle
- Ligamentous laxity
- Lateralized tibial tuberosity (↑ TT-TG distance)
- Dysplastic trochlea

CHAPTER 13

Amputation and Disarticulation

Shamim Ahmad Bhat, Simranpreet Singh, Tejpal Singh

Long Essay Questions with Answers

Q1. Classify amputations. Describe indications, techniques, complications, and rehabilitation following below-knee amputation.

(RGUHS – 2022, MUHS – 2020, DNB – 2021)

Amputation involves the removal of part or all of a limb.

Classification

- *By level:* Minor (toe, ray), major (BKA, AKA, hip disarticulation)
- *By technique:* Open (guillotine), closed (flap)
- *By cause:* Trauma, vascular, tumor, congenital

Indications for BKA

- Irreversible ischemia (PVD, Buerger's)
- Diabetic foot, chronic osteomyelitis
- Failed salvage or limb reconstruction

Technique

- Long posterior flap or skew flaps
- Tibia beveled, fibula cut shorter
- Myodesis or myoplasty
- Adequate nerve handling

Complications

- *Early:* Infection, hematoma, flap necrosis, bleeding
- *Late:* Neuroma, phantom limb pain, contractures

Rehabilitation

- *Phases:* Pre-operative, post-operative, pre-prosthetic, prosthetic, long-term
- Emphasis on stump care, strength, gait training, occupational therapy

Energy Expenditure

~25% increase compared to normal gait.

Prognosis

Better function and prosthetic adaptation compared to AKA.

Q2. Describe Syme's amputation. Discuss its indications, surgical technique, advantages, disadvantages, and prosthetic considerations.

(DNB – 2022, TNMGRMU – 2019)

Definition

Ankle disarticulation with heel pad preservation for end-bearing.

Indications

- Forefoot gangrene (e.g., diabetic foot)
- Trauma, Buerger's disease with heel sparing
- Congenital foot deformities

Surgical Technique

- Curved anterior incision, malleoli resected
- Disarticulate talus from the tibia
- Heel pad centralized and secured to the tibia

Advantages

- End-bearing stump
- Lower energy use than BKA
- Better proprioception

Disadvantages

- Bulky stump affects prosthesis
- Heel pad migration/necrosis

Prosthesis

- Requires custom bulky socket
- Suspension difficult due to short lever arm

Q3. Discuss the indications and principles of disarticulations. Describe in detail hip disarticulation with post-operative management.

(DNB – 2020, AIIMS – 2019 pattern)

Definition

Disarticulation is limb removal through a joint (e.g., hip, knee).

Indications

- Tumors (e.g., osteosarcoma, Ewing's)
- Severe infection (necrotizing fasciitis)
- Massive trauma, failed AKA

Principles

- Preserve viable soft tissue, adequate flap
- Proper nerve management, myoplasty
- Hemostasis and early rehabilitation

Surgical Technique (Hip Disarticulation)

- Extended anterior-based flap
- Femoral vessels ligated
- Femoral head disarticulated from acetabulum
- Myoplasty for coverage, tension-free closure

Post-operative Management

- Pain control, infection monitoring
- Avoid flexion contracture (proper positioning)

- Psychosocial support, stump care
- Wheelchair mobility often required

Prognosis

High morbidity, rarely used except in malignancy or sepsis

Q4. Enumerate energy expenditure at various amputation levels. Explain rehabilitation in an above-knee amputee.

(RGUHS – 2021, DNB – 2019)

Energy Expenditure by Level

- *BKA:* ~25%
- *Through-knee:* ~50%
- *AKA:* ~65%
- *Hip disarticulation:* ~100%
- *Bilateral AKA:* ~200%

Rehabilitation Phases in AKA

1. *Pre-operative*: Counseling, strength building
2. *Immediate post-operative*: Pain control, positioning to prevent contractures
3. *Pre-prosthetic*: Stump shaping, desensitization, ROM
4. *Prosthetic fitting*: Donning, gait training
5. *Community reintegration*: Mobility aids, psychological support

Challenges

- More energy needed for ambulation
- Higher rate of contractures, skin breakdown

Outcome depends on

Motivation, comorbidities, stump health

Section B: Short Essay Questions with Answers

Q1. Describe indications and technique of Syme's amputation.

(MUHS – 2021, DNB – 2020)

Indications

- Forefoot gangrene (e.g., diabetic foot)
- Trauma with distal foot loss
- Congenital deformities (e.g., clubfoot)
- Tumors limited to forefoot/midfoot
- Failed previous distal amputations

Technique

- Anterior transverse incision at ankle, posterior curved flap under heel
- Disarticulate ankle joint
- Resect malleoli, preserve heel pad
- Centralize heel pad and secure to distal tibia with sutures
- Myodesis if possible
- Tension-free closure, drain placement

Q2. Write a note on Boyd and Pirogoff amputations.

(RGUHS – 2023, TNMGRMU – 2020)

Boyd Amputation
- Disarticulation at the ankle joint
- Retain calcaneus → rotate and fuse with tibia
- Provides a stable, end-bearing stump
- Better limb length and heel pad control

Pirogoff Amputation
- Vertical osteotomy of the calcaneus → rotated upward
- Remove talus and fuse calcaneus to tibia
- Retains heel pad, allows end-bearing

Comparison
- *Boyd:* More stable, retains whole calcaneus
- *Pirogoff:* Technical complexity, better cosmesis
- Both suitable for children or low-resource settings

Q3. Discuss phantom limb and its management.

(DNB – 2021, MUHS – 2020)

Definition

Painful sensation perceived in the amputated part of the limb.

Types
- Phantom sensation (non-painful)
- Phantom limb pain (PLP)
- Stump pain (localized)

Pathophysiology
- *Peripheral:* Neuroma, ectopic discharge
- *Central:* Cortical remapping, central sensitization
- *Psychological:* Depression, stress

Management
- Mirror therapy
- TENS, CBT
- *Medications:* Gabapentin, amitriptyline, opioids (refractory)
- Nerve blocks, spinal cord stimulation (severe cases)
- *Prevention:* Good surgical technique, early rehabilitation

Q4. Describe principles of amputation surgery.

(RGUHS – 2022, DNB – 2019)

Goals
- Remove non-viable tissue
- Preserve maximum length and function
- Create stable, pain-free stump suitable for prosthesis

Principles
- *Level:* Chosen based on perfusion, soft tissue, infection extent
- *Flaps:* Posterior flap (e.g., BKA) more vascular
- *Bone:* Bevel edges, fibula shorter in BKA

- *Muscles:* Myodesis (to bone) or myoplasty (to muscle)
- *Nerves:* Pull gently, cut sharply at high level to avoid neuroma
- *Vessels:* Secure hemostasis
- *Closure:* Tension-free, layered with drain placement

Q5. Complications of amputations—early and late.

(TNMGRMU – 2021, MUHS – 2019)

Early Complications
- Hemorrhage
- Infection, flap necrosis
- DVT/PE
- Wound dehiscence
- Pain (post-operative)

Late Complications
- Phantom limb pain
- Neuroma
- Contractures
- Stump ulcers, poor prosthetic fit
- Bony overgrowth (children)
- Depression, PTSD

Q6. Disarticulations—advantages and disadvantages.

(DNB – 2021)

Advantages
- Preserve limb length
- End-bearing stump (e.g., Syme's)
- No bone cutting → lower infection risk
- Natural muscle flaps for closure

Disadvantages
- Bulky stump, difficult prosthetic fit
- Cosmetic issues
- Socket design complexity
- Less common → prosthetist experience limited

Q7. Describe myodesis and myoplasty.

(MUHS – 2022, RGUHS – 2020)

Myodesis

Muscle to bone fixation via drill holes (more stable)
- Used in healthy bone
- Improves prosthetic control

Myoplasty

Muscle to muscle suturing over bone end
- Used when bone is fragile or infected
- Easier to perform but less stable

Preference
- Myodesis preferred when possible
- Myoplasty in infected or oncological amputations

Q8. Describe the stages of rehabilitation in lower limb amputation.

(DNB – 2022, RGUHS – 2023)

1. *Pre-operative phase*:
   - Counseling, upper limb strengthening
   - Vascular assessment, comorbid optimization
2. *Immediate post-operative (0–2 weeks)*:
   - Pain management, prevent contractures
   - Proper positioning, wound care
3. *Pre-prosthetic training (2–6 weeks)*:
   - Stump shaping, desensitization
   - Balance and ROM exercises
4. *Prosthetic fitting phase (~6–8 weeks)*:
   - Fit temporary → permanent prosthesis
   - Gait training, stair climbing
5. *Community reintegration*: Vocational rehabilitation, follow-up, psychological support

Section C: Short Notes with Answers

Q1. Phantom limb pain.

(DNB – Repeated commonly)

Definition

Pain perceived in the absent limb post-amputation.

Pathophysiology

- *Peripheral:* Neuroma, ectopic discharge
- *Central:* Cortical remapping
- *Psychological:* Stress and anxiety

Features

- Burning, stabbing, electric-shock sensations
- Triggered by stress, cold, prosthesis use

Management

- Mirror therapy, CBT
- *Medications:* Gabapentin, amitriptyline
- TENS, nerve blocks, spinal cord stimulation
- Early rehabilitation and good surgical technique help prevention

Q2. Krukenberg amputation.

(DNB – 2021, RGUHS – 2019)

Definition

Forearm amputation where radius and ulna are separated longitudinally to form a pincer-like grasping stump.

Indications

- Bilateral upper limb amputation (especially blind patients)
- Low-resource settings where prosthesis not feasible

Advantages

- Preserved tactile sensation and proprioception
- Independent grasp without prosthesis

Disadvantages
- Cosmetically unacceptable
- Needs long rehabilitation
- Not suitable for unilateral amputation

Q3. Chopart amputation.

(TNMGRMU – 2020)

Definition
Midfoot amputation through talonavicular and calcaneocuboid joints.

Indications
Trauma, infection or tumors limited to forefoot/midfoot

Advantages
- Preserves hindfoot, ankle motion
- Shorter limb loss

Complications
- Equinus deformity (due to Achilles)
- Poor prosthetic fit, skin breakdown

Prevention
- Tendon transfer (e.g., tibialis anterior)
- Early orthosis fitting

Q4. Lisfranc amputation.

(MUHS – 2021)

Definition
Tarsometatarsal disarticulation removing forefoot at metatarsal bases.

Indications
Diabetic foot, trauma, infection confined to forefoot

Advantages
- Preserves hindfoot and ankle motion
- Lower energy expenditure

Complications
- Equinovarus deformity
- Skin breakdown, poor prosthetic fit

Prosthesis
- Requires custom shoe/toe filler
- May need tendon balancing

Q5. Advantages of Syme's over below-knee amputation.

(DNB – 2022)

Syme's Advantages
- Ankle disarticulation with heel pad for end-bearing
- Lower energy cost (~10–15%)
- Better proprioception and gait
- Preserved limb length

Comparison with BKA
- BKA has better cosmetic prosthesis
- Syme's needs custom bulky socket
- BKA easier for prosthetic suspension

Q6. Gait training in amputees.

(RGUHS – 2023)

Goals
Safe, symmetrical, efficient ambulation with prosthesis

Phases
1. *Pre-prosthetic*: Strengthening, balance, parallel bar walking
2. *Prosthetic fitting*: Donning, doffing, initial ambulation
3. *Advanced*: Stairs, uneven terrain, obstacle training

Focus Areas
- Stance and swing phase mechanics
- Symmetry and energy conservation

Tools
Mirror, treadmill, video feedback

Q7. Contractures in amputees—prevention and management.

(DNB – 2019)

Common Contractures
- *AKA:* Hip flexion, abduction, external rotation
- *BKA:* Knee flexion

Prevention
- Proper bed positioning (avoid pillows under joints)
- Prone lying, ROM exercises
- Early mobilization

Management
- Stretching, serial casting
- Dynamic splints
- Surgical release if severe

Q8. Pre-prosthetic training.

Aims
Prepare the patient and stump for prosthetic fitting

Components
- Stump shaping (elastic bandage, shrinker)
- Desensitization (tapping, massage)
- Strengthening of upper limbs and intact leg
- Balance and ROM exercises
- Education and motivation

Q9. Describe the key differences in diabetic amputations.

Aspect	*Diabetic amputation*	*Non-diabetic amputation*
Cause	Ischemia, infection, neuropathy, Charcot foot	Trauma, tumors, vascular diseases
Common levels	Toe, ray, transmetatarsal, BKA, Syme's	Varies (BKA, AKA, disarticulations)
Pre-operative considerations	Glycemic control, vascular assessment, infection control	General fitness, local disease extent
Flap planning	Often limited soft tissue, poor healing	Better flap options typically
Healing capacity	Delayed due to poor perfusion and infection	Usually better if systemic health is good
Complications	Higher risk of infection, wound breakdown, re-amputation	Depends on cause but generally fewer systemic complications
Prosthetic use	Challenging due to comorbidities and residual limb quality	More consistent functional outcomes
Re-amputation risk	High — due to ongoing disease and pressure ulcers	Lower if primary cause addressed
Footwear/Orthosis post-minor amputation	Custom footwear, offloading devices (e.g., total contact cast, Charcot Restraint Orthotic Walker—CROW)	Not always required

Common Types of Diabetic Foot Amputations

1. *Toe amputation*: Most common (due to infected ulcers, gangrene)
2. *Ray amputation*: Toe plus corresponding metatarsal
3. *Transmetatarsal amputation (TMA)*: For distal forefoot gangrene
4. *Lisfranc/Chopart*: Rarely performed; risk of deformity high
5. *Syme's or BKA*: When midfoot/hindfoot tissues are nonviable
6. *Initial guillotine amputation*: Life-saving in wet gangrene, followed by delayed definitive closure

Special Considerations

- *Vascular assessment:* Doppler, ABI (<0.45 predicts poor healing)
- *Glycemic optimization:* Poor control worsens outcomes
- *Infection management:* Debridement, antibiotics
- *Multidisciplinary approach:* Surgeon, diabetologist, podiatrist, vascular surgeon, rehabilitation team
- *Custom orthotics:* Prevent recurrence and ulceration

Suggested Viva Questions

Q1. Why are diabetic patients at higher risk of needing amputation?

Diabetic patients are at higher risk due to the **triad** of:

- **Peripheral neuropathy** → loss of protective sensation → unnoticed trauma
- **Peripheral vascular disease (PVD)** → poor tissue perfusion → ischemia
- **Immunosuppression** → increased susceptibility to infection

Additional risk factors:

- Repeated minor trauma due to ill-fitting footwear
- Foot deformities (Charcot foot)
- Poor glycemic control delaying wound healing

Q2. What is the role of ABI and Doppler in diabetic foot evaluation?

- *Ankle-brachial index (ABI):*
    - *Normal:* 0.9–1.3
    - ABI < 0.45 → Poor healing potential
    - ABI > 1.3 → May be falsely elevated due to arterial calcification (common in diabetics)

- *Doppler studies:*
  - Assess **arterial flow** and **identify suitable level of amputation**
  - **Triphasic signals** suggest good vascularity
  - Duplex Doppler can guide revascularization decisions

Q3. How do you manage a diabetic with wet gangrene?

Management Involves Urgent, Staged Care

Step 1: Resuscitation and infection control
- IV fluids, broad-spectrum antibiotics
- Control sepsis, glycemic control

Step 2: Surgical debridement/guillotine amputation
- Urgent guillotine amputation at the most distal viable level
- Remove all necrotic/infected tissue

Step 3: Definitive surgery
- Once infection is controlled and stump is clean
- Perform closed, flap-based definitive amputation (e.g., BKA)

Step 4: Rehabilitation and footwear
- Post-operative stump care
- *Long-term:* Glycemic control, custom footwear, regular follow-up

Q4. Compare Syme's versus BKA in diabetic foot.

Feature	*Syme's amputation*	*Below-knee amputation (BKA)*
Level	Ankle disarticulation	Tibial amputation
Heel pad	Preserved for end-bearing	Not preserved
Energy cost	Lower (~10–15%)	Higher (~25%)
Prosthetic fit	Difficult due to bulbous stump	Easier, better prosthesis options
Indication	Limited to forefoot/hindfoot with good heel pad vascularity	More extensive infection/ischemia
Healing	Depends on heel pad viability	More predictable in clean tibial stump

Syme's may fail if heel pad is ischemic; BKA preferred in extensive diabetic foot disease.

Q5. What is Charcot foot, and how is it managed?

Charcot neuroarthropathy is a progressive, destructive joint disease caused by **diabetic neuropathy**, leading to:
- Midfoot collapse
- Rocker-bottom deformity
- Risk of ulceration and infection

Management
1. *Acute stage*:
   - Immobilization (total contact cast or CROW boot)
   - Non-weight bearing
2. *Chronic stage*:
   - Custom orthotic footwear
   - Surgical correction (rare; done in deformities with ulcer risk)

Goals
Prevent ulceration, maintain ambulation, and preserve limb.

Q6. Comparison between disarticulation and amputation, including definitions, key differences, advantages, and disadvantages.

Definition

Term	Definition
Amputation	Surgical removal of a limb through the bone (e.g., below-knee amputation through tibia and fibula)
Disarticulation	Surgical removal of a limb through a joint, without cutting through bone (e.g., hip disarticulation, knee disarticulation, shoulder disarticulation)

Key Differences

Feature	Amputation	Disarticulation
Level	Through bone	Through joint
Bone cutting	Required	Not done
Examples	BKA, AKA, transmetatarsal, Pirogoff	Hip, knee, shoulder, Syme's
Stump shape	Conical, cylindrical	Bulky, often bulbous
Soft tissue coverage	Less natural, flap-based	Often more robust and natural
Prosthetic fit	Easier (especially in BKA/AKA)	More difficult (due to shape)
Use in oncology	Less commonly needed	Often used in extensive tumors
Bone overgrowth risk	In children, common	Less common (growth plate removed)

Advantages of Disarticulation
1. *Preservation of bone length*: Important in **children** to avoid growth plate disruption.
2. *Natural soft tissue coverage*: Provides **end-bearing** stump (e.g., Syme's).
3. *Lower risk of bone overgrowth*: As no bone is transected.
4. *Better hemostasis*: No medullary canal exposure.
5. *Strong muscle attachments*: Allows better myodesis and muscle balance.
6. *Less blood loss*: No cutting of bone reduces bleeding risk.

Disadvantages of Disarticulation
1. *Bulky stump*: Especially in **through-knee or elbow disarticulation** → difficult prosthetic fit.
2. *Poor cosmesis*: Stump shape affects appearance and prosthetic design.
3. *Prosthetic challenges*: Socket design more complex.
4. *Not suitable if joint is infected or involved*: E.g., osteomyelitis extending into joint.
5. *Less commonly performed*: Fewer prosthetists trained in fitting these stumps.

Q7. Forequarter amputation (interscapulothoracic amputation).

Definition
Forequarter amputation involves removal of the **entire upper limb**, including:
- Humerus
- Scapula
- Clavicle

It is also called **interscapulothoracic amputation**.

Indications
- High-grade **malignant tumors** of the shoulder girdle (e.g., sarcoma, chondrosarcoma)
- **Failed limb-salvage surgery**
- Extensive **trauma or infection**
- Recurrent tumors after limb salvage
- Intractable pain in non-functional limb

Surgical Steps
1. *Incision*: Anterior and posterior flaps including skin, muscle, and neurovascular bundles
2. *Dissection*: Removal of clavicle, scapula, and upper limb
3. *Neurovascular ligation*: Subclavian artery and vein ligated
4. *Closure*: Flap creation to cover thoracic wall

Advantages
- Oncologically safe for extensive tumors
- Reduces tumor-related pain
- Allows control of bleeding and infection

Disadvantages
- Highly disfiguring
- Requires psychological support and rehabilitation
- Complex prosthesis (often cosmetic only)

Q8. Hindquarter amputation (hemipelvectomy).

Definition
Hindquarter amputation refers to removal of the **entire lower limb**, including a portion or all of the **hemipelvis**.

Types
- *Internal hemipelvectomy:* Limb preserved; pelvic resection only
- *External hemipelvectomy:* Includes limb removal

Indications
- Large malignant tumors of pelvis/femur (e.g., osteosarcoma, chondrosarcoma)
- Severe trauma with pelvic disruption
- Advanced infection not manageable by debridement
- Vascular insufficiency with sepsis

Surgical Steps
1. *Pre-operative planning*: Vascular imaging, bowel preparation
2. *Incision*: Circumferential pelvic approach
3. Disarticulate SI joint or pubic symphysis
4. Ligation of iliac vessels and sciatic nerve
5. Myocutaneous flap closure over pelvic cavity

Advantages
- Life-saving in malignancy or infection
- Effective in eliminating non-salvageable disease

Disadvantages
- Major surgery with high morbidity
- Difficult rehabilitation
- Poor prosthetic tolerance

CHAPTER 14

Tractions, Orthosis, Prosthesis, and Braces/Splints

MD Maaz, Pankaj Spolia, Abhishek Bral

Traction

Q1. Define traction. Compare skin and skeletal traction.

(AIIMS Delhi 2021, RGUHS Karnataka 2022)

Definition

Traction is the application of a **mechanical pulling force** to a part of the body to achieve **alignment, immobilization, or reduction** of a deformity or fracture.

Comparison

Feature	*Skin traction*	*Skeletal traction*
Application	Applied over skin using adhesive straps	Involves insertion of pins/wires into bone
Weight limit	≤5–7 kg	Can withstand 10–20 kg
Indications	Temporary, preoperative	Definitive traction for unstable fractures
Risks	Skin irritation, blisters	Pin tract infection, neurovascular injury
Examples	Buck's, Bryant's	Upper tibial, distal femoral traction

Q2. Principles and complications of traction in orthopedic management.

(MUHS Maharashtra 2022, PGI Chandigarh 2021)

Principles (Laws of Traction)

1. **Line of pull** should be along the long axis of bone
2. **Countertraction** must be provided (body weight or elevation)
3. **Continuous pull** (24/7) for effectiveness
4. Use **pulleys, slings, and weights** to direct force
5. Maintain **balanced suspension** when needed

Common Complications

Skin traction	*Skeletal traction*
Skin breakdown, pressure sores	Pin tract infection
Nerve palsy (peroneal, ulnar)	Neurovascular injury
DVT due to immobility	Over-distraction or malalignment
Joint stiffness	Loosening of traction pins

Q3. Classify orthopedic traction.

Classification

1. *Based on application*:
   - **Skin traction**
   - **Skeletal traction**
2. *Based on purpose*:
   - **Static traction (continuous pull)**
   - **Dynamic traction** (spring-loaded, movement permitted)
3. *Based on region*:
   - *Upper limb*: Dunlop's, overhead
   - *Lower limb*: Buck's, Bryant's, Gallow's
   - *Spine*: Skull tongs, cervical traction
4. *Based on timeframe*:
   - Temporary (pre-operative stabilization)
   - Definitive (fracture healing)

Examples

- *Buck's traction*: Skin, static
- *Crutchfield tongs*: Skeletal, static for cervical spine
- *Bohler Braun splint*: Dynamic with skin traction

Q4. Define skeletal traction. Discuss indications, techniques, and complications.

(RGUHS, Dec 2010)

Definition

Skeletal traction involves the **insertion of a pin or wire into bone**, through which a **mechanical force** is applied using weights to maintain reduction and alignment.

Indications

- Fracture shaft femur
- Tibial fractures (comminuted)
- Cervical spine injuries
- As temporary measure before surgery

Technique (e.g., Upper Tibial Traction)

- Prepare under aseptic precautions
- Insert **Steinmann pin/K-wire** through metaphysis
- Apply **traction bow and weights (5–10% of body weight)**
- Use **pulley system** with countertraction (leg elevation)

Complications

- Pin tract infection
- Neurovascular injury (e.g., popliteal artery, peroneal nerve)
- Loosening or migration of pin
- Delayed union due to over-traction

Q5. Enumerate the types of skin traction and their clinical applications.

(RGUHS, June/July 2011)

Types of Skin Traction

Type	*Application*
Buck's traction	Fracture neck femur, hip arthritis
Bryant's traction	Pediatric femur fractures, DDH
Gallow's traction	Supracondylar fractures in children
Dunlop's traction	Elbow fractures, humerus shaft

Clinical Considerations

- Use **adhesive straps or foam boots**
- Should not exceed 5–7 kg
- Inspect skin daily
- Not suitable for high-force or long-term use

Traction Section – Questions 6 to 12 with Model Answers

Q6. Indications and contraindications of traction in orthopedics.

Indications

1. Fracture stabilization (e.g., femur, spine)
2. Pre-operative alignment before internal fixation
3. Reduction of dislocations (e.g., cervical spine injuries)
4. Correction of deformities (e.g., SCFE, DDH)
5. Immobilization during soft tissue healing
6. Pain relief in musculoskeletal injuries

Contraindications

Absolute	*Relative*
Active infection at traction site	Poor skin condition (for skin traction)
Fracture with vascular injury	Non-cooperative or neurologically impaired patient
Very young or elderly with fragile skin	Osteoporotic bone (for skeletal traction)

Q7. Complications of prolonged traction use.

Local Complications

- Pressure sores from slings or straps
- Pin tract infections in skeletal traction
- Skin abrasions/blisters (especially in children)
- Nerve palsy (peroneal, radial)

Systemic Complications

- Joint stiffness due to immobilization
- Muscle atrophy and contractures
- Hypostatic pneumonia from prolonged bed rest
- DVT and pulmonary embolism
- Psychological stress and deconditioning

Prevention

- Regular repositioning, skin inspection
- Early physiotherapy (isometric)
- Adequate hydration, anticoagulant prophylaxis if needed

Q8. What are the types of skin traction used in orthopedics?

Main Types

Traction type	***Common use case***
Buck's traction	Hip fractures, femoral neck fractures
Bryant's traction	Bilateral lower limb traction in children
Gallow's traction	Femur fractures in infants
Dunlop's traction	Elbow fractures, humeral shaft injuries

Application Method

- Adhesive/foam straps applied to skin
- Weight attached via pulley system
- Maximum 5–7 kg used

Advantages

- Non-invasive
- Easy to apply
- Useful in preoperative or pediatric care

Limitations

- Skin integrity issues
- Limited force application
- Cannot maintain reduction in unstable fractures

Q9. Limitations and complications of skin traction in children.

Limitations

- **Ineffective for unstable or displaced fractures**
- Limited to **low weights (≤10% of body weight)**
- Can not be used where **skin is compromised or fragile**
- Difficult to maintain in **uncooperative children**

Complications

Skin-related	***Neurovascular***
Blistering, excoriation	Peroneal nerve palsy (Buck's traction)
Ulcers around straps	Circulatory compromise from tight straps

Prevention

- Regular skin checks
- Padding over bony prominences
- Limit traction duration

Q10. Enumerate commonly used sites for skeletal traction pin insertion.

Common Pin Insertion Sites

Site	Purpose
Upper tibia	Femur shaft, hip fractures
Distal femur	Supracondylar or distal femur injuries
Calcaneus	Tibia, ankle, and foot fractures
Olecranon	Elbow dislocations or fractures
Metacarpals/Phalanges	Finger injuries (dynamic traction)
Skull (via tongs)	Cervical spine injuries

Key Considerations
- Aseptic technique
- Avoid neurovascular bundles
- Ensure proper alignment and support

Q11. Describe technique and precautions of applying skeletal traction.

(GMCJ 2013)

Steps
1. Prepare site aseptically
2. Local anesthesia or sedation
3. Insert **Steinmann pin or Kirschner wire** perpendicular to bone axis
4. Attach **Bohler stirrup or bow**
5. Connect to pulley with weights (5–20% body weight)
6. Maintain **countertraction** with elevation

Precautions
- Daily pin site cleaning
- Monitor for infection and loosening
- Check distal circulation, motor and sensory function
- Avoid over-traction or unequal pull
- Reassess alignment with X-rays

Q12. What is upper tibial skeletal traction? Enumerate its uses.

Definition

Skeletal traction applied through the **proximal tibia metaphysis**, often using a **Steinmann pin**, to align and stabilize lower limb fractures.

Indications
- **Fracture shaft of femur**
- **Hip fractures (intracapsular and extracapsular)**
- As pre-operative stabilization for **THA or DHS**
- **Dislocations or subluxations** of hip joint
- **Correction of deformities** in neglected cases

Technique
- Pin inserted 2–3 cm distal and medial to tibial tuberosity
- Protect **common peroneal nerve** (lateral side)
- Apply Bohler stirrup → pulley → weights (5–10 kg)

Traction Section – Questions 13 to 24 with Model Answers

Q13. Describe indications and method of femoral skeletal traction.

Indications

- Shaft femur fractures (especially mid/distal third)
- Hip fractures (as temporary pre-operative measure)
- High-energy trauma with polytrauma
- Femoral shaft fracture in children >10 years (if non-operative)

Technique

- Use **upper tibial pin** (preferred) or **distal femoral pin**
- Insert pin under **aseptic conditions**
- Attach **traction bow or stirrup**
- Use weights: typically **10–15% of body weight**
- Position limb in **Bohler Braun splint** for comfort and alignment

Precautions

- Regular neurovascular checks
- Avoid over-traction
- Monitor pin site daily for signs of infection

Q14. Discuss the complications of skeletal traction.

Complications

Local	*Systemic*
Pin tract infection	Deep vein thrombosis (DVT)
Neurovascular injury	Muscle wasting, joint stiffness
Loosening or migration of pin	Pressure sores
Bone overgrowth in children	Psychological stress (long immobilization)

Prevention

- Proper pin insertion technique
- Daily sterile dressing
- Encourage active movements of joints above and below
- Use of anticoagulants if prolonged immobilization

Q15. Discuss indications, technique, and complications of cervical traction.

(West Bengal University of Health Sciences Kolkata 2018)

Indications

- Cervical spine **dislocation or subluxation**
- **Fracture-dislocation** of cervical vertebrae
- **Traction for reduction** before definitive fixation
- Post-operative immobilization

Technique

- Use of **Crutchfield or Gardner-Wells tongs**
- Applied under local anesthesia or sedation
- Pin inserted into skull at **10–15 mm above external auditory meatus**, bilaterally
- Traction weight starts at **2.5–5 kg**, increased under radiographic control

Complications

- Skull perforation
- Pin tract infection
- Cranial nerve palsy
- Over-distraction causing cord injury

Q16. Describe types of skull tongs (crutchfield, Gardner–Wells) and their application.

Crutchfield Tongs

- Earlier generation skull tongs
- Inserted using small drill holes
- Require **sharp points and a manual torque wrench**

Gardner–Wells Tongs

- **Spring-loaded pins**, don't require drilling
- Safer and more user-friendly
- Allow **non-invasive cervical traction**

Application

- Used for **reduction of cervical dislocation/fracture**
- Traction applied via **overhead frame or pulley system**
- Allows realignment before surgery or during conservative care

Q17. Role of traction in the management of fracture shaft femur, neck of femur in children, spinal injuries, CDH, and SCFE.

Traction Indications by Condition

Condition	*Traction used*
Shaft femur (adults)	Upper tibial skeletal traction
Fracture neck femur (children)	Gallow's or Buck's traction
Spinal injuries	Skull traction with Crutchfield/Gardner–Wells tongs
Congenital dislocation of hip (CDH)	Overhead traction pre-reduction
Slipped capital femoral epiphysis (SCFE)	Skin traction before pinning

Q18. Buck's traction—indications and technique.

(MUHS Maharashtra 2023, RGUHS Karnataka 2023)

Indications

- Fracture neck of femur
- Pre-operative immobilization of hip fractures
- Post-hip surgery immobilization
- Low back pain (temporary relief)

Technique

- Skin traction using adhesive straps or foam boots
- Pulley at foot end of bed
- Weight (3–5 kg) applied over edge
- Leg should remain straight; countertraction via body weight

Precautions

- Inspect skin every 6–8 hours
- Prevent heel pressure sores
- Ensure alignment is maintained

Q19. Bryant's traction—indications and complications.

(PGI Chandigarh 2022, AIIMS Delhi 2022)

Indications
- Femoral shaft fractures in children <2 years
- Congenital dislocation of hip (CDH)—pre-operative stretching

Technique
- **Both legs suspended vertically**
- Hips flexed to 90°, knees extended
- Buttocks slightly off bed (countertraction)
- *Weight used*: 0.5–1 kg per leg

Complications
- **Compartment syndrome (rare but serious)**
- Vascular compromise
- Foot drop (if prolonged)
- Skin irritation or pressure sores

Q20. Gallow's traction—indications and method.

(JIPMER Puducherry 2022)

Indications

Also used in **femur fractures in young children**

Method
- Overhead skin traction applied to both legs
- Legs suspended with knees slightly flexed
- Buttocks elevated for countertraction
- Useful in **children under 2 years**

Caution
- Regular neurovascular checks to prevent compartment syndrome
- Limit use to **short duration (<2 weeks)**

Q21. Dunlop's traction—when and how used.

(CMC Vellore 2023)

Indications
- **Supracondylar fractures of the humerus** (flexion-type or displaced)
- Some proximal humerus fractures

Method
- **Skin traction to forearm + countertraction to arm**
- Elbow flexed to 90°, forearm suspended
- Weight applied to maintain alignment
- Used in **children with open physes**

Advantage
- Avoids surgical risks in borderline cases
- Used for initial reduction or conservative treatment

Q22. Describe the construction and application of Thomas splint.

(PGI Chandigarh 2021, RGUHS Karnataka 2022)

Construction
- **Ring at 120° angle** with inner bar (groin side) and outer bar
- Length: From groin to beyond foot
- Used with slings and traction pulleys

Application
- Limb passed through ring; padded to avoid groin pressure
- Knee slightly flexed and supported in slings
- **Used for femur fractures** with skin/skeletal traction
- Weight applied to maintain alignment and length

Advantages
- Excellent emergency stabilizer
- Useful in **field trauma care and transport**

Q23. Bohler–Braun splint—indications and features.

(MUHS Maharashtra 2022, BHU Varanasi 2022)

Indications
- Fracture shaft femur
- Tibial fractures
- Temporary immobilization pre-surgery

Features
- **Adjustable metallic frame**
- Knee kept in slight flexion
- Allows **simultaneous skin traction and elevation**
- Pulley system for multiple vectors of pull
- Supports alignment and countertraction

Benefits
- Non-invasive
- Easy access for dressing
- Promotes **better nursing care**

Q24. Perkins traction—definition and indications.

Definition

Perkins traction is a **form of skeletal traction** used to align **fracture shaft femur** using **upper tibial skeletal pin traction**, with limb supported in **Thomas splint**.

Indications
- Fracture shaft femur (closed, with soft tissue injury)
- In resource-limited or non-operative settings
- Pre-operative care before internal fixation
- Long-term traction in patients unfit for surgery

Technique
- Insert **upper tibial pin**
- Apply weights through **Bohler stirrup**
- Support limb in **Thomas splint** with slings and pulleys
- Maintain alignment and limb length

Orthoses, Splints, and Bracing

Q25. Write short notes on Dennis Browne splint.

(RGUHS, Dec 2010)

Definition

The **Dennis Browne splint** is an **abduction bar** connecting shoes or orthoses used to maintain **corrected foot position** in conditions like **CTEV (clubfoot)**.

Components

- A rigid bar with **shoes/boots** attached at each end
- Shoes set in **70° abduction on affected side**, 40° on unaffected
- Can be fixed-angle or adjustable

Indications

- Post-Ponseti correction in CTEV
- Clubfoot bracing (maintains correction)
- In **congenital foot deformities** post-manipulation

Duration of Use

- Full-time for first **3 months**
- Night-time use until **4 years of age**

Precautions

- Skin check for pressure areas
- Monitor for recurrence
- Parental education is key

Q26. Describe indications and types of ankle foot orthosis (AFO).

(AIIMS Delhi 2022, JIPMER Puducherry 2023)

Definition

Ankle foot orthosis (AFO) is a **brace that spans from below the knee to the foot**, used to support ankle motion, improve alignment, or prevent deformity.

Indications

- Foot drop (e.g., peroneal nerve palsy)
- Spastic cerebral palsy
- Stroke and hemiplegia
- Polio, post-operative orthopedic rehabilitation
- Charcot–Marie–Tooth disease

Types

Type	***Function***
Solid AFO	Total ankle immobilization
Hinged AFO	Allows dorsiflexion, restricts plantar flexion
Posterior leaf spring (PLS)	Dynamic assist for foot drop
Floor reaction AFO	Assists in knee extension (for crouch gait)

Q27. Discuss KAFO—indications and advantages.

(MUHS Maharashtra 2023, RGUHS Karnataka 2023)

Definition

Knee-ankle-foot orthosis (KAFO), a full-leg brace used to **stabilize the knee and ankle**, often in **paralysis or deformity** cases.

Indications

- Post-polio residual paralysis (PPRP)
- Paraplegia (incomplete spinal cord injury)
- Post-fracture rehabilitation (e.g., femur or tibia)
- Multiple deformities in knee and ankle (genu recurvatum, foot drop)

Components

- Metal or plastic uprights
- Knee joint lock (drop lock, dial lock)
- AFO incorporated at the bottom

Advantages

- Prevents knee buckling
- Allows **standing and short-distance walking**
- Helps in **joint alignment correction**
- Improves **functional independence**

Q28. Role of orthosis in the treatment of clubfoot.

(DNB, Dec 2010)

Role of Orthoses Post-correction (Ponseti Protocol)

Device	*Purpose*
Dennis Browne splint	Maintains foot abduction
Foot abduction brace (FAB)	Used 23 h/day initially
AFO/SMO (in mild cases)	Provide passive support

Duration of Use

- 23 h/day for 3 months
- Then **night-time** till 4 years of age

Importance

- Prevents **relapse of deformity**
- Maintains **alignment post-serial casting**

Q29. Indications and types of spinal orthoses.

(NTR University, Nov 2016)

Indications

- Vertebral fractures (compression, burst)
- Post-operative stabilization (spinal instrumentation)
- Scoliosis/bracing in adolescents
- Spondylolisthesis
- Tuberculosis spine (immobilization)

Types of Spinal Orthoses

Region	Examples
Cervical	Philadelphia collar, SOMI brace
Thoracolumbar	Taylor brace, TLSO, Jewett brace
Lumbosacral	Knight's brace, LS belt
Full spine	Milwaukee brace (for scoliosis)

Q30. Role of orthoses in neuromuscular disorders.

(Manipal University, 2011)

Neuromuscular Disorders Needing Orthoses

- Post-polio residual paralysis
- Muscular dystrophies
- Cerebral palsy
- Spinal cord injury
- Peripheral neuropathies (e.g., CMT)

Common Orthoses Used

Disorder	Orthosis
Foot drop	AFO or PLS brace
Knee instability	KAFO with locking joint
Crouch gait (CP)	Floor reaction AFO
Flail limb (SCI)	HKAFO + crutches

Benefits

- Prevent contractures
- Improve ambulation
- Maintain limb alignment
- Assist in ADLs

Q31. Orthotic management in post-polio residual paralysis (PPRP).

(DNB, June 2012)

Background

Post-polio residual paralysis (PPRP) results in **asymmetric muscle weakness** or flaccid paralysis, often affecting the **lower limbs**, requiring customized orthotic solutions for **ambulation and deformity prevention**.

Goals of Orthosis in PPRP

- Improve **gait** and functional mobility
- Prevent/correct **deformities** (e.g., equinus, genu recurvatum)
- Enhance **stability and balance**
- Facilitate **independence**

Common Orthoses by Deficit

Deficit	Orthosis
Isolated foot drop	AFO or PLS orthosis
Quadriceps weakness (knee instability)	KAFO with locking joint
Hip and knee involvement	HKAFO
Fixed deformity	Custom-molded brace or surgery + brace

Add-on Aids
- Crutches or canes for balance
- Shoe modifications for LLD (if present)

Q32. Principles and applications of functional bracing in fracture management.

(DNB, 2019)

Definition

Functional bracing is a technique of fracture care that **allows early joint motion** while maintaining **fracture alignment and stability**, primarily using **cast braces or prefabricated shells**.

Principles (Sarmiento's Concept)
1. Fracture healing by **secondary (callus) healing**
2. Controlled micromotion at fracture site
3. Circumferential compression improves stability
4. Allows **joint mobilization above and below**

Applications

Fracture site	*Brace used*
Tibial shaft fracture	PTB cast or shell brace
Humeral shaft fracture	Functional humeral brace
Radius/Ulna	Forearm brace

Benefits
- Avoids surgery in selected cases
- Preserves joint ROM
- Reduces cost and hospital stay

Limitations
- Not suitable for displaced/comminuted fractures
- Requires patient compliance

Q33. Orthotic management in cerebral palsy.

(DNB, Dec 2011)

Goals in CP Orthotics
- Prevent/treat **contractures** and deformities
- Facilitate **functional movement patterns**
- Improve **balance and posture**
- Support **ambulation** and assistive transitions

Commonly Used Orthoses

Condition	*Orthosis*
Equinus gait	Solid AFO or Hinged AFO
Crouch gait	Floor reaction orthosis (FRO)
Scissoring gait	Hip abduction bar
Hemiplegic CP	PLS brace or dynamic AFO
Scoliosis	TLSO (in adolescents)

Selection Criteria
- Type of CP (spastic, athetoid, ataxic)
- Ambulatory status (GMFCS level)
- Contractures or fixed deformities

Q34. Indications and design considerations for KAFOs.

(RGUHS, June/July 2010)

Indications
- Flaccid or spastic knee instability
- Quadriceps paralysis (e.g., PPRP, SCI)
- Post-operative stabilization (fractures or osteotomies)
- Multiplanar deformity correction
- Foot drop + knee hyperextension

Design Considerations

Component	Design options
Knee joint	Drop lock, dial lock, posterior offset
Uprights	Metal bars or thermoplastic shell
Foot section	Incorporate AFO for ankle control
Straps and bands	Calf, thigh, and patellar straps for stability

Functional Considerations
- Must be lightweight but strong
- Should allow **easy donning/doffing**
- Fit must avoid pressure points

Q35. Role of orthoses in spinal cord injury rehabilitation.

(Manipal University, 2012)

Orthoses by Neurological Level

Level	Orthosis used
Thoracic (T6–T12)	HKAFO with walker/crutches
Lumbar (L1–L3)	KAFO or AFO based on deficit
Cervical	Philadelphia collar, SOMI, Halo vest

Goals
- Enable **standing and walking (if feasible)**
- Prevent **contractures and deformities**
- Assist with **trunk balance**
- Maintain **bone health and prevent falls**

Additional Support
- Wheelchairs
- Transfers and pressure relief training
- Regular skin checks with brace use

Q36. Orthotic management strategies for genu valgum in children.

(NTR University, Oct 2015)

When to Treat Orthotically
- Age 2–5 years (mild deformity)
- Intermalleolar distance >7.5 cm
- Functional or cosmetic concern
- No bony deformity on X-ray

Orthotic Options

Brace type	Function
Medial pull knee brace	Applies valgus correction force
Night-time positioning splints	Maintains straight leg alignment
Corrective footwear	Supports arch, redirects mechanical axis

Duration
- Minimum 6–12 months
- Regular monitoring of **growth plates and alignment**

Limitations
- Less effective in moderate/severe cases
- Surgical intervention needed if persistent after age 10

Q37. Define splints and classify them.

Definition
A **splint** is a device used to **immobilize, support, or protect** a limb or body part, typically used for **temporary stabilization**, especially in trauma or post-operative care.

Classification
1. *By purpose*:
   - Immobilization (e.g., Thomas splint)
   - Functional support (e.g., dynamic splints)
2. *By material*:
   - Plaster of Paris (POP)
   - Thermoplastics
   - Prefabricated foam/metal
3. *By region*:
   - *Upper limb*: Volar splint, sugar-tong
   - *Lower limb*: Posterior slab, Bohler-Braun splint
   - *Spine*: Philadelphia collar, TLSO

Q38. Enumerate the indications of splints in orthopedic practice.

Indications
- **Fracture immobilization** (initial or definitive)
- **Post-operative protection**
- **Soft tissue injuries** (ligament sprain, tendon rupture)
- **Correction/prevention** of deformities (e.g., CTEV)
- Support in **neurological conditions** (CP, PPRP)
- Pain relief and joint rest in arthritis
- Burn contracture prevention

Q39. Compare splints versus orthosis versus braces.

General

Parameter	Splint	Orthosis	Brace
Purpose	Immobilize/support temporarily	Assist/replace musculoskeletal function	Provide support/compression
Duration	Usually short-term	Long-term (can be permanent)	Intermediate (sports, instability)

Continued

Continued

Parameter	Splint	Orthosis	Brace
Example	Thomas splint, POP slab	AFO, KAFO, TLSO	Hinged knee brace, elastic lumbar belt
Customization	Often generic or quickly made	Usually custom-fitted	Ready-made or semi-customized

Q40. Indications of thomas splint.

General

Indications

- Fracture shaft femur
- Hip dislocations/fractures (temporary support)
- Transport splint for lower limb trauma
- Combined with traction (e.g., Perkins traction)
- Support during **field immobilization** in war or disaster settings

Advantages

- Allows **traction and immobilization**
- Provides **alignment and pain relief**
- Reduces risk of further soft tissue damage

Q41. Principles of traction weight calculation.

General Rule

Traction weight = 1/7th to 1/10th of the patient's body weight

This ensures **adequate pull** without tissue damage.

Examples

- For **50 kg patient**, traction weight ≈ **5–7 kg**
- *Femoral fracture*: 10–15% of body weight
- *Cervical spine*: Start at 2.5 kg and increase by 1–2 kg under X-ray control

Factors Affecting Weight

- Muscle mass and tone
- Friction (bed/pulley system)
- Need for countertraction
- Fracture site and bone involved

Q42. Balanced suspension traction.

Definition

A method where the **limb is suspended in slings** and pulleys, allowing **free mobility while maintaining traction.**

Components

- **Thomas splint + Pearson attachment**
- Slings for thigh and leg
- Pulley system allowing limb motion in all planes
- Used with **skin or skeletal traction**

Indications

- Fracture shaft femur
- Long-term immobilization
- Where motion at hip/knee needs to be preserved

Q43. Countertraction and its significance.

Definition

Countertraction is the **opposing force** that balances the applied traction to keep the **bone ends aligned**.

How It's Achieved

Traction site	*Countertraction method*
Femur (skin/skeletal)	Elevating foot end of bed
Thomas splint	Body weight and groin support
Cervical spine	Weight of the trunk

Importance

- Prevents **sliding of patient**
- Ensures **effective alignment and reduction**
- Reduces **soft tissue strain**

Q44. Role of traction in tuberculosis spine.

Historical Use

- **Pre-operative immobilization**
- Reduction of **kyphosis in active TB spine**
- Relief of **muscle spasm** and pain
- Correction of **subluxation** (especially in cervical region)

Modern Practice

- Less common with **early surgical decompression**
- Still used in **developing regions or resource-limited settings**

Devices

- **Cervical traction** (Gardner–Wells tongs)
- **Pelvic traction** for lumbar TB

Q45. Splints used in brachial plexus injury.

Purpose of Splinting

- Prevent contractures
- Maintain **functional position** of hand and elbow
- Allow **nerve regeneration** and rehabilitation without deformity

Common Splints

Splint	*Use*
Cock-up splint	Wrist support in radial nerve palsy
Elbow flexion-extension splint	Prevent contractures during recovery
Airplane splint	Maintain **abduction + external rotation** of shoulder
Resting hand splint	Functional positioning at night

Q46. Functional cast brace—definition and indications.

Definition

A **functional cast brace** is a modified plaster or thermoplastic brace that allows **controlled joint movement** while maintaining **fracture alignment**, used during the **healing phase of long bone fractures**.

Indications
- Shaft of femur fractures
- Humerus shaft fractures
- Tibial shaft fractures
- Post-initial immobilization (after 3–4 weeks)

Features
- Made of **rigid outer shell** with straps
- **Open design** for limb inspection
- Allows **weight-bearing and movement**

Advantages
- Promotes early mobilization
- Enhances callus formation
- Reduces joint stiffness

Q47. SACH foot—features and indications.

[Dr Ram Manohar Lohia Institute of Medical Sciences (RMLIMS) Lucknow 2014]

Full Form
SACH: Solid Ankle, Cushion Heel

Features
- No ankle joint (rigid core)
- **Heel cushion** to absorb shock
- **Toe lever** allows toe-off
- Lightweight, maintenance-free

Indications
- **Below-knee amputees**
- Low to moderately active users
- Early prosthetic fitting phase
- Budget-limited patients

Limitations
- No active push-off
- Not ideal for high-performance users

Q48. Floor reaction orthosis (FRO)—use in gait management.

Definition
A type of AFO that uses **ground reaction force** to assist **knee extension** during gait.

Indications
- **Crouch gait in cerebral palsy**
- **Quadriceps weakness**
- Spina bifida
- SCI with partial motor recovery

Mechanism
- Rigid anterior shell transmits GRF to **stabilize knee**
- Prevents excessive **knee flexion** during stance phase

Q49. HKAFO—definition and indications.

Full Form

HKAFO: Hip-knee-ankle-foot orthosis

Definition

A long leg orthosis extending from the **pelvis to the foot**, used in patients with **hip and lower limb paralysis** or instability.

Indications

- Spinal cord injury (T10–L2)
- Myelomeningocele
- Bilateral **PPRP**
- Hip dislocation instability

Features

- Hip joint with lock mechanism
- KAFO integrated below
- Often combined with **crutches or walker**

Q50. Plaster of paris (POP)—properties and uses.

Properties

- **Exothermic setting reaction**
- Sets in 5–15 minutes
- **Malleable**, excellent molding capacity
- Strong when dry, but **brittle if wet**

Uses in Orthopedics

- Immobilization (casts, slabs)
- **Moulding splints and braces**
- Back slabs for fractures
- **Spinal jackets and body casts**
- As a **template in prosthesis manufacturing**

Q51. CTEV shoe—indications and design.

Definition

Custom-made shoes used post-correction in **congenital talipes equinovarus (clubfoot)** to maintain **foot abduction and alignment**.

Indications

- Post **Ponseti casting**
- After soft tissue release
- Following Dennis Browne bar or FAB protocol

Design

- Straight medial border
- Broad toe box
- Shoe holds foot in **external rotation** (60°–70°)
- Reinforced counter for support

Q52. Dennis Brown splint—components and role.

(Previously covered in Q25, but summarising here for completeness)

Components
- Rigid bar connecting two open-toe boots
- Boots fixed in **external rotation**
- Optional spring or hinged bar

Role
- Maintains **corrected position in clubfoot**
- Part of **Ponseti protocol maintenance phase**
- Worn **23 h/day for 3 months**, then nights till age 4

Q53. Crutchfield tongs—application and indications.

Definition
Skull traction device with **sharp pins** applied to the outer table of the skull to treat **cervical spine injuries**.

Application
- Inserted ~1 cm above ear, bilaterally
- Connected to overhead frame
- Weight applied to achieve reduction/alignment

Indications
- **Cervical spine dislocation**
- **Fracture-dislocation** C5–C7
- Temporary immobilization pre-surgery

Q54. Jaipur foot—features and benefits.

[All India Institute of Medical Sciences (AIIMS) New Delhi 2016]

Definition
A **low-cost, prosthetic foot** designed in India for **below-knee amputees**, allowing walking **barefoot or with shoes**.

Features
- Made from **rubber, wood, and vulcanized material**
- Lightweight and waterproof
- Can **squat, run, and walk on uneven ground**
- *Cost*: Less than ₹2,000 (~$25)

Benefits
- Highly **functional for rural users**
- No cosmetic compromise
- Easily replaceable and repairable

Q55. Pavlik harness—indications and fitting.

Indications
- **Developmental dysplasia of the hip (DDH)** in infants
- Best for age **<6 months**

Fitting Principles
- Maintains **hip flexion (90–110°)** and **abduction (~45°)**
- Straps adjust shoulder and leg positions
- **Never force abduction** (risk of avascular necrosis)

Duration
- Worn **23 h/day for 6–12 weeks**
- Regular ultrasound monitoring

Q56. Types of crutches—features and indications.

Types of Crutches

Type	*Features*	*Indications*
Axillary crutch	Underarm support	Short-term weight-bearing aid
Elbow/Lofstrand	Forearm cuff, used with hand grip	Long-term use, better for stairs
Gutter crutch	Forearm support tray	Post wrist/elbow surgery
Platform crutch	Used when grip strength is absent	Arthritis, neuro conditions

Selection
- Based on **patient stability, strength**, and duration of use
- Always measure and fit correctly to avoid **nerve palsy**

Q57. Crutch walking—gait patterns.

Gait Patterns

Pattern	*Use case*
Two-point gait	Partial weight bearing both legs
Three-point gait	NWB on one leg
Four-point gait	Maximal stability needed
Swing-to gait	Bilateral LE weakness
Swing-through gait	Paralysis, SCI

Training Steps
- Measure crutch height properly
- Teach **weight transfer**
- Supervise practice on stairs and slopes

Q58. Fisk splint—indications.

Definition
A hand splint used to **immobilize the thumb and wrist**, especially after tendon repair.

Indications
- **Flexor tendon injury (Zone II)**
- **Post-operative care** after tendon grafting
- Thumb injuries requiring neutral positioning

Features
- Keeps **MCP and IP joints slightly flexed**
- Prevents overstretching repaired structures
- Often made from **low-temperature thermoplastics**

Q59. Orthosis in DDH—devices and role.

Common Orthotic Devices

Age group	*Device*
<6 months	Pavlik harness
6–18 months	Rhino cruiser brace
>18 months (post-operative)	Abduction orthosis

Role

- Maintain hip in **flexion and abduction**
- Promote **acetabular remodeling**
- Avoid need for surgery (if early)

Monitoring

- Periodic **USG or X-ray**
- Adjust as baby grows

Q60. Below knee prosthesis—components and function.

[Assam Medical College (affiliated to Srimanta Sankaradeva University of Health Sciences) 2023]

Main Components

1. **Socket**: Custom-fit to residual limb
2. **Pylon**: Connects socket to foot, often aluminum
3. **Foot** – e.g., SACH foot or energy-return foot
4. **Suspension system**: Belt, sleeve, or pin-lock

Functions

- Allow **stable stance and ambulation**
- Absorb shock and return energy
- Improve **mobility and body symmetry**
- Restore **functional independence**

Q61. Patellar tendon bearing prosthesis—design and utility.

(DNB, Dec 2010)

Definition

The **Patellar Tendon Bearing (PTB) prosthesis** is a type of **below-knee prosthetic socket** that **distributes body weight through the patellar tendon**, thereby relieving pressure from distal limb tissues.

Design Features

Component	*Function*
PTB socket	Custom-molded socket, indents at patellar tendon
Relief areas	For tibial crest, fibular head, tibial condyles
Weight-bearing areas	Patellar tendon, popliteal area, medial tibial flare
Supracondylar/suprapatellar suspension	Provides additional grip and control
Soft liner	Cushions stump and prevents shear forces

Utility

- **Improved comfort** and limb fit
- Allows **partial weight-bearing** through proximal structures
- Reduces pressure on distal end—especially in **short or sensitive stumps**
- Enhances **gait control** and socket suspension

Q62. Rehabilitation after below knee amputation.

(RGUHS, June/July 2010)

Goals of Rehabilitation

- Wound healing and residual limb care
- Prevention of contractures
- Strengthening of proximal muscles
- Functional independence in transfers, ambulation
- Psychological adaptation and community reintegration

Phases of Rehabilitation

Phase	*Key activities*
Immediate post-operative (0–2 weeks)	Wound care, pain control, shrinker bandaging
Pre-prosthetic (2–6 weeks)	Stump shaping, ROM exercises, desensitization
Prosthetic training	Gait training with PTB or modular prosthesis
Community reintegration	ADLs, home/workplace adaptation, long-term monitoring

Preventive Measures

- Avoid **knee flexion contracture** (keep leg extended)
- Use of **rigid dressing or shrinker sock**
- Daily inspection of residual limb
- Psychological counseling

Q63. Recent advancements in prosthetic limbs.

(Vinayaka Missions University, 2015)

Key Recent Advancements

1. *Microprocessor-controlled prostheses*:
    - C-leg (by Otto Bock), Genium, Rheo knee
    - Sensors adjust gait in real-time
    - Better for **variable terrain and stair descent**
2. *Myoelectric arms*:
    - Use EMG signals to power movements
    - More intuitive and **multi-joint** control
    - Advanced versions can **sense grip force and position**
3. *Osseointegration*:
    - Titanium implant directly integrated with bone
    - Eliminates socket; allows **better proprioception and stability**
4. *3D printing of prostheses*:
    - **Low-cost**, customizable prosthetic limbs
    - Lightweight materials; great for **pediatric use**
5. *Sensory feedback and neural integration*:
    - Ongoing research in **brain-machine interfaces**
    - Goal: allow patients to "feel" and control limbs like a natural extension

Conclusion

Modern prosthetics are **smarter, lighter, and more lifelike**, focusing on **user comfort, control, and feedback**, drastically improving quality of life.

CHAPTER 15

Gait Analysis and Disorders

Sajal Maingi, Varun Gupta, Naresh V

Commonly Asked Theory Questions

Q1. Define gait and describe phases of normal gait cycle.

(Rajasthan University of Health Sciences Jaipur 2017)

- *Universities*:
  - *RGUHS*: 2020
  - *MUHS*: 2019
  - *DNB*: 2021

Definition of Gait

- **Gait** is the **pattern of movement of the limbs during locomotion** over a solid surface.
- It involves a **cyclical and coordinated sequence of motions** that result in forward propulsion of the body.

Gait Cycle

- One complete gait cycle is from **heel strike of one foot to the next heel strike of the same foot**.
- Divided into two main **phases**

1. Stance Phase (60% of Gait Cycle)

Period during which the foot is in contact with the ground.

Subphases

Subphase	*Description*
Heel strike	Initial contact of heel with ground
Foot flat	Entire plantar surface contacts ground
Mid-stance	Body weight is directly over supporting foot
Heel-off	Heel lifts off the ground
Toe-off	Toes push off to propel body forward

2. Swing Phase (40% of Gait Cycle)

Period when the foot is **not in contact with the ground**.

Subphases

Subphase	*Description*
Acceleration	Foot leaves the ground
Mid-swing	Foot passes beneath the body
Deceleration	Leg slows down in preparation for heel strike

Double Support Phase

- Occurs **twice in each gait cycle** (when both feet are on the ground)
- Accounts for ~20–25% of the total cycle

Q2. Enumerate determinants of gait and explain their significance.

- *Universities*:
  - *RGUHS*: 2022
  - *DNB*: 2020

Definition

Determinants of gait are **biomechanical adjustments** that minimize the **vertical and lateral displacement** of the centre of gravity (COG), making gait more **efficient and energy-conserving**.

Six Determinants of Gait

Determinant	Function
1. Pelvic rotation	~4° forward rotation of pelvis reduces vertical drop
2. Pelvic tilt	Downward tilt of swing-side pelvis reduces vertical rise
3. Knee flexion in stance phase	Lowers apex of vertical COG rise
4. Ankle mechanisms	Dorsiflexion at heel strike and plantarflexion at toe-off smoothens vertical displacement
5. Foot mechanisms	Foot pronation and supination reduce shock and stabilize limb
6. Lateral displacement of pelvis	Balances weight during single-limb support

Significance

- Helps **reduce energy expenditure** during walking.
- Promotes **smooth and rhythmic gait**.
- Assists in maintaining **stability and balance**.

Q3. Discuss abnormal gait patterns and their causes.

- *Universities*:
  - *MUHS*: 2021
  - *DNB*: 2019

Definition

Abnormal gait results from **neurological, muscular, skeletal, or pain-related impairments** that alter the **normal walking pattern**.

Common Abnormal Gait Patterns

Gait type	Features	Causes
Antalgic gait	Shortened stance phase on painful side	Trauma, arthritis
Trendelenburg gait	Pelvic drop on swing side	Gluteus medius weakness, DDH
High stepping/Steppage gait	Foot drop with exaggerated hip/knee flexion	Common peroneal nerve palsy
Circumduction gait	Lateral swing of leg	Stiff knee, long limb, prosthesis
Vaulting gait	Rise on contralateral toe	Prosthetic limb too long
Scissoring gait	Legs cross during swing	Spasticity (e.g., cerebral palsy)
Ataxic gait	Wide base, unsteady, irregular steps	Cerebellar lesions
Spastic gait	Stiff-legged, scissoring motion	Hemiplegia, upper motor neuron lesion
Waddling gait	Bilateral pelvic drop	Muscular dystrophy, bilateral hip weakness

Approach to Diagnosis
- *History*: Pain, trauma, neurological illness
- *Physical exam*: Muscle power, joint ROM, balance
- *Imaging/EMG*: As needed

Q4. Trendelenburg gait—causes and clinical significance.

- *Universities*:
  - *TNMGRMU*: 2020
  - *RGUHS*: 2023

Definition

Trendelenburg gait is a compensatory gait seen due to **weakness/paralysis of the hip abductors**, mainly the **gluteus medius and minimus**.

Mechanism
- During the **stance phase**, the **gluteus medius on the stance side** contracts to maintain **pelvic stability**.
- If weak, the **pelvis drops on the swing side**, resulting in:
  - *Uncompensated gait*: Pelvic drop
  - *Compensated gait*: Patient leans toward the affected side

Causes

Category	*Examples*
Neurological	Superior gluteal nerve injury, polio
Muscular	Gluteus medius/minimus weakness (myopathies)
Skeletal	DDH, coxa vara
Post-surgical	Following total hip arthroplasty or hip surgery

Clinical Significance
- Indicates **hip abductor weakness**
- Can lead to **lurching, fatigue, and poor balance**
- *Evaluated using Trendelenburg test*:
  - Positive if pelvis drops on **contralateral side** when standing on affected leg

Diagram (Recommended)
- Pelvic tilt with gluteus medius action
- Leaning posture in compensated gait

Q5. Draw and describe the stance and swing phases of gait.

- *Universities*:
  - *DNB*: 2021
  - *MUHS*: 2022
- *Expected*: Labelled diagram + temporal components.

Q6. Discuss muscle actions in various phases of gait.

- *Universities*:
  - *PGIMER pattern*: Frequently asked in viva
  - *DNB*: 2020

Muscle activation during gait is **phasic and coordinated** to ensure smooth, energy-efficient walking. Different muscle groups act during different phases of **stance and swing**.

Key Muscle Activity During Gait Phases

Gait phase	*Muscles active*	*Function*
Heel strike	Tibialis anterior	Ankle dorsiflexion to prevent foot slap
Foot flat	Quadriceps	Eccentric control to prevent knee collapse
Mid-stance	Gluteus medius/minimus	Pelvic stabilization
Heel-off	Gastrocnemius-soleus	Plantar flexion for push-off
Toe-off	Flexor hallucis longus, intrinsic foot muscles	Propel body forward
Acceleration	Iliopsoas, rectus femoris	Hip flexion
Mid-swing	Tibialis anterior	Maintain dorsiflexion to clear foot
Deceleration	Hamstrings	Control hip and knee extension

Clinical Relevance

- Helps localize **nerve or muscle lesions** (e.g., foot drop will lead to weak dorsiflexors)
- Essential in designing **rehabilitation and orthotic strategies**

Q7. Discuss pathologic gait patterns in polio.

(Bihar University 2018)

- *Universities*:
  - *MUHS*: 2021
  - *TNMGRMU*: 2022

Introduction

Poliomyelitis causes **lower motor neuron lesions** leading to **muscle weakness and paralysis**, resulting in **compensatory gait abnormalities**.

Common Gait Patterns in Polio

Gait type	*Cause*	*Features*
Hand-to-knee gait	Weak **quadriceps**	Patient pushes thigh with hand to prevent knee collapse during stance
Waddling gait	Bilateral **gluteus medius weakness**	Pelvic drop on both sides; trunk sways laterally
Equinus gait	Weak dorsiflexors/plantarflexor spasticity	Walks on toes, heel does not contact ground
Steppage gait	Foot drop due to **anterior tibial group weakness**	High hip/knee flexion to prevent toe drag
Circumduction gait	Knee or ankle stiffness	Swing leg is abducted in arc to clear ground
Lurch gait	**Gluteus maximus weakness**	Backward trunk lurch during heel strike

Management Implications

- **Orthoses** (e.g., KAFO, AFO)
- **Tendon transfers**
- **Rehabilitation and gait training**
- Corrective surgeries (e.g., triple arthrodesis, osteotomies)

Q8. What is antalgic gait? List common causes.

- *Universities*: DNB—2019

Definition

An **antalgic gait** is a **compensatory gait** where the **stance phase of the affected limb is shortened** to avoid pain.

Features

- Reduced time on painful limb (stance phase)
- Increased swing phase on affected side
- Asymmetrical step length
- May have a limp or lateral sway

Common Causes

Lower limb pain sources

Region	Examples
Hip	Osteoarthritis, septic arthritis
Knee	Meniscal tear, ligament injury, OA
Ankle/Foot	Plantar fasciitis, fracture, sprain
Bone	Tumors, infections, stress fractures
Soft tissue	Bursitis, tendinitis

Diagnosis and Management

- **Identify and treat** the pain source
- Use of **walking aids**, pain management, and **rehabilitation**

Q9. Classification of gait abnormalities.

- *Universities*:
  - *RGUHS*: 2021
  - *DNB*: 2023

Gait abnormalities can be classified based on etiology, biomechanical basis, or clinical pattern.

I. Based on Biomechanics

Type	Example
Antalgic	Shortened stance (painful limb)
Trendelenburg	Gluteus medius weakness
Vaulting	Long prosthesis or stiff knee
Steppage	Foot drop
Circumduction	Stiff knee/long limb
Scissoring	Spastic cerebral palsy

II. Based on Etiology

Cause	Gait type
Neurological	Ataxic, hemiplegic, steppage
Muscular	Trendelenburg, lurch, waddling
Orthopedic	Antalgic, circumduction
Prosthetic	Vaulting, unequal limb gait

III. Based on Neurologic Pattern

Pattern	Lesion type
Spastic gait	UMN lesion (e.g., stroke)
Flaccid gait	LMN lesion (e.g., polio)
Ataxic gait	Cerebellar dysfunction
Festinating gait	Parkinson's disease

Q10. Steppage gait—causes and associated nerve lesion.

- *Universities*:
  - *MUHS*: 2020
  - *DNB*: 2021

Definition

Steppage gait is characterized by **exaggerated hip and knee flexion** during the swing phase to **clear the foot**, due to **foot drop**.

Mechanism

- Weakness of **ankle dorsiflexors** leads to inability to lift the forefoot.
- Compensation by **lifting the knee and hip** higher.

Causes

Type	*Examples*
Peripheral nerve	Common peroneal nerve palsy, sciatic nerve palsy
Root lesion	L5 radiculopathy
Neuromuscular	Charcot–Marie–Tooth disease, muscular dystrophy
CNS disorders	Less common (ALS, syringomyelia)

Associated Nerve Lesion

- *Common peroneal nerve*:
  - Supplies **tibialis anterior, EHL, EDL** (dorsiflexors)
  - Most commonly injured at the **fibular neck**

Clinical Exam

- Foot drop
- Weak dorsiflexion/toe extension
- Positive foot slap during heel strike

Q11. Describe energy expenditure during different types of gait or with prostheses.

(Rajasthan University of Health Sciences Jaipur 2018)

- *Universities*: *DNB*—2022

Normal Gait

Baseline energy requirement for walking is set at **100%**.

Energy Expenditure in Various Amputation Levels

Amputation type	*Increase in energy (%)*
Below-knee (BKA)	~25%
Through-knee	~50%
Above-knee (AKA)	~65%
Hip disarticulation	~100–125%
Bilateral AKA	~200–300%

Factors Affecting Energy Cost

- Level of amputation
- Muscle strength and control
- Prosthetic design (e.g., energy-storing feet)
- Gait training and rehabilitation quality

Energy-efficient Gait Aids

- Lightweight prostheses
- Dynamic response feet (e.g., flex-foot)
- Proper socket alignment
- Physiotherapy and endurance training

Q12. Difference between spastic and ataxic gait.

- *Universities*:
  - *TNMGRMU*: 2021
  - *DNB*: 2020

Definition

- *Spastic gait*: Gait pattern resulting from **upper motor neuron (UMN) lesions**, characterized by **stiff, scissoring leg movements.**
- *Ataxic gait*: Gait due to **cerebellar dysfunction**, marked by **wide-based, unsteady, and irregular steps.**

Comparison Table Spastic versus Ataxic Gait

Feature	*Spastic gait*	*Ataxic gait*
Cause	UMN lesions (e.g., stroke, cerebral palsy)	Cerebellar lesion (tumor, infarct, alcohol)
Base of support	Narrow	Wide-based
Step pattern	Short, stiff steps	Irregular, variable stride
Leg posture	Extended knees, adducted thighs	No specific posturing
Arm swing	Reduced or absent	May be normal
Balance	Generally preserved unless bilateral	Poor – frequent veering, instability
Characteristic	"Scissoring" gait	"Drunken", "Lurching" gait
Romberg test	Negative	Often positive

Q13. Cerebellar gait—features and clinical significance.

- *Universities*: *RGUHS—2022*

Definition

A **cerebellar gait** is a type of **ataxic gait** characterized by **poor coordination and balance**, due to lesions of the **cerebellum.**

Features

- Wide-based gait
- Unsteady, irregular steps
- Lateral swaying of trunk (truncal ataxia)
- Staggering/lurching movements
- Difficulty walking in tandem (heel-to-toe)
- Frequent veering, especially toward side of lesion
- May have dysmetria, intention tremor, or nystagmus on exam

Causes

Category	*Examples*
Stroke	Cerebellar infarcts or hemorrhage
Tumor	Medulloblastoma, astrocytoma
Degeneration	Alcoholic cerebellar degeneration
Demyelination	Multiple sclerosis

Clinical Relevance

- Seen in **neurology and orthopedic clinics** (fall-risk assessment)
- May mimic orthopedic disorders if not recognized
- Requires **neuroimaging** for diagnosis

Q14. Gait abnormalities in cerebral palsy.

- *Universities*:
    - *DNB*: 2021
    - *MUHS*: 2019

Introduction

Cerebral palsy often causes **spasticity and muscle imbalance**, leading to a variety of **abnormal gait patterns**, particularly in **diplegic and hemiplegic types**.

Common Gait Patterns in CP

Gait type	*Cause/Mechanism*
Toe-walking	Gastrocnemius-soleus spasticity
Scissoring gait	Spastic hip adductors causing legs to cross
Crouch gait	Excessive hip and knee flexion + ankle dorsiflexion (common in diplegic CP)
Jump gait	Hip and knee flexion with equinus at ankle
Hemiplegic gait	Stiff-legged gait, circumduction on affected side

Contributing Factors

- Spasticity
- Muscle contractures (especially hamstrings, adductors)
- Bony deformities (e.g., femoral anteversion)
- Poor trunk control

Management

- **Physiotherapy**
- *Orthoses*: AFO, KAFO, floor reaction orthosis
- **Botulinum toxin injections** (spasticity management)
- *Surgical interventions*: Tendon lengthening, osteotomies (e.g., SEMLS – single event multilevel surgery)
- *Gait analysis*: Instrumented gait labs help plan treatment

Q15. What is hand-to-knee gait?

(Madras Medical College Chennai Tamil Nadu 2017)

Definition

A **compensatory gait** seen in **quadriceps paralysis**, where the patient **uses their hand to push the thigh anteriorly** during stance to prevent **knee buckling**.

Mechanism

- **Quadriceps weakness** → knee cannot be stabilized in extension during weight-bearing.
- Patient **applies external force using hand** to prevent knee collapse.

Seen in

- **Poliomyelitis**
- Femoral nerve palsy
- Post-total knee arthroplasty (early quadriceps inhibition)

Q16. What is equinus gait?

Definition

A gait pattern where the patient **walks on their toes** due to **ankle plantar flexion contracture or spasticity**.

Features

- **Heel does not touch the ground**
- Premature toe contact
- May result in **early heel rise**, poor push-off, or compensations like knee hyperextension

Seen in

- **Spastic diplegic cerebral palsy**
- Clubfoot (CTEV)
- Contracture of **gastrocnemius-soleus** complex

Q17. How do orthoses affect gait patterns?

Role of Orthoses

Orthoses can **correct, support, assist, or restrict** movement in a limb, improving **gait mechanics and energy efficiency**.

Examples

Orthosis	*Effect on gait*
Ankle-foot orthosis (AFO)	Prevents foot drop, improves toe clearance and heel strike
Floor reaction orthosis (FRO)	Assists in knee extension in crouch gait
Knee-ankle-foot orthosis (KAFO)	Stabilizes weak knee during stance (e.g., polio)
HKAFO	Enables standing and swing-through gait in paraplegia

Benefits

- Prevents deformity
- Enhances balance and stability
- Reduces energy cost

Q18. What is vaulting gait?

Definition

A **compensatory gait** where the patient **rises on the toes of the unaffected leg** during **swing phase** of the affected leg.

Mechanism

- Used to **help clear the contralateral limb** which is:
    - Too long
    - Stiff knee or ankle
    - Prosthesis that is poorly aligned or too long

Seen in

- **Prosthetic limb users**
- Knee fusion
- Limb length discrepancy

Q19. What is circumduction gait and when is it seen?

Definition

A gait pattern where the **affected limb swings outward in an arc** during swing phase to compensate for **inability to flex knee or dorsiflex ankle.**

Features
- **Semi-circular movement** of the leg during swing
- Often accompanied by **hip hike** or trunk lean

Seen in
- **Knee extension contracture**
- Long leg prosthesis
- **Stiff knee gait**
- Foot drop (if no AFO used)

Summary Table

Gait type	*Key feature*	*Common cause*
Hand-to-knee gait	Hand stabilizes knee in stance	Quadriceps paralysis (e.g., polio)
Equinus gait	Toe walking, heel not contacting ground	CP (spastic diplegia), contracture
Vaulting gait	Tiptoe stance on normal limb	Long/stiff opposite limb or prosthesis
Circumduction gait	Outward arc of limb during swing	Stiff knee, long leg, foot drop

Q20. Biomechanics of normal gait.

Key Principles
- Gait is a **cyclical movement** involving alternating limb motions to produce locomotion.
- **Energy-efficient**, requires minimal muscle activity due to **inverted pendulum mechanics**.

Kinematics (Motion)
- *Pelvis*: Rotates ~4°, tilts ~5°
- *Hip*: Flexion (30°) to extension (10°)
- *Knee*: Flexion (60° in swing), extension (0° at heel strike)
- *Ankle*: Dorsiflexion (10°) and plantarflexion (20°)

Kinetics (Forces)
- Joint moments and muscle contractions counteract **GRF** (ground reaction forces)
- **Center of mass** oscillates vertically and laterally

Q21. What is antalgic gait? Mention its features and causes.

Antalgic gait is a **pain-avoidance pattern**.

Features
- **Shortened stance phase** on affected limb
- May limp or shift weight quickly to opposite side

Causes
- Osteoarthritis
- Fracture
- Infection (osteomyelitis, septic arthritis)
- Tumor
- Soft tissue injuries

Q22. How do you assess gait clinically?

Clinical Gait Analysis
1. *Observation*: From front, side, and back
2. Check **stride length, cadence, arm swing, step width**

3. **Look for asymmetry**, deviations, foot position
4. *Specific tests*:
   - Heel walking (L5)
   - Toe walking (S1)
   - Trendelenburg test
   - Foot drop assessment (ask to dorsiflex ankle during swing)

Q23. What is the role of gait analysis in orthopedics?

(Narayana Medical College Nellore Andhra Pradesh 2018)

Uses

- **Diagnosis** of neuromuscular and musculoskeletal disorders
- **Preoperative planning** (especially in CP and post-polio cases)
- **Postoperative outcome evaluation** (e.g., THR, ACL reconstruction)
- Design of **orthotic and prosthetic devices**

Tools

- Observational gait assessment
- *Instrumented gait analysis*: Markers, force plates, EMG

Q24. What is foot drop gait and what are its orthopedic causes?

Foot drop gait leads to **high-stepping gait**

Cause

Weakness or paralysis of **dorsiflexors** (tibialis anterior)

Orthopedic Causes

- **Common peroneal nerve injury** (e.g., fibular neck fracture)
- **L5 radiculopathy**
- Compartment syndrome (anterior)
- Poliomyelitis
- Post-surgical nerve injury (e.g., TKR)

Compensation

Excessive hip and knee flexion during swing to clear the foot.

Q25. Describe ataxic gait and its relevance in orthopedics.

Ataxic gait is an **unsteady, uncoordinated walking pattern** with a broad base.

Causes

- **Cerebellar disorders** (e.g., tumor, stroke)
- **Sensory ataxia**—posterior column lesions (e.g., tabes dorsalis)
- **Peripheral neuropathy**

Orthopedic relevance

- May mimic or coexist with **structural deformities**
- Important to differentiate from **mechanical or muscular gaits**

Q26. Write short note on compensatory mechanisms in abnormal gait.

To overcome deficits in power, pain, or range of motion, the patient may:
- Lateral trunk lean (toward weak abductors—Trendelenburg compensation)
- Increased pelvic rotation (for limited hip flexion)
- Knee hyperextension (to compensate quadriceps weakness)
- Vaulting on opposite limb (to assist with clearance of a long or stiff limb)

Suggested Viva Questions

Q1. What is double support phase in gait?

The **period when both feet are in contact with the ground** during the gait cycle.
- Occurs **twice per gait cycle** (initial contact and terminal stance).
- Accounts for approximately **20–25%** of the cycle in normal walking.

Q2. What is step length and stride length?

Term	*Definition*
Step length (e.g., right to left heel strike)	Distance between the **heel strikes of opposite feet**
Stride length (e.g., right to next right heel strike)	Distance between **two successive heel strikes of the same foot**

- Stride length = 2 × step length

Q3. Most energy-consuming phase of gait?

Heel-off to toe-off phase (also called **push-off phase**).
- Involves **plantar flexion of ankle**, activation of **calf muscles (gastrocnemius–soleus)**.
- Requires **highest muscular effort** to propel body forward.

Q4. What is festinating gait?

A gait seen in **Parkinson's disease**, characterized by:
- **Short, rapid, shuffling steps**
- **Forward flexed posture**
- Patient appears as if they're trying to **"catch up" with their center of gravity**
- May also have **difficulty initiating movement (freezing)**

CHAPTER 16

Common Surgical Approaches and Procedures

Mohammed Farooq Butt, Amit Kumar

Section 1: General Principles and Soft Tissue Handling

Q1. Enumerate principles of surgical exposure in orthopedics. Describe methods to protect neurovascular structures during open surgery.

(RGUHS 2021, DNB 2020)

Principles of Surgical Exposure in Orthopedics

1. *Adequate exposure:* Incision should provide a **clear, extensile view** of the operative field.
2. *Layered dissection:* Respect **anatomical planes** and preserve tissue integrity.
3. *Preserve blood supply:* Avoid indiscriminate stripping of **periosteum and muscle**.
4. *Minimize soft tissue damage:* Use **sharp dissection** where possible; avoid crushing or tearing.
5. *Gentle tissue handling:* Use **atraumatic instruments**, keep tissues moist.
6. *Respect internervous and intermuscular planes:* Prevents denervation and preserves function (e.g., **deltopectoral plane** in shoulder surgery).
7. *Adequate retraction:* Use appropriate retractors with minimal pressure and proper padding.
8. *Maintain hemostasis:* Use **bipolar cautery** and ligatures to reduce bleeding.
9. *Exposure should be reversible:* Allows easy closure and anatomical restoration.
10. *Planning for extensile access:* Incisions should be extendable if required (e.g., **Kocher's** to **Boyd's** for elbow).

Protection of Neurovascular Structures

1. *Knowledge of surgical anatomy:* Preoperative review of **danger zones** (e.g., radial nerve in posterior humerus approach).
2. *Marking anatomical landmarks:* Surface marking of nerves and vessels pre-operative when feasible.
3. *Use of nerve stimulator or magnification:* Especially useful in **nerve exploration or re-do surgeries**.
4. *Blunt dissection near neurovascular bundles:* Prevents inadvertent cuts; retract structures medially/laterally as needed.
5. *Use of vessel loops or silastic slings:* To safely retract nerves and vessels during deep dissection.
6. *Avoiding prolonged retraction:* Especially over nerves (e.g., avoid brachial plexus stretch during shoulder surgeries).
7. *Intraoperative neuromonitoring (IONM):* Optional in spine surgery or complex tumor resections.

Q2. Principles of soft tissue dissection and handling during open orthopedic procedures.

(MUHS 2022)

Why It Matters?

Soft tissue injury increases risk of:

- Infection
- Delayed healing
- Scarring
- Neurovascular complications
- Poor functional outcome

Principles of Soft Tissue Dissection

1. *Respect tissue planes:* Follow **natural cleavage planes** (internervous/intermuscular).
2. *Minimal use of electrocautery in muscles:* Avoids thermal necrosis; prefer **sharp dissection**.
3. *Atraumatic instruments:* Use **skin hooks, blunt retractors** to prevent crush injuries.
4. *Avoid undue retraction or tension:* Use **self-retaining retractors** gently; pad nerves.
5. *Preserve periosteum and vascular supply:* Particularly important in fractures and tumor surgeries.
6. *Avoid muscle devitalization:* Do not strip or over-dissect; it reduces bleeding and necrosis.
7. *Keep tissues moist:* Use **saline-soaked gauze** to prevent desiccation.
8. *Use of suction judiciously:* Avoid negative pressure injury to nerves/vessels.
9. *Meticulous layered closure:* Restore anatomy; avoids dead space and seromas.
10. *Hemostasis throughout:* Reduces hematoma formation and infection risk.

Q3. Describe Halsted's principles. How do they apply in orthopedic surgery?

(DNB 2023)

Halsted's Principles of Surgery (Established in Late 19th Century)

1. Gentle handling of tissues
2. Meticulous hemostasis
3. Preservation of blood supply
4. Strict aseptic technique
5. Minimization of tissue tension
6. Accurate tissue apposition
7. Obliteration of dead space

Application in Orthopedics

Principle	*Orthopedic relevance*
Gentle tissue handling	During flap elevation, nerve protection, and exposure
Meticulous hemostasis	Prevents hematoma in deep tissues or under implants
Preserve blood supply	Important in periosteal stripping, joint capsule handling
Asepsis	Reduces post-operative wound infections and implant-related sepsis
Minimize tension	In skin closure, especially in trauma and tumor resections
Accurate apposition	Ensures proper wound healing and functional restoration
Obliterate dead space	Prevents fluid accumulation → infection, delayed healing

Q4. Enumerate basic principles of surgical wound closure in orthopedics.

(RGUHS 2020)

Key Principles

1. *Anatomic layer-by-layer closure:* Skin, fascia, muscle, and subcutaneous tissue must be closed separately when possible.
2. *Minimize tension:* Tension-free closure promotes healing and prevents ischemia or necrosis.
3. *Use appropriate suture material:* Non-absorbable for skin (e.g., nylon), absorbable for deeper layers (e.g., vicryl).
4. *Preserve vascularity:* Avoid strangulation of flaps or crushing tissues.
5. *Avoid dead space:* Close in layers and consider drains if necessary.
6. *Handle tissue gently:* Use fine instruments and avoid forceful pulling.
7. *Aseptic technique:* Ensure sterility during closure to reduce infection risk.
8. *Alignment with skin creases (Langer's lines):* For better cosmesis and reduced tension.
9. *Secure hemostasis before closure:* Avoid closing over active bleeds.
10. *Post-closure dressing:* Use sterile, pressure-appropriate dressing to support healing.

Q5. Describe surgical approach to humerus shaft—anterior and posterior. Add a note on radial nerve protection.

(DNB 2022, RGUHS 2021)

Anterior Approach to Humeral Shaft

Indications:

- Midshaft humeral fractures (anterolateral plate)
- Anterior neurovascular exploration

Landmarks:

- Deltoid insertion
- Biceps brachii
- Brachialis

Steps:

1. **Patient in supine** or beach chair position.
2. **Skin incision** along lateral biceps border.
3. Retract **biceps medially** to expose **brachialis.**
4. **Split brachialis longitudinally**—lateral part is innervated by radial nerve, medial by musculocutaneous nerve.
5. **Fracture site exposed**—preserve periosteum as needed.

Radial Nerve Risk

Crosses from **medial to lateral in the spiral groove** → avoid deep dissection posteriorly.

Posterior Approach to Humeral Shaft

Indications:

- Mid to distal third humerus fractures (especially posterior plating)
- Radial nerve exploration

Steps:

1. Lateral decubitus or prone position.
2. *Skin incision*: Posterior midline from acromion to olecranon.

3. Incise **fascia**, identify and **reflect triceps** (split or lift entire muscle).
4. Radial nerve lies in spiral groove (crosses ~10–14 cm from lateral epicondyle).
5. Nerve identified, mobilized gently.

Radial Nerve Protection

- Use vessel loops
- Avoid retraction trauma
- Avoid sharp dissection in nerve area
- Identify early if nerve exploration is planned

Diagram

Draw **cross-section of mid-humerus** showing nerve course or approach.

Q6. Discuss deltopectoral approach to the shoulder joint—anatomical boundaries and structures encountered.

(TNMGRMU 2021, MUHS 2020)

Indications

- Shoulder arthroplasty (excluded here)
- Proximal humerus fracture fixation
- Shoulder dislocation open reduction
- Tumor exposure

Anatomical Boundaries

Landmark	*Structure*
Medial	Clavicular head of deltoid
Lateral	Pectoralis major (deltopectoral groove)
Floor of interval	Cephalic vein (preserve or lateralize)

Steps

1. Patient supine, **arm on arm board**.
2. Skin incision from **coracoid to deltoid insertion**.
3. Identify and **preserve cephalic vein**.
4. Retract **deltoid laterally**, **pec major medially**.
5. *Deep dissection to access*:
    - Subscapularis
    - Anterior capsule
    - *Biceps tendon (long head)*: Inspect or tenotomize if needed

Structures at Risk

- Cephalic vein
- Axillary nerve (inferior capsule)
- Musculocutaneous nerve (medial retraction)

Advantages

- Preserves deltoid
- Extensible proximally and distally

Q7. Write in detail about posterior approach to the elbow joint—indications and complications.

(RGUHS 2020, DNB 2021)

Indications

- *ORIF of*:
  - Olecranon fractures
  - Distal humerus fractures
- Total elbow arthroplasty (excluded here)
- Tumor excision

Steps (Triceps-splitting Approach)

1. **Prone or lateral** position with arm over bolster.
2. Posterior midline incision from **mid-arm to ulna shaft**.
3. Identify and **isolate ulnar nerve** (medial to triceps, posterior to medial epicondyle).
4. **Split triceps** or use **olecranon osteotomy** for better exposure.
5. Reflect triceps to expose **olecranon, distal humerus, and joint**.

Modifications

- Bryan–Morrey (triceps reflecting)
- Campbell (triceps splitting)
- Olecranon osteotomy (best exposure for distal humerus)

Structures at Risk

- Ulnar nerve—must be isolated and protected
- Medial and lateral collateral ligaments
- Posterior interosseous nerve (laterally)

Complications

- Ulnar nerve palsy
- Triceps weakness (in splitting or reflecting)
- Non-union of osteotomy
- Elbow stiffness

Q8. Describe the Kocher and Boyd approaches to the radial head and proximal ulna.

(MUHS 2022)

Kocher Approach (Lateral Elbow)

Indications:

- Radial head ORIF/excision
- Radial neck fractures
- Lateral capsule release

Interval: Between **anconeus** and **extensor carpi ulnaris**

Steps:

1. Lateral elbow incision (~2 cm distal to lateral epicondyle).
2. Develop interval between anconeus and ECU.
3. Retract tissues to expose **capsule and radial head**.

At risk:
- *Posterior interosseous nerve (PIN)*: Lies deep, anterior to radial neck
- Supinator if extended too far distally

Boyd Approach (Posterior Proximal Ulna)
Indications:
- ORIF of **proximal ulna**
- Combined elbow fracture-dislocation

Interval:
- Between **anconeus and extensor carpi ulnaris**
- More posterior and extensile than Kocher

Steps:
1. Posterolateral incision along ulna.
2. Reflect anconeus and ECU laterally.
3. Expose **proximal ulna and radial head/neck**.

At risk:
- **Ulnar nerve (medially)**
- Triceps insertion (if extended too proximally)

Section 2: Surgical Approaches to Lower Limb

Q1. Describe anterior and lateral approaches to femoral shaft. Discuss precautions to avoid neurovascular injury.

(DNB 2019, MUHS 2020)

A. Anterior Approach to Femoral Shaft
Indications:
- ORIF of femoral shaft fractures (especially midshaft)
- Exposure for tumor resection
- Vascular access procedures

Landmarks and interval:
- *Skin incision*: Along line between **ASIS and lateral patella.**
- *Interval*: **Between sartorius (medial)** and **rectus femoris/vastus lateralis (lateral)**.

Steps:
1. Supine position, thigh externally rotated.
2. Incise skin and fascia lata.
3. Retract sartorius medially and rectus laterally.
4. Dissect deep to expose femoral shaft.
5. Protect **femoral artery/vein/nerve** (medially).

Advantages: Good access to **mid to proximal femoral shaft**.

Neurovascular precautions:
- Avoid deep dissection **medial to sartorius** to protect femoral neurovascular bundle.
- Gentle retraction and use of vessel loops if exposure extended proximally.

B. Lateral Approach to Femur (Direct Lateral/Vastus Split)
Indications:
- Most commonly used for **plating of femoral shaft fractures**.
- ORIF of subtrochanteric and mid-shaft fractures.

Steps:

1. Lateral incision over femur (proximal to distal).
2. Incise fascia lata, identify **vastus lateralis**.
3. Retract vastus anteriorly or **split along fibers**.
4. Avoid injuring **perforating branches** of profunda femoris (posterior).

Neurovascular structures at risk:

- Perforators from profunda femoris artery (cause hematoma)
- Lateral femoral cutaneous nerve (at ASIS region, if incision is too anterior)

Q2. Posterolateral approach to the hip joint—indications, technique, and complications.

(TNMGRMU 2019)

Indications

- Open reduction of hip dislocation
- ORIF of **acetabular posterior wall/column fractures**
- Tumor excision
- *Excluded*: Arthroplasty

Landmarks

- Posterior iliac crest
- Greater trochanter
- Lateral femoral shaft

Steps

1. **Lateral or prone** position.
2. Skin incision centered over **posterior greater trochanter**.
3. Incise fascia lata in line with skin.
4. **Split gluteus maximus** in line of fibers.
5. Identify **short external rotators (piriformis, obturator internus, gemelli)**.
6. Tag and release external rotators and **posterior capsule**.
7. Retract gluteus medius superiorly to expose **posterior hip joint**.

Structures at Risk

- Sciatic nerve (runs medial to external rotators)
- Medial femoral circumflex artery

Complications

- **Posterior dislocation** (if rotators not repaired)
- Sciatic nerve injury
- Hematoma, infection

Q3. Describe posterolateral approach to tibia and its relevance in tibial plateau fractures.

(RGUHS 2022)

Indications

- **Posterolateral tibial plateau fractures**
- Combined bicondylar tibial plateau fractures
- Avulsion fractures involving the posterior horn of lateral meniscus

Landmarks

- Head of fibula
- Lateral border of gastrocnemius
- Posterior aspect of fibula and tibia

Steps

1. Patient prone or lateral decubitus.
2. Skin incision posterior to fibula.
3. Identify and protect **common peroneal nerve** near fibular neck.
4. Retract peroneal muscles and lateral head of gastrocnemius.
5. Access **posterolateral tibial plateau** between popliteus and fibula.

Structures at Risk

- Common peroneal nerve
- Popliteal vessels if dissection is too deep

Advantages

- Direct visualization and reduction of **posterolateral fragments**
- Enables **buttress plating**

Q4. Describe surgical approach to distal femur fractures.

(MUHS 2021)

Indications

- **Supracondylar or intercondylar distal femur fractures**
- Tumor resection
- Periprosthetic fractures (excluding arthroplasty)

Approaches

A. Lateral Approach (Standard)

Steps:

1. Patient **supine with bump under knee**.
2. Lateral incision from vastus lateralis to lateral epicondyle.
3. Split or elevate vastus lateralis from lateral intermuscular septum.
4. Expose distal femur; reduce and fix fracture.

Structures at risk:

- Genicular vessels
- Perforators from profunda femoris

B. Medial Parapatellar (for Intra-articular)

- Used for **intercondylar extension**
- Medial arthrotomy may be combined with lateral incision

Q5. Lateral approach to fibula—indications and steps.

(DNB 2022)

Indications

- ORIF of **distal fibula fractures**
- Fixation of **Weber B and C** ankle fractures
- Harvesting fibular graft (midshaft)

Steps

1. Supine position, leg internally rotated.
2. Longitudinal incision **posterior to fibular crest**, over lateral malleolus.
3. Dissect subcutaneous tissue carefully.
4. Protect **superficial peroneal nerve** (crosses ~10 cm above lateral malleolus).

5. Incise periosteum and expose fibula.
6. **Reduce fracture** and apply lateral plate.

Structures at Risk
- Superficial peroneal nerve (anterior to incision)
- Short saphenous vein and sural nerve (posterior)

For Midshaft Fibular Graft
- Incision centered over fibular shaft
- Avoid **peroneal artery and muscles**
- Minimum 6 cm left proximally and distally for stability

Section 3: Spine Approaches

Q1. Describe posterior midline approach to the lumbar spine—steps and precautions.

(RGUHS 2023)

Indications
- Lumbar decompression (laminectomy, discectomy)
- Posterior spinal instrumentation/fixation
- Tumor or infection involving posterior elements
- Access for **spinal osteotomies** (e.g., for deformity correction)

Positioning
- Patient in **prone position** with abdomen free to reduce venous pressure.
- Padding for pressure points (chest, pelvis, knees).

Landmarks
- Spinous processes
- Posterior iliac crest (guides L4 level)
- Midline skin incision

Steps
1. *Skin incision*: Midline incision over desired levels (e.g., L3–L5).
2. *Subcutaneous dissection*: Blunt dissection to expose thoracolumbar fascia.
3. *Paraspinal muscle elevation*: Detach **erector spinae** muscles (longissimus, iliocostalis) from spinous process and lamina using monopolar cautery or periosteal elevator.
4. *Exposure*:
   - Lamina, spinous processes, transverse processes exposed.
   - Extend laterally to facet joints and transverse processes as needed.
5. *Procedure performed*: Decompression, fixation, osteotomy, biopsy, etc.
6. *Wound closure*: Layered closure ensuring muscle reapproximation and drain placement.

Precautions and Structures at Risk
- *Dural tear*: Use meticulous dissection near lamina
- *Nerve roots*: Retract carefully if performing foraminotomy
- *Muscle denervation*: Excessive lateral dissection injures dorsal rami
- Avoid excessive cautery in muscles (prevents necrosis)

Advantages
- Familiar approach
- Access to multiple segments
- Easily extensile cranially/caudally

Q2. Describe anterior cervical approach—structures encountered and complications.

(DNB 2021, MUHS 2020)

Indications

- Cervical disc prolapse (anterior cervical discectomy and fusion—ACDF)
- Vertebral body pathology (tumor, trauma)
- Infection (TB), decompression

Positioning

- Supine with **neck extended** (shoulder roll).
- **Head supported**, slight traction with head holder (if needed).

Landmarks

- Sternocleidomastoid (SCM)
- Thyroid cartilage (C4 level)
- Hyoid bone (C3 level)
- Cricoid cartilage (C6 level)

Steps

1. **Transverse skin incision** parallel to skin crease, over level of interest.
2. Blunt dissection through platysma.
3. Identify **interval between SCM (laterally)** and **strap muscles/trachea/esophagus (medially)**.
4. **Retract carotid sheath laterally, trachea/esophagus medially**.
5. Prevertebral fascia opened to expose **longus colli.**
6. Retract longus colli to visualize **anterior vertebral body and disc**.

Structures Encountered/at Risk

Structure	***Risk/Note***
Carotid sheath (lateral)	Must retract gently
Recurrent laryngeal nerve	*Right side*: More oblique, deeper; injury can cause hoarseness
Esophagus	Risk of injury → dysphagia, fistula
Trachea	Risk of airway injury or swelling
Vertebral artery	Injury if dissection is extended laterally
Thyroid vessels	May require ligation in low cervical levels

Complications

- Hoarseness (recurrent laryngeal nerve palsy)
- Dysphagia, esophageal perforation
- Hematoma → airway compression
- Vertebral artery injury
- Pseudoarthrosis/non-union
- Infection

Q3. Posterior approach to thoracic spine—indications and complications.

(RGUHS 2022, TNMGRMU 2021)

Indications

- **Thoracic decompression** (laminectomy for stenosis or tumor)
- Posterior instrumentation for:
    - Fractures
    - Infection (TB)
    - Deformity correction (kyphosis/scoliosis)
- **Tumor resection**

Positioning
- **Prone** on spinal frame
- Padding under iliac crest and chest

Landmarks
- Spinous processes
- Rib angles
- Scapular spine (T3 level)

Steps
1. Midline skin incision over desired levels.
2. Dissect subcutaneous tissue and open **thoracolumbar fascia**.
3. Elevate **paraspinal muscles** (erector spinae) bilaterally from spinous process and lamina.
4. Expose lamina, transverse processes, and facets.
5. Perform **laminectomy**, **pedicle screw fixation**, or **posterior osteotomies** as required.

Structures at Risk
- Spinal cord (especially narrow thoracic canal)
- *Dura mater*: Risk of tear during decompression
- Segmental arteries (risk of bleeding if exposed too laterally)
- Lung injury if dissection is aggressive near costovertebral junction

Complications
- Neurological deficit (cord injury)
- Dural tear and CSF leak
- Hematoma formation
- Wound infection
- Paraspinal muscle necrosis can lead to chronic pain

Summary Comparison Table

Approach	*Level*	*Key structures at risk*	*Main indications*
Posterior lumbar midline	L1–L5	Dura, nerve roots	Decompression, instrumentation
Anterior cervical	C3–C7	RLN, esophagus, carotid, vertebral a.	ACDF, tumor, TB
Posterior thoracic	T1–T12	Spinal cord, segmental vessels	Trauma, TB, deformity correction

Section 4: Open Reduction and Fixation Procedures

Q1. Describe the steps of open reduction and internal fixation (ORIF) of both bones forearm fracture.

(DNB 2021, MUHS 2020)

Indications
- Displaced fractures of both **radius and ulna**
- **Unstable fractures**, segmental or comminuted
- Failure of closed reduction
- Fractures with **neurovascular injury**

Preoperative Planning
- X-rays of **forearm with wrist and elbow**
- Decide approach (volar/dorsal)
- **AO classification** consideration
- Prepare both **2.7/3.5 mm plates**, appropriate screws

Surgical Approaches

- *Radius*: Volar Henry approach (mid to distal) or dorsal Thompson (proximal)
- *Ulna*: Direct subcutaneous approach (posterior)

Steps

1. **Patient supine**, arm on hand table, tourniquet inflated.
2. **Radius fixed first** (restores length and alignment).
   - Volar approach → retract FCR, pronator teres.
   - Expose fracture, **reduce and fix with plate** on volar aspect.
3. **Ulna fixed next** via posterior longitudinal incision.
   - Subcutaneous border is directly accessible.
   - Reduce and apply **plate on posterior surface**.
4. Check **rotation**, pronation/supination intraoperatively.
5. Wound irrigation and layered closure.
6. **Post-operative immobilization** for pain, followed by physiotherapy.

Complications

- Cross-union (radius-ulna synostosis)
- Non-union or malunion
- Implant failure
- Compartment syndrome
- Nerve injury (posterior interosseous nerve in radius approach)

Q2. Write in detail about surgical fixation of intertrochanteric fracture using DHS.

(TNMGRMU 2022, RGUHS 2020)

Indications

- **Stable intertrochanteric fracture (AO 31-A1, A2)**
- **Elderly patients** with good bone stock
- Excludes reverse obliquity fractures

Implant

- **Dynamic Hip Screw (DHS)** with 135° barrel plate
- 4-hole or longer side plate depending on comminution

Surgical Steps

1. *Position*: Supine on **fracture table**, foot secured in boot.
2. Apply **traction with internal rotation** to reduce fracture.
3. Confirm reduction with **C-arm**.
4. **Lateral incision** over greater trochanter.
5. Expose **lateral femoral cortex**; drill guide inserted into neck.
6. Guidewire passed into **center–center** of femoral head.
7. Ream for lag screw; insert lag screw to subchondral bone (~1 cm short of joint).
8. **Barrel plate slid over lag screw**, side plate fixed with cortical screws.
9. Confirm position (tip–apex distance <25 mm).
10. Irrigation, drain placement, and layered closure.

Postoperative Care

- Mobilization begins **within 24–48 hours**
- Early **weight-bearing as tolerated** (if fixation stable)
- DVT prophylaxis, calcium/vitamin D, osteoporosis management

Complications

- Cut-out of lag screw (Z-effect)
- Varus malreduction
- Infection
- Limb shortening
- Nonunion (rare)

Q3. Describe surgical technique for ORIF of displaced supracondylar fracture humerus in children.

(DNB 2022)

Indications

- **Gartland type II and III** fractures
- Displaced supracondylar fracture in child >5 years
- Vascular compromise or failed closed reduction

Preferred Fixation

- **Closed reduction + percutaneous K-wire fixation**
- **Open reduction** only if closed reduction fails or neurovascular structures need exploration

Surgical Approach (Open Reduction)

- **Posterior (triceps-splitting)** or **lateral** approach
- Posterior is common for open reduction

Steps (Posterior Approach)

1. **Prone or lateral position** under GA.
2. Posterior midline skin incision ~6–8 cm.
3. Split **triceps muscle** in midline.
4. Expose and reduce fracture fragments anatomically.
5. Fix with **crossed K-wires** (one from medial, one lateral) or **2 lateral divergent K-wires.**
6. Confirm under **C-arm.**
7. Cut and bend wires, apply sterile dressing.
8. **Above-elbow posterior slab** in 90° flexion applied.

Precautions

- Protect **ulnar nerve** when placing **medial pin.**
- Avoid hyperflexion if **vascularity compromised.**

Postoperative Protocol

- Check circulation and nerve function
- X-ray at 1 week
- K-wires removed at 3–4 weeks
- Begin ROM exercises after wire removal

Complications

- **Cubitus varus deformity** (malunion)
- Ulnar nerve injury
- Pin tract infection
- Stiffness
- Myositis ossificans (rare)

Q4. ORIF of olecranon fracture—approach, steps, fixation options.

(MUHS 2021)

Indications
- Displaced olecranon fracture (>2 mm gap)
- Involvement of **articular surface**
- Tension failure pattern

Surgical Approach
- **Posterior midline incision** over olecranon.
- Ulnar nerve not usually exposed unless extended proximally.

Fixation Options

Type	*Indication*
Tension band wiring (TBW)	Transverse fractures (Mayo I or II)
Plate fixation	Comminuted or oblique fractures
Intramedullary screw	Rarely used now

TBW Technique Steps
1. Supine or lateral position, elbow flexed.
2. Expose fracture, clean hematoma.
3. Reduce and hold with **K-wires across fracture site**.
4. Drill transverse hole distal to fracture.
5. Pass **18G SS wire** in figure-of-eight fashion and tighten.
6. Cut and bend K-wires.
7. Confirm under C-arm, close wound in layers.

Complications
- Wire prominence
- Infection
- Non-union
- Loss of reduction
- Hardware irritation

Q5. Describe lateral approach and steps of fixation of tibial plateau fractures.

(RGUHS 2021)

Indications
- Lateral split or depressed **tibial plateau fractures (Schatzker Type I–III)**
- Bicondylar fractures (with separate medial approach)

Surgical Approach

Anterolateral approach to proximal tibia.

Steps
1. Supine position with knee support.
2. Incision from **lateral condyle to midshaft of tibia**.
3. Dissect through skin and fascia.
4. Retract **iliotibial band and anterior compartment muscles**.
5. Elevate **lateral meniscus if needed**.
6. Reduce fracture with bone tamp or elevator.

7. Use **elevators, subchondral support (bone graft, void filler)**.
8. Apply **buttress or locking plate** on lateral surface.
9. Confirm alignment with **C-arm**.

Precautions
- Protect **common peroneal nerve** (posterior to fibular neck).
- Avoid intra-articular screw placement.

Section 5: Tendon Surgery and Nerve Exploration

Q1. Describe the technique of flexor tendon repair in zone II. What are the post-operative protocols?

(TNMGRMU 2021)

Zone II – "No Man's Land"
- From **distal palmar crease to insertion of FDS on middle phalanx**
- Challenging due to **FDS and FDP** sheaths, poor blood supply

Surgical Technique
Approach:
- **Bruner (zigzag)** or midlateral incision
- Careful dissection of **tendon sheath and pulleys**
- Preserve **A2 and A4 pulleys** if possible

Repair technique:
- **Core suture repair** (e.g., modified Kessler, 4-strand technique)
- **Epitendinous running suture** for reinforcement
- Use **non-absorbable 4-0 or 5-0** monofilament suture

Postoperative Protocols

Timeline	*Management*
0–4 weeks	Passive flexion–active extension (Kleinert protocol) with dorsal blocking splint
4–6 weeks	Gradual active ROM initiated
6–8 weeks	Strengthening exercises
12 weeks	Full unrestricted activity (if no complications)

Complications
- Adhesion formation
- Rupture of repair
- Joint stiffness
- Flexion contracture

Conclusion
Zone II repairs require **meticulous technique and a well-structured rehabilitation protocol** to restore finger function while minimizing adhesions and rupture.

Q2. Write a note on extensor tendon repair over dorsum of the hand.

(MUHS 2020)

Extensor Zones Involved
Most common: **Zone V–VII** (dorsum of hand/wrist)

Surgical Technique

1. **Longitudinal dorsal incision**
2. Identify retracted tendon ends
3. Debride frayed edges
4. *Perform repair*:
    - Modified Bunnell or interrupted figure-of-eight suture
    - Use non-absorbable suture (e.g., 4-0 Prolene)
5. If >50% lacerated → repair indicated
6. *If tendon loss*: **Graft or tendon transfer**

Post-Operative Protocol

Timeline	Protocol
0–4 weeks	Static splinting with wrist at 30° extension, MCP in 30–40° flexion
4–6 weeks	Controlled passive mobilization
6–8 weeks	Active ROM begins
>8 weeks	Strengthening, function restoration

Complications

- Tendon rupture
- Extensor lag
- Adhesions
- Boutonnière deformity (if central slip injury)

Conclusion

Extensor tendon repair is **less technically demanding** than flexor repairs but must be followed by **controlled splinting and rehabilitation** to ensure function.

Q3. Describe surgical technique of posterior tibial tendon transfer for foot drop.

(DNB 2020)

Indications

- **Irreparable peroneal nerve palsy**
- Chronic foot drop >6–12 months
- Intact and strong **posterior tibial tendon**

Principle

Redirect **posterior tibial tendon (PTT)** to **dorsum of foot** to compensate for dorsiflexor weakness

Surgical Steps (Brunelli Technique or its variants)

1. **Medial approach** behind tibia—harvest **PTT**.
2. Create tunnel through **interosseous membrane** into anterior compartment.
3. Re-route tendon to **dorsum of foot**.
4. *Fix to*:
    - **Tibialis anterior**
    - Or into **cuneiforms or intermediate cuneiform bone**
5. Use **bone tunnel or suture anchor** fixation.

Postoperative Care

- Below-knee cast in dorsiflexion for 4–6 weeks
- Then initiate passive → active rehabilitation
- Full return to walking in 10–12 weeks

Complications

- Under/Overcorrection
- Infection
- Donor site weakness
- Incomplete dorsiflexion

Q4. Indications and technique of radial nerve exploration in humerus shaft fracture.

(RGUHS 2021)

Indications

Timing	*Indications*
Primary exploration	Open fracture, nerve caught between fragments, vascular injury
Early exploration (3–4 weeks)	No recovery, EMG shows complete denervation
Delayed (>3 months)	No functional recovery despite conservative management

Approach

- **Posterior humeral approach** (triceps-splitting or triceps-reflecting)
- Identify **radial nerve in spiral groove**

Steps

1. Posterior incision along lateral arm
2. Split or reflect triceps
3. Identify **nerve proximally**, trace distally
4. *Look for*:
   - Neuroma
   - Scar entrapment
   - Nerve discontinuity
5. If nerve intact but in scar → neurolysis
   If severed → **nerve repair or grafting**

Post-operative Management

- Splinting in wrist/finger extension
- Monitor nerve recovery clinically and with EMG

Section 6: Bone Biopsy and Tumor Exposure

Q1. Describe principles and technique of open bone biopsy in suspected malignant lesion.

(DNB 2022, RGUHS 2021)

Indications

- **Radiologically aggressive bone lesion** with suspicion of malignancy
- Lesions not accessible by core needle or inconclusive report

Principles (Crucial for Exam)

1. **Biopsy tract in line with future incision**
2. Avoid **crossing multiple compartments**
3. Prevent **hematoma spillage**
4. Sample **viable part** of tumor (not necrotic)

5. Use **separate instruments** (no contamination)
6. Close biopsy tract in layers and mark it

Technique
1. Pre-operative imaging (MRI, CT) to plan **safe corridor**
2. Small incision, just enough to reach lesion
3. Cut **cortex with burr or osteotome**
4. Curette or scoop out sample
5. Place **tissue in formalin/saline**
6. Irrigation, **no drain**, layered closure
7. Send sample for **HPE, IHC, culture (if required)**

Complications
- Tumor seeding
- Inadequate diagnosis
- Infection
- Fracture

Q2. What are the precautions during biopsy of a bone tumor? Describe the safe biopsy principles.

(MUHS 2020)

Safe Biopsy Principles (Enneking Guidelines)

Principle	*Explanation*
Minimal incision	Just enough to access target tissue
Longitudinal incision	In line with limb axis; facilitates future excision
Same compartment	Avoid traversing multiple tissue planes
No contamination of healthy tissue	Isolate instruments; no excess irrigation
Avoid neurovascular bundles	Do not expose or dissect unnecessary structures
Biopsy tract excisable	Plan so entire tract can be removed during tumor surgery
Single pass	Avoid multiple re-entries, which increase seeding
Experienced team involvement	Preferably at a tertiary tumor center

Q3. Discuss incisional versus excisional biopsy. How do you plan approach in musculoskeletal tumors?

(TNMGRMU 2021)

Definitions

Type	*Definition*
Incisional biopsy	Small sample taken from tumor for diagnosis
Excisional biopsy	Entire tumor mass is removed with margin

Indications
- *Incisional*:
  - Most **bone sarcomas and deep tumors**
  - Tumors >3 cm or in critical location
- *Excisional*:
  - Small, superficial, **clearly benign** soft tissue lesions
  - Lipomas, ganglion cysts

Planning Approach

1. Use MRI to **define compartments** and tumor extent
2. Select site that **does not compromise future surgery**
3. Coordinate with oncologic surgeon for limb salvage
4. Pre-operative biopsy should be routed through the future **definitive surgery incision**

Section 7: Pediatric Orthopedic Procedures

Q1. Describe surgical steps of open reduction in congenital dislocation of hip (CDH).

(DNB 2022, MUHS 2019.)

Indications

- Failed closed reduction
- Late presentation (>18 months)
- Obstructing structures preventing closed reduction
- Residual subluxation after conservative treatment

Preferred Approach

Anterior Smith–Petersen approach.

Surgical Steps (Smith–Petersen)

1. *Position*: Supine with sandbag under pelvis
2. *Incision*: Bikini or vertical incision centered over ASIS
3. Dissect through **subcutaneous tissue and fascia**
4. Identify and retract **sartorius laterally**, **rectus femoris medially**
5. Protect **lateral femoral cutaneous nerve**
6. Incise **joint capsule (T-shaped capsulotomy)**
7. Excise **pulvinar tissue**, **ligamentum teres**, and **inverted labrum (limbus)**
8. **Release iliopsoas tendon** (if obstructing)
9. Reduce femoral head into acetabulum
10. **Capsulorrhaphy** if needed
11. Close in layers

Postoperative Care

- **Hip spica** cast in **human position (flexion, abduction, external rotation)**
- *Duration*: 6–12 weeks, then abduction brace

Complications

- Avascular necrosis of femoral head
- Redislocation
- Growth disturbances
- Joint stiffness

Q2. Describe medial approach to hip in infants and its advantages.

(RGUHS 2021)

Indications

- Children <1 year with **failed closed reduction**
- Obstructing soft tissues causing irreducibility

Surgical Steps (Ludloff's Medial Approach)

1. Child in **supine position**, frog-leg position
2. Curvilinear **medial incision** along adductor longus
3. Divide adductor longus and brevis
4. Retract **psoas tendon laterally**, **gracilis medially**
5. Expose and open **hip capsule anterior to obturator nerve**
6. Excise **ligamentum teres**, **pulvinar**, and **limbus**
7. Reduce femoral head into acetabulum

Advantages

- **Minimal soft tissue dissection**
- Low incidence of **AVN**
- Avoids anterior structures (femoral neurovascular bundle)
- Suitable for **younger infants (<12 months)**

Disadvantages

- Limited exposure
- Not suitable for older children or when bony correction is needed

Q3. Open reduction in neglected clubfoot (CTEV)—surgical release and complications.

(TNMGRMU 2020)

Indications

- **Rigid CTEV deformity** unresponsive to Ponseti method
- Age >2 years
- Neglected/unmanaged cases

Goals of Surgery

- *Correct all four deformities*:
  i. Cavus
  ii. Adduction
  iii. Varus
  iv. Equinus

Common Procedures

- **Posteromedial soft tissue release (PMSTR)**
- Z-lengthening of **Achilles tendon**
- Release of **plantar fascia, tibialis posterior, FDL, FHL**
- **Capsulotomy** of subtalar, talonavicular joints
- Correction of **bony deformities** (e.g., cuboid decancellation) if needed

Surgical Steps (PMSTR)

1. *Incision*: Cincinnati or Turco's curved posteromedial incision
2. *Sequential release of*:
   - *Posterior structures*: Achilles tendon, posterior capsule
   - *Medial structures*: Talonavicular joint capsule, tibialis posterior, FDL
   - *Plantar fascia*: For cavus
3. Realign talus and navicular
4. K-wire fixation across talonavicular joint (if needed)
5. **Layered closure**, below-knee cast in corrected position

Postoperative Protocol

- Cast for 6–8 weeks

- Gradual rehabilitation with bracing or **CTEV shoes**
- Regular follow-up for growth/deformity recurrence

Complications
- Overcorrection or undercorrection
- Stiffness
- Neurovascular injury
- Recurrence
- AVN of talus (rare)

Summary Table: Common Pediatric Orthopedic Procedures

Procedure	***Approach***	***Ideal age***	***Key risks***
Open reduction in CDH	Smith–Petersen (anterior)	>12–18 months	AVN, redislocation
Medial hip approach	Ludloff (medial)	<12 months	Limited exposure
CTEV open release	Posteromedial (Turco)	>2 years/neglected	Stiffness, recurrence

16.1 Arthroplasty, Arthroscopy, Arthrodesis, and Minimally Invasive Surgery (MIS)

Vijay Kumar, Heemanshu Bhat, Pardeep Singh

Arthroplasty

Q1. Define arthroplasty. Enumerate types. Indications and contraindications.

Source: RGUHS 2021, DNB 2022

Type: Long essay

Definition

Arthroplasty is a **surgical procedure to restore joint function** by resurfacing the joint or replacing it with an artificial prosthesis.

Types of Arthroplasty

Type	*Description*	*Examples*
Hemiarthroplasty	Replacement of one joint surface only	Bipolar for NOF fracture
Total arthroplasty	Replacement of both articular surfaces	THA, TKA
Unicompartmental	Replacement of one compartment	UKA—medial or lateral knee
Resurfacing arthroplasty	Minimal bone removal; cap-like implants	Hip resurfacing (BHR)
Reverse arthroplasty	Glenoid becomes convex, humerus concave	Reverse shoulder arthroplasty
Interpositional	Soft tissue/membrane between joint ends	Elbow arthroplasty (historical)

Indications

- Advanced osteoarthritis
- Rheumatoid arthritis
- Ankylosing spondylitis
- Avascular necrosis (late stage)
- Fractures (NOF, proximal humerus in elderly)
- Failed internal fixation or arthrodesis
- Severe post-traumatic arthritis

Contraindications

Absolute	*Relative*
Active infection (e.g., PJI)	Poor bone stock
Neuropathic arthropathy	Severe vascular insufficiency
Poor general health	Uncontrolled diabetes, obesity
Non-compliant patient	Dementia or psychosis

Q2. Enumerate bearing surface combinations in THA and describe their pros and cons.

Source: MUHS 2022, DNB 2021

Total hip replacement (THR), the **bearing surfaces** are the materials that articulate against each other to mimic the natural hip joint motion—typically the **femoral head** and the **acetabular liner**. The choice of bearing surface impacts wear, longevity, and complication rates.

Main Types of Bearing Surfaces in THR

- **Femoral head**
- **Acetabular liner**
- Metal
- Polyethylene
- Ceramic
- Polyethylene

1. Metal-on-Polyethylene (MoP)

Description: Metal femoral head articulates with a polyethylene (plastic) liner.

Pros:

- Most commonly used; well-studied.
- Cost-effective.
- Good long-term results in older, less active patients.

Cons:

- Polyethylene wear particles → osteolysis and aseptic loosening.
- Less ideal for young, active patients.

2. Ceramic-on-Polyethylene (CoP)

Description: Ceramic femoral head with a polyethylene liner.

Pros:

- Less wear than metal-on-polyethylene.
- Reduced risk of osteolysis.
- Good biocompatibility.

Cons:

- More expensive than MoP.
- Ceramic heads can still fracture (rare with newer ceramics).

3. Ceramic-on-Ceramic (CoC)

Description: Both the head and liner are ceramic.

Pros:

- Lowest wear rate.
- Excellent biocompatibility.
- Suitable for young, active patients.

Cons:

- Risk of ceramic fracture (though rare with modern materials).
- Can produce squeaking noise.
- Expensive

4. Metal-on-Metal (MoM)

Description: Both components are metal (usually cobalt-chrome alloy).

Pros:

- Very low wear (initially appealing for young, active patients).
- Large head sizes reduce dislocation risk.

Cons:

- Metal ion release → systemic toxicity (cobalt/chromium).
- Risk of adverse local tissue reaction (ALTR).
- Rarely used today due to high complication rates.

5. Ceramic-on-Metal (CoM)
Description: Ceramic femoral head with metal liner (rare, experimental).

Pros: Theoretical benefits of low wear + durability.

Cons:
- Insufficient long-term data.
- Unpredictable ion release.
- Not widely used.

Summary Table

Bearing type	*Wear rate*	*Fracture risk*	*Cost*	*Noise risk*	*Ion release*	*Suitability*
MoP	Moderate	No	Low	No	No	Older/Less active
CoP	Low	Very low	Medium	No	No	Broad usage
CoC	Very low	Low (rare)	High	Yes	No	Young/Active
MoM	Low	No	Medium	No	Yes (high)	Mostly discontinued
CoM	Unknown	Unknown	High	Possible	Possible	Experimental

Q3. What are the types and objectives of THR?

Objectives
- Pain relief
- Restoration of mobility and function
- Correction of deformity
- Improvement in quality of life

Common Bearing Surface Combinations in THA

Acetabular cup	*Femoral head*	*Type*
UHMWPE	Metal	Metal-on-polyethylene
UHMWPE	Ceramic	Ceramic-on-polyethylene
Ceramic	Ceramic	Ceramic-on-ceramic
Metal	Metal	Metal-on-metal (historical)

Comparison of Bearing Surfaces

Type	*Advantages*	*Disadvantages*
Metal-on-polyethylene	Inexpensive, proven track record	Poly wear debris → osteolysis
Ceramic-on-polyethylene	Lower wear than MoP	Expensive, risk of fracture
Ceramic-on-ceramic	Least wear, good for younger patients	Expensive, squeaking, fracture risk
Metal-on-metal (MoM)	Historical use, low wear rate	Metal ion release, not recommended anymore

Q4. Describe biomechanics and components of total hip arthroplasty (THA).

Source: RGUHS 2022

Type: Short essay

Biomechanical Goals of THA
- Restore **hip center**
- Maintain **limb length**
- Preserve **offset** (distance from center of femoral head to axis of femur)
- Ensure **joint stability** and range of motion
- Minimize **wear and loosening**

THA Components

Component	*Material options*
Acetabular cup	Titanium shell + polyethylene/ceramic insert
Femoral stem	Titanium or stainless steel
Femoral head	Ceramic, cobalt-chrome, or metal

Fixation Types

- *Cemented*: Older, osteoporotic patients
- *Cementless (press-fit)*: Younger patients with good bone
- *Hybrid*: Cemented stem + uncemented cup

Q5. Discuss indications, technique, and advantages of uncemented total hip arthroplasty.

[Kasturba Medical College (KMC) Manipal Karnataka 2017]

Source: DNB 2021

Type: Short essay

Indications

- Young, active patients (<60 years)
- Good bone stock (Dorr type A or B femur)
- Revision THA (if bone quality permits)

Technique Overview

1. *Acetabulum*: Ream to bleeding bone → press-fit shell → liner inserted
2. *Femur*: Ream and broach canal → press-fit stem → head inserted
3. Trial reductions before final components
4. Bone ingrowth ensures **biological fixation** (typically porous-coated implants)

Advantages

- No cement complications (e.g., cement disease, thermal necrosis)
- Long-term biologic fixation
- Better survival in young patients
- Easier revision

Disadvantages

- Requires good bone quality
- Higher risk of **early micromotion** → loosening
- Costlier

Q6. Complications of THA—enumerate and discuss management.

Source: TNMGRMU 2022, RGUHS 2020

Type: Short essay

Early Complications

Complication	*Management*
Infection (superficial/deep)	Debridement ± revision ± antibiotics
Dislocation	Closed reduction → brace → revision if recurrent
DVT/PE	LMWH, early mobilization, stockings
Nerve injury (sciatic)	Usually resolves; supportive therapy

Late Complications

Complication	*Management*
Aseptic loosening	Revision arthroplasty
Periprosthetic fracture	ORIF or revision stem based on fracture
Heterotopic ossification	Indomethacin prophylaxis, radiation (rare)
Wear and osteolysis	Polyethylene exchange, revision
Leg length discrepancy	Shoe raise, revision if severe

Summary Table: THA Quick Reference

Topic	*Key points*
Types of arthroplasty	Total, hemi, resurfacing, unicompartemental, reverse
Bearing surfaces	MoP, CoC, CoP—chosen based on age/activity
Cemented versus uncemented	Uncemented for young/good bone, cemented for elderly
Key biomechanics	Center of rotation, offset, stability, limb length
Common complications	Dislocation, infection, aseptic loosening, DVT

Q7. Hip resurfacing arthroplasty (HRA)—short note.

Definition

Bone-conserving arthroplasty where femoral head is capped with a metal prosthesis and acetabular cup is placed, preserving native bone.

Indications

Young, active patients with good bone quality; early AVN or osteoarthritis.

Advantages

- Preserves femoral bone
- Large head → less dislocation risk
- Easier revision to THR

Disadvantages

- Risk of femoral neck fracture
- Metal-on-metal wear complications (e.g., metallosis)

Contraindications

Osteoporosis, femoral head cysts, renal impairment.

Q8. Evolution of total hip replacement (THR)—short note.

- *Early 20th century:* Ivory and mold arthroplasty (Glück, Smith-Petersen)
- *1950s:* Charnley's low-friction arthroplasty using polyethylene, metal, and bone cement
- *1970s-1980s:* Cementless designs, porous coating, modularity
- *1990s-2000s:* Introduction of ceramic heads, highly cross-linked polyethylene
- *Present:* Robotic-assisted THR, dual mobility cups, improved tribology

Q9. Tribology—short note.

Definition

Science of friction, wear, and lubrication between moving surfaces—critical in arthroplasty.

Bearing Surfaces

- *Metal-on-polyethylene (MoP):* Proven, but wear debris risk

- *Ceramic-on-ceramic (CoC):* Least wear, risk of squeaking/fracture
- *Metal-on-metal (MoM):* Low wear, high risk of metal ion release

Lubrication Types
Boundary and fluid film; fluid film preferred.

Recent Advances
Highly cross-linked polyethylene, delta ceramics, oxinium.

Q10. Describe the biomechanics and replacement types of total knee arthroplasty (TKA).

[Rajiv Gandhi University of Health Sciences (RGUHS) Bangalore Karnataka 2015]

Biomechanics
- The knee acts as a **modified hinge joint** with 6 degrees of motion (flexion-extension, internal-external rotation, translation).
- *Load transmission:* Mostly across the **medial compartment**
- Ligaments (ACL, PCL, collaterals) provide **stability**

TKA Types
1. *Cruciate-retaining (CR)*: PCL preserved
2. *Posterior-stabilized (PS)*: PCL sacrificed; cam-post mechanism used
3. **Mobile-bearing versus fixed-bearing designs**
4. *Constraint level*: Unconstrained → semi-constrained → constrained (hinged)

Indications
Osteoarthritis, RA, post-traumatic arthritis, AVN of femoral condyle

Implant Components
- Femoral (usually cobalt-chromium)
- Tibial baseplate + polyethylene insert
- Patellar button (optional)

Approach
Medial parapatellar arthrotomy is most common

Q11. Enumerate complications of total knee arthroplasty (TKA) and their management.

Source: DNB 2022, TNMGRMU 2021

Type: Short essay

Early Complications

Complication	*Management*
Infection	*Superficial*: Antibiotics ± debridement
Deep: Staged revision	
DVT/PE	LMWH, mobilization, compression devices
Hemarthrosis	Aspiration if needed; rest, ice, elevation
Nerve injury (peroneal)	Observation/supportive; surgery if persistent

Late Complications

Complication	*Management*
Loosening (aseptic)	Revision TKA
Instability	Polyethylene exchange or constrained prosthesis
Patellar maltracking	Realignment or revision of patellar component

Continued

Continued

Complication	*Management*
Stiffness (arthrofibrosis)	Manipulation under anesthesia or arthrolysis
Periprosthetic fracture	ORIF or revision prosthesis

Q12. Explain total ankle arthroplasty (TAA) and its key principles.

Indications
- End-stage ankle arthritis (OA, RA, post-traumatic)
- Pain and stiffness unresponsive to conservative therapy

Contraindications
Severe deformity (>15° varus/valgus), infection, neuropathy (Charcot), poor bone stock

Biomechanics
- Ankle bears 4–5 times body weight during walking
- Requires preservation of subtalar and midfoot mobility

Implant Design
- 2-component (fixed-bearing)
- 3-component (mobile-bearing with polyethylene insert)

Fixation
Cemented or cementless (press-fit or porous coated)

Challenges
- Higher failure rate than knee/hip
- Difficult revision
- Long learning curve

Q13. Describe the biomechanics and surgical approach to total shoulder arthroplasty (TSA).

Biomechanics
- **Ball-and-socket joint** with wide ROM
- Stability from **rotator cuff and glenoid labrum**

Types
1. *Anatomic TSA*: Requires intact rotator cuff
2. *Reverse shoulder arthroplasty (RSA)*: Used when cuff is torn/deficient
    - Glenoid will become ball and humeral head will become the socket in this case, which is the reverse of normal anatomy
    - Relies on deltoid for function

Implant Components
- Humeral stem (usually cementless)
- Glenoid component (PE or metal-backed)

Approach
- Deltopectoral approach is standard
- Subscapularis often detached and later repaired

Indications
- Advanced glenohumeral arthritis
- Cuff tear arthropathy
- Complex proximal humerus fractures (elderly)

Q14. Discuss total elbow arthroplasty (TEA) and its considerations.

Indications

- Advanced RA
- Complex distal humerus fractures in elderly
- Ankylosis with severe functional limitation
- Tumor resection

Biomechanics

Elbow is a **hinge joint** with valgus/varus stability from collateral ligaments

Types of Implants

1. *Linked (semiconstrained):* Most common; mechanical link between components
2. *Unlinked:* Requires good soft-tissue stability

Fixation

- Often **cemented** due to poor bone stock
- *Components*: Humeral and ulnar stem, polyethylene hinge

Limitations

- Weight-lifting restrictions post-operative
- Risk of loosening and infection

Approach

Posterior approach with triceps-sparing or triceps-reflecting technique

Q15. Compare arthroplasty of knee, ankle, shoulder, and elbow.

(Kashmir University 2018)

Joint	*Common indications*	*Design types*	*Key challenges*
Knee	OA, RA, post-trauma	CR, PS, hinged	Flexion contracture, instability
Ankle	Post-traumatic arthritis	2/3 component designs	High failure rate, limited revision
Shoulder	OA, cuff tear arthropathy	Anatomic/Reverse	Rotator cuff dependence
Elbow	RA, elderly fractures	Linked/Unlinked TEA	Limited load tolerance, loosening

FREQUENTLY ASKED VIVA QUESTIONS

Q: What is the gold standard for knee arthritis in elderly?
A: Total Knee Arthroplasty
Q: Indication for reverse shoulder arthroplasty?
A: Cuff tear arthropathy or irreparable rotator cuff with arthritis
Q: Why is elbow arthroplasty avoided in young patients?
A: High complication and loosening rate; better preserved with ORIF or osteotomy
Q: What is the most common complication of ankle arthroplasty?
A: Aseptic loosening and implant failure

Arthroscopy—Principles, Indications, and Procedures

Q16. Define arthroscopy. List indications and contraindications.

Source: RGUHS 2021, DNB 2020

Type: Short essay

Definition

Arthroscopy is a **minimally invasive surgical technique** used to visualize, diagnose, and treat joint pathologies using a small **camera (arthroscope)** inserted through portals.

Common Joints for Arthroscopy

- **Knee** (most common)
- Shoulder
- Ankle
- Wrist
- Hip
- Elbow

Indications

Diagnostic	*Therapeutic*
Unexplained joint pain/swelling	Meniscal tear repair/removal
Chronic synovitis	ACL/PCL reconstruction
Suspected loose bodies	Synovectomy
Suspected cartilage lesion	Chondroplasty, microfracture
Recurrent dislocation (e.g., shoulder)	Rotator cuff repair, labral repair

Contraindications

Absolute	*Relative*
Active joint infection	Severe joint stiffness or ankylosis
Advanced osteoarthritis	Poor patient compliance
Coagulopathy (uncontrolled)	Excessive soft tissue swelling

Conclusion

Arthroscopy is a **diagnostic and therapeutic tool** offering **faster recovery, less morbidity**, and **excellent joint visualization**.

Q17. Describe instruments and basic setup used in knee arthroscopy.

Source: DNB 2021, MUHS 2020

Type: Short essay

Basic Instruments in Arthroscopy

Instrument	*Function*
Arthroscope (4 mm 30°)	Visualization
Light source and camera	Illumination and image projection
Cannula and trocar	Port access and fluid inflow
Shaver	Debridement of soft tissues or meniscus
Probe	Palpation, meniscus testing
Punch/Biter	Meniscectomy
Electrocautery/RF wand	Synovial ablation, hemostasis
Fluid pump system	Maintains intra-articular distension

Arthroscopy Setup

1. **Tourniquet on thigh** (usually inflated after exsanguination)
2. Leg holder or side post to stabilize the limb

3. Saline used as irrigation fluid
4. Monitors display real-time intra-articular visuals

Q18. Enumerate portals used in knee arthroscopy and structures seen through them.

Source: TNMGRMU 2021

Type: Short note

Standard Portals in Knee Arthroscopy

Portal	*Location*	*Structures visualized*
Anterolateral	Lateral to patellar tendon	Medial meniscus, intercondylar notch
Anteromedial	Medial to patellar tendon	Lateral meniscus, patellofemoral joint
Superolateral	Above patella (for fluid outflow/inflow)	Suprapatellar pouch
Posteromedial	Medial to medial head of gastrocnemius	Posterior horn of medial meniscus
Posterolateral	Lateral to lateral head of gastrocnemius	Posterior horn of lateral meniscus

Accessory Portals
Used for meniscal repair, PCL reconstruction, loose body retrieval, etc.

Conclusion
Correct **portal placement** is essential for **complete visualization, triangulation, and safe instrumentation** in arthroscopy.

Q19. Indications and steps of arthroscopic meniscectomy.

Source: RGUHS 2022

Type: Short essay

Indications
- Irreparable meniscal tear (complex, degenerative)
- Locked knee due to bucket handle tear
- Flap tear causing mechanical symptoms
- Meniscal cyst with torn segment

Steps of Meniscectomy
1. **Diagnostic arthroscopy** via anterolateral portal
2. Use probe to assess meniscal integrity
3. Use punch and shaver via anteromedial portal
4. Remove loose or torn fragment (**partial meniscectomy preferred**)
5. Smoothen edges (debride ragged meniscus)
6. Irrigate and close portals

Precautions
- Preserve as much meniscus as possible
- Avoid iatrogenic cartilage damage
- Early mobilization post-operative

Q20. Arthroscopic procedures in shoulder—indications and commonly performed surgeries.

Source: DNB 2022, MUHS 2021

Type: Short essay

Indications

Diagnostic	*Therapeutic*
Chronic unexplained shoulder pain	Rotator cuff tear repair
Recurrent dislocations	Bankart repair
Labral pathology (SLAP lesions)	Labral repair
Impingement	Subacromial decompression
Loose bodies	Debridement
Stiffness/Adhesive capsulitis	Capsular release

Common Arthroscopic Shoulder Procedures

- Subacromial decompression
- Rotator cuff tear repair (supraspinatus most common)
- Bankart repair (for anterior instability)
- SLAP lesion repair
- Biceps tenotomy or tenodesis
- Capsule release (frozen shoulder)
- Synovectomy, debridement

Portals

- *Posterior portal*: Standard viewing portal
- *Anterior and lateral portals*: For instrumentation
- *Anterosuperior*: For labral work or rotator cuff access

Summary Table: Arthroscopy Essentials

Topic	*Key points*
Indications	Meniscus tears, ACL injury, impingement, dislocations
Common joints	Knee > Shoulder > Ankle, wrist, elbow
Portals (knee)	Anteromedial, anterolateral, posteromedial, posterolateral
Common procedures	Meniscectomy, ACL reconstruction, rotator cuff repair
Advantages	Minimally invasive, fast recovery, diagnostic and therapeutic combined

Q21. Arthroscopic procedures in hip—indications and commonly performed surgeries.

Indications for Hip Arthroscopy

- Femoroacetabular impingement (FAI)
- Labral tears
- Loose bodies
- Chondral lesions (cartilage damage)
- Snapping hip syndrome
- Ligamentum teres injuries
- Hip instability
- Septic arthritis (diagnostic/therapeutic washout)
- Early osteoarthritis (limited role)

Common Hip Arthroscopic Surgeries

1. *Labral repair or debridement*: Refixation or trimming of torn labrum to restore joint seal and function.
2. *FAI correction (osteoplasty)*: Cam or pincer lesion resection to improve joint clearance.
3. *Chondroplasty/Microfracture*: Treatment of cartilage defects to promote fibrocartilage healing.
4. *Loose body removal*: Extraction of intra-articular fragments causing mechanical symptoms.

5. *Synovectomy*: Resection of inflamed synovium (e.g., in PVNS or inflammatory arthritis).
6. *Iliopsoas release*: For internal snapping hip syndrome.
7. *Ligamentum teres debridement or reconstruction*: For tears contributing to pain or instability.

The main portals used in hip arthroscopy, along with their locations and uses:

1. *Anterolateral portal*:
   - *Location*: Just anterior to the greater trochanter.
   - *Use*: Standard viewing portal.
   - Most commonly used initial portal.
2. *Anterior portal*:
   - *Location*: 1–2 cm distal and 2 cm lateral to the ASIS.
   - *Use*: Instrumentation, labral work, FAI treatment.
   - *Risk*: Close to lateral femoral cutaneous nerve—careful placement needed.
3. *Posterolateral portal*:
   - *Location*: Posterior to the greater trochanter.
   - *Use*: Optional viewing portal, access to posterior joint or lesions.
4. *Mid-anterior portal (MAP)*:
   - *Location*: Between anterior and anterolateral portals.
   - *Use*: Instrument access for labral repair, FAI correction.
   - Becoming more common.
5. *Distal anterolateral accessory (DALA) portal*:
   - *Location*: Distal and anterior to anterolateral portal.
   - *Use*: Better angle for femoral osteoplasty (cam resection).

Optional/Less Common Portals

- *Proximal mid-anterior portal*: For improved access in complex cases.
- *Peritrochanteric portals*: For work around the greater trochanter (e.g., bursectomy, tendon repairs).

Arthrodesis—Indications, Techniques, and Site-specific Fusion

Q22. Define arthrodesis. Enumerate indications and contraindications.

(Goa Medical College Bambolim Goa 2011)

Source: RGUHS 2021, DNB 2020

Type: Short essay

Definition

Arthrodesis is a **surgical fusion of a joint** to eliminate movement and provide **pain relief, stability, and alignment**, often used when joint preservation or arthroplasty is not an option.

Indications

Joint pathology	*Reason for arthrodesis*
Advanced joint arthritis	When arthroplasty not feasible (e.g., ankle, wrist)
Septic arthritis (healed infection)	Pain relief and prevent recurrence
Charcot joint (neuropathic)	Provide stability (especially foot/ankle)
Post-traumatic joint instability	Unreconstructable joints
Failed joint replacement	As salvage after THA/TKA failure
Paralytic deformities	Polio, cerebral palsy—e.g., hip or knee instability

Contraindications

Absolute	*Relative*
Active infection	Contralateral joint pathology
Poor vascularity	High functional demand for motion
Non-compliance	Poor bone stock or severe osteoporosis

Q23. Enumerate types of arthrodesis techniques with examples.

Source: MUHS 2022, DNB 2021

Type: Short essay

Types of Arthrodesis Techniques

Category	*Technique*	*Example*
Open (surgical)	Open joint exposure, cartilage removal	Knee, ankle, wrist arthrodesis
Closed	Percutaneous pinning without full exposure	C1–C2 fusion using wires or screws
External fixation	Ilizarov ring fixator, uniplanar frames	Complex foot/ankle arthrodesis
Internal fixation	Screws, plates, intramedullary nails	Subtalar fusion, knee fusion
Bone graft-assisted	Autograft/allograft for nonunion or infection	Post-infective arthrodesis

Grafting is often needed to promote fusion in infection or poor biology.

Q24. Describe technique and functional outcome of ankle arthrodesis.

Source: DNB 2022, RGUHS 2021

Type: Short essay

Indications
- End-stage arthritis (post-traumatic, inflammatory)
- Failed ankle replacement
- Neuropathic joints (Charcot)
- Severe deformities or instability

Surgical Technique (Open Anterior Approach)
1. Expose joint via anterior incision
2. Remove articular cartilage from **tibia and talus**
3. Prepare raw bleeding surfaces
4. Position ankle in **neutral dorsiflexion**, 5° valgus
5. Internal fixation with **two cannulated screws** or anterior plate
6. Bone grafting if needed
7. Cast immobilization for 6–12 weeks

Alternative Techniques
- Transfibular approach
- Ilizarov or external fixator in infection
- Arthroscopic fusion in selected cases

Outcomes
- Pain relief and stability
- Loss of ankle motion; patients compensate via **subtalar and midfoot joints**
- Difficulty with uneven terrain or running

Q25. Write short note on triple arthrodesis—indication, technique, and outcome.

Source: TNMGRMU 2022

Type: Short note

Definition

Triple arthrodesis involves fusion of the **subtalar, talonavicular, and calcaneocuboid joints.**

Indications

- Rigid hindfoot deformity (e.g., pes planus, cavus)
- Post-polio, CP, spina bifida
- Tibialis posterior tendon dysfunction
- Arthritic or painful flatfoot
- Charcot foot

Surgical Technique

- Incision over **lateral and medial hindfoot**
- Removal of cartilage from three joints
- Bone grafting as needed
- Fixation with screws or staples
- Immobilization in cast

Functional Outcome

- Stable hindfoot
- Good relief from deformity/pain
- Loss of inversion–eversion
- May alter gait in high-demand athletes

Q26. Compare arthroplasty versus arthrodesis—indications and outcomes.

(AIIMS Delhi 2018)

Source: RGUHS 2020, DNB 2021

Type: Short essay

Comparison Table

Aspect	*Arthrodesis*	*Arthroplasty*
Definition	Surgical joint fusion	Joint replacement with prosthesis
Motion	Lost completely	Preserved/Restored
Stability	Excellent	Depends on implant and soft tissue
Indications	Infection, instability, failed arthroplasty	Primary arthritis, AVN, functional demand
Sites commonly used	Ankle, wrist, spine, small joints	Hip, knee, shoulder
Complications	Adjacent joint overload, stiffness	Loosening, infection, dislocation
Cost	Generally lower	High (implant, revision potential)
Outcome	Pain relief, stable joint	Better function and range if successful

Q27. What are the general principles of arthrodesis?

1. Adequate **exposure and debridement**
2. Correct **alignment and positioning**
3. Secure **internal or external fixation**
4. Use of **bone grafts** (autograft, allograft, or bone substitutes)

5. Ensure **compression across the joint surfaces**
6. **Immobilization** until bony fusion

Q28. Describe common types of lower limb arthrodesis.

Knee Arthrodesis

- *Indications*: Failed TKA, post-infective arthritis, tumor resections
- *Position*: 5–10° flexion, 5–7° valgus
- *Fixation*: Intramedullary nail, plate + screws, external fixator
- Alternative to amputation in **non-salvageable knees**

Ankle Arthrodesis

- *Indications*: Post-traumatic arthritis, neuropathic joints, TB
- *Position*: Neutral dorsiflexion, 5° valgus, 10° external rotation
- *Fixation*: Screws, plates, external fixators
- *Goal*: Pain-free plantigrade foot

Subtalar Arthrodesis

- *Indications*: Arthritis following calcaneal fracture, hindfoot instability
- Often combined with triple arthrodesis
- *Fixation*: Cannulated screws

Q29. Describe hip arthrodesis—indications, technique, and position.

Indications

- Young patients with unilateral end-stage arthritis
- TB hip in children and adolescents
- Failed hip arthroplasty (in limited settings)

Preferred Position

- 20–30° flexion
- 0–5° adduction
- 5–10° external rotation

Techniques

- Charnley compression arthrodesis (external fixator)
- Plate fixation with bone graft
- Intramedullary nailing

Complications

- Adjacent joint degeneration (lumbar spine, knee)
- Limb length discrepancy
- Difficulty converting to THR

Q30. What are the commonly performed upper limb arthrodesis procedures?

Shoulder Arthrodesis

- *Indications*: Brachial plexus injury, failed arthroplasty, instability
- *Position*: 30° flexion, 30° abduction, 30° internal rotation
- *Fixation*: Plates or screws

Elbow Arthrodesis

- Rarely done due to functional loss
- Indicated in infection or severe destruction
- *Position*: ~90° flexion

Wrist Arthrodesis

- *Indications*: RA, failed wrist salvage, instability
- *Position*: 10–15° extension, slight ulnar deviation
- *Fixation*: DCP plate or pinning
- Fusion may be partial or total

Thumb CMC Arthrodesis

- Indicated in young manual workers with CMC arthritis
- *Fixation*: K-wires or screws

Q31. Describe spinal arthrodesis—indications and techniques.

(AIIMS Delhi 2018)

Indications

- Spinal instability (trauma, spondylolisthesis)
- Spinal deformities (scoliosis, kyphosis)
- Degenerative disc disease
- TB spine with instability or deformity
- Tumor resection

Techniques

- Posterior spinal fusion (PSF)
- Anterior spinal fusion (ASF)
- *Interbody fusion*: PLIF (posterior), TLIF, ALIF
- *Instrumentation*: Pedicle screws, rods, cages
- *Bone graft*: Autograft (iliac crest), allograft, synthetic

VIVA POINTERS

Q: What is triple arthrodesis?
A: Fusion of subtalar, talonavicular, and calcaneocuboid joints.
Q: Position for shoulder fusion?
A: 30° flexion, 30° abduction, and 30° internal rotation.
Q: Most common complication of spinal fusion?
A: Adjacent segment degeneration
Q: Most preferred site for hip arthrodesis today?
A: Not commonly done due to THR being preferred; only in selected young manual laborers.

Minimally Invasive Surgery (MIS) in Orthopedics

Q32. Define minimally invasive surgery in orthopedics. List its advantages and limitations.

Source: DNB 2022, RGUHS 2021

Type: Short essay

Definition

Minimally invasive surgery (MIS) refers to orthopedic procedures performed using **small incisions, specialized instruments**, and **imaging guidance**, with **minimal soft tissue disruption** compared to traditional open surgery.

Examples

- MIS total knee replacement
- MIS spine fixation (TLIF, PLIF with tubular retractors)
- Closed intramedullary nailing
- Percutaneous screw fixation (e.g., sacroiliac joint)

Advantages

Category	*Benefit*
Surgical trauma	Less soft tissue damage
Recovery	Faster mobilization, reduced hospital stay
Pain and blood loss	Reduced compared to open procedures
Aesthetics	Smaller scar
Infection risk	Lower with reduced exposure

Limitations

Limitation	*Explanation*
Steep learning curve	Requires specialized training
Expensive equipment	Endoscopic towers, fluoroscopy, navigation
Limited exposure	Risk in complex or revision cases
Imaging dependency	Radiation exposure, navigation errors

Q33. MIS in total knee arthroplasty—indications, advantages, limitations.

Source: MUHS 2022, DNB 2020

Type: Short essay

Definition

MIS-TKA is a technique where total knee replacement is performed using **smaller incisions (~8–10 cm)** and **reduced soft tissue dissection**, often with **quad-sparing or subvastus approaches**.

Indications

- Primary osteoarthritis
- BMI <30
- No severe deformity (<15° varus/valgus)
- Younger, active patients
- High demand for early return to activity

Advantages

- Less postoperative pain
- Quicker return of quadriceps function
- Early ambulation and hospital discharge
- Better cosmetic results

Limitations

- Technically demanding
- Increased risk of malalignment or component malposition
- Not ideal for severe deformity, obesity, or revision cases
- Requires **special instruments and training**

Q34. Describe role of MIS in spine surgery.

Source: TNMGRMU 2021, DNB 2022

Type: Short essay

Common MIS Spine Procedures

Procedure	*Indication*
Microdiscectomy	Lumbar disc herniation
MIS TLIF/PLIF	Spondylolisthesis, disc degeneration

Continued

Continued

Procedure	Indication
Percutaneous pedicle screws	Spinal fixation in trauma, degenerative spine
Vertebroplasty/Kyphoplasty	Osteoporotic vertebral fractures

Advantages
- Less muscle dissection (preserves multifidus)
- Reduced blood loss and pain
- Faster recovery and ambulation
- Smaller scar and reduced infection rates

Limitations
- Fluoroscopy/Navigation dependent
- Steep learning curve
- Limited field of vision
- Challenging in deformities or revisions

Q35. Short note on percutaneous fracture fixation.

Source: RGUHS 2022

Type: Short note

Definition
Percutaneous fracture fixation involves **minimal incisions**, **indirect reduction**, and **implant placement** under fluoroscopic guidance, often used in **closed or minimally displaced fractures**.

Examples
- Percutaneous K-wiring in metacarpal fractures
- Percutaneous screw fixation of scaphoid
- CRIF of lateral malleolus
- Sacroiliac screw fixation
- Minimally invasive percutaneous plate osteosynthesis (MIPPO) technique

Advantages
- Preservation of fracture hematoma → biological healing
- Less soft tissue trauma
- Shorter operative time and hospitalization
- Early mobilization

Summary Table: MIS in Orthopedics

Procedure	MIS benefit	Notes
MIS TKA	Less pain, faster recovery	Ideal in mild deformity, young patients
MIS THA (mini-posterior/anterolateral)	Less muscle damage	Limited in obese or deformed hips
Spine (TLIF, pedicle screws)	Less bleeding, quicker ambulation	Needs imaging and training
Percutaneous trauma fixation	Preserves biology, minimal incision	Fluoro-guided, ideal for simple fractures

Recent Advances in Arthroplasty and Arthroscopic Techniques

Q36. Robotic-assisted total knee arthroplasty—advantages and limitations.

Source: DNB 2022

Type: Short note

Definition
Robotic-assisted TKA uses **computerized robotic systems** to help surgeons perform precise bone cuts and implant positioning based on a **preoperative or intraoperative plan**.

Advantages
- Greater accuracy of alignment
- Precise bone resection (≤1 mm deviation)
- Less soft tissue balancing error
- Better postoperative functional scores (early phase)

Limitations
- Expensive (capital + disposable costs)
- Requires specific training and planning software
- Longer operative time in early learning curve
- Not suitable for severe deformities or bone loss

Systems in Use
- MAKO (Stryker)
- ROSA (Zimmer–Biomet)
- NAVIO, CORI (Smith and Nephew)

Q37. What are patient-specific instrumentation (PSI) and its role in arthroplasty?

Source: MUHS 2021

Type: Short note

Definition
Patient-specific instrumentation (PSI) uses **preoperative imaging (MRI/CT)** to create **customized cutting blocks and alignment jigs**, tailored to a patient's anatomy.

Applications
- Primarily used in **TKA and THA**
- Ideal in **extra-articular deformities**, previous surgeries, or bony anomalies

Benefits
- Better alignment accuracy
- Reduced intraoperative decision-making
- May reduce surgical time and instrument trays
- Minimizes soft tissue releases

Limitations
- Requires **pre-operative CT or MRI** → cost, time
- Delayed surgical planning
- May not fit intraoperatively (mismatch risk)

Q38. Mention recent advances in shoulder arthroscopy.

Source: TNMGRMU 2021

Type: Short note

Recent Innovations

Advancement	*Use/Benefit*
All-suture anchors	Smaller footprint, better bone preservation
Knotless suture techniques	Faster, easier fixation of rotator cuff/labrum

Continued

Continued

Advancement	Use/Benefit
Biologic augmentation	Use of patches, PRP for massive cuff repair
Arthroscopic Latarjet	Minimally invasive bone block procedure for instability
3D intra-operative navigation	Labral tear localization and bony glenoid assessment

Q39. What is single portal arthroscopy? Compare with conventional arthroscopy.

Source: RGUHS 2022

Type: Short note

Definition

Single-portal arthroscopy uses **one working portal** (vs. standard 2–3) for both **visualization and instrumentation**, often assisted by **special cannulas** and **angled devices**.

Advantages

- Smaller incision
- Lower infection risk
- Better cosmetic outcomes
- Less post-operative pain

Disadvantages

- Technically demanding
- Limited access to complex intra-articular regions
- Instrument crowding possible
- Requires special training and tools

Applications

- Diagnostic arthroscopy
- Meniscectomy
- Loose body removal
- Subacromial decompression

Summary Table: Recent Advances in Arthroplasty and Arthroscopy

Advance	Area	Benefit
Navigation and robotics	Arthroplasty	Precision alignment, improved kinematics
PSI (custom blocks)	Arthroplasty	Personalized implant positioning
Knotless anchors and biologics	Shoulder arthroscopy	Better healing, reduced operative time
Single-portal arthroscopy	Arthroscopy	Minimally invasive, cosmetic
Augmented reality and AI planning	Arthroplasty (emerging)	Enhanced planning and intra-operative feedback

Post-operative Rehabilitation and Complications in Arthroplasty and Arthroscopy

Q40. Describe rehabilitation protocol following total knee arthroplasty (TKA).

Source: RGUHS 2022, DNB 2021

Type: Short essay

Goals

- Regain full **ROM**, **quadriceps strength**, and **independent ambulation**
- Prevent **complications** (DVT, stiffness, infection)

Timeline-based Protocol

Phase	*Time*	*Rehabilitation components*
Immediate (POD 0–2)	Bed mobility, ankle pumps, static quads/glutes, cryotherapy	
Early (week 1–2)	Assisted ambulation (walker), CPM for ROM, ROM goal: 0–90°	
Intermediate (week 2–6)	Full WB (if cemented), stair climbing, balance training	
Late (6–12 weeks)	Strengthening, proprioception drills, ROM >110°	
>3 months	Return to low-impact activities (cycling, swimming)	

Precautions

- Avoid pillow under knee → flexion contracture
- Infection surveillance
- Ensure proper wound care and compliance with anticoagulants

Q41. Outline rehabilitation after total hip arthroplasty (THA).

Source: MUHS 2021

Type: Short essay

Key Objectives

- Early mobilization
- Joint protection (especially against dislocation)
- Regain strength and gait

Phase-wise Protocol (Posterior Approach)

Timeframe	*Rehabilitation focus*
POD 1–3	Ambulation with walker, ankle pumps, isometrics
Week 1–2	Avoid hip flexion >90°, adduction, internal rotation
Week 3–6	Progress WB, stair practice, hip strengthening
Week 6–12	Gait correction, balance training
>3 months	Return to ADLs, gradual resumption of low-impact sports

Hip Precautions (Posterior THA)

- No low chairs
- Avoid bending to pick up objects
- Sleep with abduction pillow (initial 4–6 weeks)

Q42. Write a note on post-arthroscopy rehabilitation of the knee.

Source: RGUHS 2021

Type: Short note

Depends on Procedure

Procedure	*Rehabilitation approach*
Meniscectomy	WBAT (weight bearing as tolerated) from day 1, full ROM in 1–2 weeks
Meniscal repair	NWB or PWB × 4–6 weeks, ROM restricted to 0–90° initially
ACL reconstruction	Brace for 4–6 weeks, early ROM, WB as tolerated (often with support)

General Components
- Cryotherapy to reduce swelling
- Quadriceps and hamstring strengthening
- Patellar mobilization
- Proprioception and balance drills
- Return to sport after 4–6 months (for ligament reconstructions)

Q43. Enumerate causes of poor outcomes after arthroplasty.

Source: DNB 2021, MUHS 2022

Type: Short note

Patient Factors
- Poor compliance with rehabilitation
- Obesity
- Comorbidities (e.g., diabetes, RA)
- Osteoporosis

Surgical Factors
- Malalignment of components
- Improper soft tissue balancing
- Suboptimal implant sizing
- Infection

Post-operative Factors
- Inadequate rehabilitation
- Stiffness (due to delayed mobilization)
- Persistent pain
- Instability or loosening

Revision Arthroplasty, Periprosthetic Fractures, and Salvage Procedures

This section is especially important for **MS Orthopedics and DNB exams** under:
- Complications of arthroplasty
- Salvage techniques in failed joint replacement
- Management of periprosthetic fractures
- Long-case discussions and theory essays

Q44. Indications for revision total hip arthroplasty (THA).

Source: RGUHS 2021, DNB 2022

Type: Short essay

Definition
Revision THA refers to **replacement or reconstruction of a failed primary total hip prosthesis**, either partially (head/liner) or completely.

Indications

Mechanical	*Infective*	*Other*
Aseptic loosening	Periprosthetic joint infection (PJI)	Recurrent dislocation
Implant wear	Late hematogenous infection	Leg length discrepancy

Continued

Continued

Mechanical	Infective	Other
Periprosthetic fracture		Malalignment or instability
Osteolysis due to debris		Metal-on-metal complications
Implant breakage		Pseudotumor (MoM THA)

Q45. Write short note on vancouver classification of periprosthetic femoral fractures.

Source: DNB 2021, TNMGRMU 2022

Type: Short note

Purpose
To classify periprosthetic **femoral fractures around a hip prosthesis**, guiding treatment.

Vancouver Classification

Type	Location	Implant stability	Bone stock	Management
A	Trochanteric (AG/AL)	Stable	Good	ORIF or conservative
B1	Around stem	Stable stem	Good	ORIF
B2	Around stem	Loose stem	Good	Revision THA
B3	Around stem	Loose stem	Poor	Revision THA + bone graft/augment
C	Distal to stem	Irrelevant	May vary	ORIF (standard fracture care)

Q46. Discuss management of periprosthetic infection in THA.

Source: RGUHS 2020, DNB 2021

Type: Short essay

Types of Infection

Category	Timeline
Acute	Within 4 weeks of surgery or <4 weeks of symptoms
Chronic	>4 weeks, indolent course
Hematogenous	Remote infection seeds joint

Diagnosis
- CRP, ESR
- Synovial WBC count, alpha-defensin
- Aspiration and culture
- Intraoperative frozen section, sonication

Management Options

Approach	Indication
Debridement, antibiotics, implant retention (DAIR)	Acute infections, stable implant, healthy soft tissue
1-stage revision	Select chronic cases (low virulence, good bone)
2-stage revision	Gold standard for chronic infection
Suppressive antibiotics	High-risk, non-operative candidates

Q47. What are the options for salvage after failed TKA?

Source: MUHS 2022

Type: Short note

Reasons for TKA Failure
- Infection
- Instability
- Stiffness
- Loosening
- Periprosthetic fracture

Salvage Options

Scenario	*Salvage approach*
Recurrent infection	2-stage revision or arthrodesis
Massive bone loss	Hinged prosthesis or megaprosthesis
Non-reconstructable knee	Knee arthrodesis
Non-ambulatory elderly patient	Girdlestone-type excision arthroplasty
Repeated dislocation/instability	Constrained prosthesis or revision alignment

Q48. Define girdlestone procedure. When is it indicated?

Source: DNB 2020

Type: Short note

Definition
The **Girdlestone procedure** (also called excision arthroplasty of the hip) involves **removal of the femoral head and neck**, creating a **flail pseudo-joint**.

Indications
- Chronic or intractable periprosthetic infection
- Failed THA with poor bone stock
- Non-ambulatory or debilitated patients
- Neuropathic hip
- Low-demand patients (non-reconstructable cases)

Functional Outcome
- Pain relief
- Limb shortening (4–5 cm)
- Loss of hip stability
- Wheelchair-bound or limited ambulation with walking aid

CHAPTER 17

Complications in Orthopedics

Dev Kant Meena, Niaz Ahmed, Bhaarath KS, Shubam Surmal

Nonunion and Delayed Union—Model Answers

Q1. Define nonunion. Describe types, causes, and management.

(AIIMS Delhi 2022, PGI Chandigarh 2022)

Definition

Nonunion is defined as a fracture that **fails to show any evidence of healing** for at least **9 months** from injury and shows **no progression of healing for three consecutive months**, as per **FDA and AAOS criteria.**

Types of Nonunion (Based on Radiology and Biology)

Type	*Features*	*Bone activity*
Hypertrophic	Abundant callus, failure due to instability	Good biological activity
Oligotrophic	Minimal callus, poor alignment	Reduced activity
Atrophic	No callus, tapered bone ends	Poor biological activity
Infected (septic)	Sinus or abscess present	Variable

Causes

Biological:
- Poor blood supply
- Infection
- Soft tissue interposition
- Corticosteroid use
- Smoking, malnutrition

Mechanical:
- Inadequate fixation
- Excessive movement
- Large fracture gap

Management Principles (Based on "Diamond Concept")

1. *Mechanical stability*: Rigid internal fixation or external fixator
2. *Biological stimulation*: Autograft/allograft, BMPs, PRP
3. Debridement (if infected)
4. Alignment restoration
5. *Host optimization*: Nutrition, diabetes control, smoking cessation

Q2. Difference between hypertrophic and atrophic nonunion—management strategies.

(MUHS Maharashtra 2022, RGUHS Karnataka 2022)

Feature	*Hypertrophic nonunion*	*Atrophic nonunion*
Callus formation	Abundant ("elephant foot" or "horse hoof")	Absent, bone ends appear tapered
Cause	Instability (mechanical failure)	Poor biology or blood supply
X-ray appearance	Radiodense, callus around fracture site	Osteopenic bone ends, no callus
Treatment focus	Improve stability	Enhance biology + stability
Surgical approach	Exchange nailing, compression plating	Bone grafting + stable fixation (LCP/Ilizarov)

Management Summary
- *Hypertrophic*: Internal fixation with compression (e.g., dynamic compression plate), or exchange nailing
- *Atrophic*: Debridement, bone grafting (autograft preferred), and stable fixation (e.g., locking plate, Ilizarov)

Q3. Enumerate complications of fractures. Describe classification and management of non-union.

(RGUHS 2021, DNB 2022)

Fracture Complications (General)
- *Immediate*: Hemorrhage, neurovascular injury, compartment syndrome
- *Early*: Infection, fat embolism, DVT, skin necrosis
- *Late*: **Nonunion**, malunion, joint stiffness, CRPS, osteomyelitis

Nonunion Classification (Weber and Cech)

Biological type	*Subtype*
Viable (80%)	Hypertrophic, oligotrophic
Non-viable (20%)	Atrophic, torsion wedge, comminuted, defect

Management Principles
1. *Stabilization*: Improve mechanical environment
2. *Biological support*: Bone grafting (autograft, BMPs, PRP)
3. *Infected nonunion*: Two-stage surgery (debridement → bone graft/fixation)
4. *Ilizarov fixator*: Excellent for complex/segmental nonunions

Q4. Enumerate types of delayed union and non-union. Describe principles of treatment.

(TNMGRMU 2020, RGUHS 2022)

Types of Delayed/Nonunion
- *Delayed union*: Healing is slower than expected, but ongoing
- *Types of nonunion*: Hypertrophic, atrophic, oligotrophic, infected

Treatment Principles (Same as "Diamond Concept")
1. *Stabilization*: For example, exchange nailing, LCP
2. *Stimulation*: Bone graft, BMPs, PRP
3. *Correction of alignment*: Especially in oligotrophic or malalignment
4. *Host optimization*: Smoking, nutrition, comorbidities
5. *Monitoring*: Serial X-rays, infection markers if needed

Q5. Management of infected nonunion.

(DNB 2021, MUHS 2020)

Definition

Nonunion in the presence of **clinical or microbiological evidence of infection**, commonly seen after **open fractures or failed internal fixation**.

Clinical Features

- Sinus discharge
- Implant loosening
- Pain, swelling, erythema
- Elevated ESR/CRP, positive cultures

Management: 2-stage Approach

Stage 1: Infection control

- Radical **debridement** of necrotic bone
- **Implant removal** (if loose/infected)
- Antibiotic cement beads/spacers
- External fixation for stabilization
- Targeted IV antibiotics (6 weeks)

Stage 2: Reconstruction

- Bone defect management (graft, transport, Masquelet technique)
- Definitive stable fixation (Ilizarov preferred in infected bone)
- Soft tissue cover if needed

Malunion

Q6. Define malunion. Enumerate causes and principles of treatment.

(RGUHS 2021, DNB 2021)

Definition

Malunion is defined as a **fracture that has healed in an abnormal anatomical position**, resulting in **functional impairment or cosmetic deformity**.

Causes

Patient-related	***Surgeon/Technique-related***
Non-compliance	Inadequate reduction/fixation
Osteoporosis	Premature weight-bearing
Smoking, diabetes	Wrong implant selection
Infection during healing	Absence of monitoring

Types of Malunion

- Angular deformity (varus/valgus, recurvatum/procurvatum)
- Rotational malalignment
- Translational deformity
- Shortening (limb length discrepancy)
- Intra-articular malunion (e.g., malunited distal radius)

Principles of Treatment

1. *Identify deformity*: Clinical and radiological assessment (CT for rotational issues)
2. *Determine indication for correction*: Functional or cosmetic need
3. *Correct the deformity*:
   - *Acute correction*: Osteotomy + plate fixation
   - *Gradual correction*: Ilizarov fixator/hexapod (e.g., Taylor Spatial Frame)
4. Restore length, rotation, axis, and alignment
5. *Rehabilitation*: Physical therapy post correction

Q7. Classification of malunion and its impact on function.

(MUHS 2022, TNMGRMU 2021)

Classification Based On

Parameter	*Types*
Plane	Angular, rotational, translational, shortening
Bone involved	Long bone vs. intra-articular malunion
Severity	Mild (<5°), moderate (5–15°), severe (>15°)
Joint vs. shaft	Intra-articular (e.g., distal radius), diaphyseal

Impact on Function

Deformity	*Functional consequence*
Angular deformity (e.g. varus femur)	Abnormal gait, limb length discrepancy
Rotational deformity	Gait disturbance, decreased strength (especially femur/tibia)
Intra-articular malunion	Joint incongruity → arthritis, stiffness
Shortening >2 cm	Pelvic tilt, scoliosis, back pain

Q8. Management of distal radius malunion.

(DNB 2021, RGUHS 2020)

Common Malunion Patterns

- Dorsal tilt of distal fragment
- Radial shortening
- Loss of radial inclination
- Distal radioulnar joint (DRUJ) incongruity

Indications for Correction

- Pain and stiffness
- DRUJ instability
- Weak grip strength
- Functional limitation (especially pronation/supination)

Treatment Options

Type of deformity	*Correction strategy*
Extra-articular malunion	Corrective opening wedge osteotomy + volar plate
Intra-articular step-off	Intra-articular osteotomy (if early) or salvage procedures (late)
Severe DRUJ dysfunction	Darrach/Sauve–Kapandji procedures
Early cases (<6 weeks)	Remanipulation, revision fixation

Q9. Management of cubitus varus deformity in children.

IIMS 2022, PGI Chandigarh 2022)

Definition

Cubitus varus is a **medial angular deformity** of the elbow, most commonly a sequela of **malunited supracondylar humerus fracture** in children.

Clinical Features

- Medial elbow deviation
- "Gunstock deformity"
- Cosmetic deformity > functional loss
- Possible tardy ulnar nerve palsy (rare)

Radiology

- Baumann's angle decreased
- Compare with opposite side
- CT if rotational component suspected

Surgical Correction Options

Osteotomy type	*Key point*
Lateral closing wedge osteotomy	Most commonly used, simple and reliable
Dome osteotomy	Allows angular + rotational correction
Step-cut osteotomy	More stable, allows controlled correction
3D-corrective osteotomy	For multi-planar deformity (rare)

Fixation Methods

- K-wires (small kids)
- Plates (adolescents)
- Cast post-operative

Complications of Internal Fixation

Q10. Enumerate complications of internal fixation. Describe their classification and management.

(RGUHS 2022, DNB 2021)

General Classification of Complications

Timing	*Examples*
Intraoperative	Iatrogenic fracture, nerve or vessel injury, implant breakage
Early Post-operative	Infection, hematoma, implant back-out, compartment syndrome
Late Post-operative	Nonunion, implant failure, metal allergy, stress shielding
Delayed	Refracture after implant removal, osteopenia under plate

Implant-specific Complications

Plates (e.g., DCP/LCP)	*Intramedullary nails*	*Screws/Wires*
Plate pull-out or breakage	Malalignment (rotation, shortening)	Wire migration, screw cut-out
Stress shielding	Nail breakage	Loosening, neurovascular impingement
Peri-implant fracture	Entry-site cortical cracks	Difficult hardware removal

Management Principles

1. *Assess the failure type*: Mechanical versus biological
2. *Infection control*: If infection suspected, culture and debridement
3. *Implant revision or removal*: Replace with appropriate hardware
4. *Bone support*: Add grafting (if delayed union or atrophic bone)
5. *Rehabilitation*: Restore function through guided physiotherapy

Q11. Causes and management of implant failure.

(MUHS 2021, DNB 2022)

Causes of Implant Failure

Mechanical factors	*Biological factors*
Inadequate fixation	Poor bone quality (osteoporosis)
Improper load-sharing	Infection leading to loosening
Fatigue from delayed union	Atrophic or avascular bone ends
Inappropriate implant selection/length	Smoking, malnutrition

Types of Implant Failure

- Plate breakage (usually at screw hole or stress riser)
- Screw loosening or pull-out
- Nail breakage (at fracture site)
- Backing out of screws or pins
- Wire migration (especially K-wires in clavicle, patella)

Management Strategy

1. Rule out infection (ESR, CRP, aspiration)
2. Debride if infected, remove failed implant
3. Re-fixation with stronger or longer implant
4. *Augment biology*: Bone grafting, BMPs
5. *External fixation*: Temporary or definitive, especially in infection
6. Patient education on weight-bearing and compliance

Q12. Describe causes and prevention of plate breakage and screw loosening.

(TNMGRMU 2021, RGUHS 2020)

Plate Breakage

Causes:

- Cyclic loading (fatigue failure)
- Improper plate length (too short plate leads to stress riser)
- Eccentric drilling or excessive torque
- Nonunion leading to stress concentration
- Repeated instrumentation (during surgery)

Screw Loosening

Causes:

- Poor purchase in osteoporotic bone
- Infection (causes bone lysis around screw)
- Micromotion at screw-bone interface
- Inappropriate screw length or angle

Prevention Strategies

For plate breakage	*For screw loosening*
Use long plates for bridging	Bicortical screws in osteoporotic bone
Avoid stress risers (e.g., empty holes near fracture)	Locking screws in poor-quality bone
Ensure fracture stability	Augment screw with cement or bone
Encourage proper rehabilitation	Avoid early, unsupported loading

Q13. Discuss implant removal—indications, timing, and complications.

(DNB 2021, RGUHS 2022)

Indications for Implant Removal

- Pain or prominence of implant
- Infection (even if quiescent)
- Broken/failed hardware
- Pediatric fractures (to prevent growth disturbance)
- Functional limitation due to hardware
- Prior to MRI (if incompatible) or for prosthesis planning

Timing

Implant	*Recommended time of removal*
Plates (adults)	≥18 months post-fixation (if required)
IM nails	≥18–24 months, only if symptomatic
Pediatric implants	After skeletal maturity or union
K-wires	6–8 weeks or once healing confirmed

Complications of Removal

- Iatrogenic fracture (due to stress riser or poor healing)
- Neurovascular injury
- Implant breakage during removal
- Bleeding or infection
- Refracture if healing incomplete or inadequate bone remodeling

Complications of Joint Replacement—Model Answers

Q14. Enumerate complications of total hip arthroplasty (THA). Describe management of dislocation after THA.

(RGUHS 2021, DNB 2022)

Complications of THA

Timeframe	*Complications*
Immediate	Bleeding, nerve injury (sciatic), DVT, PE
Early	Infection, dislocation, leg length discrepancy (LLD)
Late	Aseptic loosening, wear, periprosthetic fracture, HO
Very late	Metallosis, pseudotumor, component migration

Dislocation after THA—Key Points

- Most common in posterior approach
- *Risk factors*: Malpositioned components, weak abductors, neuromuscular disorders, noncompliance

Management

1. *Acute dislocation (within 6 weeks)*:
   - Closed reduction under sedation/anesthesia
   - Immobilization in abduction brace
   - Identify cause (X-ray, CT)
2. *Recurrent dislocation*:
   - Component malposition → Revision THA
   - Soft tissue laxity → Use of **constrained liner or dual mobility cup**
   - Address patient education and compliance

Q15. Enumerate causes and management of aseptic loosening in TKA.

(MUHS 2022, DNB 2021)

Definition

Aseptic loosening is **non-infective mechanical failure** of the prosthesis-bone interface, leading to **implant instability and failure**.

Causes

Mechanical	*Biological*
Malalignment of components	Osteolysis due to wear particles
Inadequate cementing	Host factors (osteopenia, comorbidities)
High BMI or overuse	Stress shielding

Diagnosis

- *Clinical*: Pain, instability, swelling
- *X-ray*: Radiolucent lines, subsidence, osteolysis
- *Rule out infection*: CRP, ESR, joint aspiration

Management

- *Early loosening*: May attempt bone graft + liner change (rare)
- *Established loosening*: **Revision TKA** with longer stemmed prosthesis, possibly using augments or cones for bone defects
- Cemented or cementless revision depending on bone stock

Q16. Describe classification and management of periprosthetic femoral fractures.

(DNB 2022, RGUHS 2021)

Vancouver Classification (THA)

Type	*Location*	*Implant Stability*	*Management*
A	Trochanteric (AG/AL)	Stable	ORIF or conservative
B1	Around stem	Stem stable	ORIF with plate
B2	Around stem	Stem loose	Revision stem with fixation
B3	Around stem	Stem loose + bone loss	Revision + bone graft/augment
C	Distal to implant	Irrelevant	Standard fracture fixation (e.g., LCP, nail)

Key Management Principles

- Assess implant stability (radiologically or intraoperatively)
- Bone quality and comminution dictate fixation method
- Consider **locking plates or dual plating** in osteoporotic patients
- If stem is loose → **revision THA mandatory**

Q17. Write a note on leg length discrepancy (LLD) after THA.

(TNMGRMU 2021, DNB 2021)

Causes

Intraoperative	*Preoperative factors*
Excessive offset or stem length	Fixed flexion or adduction deformities
Cup malposition (inclination/anteversion)	Preexisting LLD
Inadequate templating	Pelvic obliquity or spinal imbalance

Clinical Significance

- Patient dissatisfaction
- Limp, back pain
- Nerve palsy (especially sciatic or femoral stretch)
- Pelvic tilt, compensatory scoliosis

Management

- *Mild (<1.5 cm)*: Shoe raise
- *Moderate (1.5–2.5 cm)*: Conservative or corrective osteotomy (rare)
- *Significant intraoperative mismatch*: May revise component or adjust modular head

Prevention

- Proper **templating and intra-operative leg length checks**
- Use of **reference points** (e.g., lesser trochanter)
- **Digital devices** (e.g., leg length calipers, navigation tools)

Q18. Management of post-TKA joint stiffness.

(RGUHS 2022, DNB 2020)

Definition

Post-TKA stiffness is defined as knee flexion <90° or flexion contracture >10–15° beyond 6 weeks post-operative.

Etiology

- Preoperative stiffness (OA, RA)
- Inadequate rehabilitation
- Excessive scar tissue or fibrosis
- Component malrotation
- Overstuffing of joint (large polyethylene insert)

Management

Timeline	*Strategy*
0–6 weeks	Aggressive physiotherapy + analgesia
6–12 weeks	Manipulation under anesthesia (MUA)
>3 months	Arthroscopic or open lysis of adhesions
Structural issue	Revision TKA if malalignment/component issue

Prevention

- Prehabilitation before surgery
- Early mobilization
- Adequate pain control
- Avoid overstuffing or imbalance during surgery

Vascular Complications

Q19. Vascular injuries in orthopedics—enumerate and describe management.

(DNB 2022, RGUHS 2021)

Common Sites and Causes

Injury site	*Orthopedic association*
Popliteal artery	Knee dislocation, distal femur fracture
Axillary artery	Shoulder dislocation, proximal humerus fracture
Brachial artery	Supracondylar humerus fracture (children)
Femoral artery	Acetabular or pelvic trauma
Anterior tibial artery	Tibial nailing, leg trauma

Signs of Vascular Injury ("5 P's")

- *P*ain
- *P*allor
- *P*ulselessness
- *P*aresthesia
- *P*aralysis

Also expanding hematoma, bruit, thrill

Diagnosis

- *Doppler ultrasound*: bedside
- *CT angiography*: gold standard
- Compartment pressure monitoring (if suspecting ACS)

Management Principles

Step	*Details*
Urgent reduction	For example, dislocation (especially knee)
Vascular repair	End-to-end anastomosis or interposition graft
Fasciotomy	If prolonged ischemia or compartment syndrome
Orthopedic stabilization	External fixator preferred in acute phase

Infection

Q20. Classify surgical site infection (SSI). Discuss management in joint replacement.

(DNB 2022, RGUHS 2021)

CDC Classification of SSI

Type	*Timing*	*Location*
Superficial incisional	Within 30 days	Skin and subcutaneous tissue
Deep incisional	30–90 days (implant surgery)	Fascia and muscle
Organ/space infection	Up to 1 year (implant)	Bone or joint cavity (PJI)

Management of SSI after Arthroplasty (THA/TKA)

Acute infection (<4 weeks):

- *DAIR procedure*:
  - Debridement

- *A*ntibiotics
- *I*mplants *R*etained
- Exchange polyethylene liner

Chronic infection (>4 weeks):

- *Two-stage revision*:
  1. Remove implant, place antibiotic spacer
  2. IV antibiotics (6 weeks)
  3. Re-implantation after CRP/ESR normalize

Suppression only (non-surgical candidates):

- Long-term oral antibiotics
- Functional braces

Q21. What is the role of antibiotic-loaded bone cement?

(TNMGRMU 2021, DNB 2021)

Definition

Antibiotic-loaded bone cement (ALBC) is **PMMA** cement mixed with antibiotics like **gentamicin or vancomycin** to **elute locally at high concentrations**, preventing or treating infection.

Indications

- **Prophylactic use** in joint replacement
- **Therapeutic use** in infected joint revisions
- Antibiotic spacers during **2-stage revisions**
- Used in infected nonunions or trauma cases

Advantages

- High local antibiotic concentration
- Low systemic toxicity
- Can be molded into spacers (temporary prosthesis)

Limitations

- Antibiotic resistance risk
- Thermal degradation of some antibiotics
- Reduced mechanical strength if mixed in excess

Q22. What is a sinus tract in chronic osteomyelitis? How is it managed?

(DNB 2020, RGUHS 2020)

Definition

A **sinus tract** is an abnormal epithelialized channel that connects an underlying **chronic focus of infection** (usually bone) to the skin surface.

Causes

- Chronic osteomyelitis
- Infected implant or nonunion
- Sequestrum not removed completely

Diagnosis

- Clinical exam (intermittent pus discharge)
- MRI—to trace the sinus and identify sequestrum
- Sinogram—may help in complex tracts
- Culture/sensitivity from deep tract

Management
- Wide **excision of the sinus tract**
- **Sequestrectomy + saucerization**
- **Debridement + antibiotics**
- If implant present → removal and stabilization (external fixator)
- Ensure **adequate soft tissue cover**

CRPS, DVT, and Other Systemic Complications

Q23. Define complex regional pain syndrome (CRPS). Discuss its diagnosis and management.

(DNB 2021, RGUHS 2022)

Definition

Complex regional pain syndrome (CRPS) is a chronic pain condition usually occurring **after trauma or surgery**, characterized by **disproportionate pain**, **autonomic dysfunction**, and **trophic changes**, without any nerve injury (CRPS-I) or with identifiable nerve injury (CRPS-II).

Types (Budapest Criteria)

CRPS type	*Cause*
Type I	No identifiable nerve lesion
Type II	Associated with nerve injury

Diagnostic Features (Budapest Criteria)
- Pain **disproportionate to inciting event**
- *At least one symptom in three of four categories*:
  - Sensory (allodynia, hyperalgesia)
  - Vasomotor (temperature, skin color changes)
  - Sudomotor (sweating, edema)
  - Motor/Trophic (weakness, tremor, nail/skin changes)

Investigations
- *X-ray*: **Patchy osteoporosis** (late)
- *Bone scan (3-phase)*: Increased uptake
- Thermography (optional)

Management

Modality	*Example*
Pharmacologic	NSAIDs, pregabalin, amitriptyline, bisphosphonates
Physiotherapy	Desensitization, ROM exercises
Psychological	CBT, reassurance
Interventional	Sympathetic block, spinal cord stimulation (severe)

Q24. Deep vein thrombosis (DVT)—risk factors, diagnosis, and prophylaxis.

(MUHS 2022, DNB 2020)

Risk Factors

Patient-related	*Surgery-related*
Age >60, obesity, varicose veins	Joint replacement, prolonged immobilization
Oral contraceptives, malignancy	Use of tourniquet, spinal injury
Previous DVT/PE	Pelvic or lower limb trauma

Clinical Features
- Calf pain, swelling
- **Positive Homan's sign** (pain on dorsiflexion)
- Warmth, redness

Diagnosis
- **Doppler ultrasound** (first-line)
- D-dimer (screening)
- Venography (gold standard, rarely used)

Prophylaxis and Treatment

Mechanical	*Pharmacological*
Compression stockings	LMWH (e.g., enoxaparin)
Intermittent pneumatic compression	Rivaroxaban, apixaban (oral)
Early mobilization	Aspirin (low risk patients)

Duration
- *Post-THA*: ≥35 days
- *Post-TKA*: 10–14 days minimum
- Treat DVT for **3–6 months**

Q25. Pulmonary embolism (PE)—Clinical features and management.

(DNB 2020, TNMGRMU 2021)

Etiology
- Complication of DVT (femoral, iliac vein thrombi)
- Can occur after trauma, surgery, immobilization

Clinical Features
- Sudden dyspnea, tachypnea
- Chest pain, hemoptysis
- Syncope or hypotension (massive PE)
- Raised JVP (acute cor pulmonale)

Diagnosis
- **CT pulmonary angiography** (gold standard)
- *ECG*: S1Q3T3 pattern (classic, rare)
- D-dimer elevated
- V/Q scan (if contrast contraindicated)

Management

Type of PE	*Treatment*
Stable PE	Anticoagulation (LMWH, rivaroxaban)
Massive PE	Thrombolysis (e.g., alteplase), oxygen, ICU support
Recurrent PE	IVC filter (in selected cases)

Duration of Anticoagulation
- *First event*: 3–6 months
- *Recurrent or unprovoked*: Lifelong

Bone Tumor–related Complications

Q26. Enumerate complications of limb salvage surgery in bone tumors.

(DNB 2021, RGUHS 2022)

Definition

Limb salvage surgery (LSS) refers to the **preservation of limb function** while ensuring **oncological safety** during tumor resection.

Complications of LSS

Category	*Examples*
Local	Wound dehiscence, flap necrosis, infection
Mechanical	Prosthesis loosening, stem breakage, periprosthetic fracture
Oncological	Local recurrence, positive margins
Neurological	Nerve injury, sensory loss
Vascular	Bleeding, ischemia, DVT
Functional	Limb length discrepancy, reduced ROM, joint stiffness
Systemic	Chemotherapy-related (neutropenia, cardiotoxicity)

Q27. What are the causes of local recurrence in bone tumors? Management.

(MUHS 2022, DNB 2020)

Causes of Local Recurrence

Cause	*Details*
Inadequate surgical margin	Intralesional or marginal excision
Violation of tumor pseudocapsule	Spillage during surgery
Poor chemo/radiotherapy response	In aggressive tumors (e.g., Ewing's, osteosarcoma)
Skip metastases	Undetected at diagnosis
Wrong histological diagnosis	Under-staged tumor

Management Based on Scenario

Scenario	*Treatment*
Recurrence in soft tissue	Wide local re-excision
Recurrence with prosthesis	Revision LSS or amputation
Positive margin with high-grade tumor	Chemotherapy ± radiation
Recurrent GCT	Extended curettage + PMMA or phenol, resection

Prevention

- Strict adherence to **Enneking's surgical margins**
- Neoadjuvant therapy in malignant tumors
- Proper pre-operative staging (MRI, PET-CT)

Q28. Enumerate complications of megaprosthesis reconstruction.

(DNB 2022, TNMGRMU 2021)

Definition

Megaprosthesis refers to **large-segment joint or bone replacement prostheses** used after **oncologic resections**.

Complications

Early	*Late*
Wound infection	Aseptic loosening
Joint stiffness	Periprosthetic fracture
Nerve palsy	Mechanical failure (hinge/locking)
Dislocation (hip/knee)	Leg length discrepancy
Skin necrosis, hematoma	Tumor recurrence

Risk Factors

- Large resection volume
- Immunosuppression (chemotherapy)
- Poor soft tissue cover
- Pediatric cases with expandable prostheses

Management

- *Infection* → Debridement, antibiotics, two-stage revision
- *Mechanical failure* → Revision of components
- *Fractures* → ORIF or prosthetic revision
- *Recurrence* → Imaging + MDT review; possible revision surgery

Q29. Discuss chemotherapy-related complications in orthopedic oncology.

(RGUHS 2021, DNB 2020)

Chemotherapy Agents Commonly Used

- Doxorubicin
- Methotrexate
- Cisplatin
- Ifosfamide
- Vincristine

Complications (Organ-system Wise)

System	*Complication*
Hematologic	Pancytopenia, neutropenic fever
GI	Nausea, vomiting, mucositis, diarrhea
Renal	Nephrotoxicity (cisplatin, methotrexate)
Cardiac	Cardiomyopathy (doxorubicin)
Nervous system	Peripheral neuropathy (vincristine)
Musculoskeletal	Growth arrest in children, osteopenia
Immune system	Delayed wound healing, infection risk

Management

- Routine monitoring (CBC, ECG, renal panel)
- Dose adjustments and hydration
- Growth factor support (e.g., G-CSF)
- Delay/reduction of surgery if marrow suppression present

Q30. Explain expandable prosthesis in pediatric bone tumors—mechanism and complications.

(DNB 2022, MUHS 2021)

Definition

An expandable prosthesis is a **custom-designed, growing implant** used after resection of tumors in skeletally immature patients to prevent **limb length discrepancy**.

Mechanism

Type	*Expansion method*
Invasive	Requires surgical reopening
Non-invasive	Uses magnetic remote-controlled system (e.g., Stanmore)

Indications

- Pediatric osteosarcoma, Ewing's sarcoma
- Tumors around knee (distal femur/proximal tibia)
- Anticipated growth >3–5 cm

Complications

- Mechanical failure (expansion lock, hinge)
- Infection (especially with repeated surgery)
- Implant fatigue and fracture
- High cost and limited availability
- Loss of ROM or stiffness
- Leg length discrepancy if growth under-corrected

CHAPTER 18

Rehabilitation in Trauma and Orthopedics

Amandeep Singh Bakshi, Tejpal Singh, Deepali Gupta

General Principles of Rehabilitation in Orthopedics and Trauma

Q1. Enumerate principles of orthopedic rehabilitation.

Source: RGUHS 2021, DNB 2020

Type: Long essay

Definition

Rehabilitation is a coordinated set of **medical, physical, psychological, and vocational interventions** aimed at restoring function and improving quality of life after orthopedic injury or surgery.

Core Principles of Orthopedic Rehabilitation

1. *Early mobilization*: Reduces joint stiffness, muscle atrophy, DVT risk
   - Promotes circulation and healing
2. *Individualized protocols*: Based on injury type, patient comorbidities, and surgical method
3. *Multidisciplinary approach*: Collaboration between **orthopedicians**, **physiotherapists**, **occupational therapists**, **psychologists**, and **orthotists**
4. *Progressive loading*: Gradual increase in weight bearing or ROM to restore function
5. *Functional restoration*: Focus on **activities of daily living (ADLs)**, gait, and coordination
6. *Patient education*: Importance of **home exercises**, adherence, and ergonomics
7. *Pain and swelling management*: Cryotherapy, TENS, medication support
8. *Monitoring and outcome assessment*: Use of scores (e.g., DASH, Harris Hip Score)

Q2. Write briefly on stages of rehabilitation following orthopedic trauma.

Source: MUHS 2021

Type: Short essay

Phases of Rehabilitation

Phase	*Timeline*	*Objectives*
Acute phase	0–5 days	Pain control, swelling reduction, protect injury
Subacute phase	1–3 weeks	Begin ROM, gentle strengthening, prevent stiffness
Early functional phase	3–6 weeks	Improve mobility, initiate weight bearing (as per protocol)
Late functional phase	6–12 weeks	Restore strength, proprioception, balance
Return to function	3–6 months and beyond	Full return to activity, sports, work

Key Goals in Each Phase
- Maintain **joint integrity and alignment**
- Prevent **complications** like contractures, myositis ossificans
- **Tailor progression** to healing stage and surgical considerations

Q3. Multidisciplinary approach to orthopedic rehabilitation—discuss.

Source: TNMGRMU 2022

Type: Short essay

Definition
A **multidisciplinary approach** integrates input from various professionals to address the **physical, psychological, and social aspects** of rehabilitation.

Key Team Members and Their Roles

Professional	*Role in rehabilitation*
Orthopedic surgeon	Surgical management, protocol guidance
Physiotherapist	ROM, strength, mobility training
Occupational therapist	ADLs, hand function, splints
Psychologist	Coping skills, motivation, depression management
Orthotist/Prosthetist	Design of braces, orthoses, prostheses
Social worker/vocational therapist	Return to work planning, community reintegration
Nurse	Wound care, support, patient education

Benefits
- **Holistic care**
- **Improved compliance and outcomes**
- Faster **return to independence**

Q4. Role of physiotherapist in post-operative orthopedic care.

Source: RGUHS 2022

Type: Short essay

Key Responsibilities of a Physiotherapist Post-surgery
1. *Pain and swelling management*: Cryotherapy, TENS, positioning
2. *Respiratory care (especially in spinal or polytrauma)*: Breathing exercises to prevent atelectasis
3. *Joint mobilization*: Early passive and active ROM to prevent stiffness
4. *Strengthening exercises*: Isometrics early; progressive resistance later
5. *Gait training*: Use of **crutches, walkers, orthoses**
6. *Education and motivation*: Home programs, precautions, ergonomics
7. *Monitoring recovery*: Regular evaluation using functional scores

Surgeries Where Physio is Vital
- THA/TKA
- Rotator cuff repair
- ACL reconstruction
- Spinal instrumentation
- Fracture fixations

Q5. Goals of rehabilitation in orthopedic surgery and trauma.

Source: DNB 2021

Type: Short note

Key Goals

1. Pain relief and swelling control
2. Restoration of joint ROM and muscle strength
3. Return to independent mobility and ADLs
4. *Prevent complications*: DVT, joint stiffness, contractures
5. Promote psychological well-being
6. Prevent recurrence or reinjury
7. Assist return to work or sports (if applicable)

SMART Goal Approach

S: Specific	Targeted area (e.g., knee flexion ≥90°)
M: Measurable	Use scores like DASH, Harris Hip, Lysholm
A: Achievable	Realistic timelines
R: Relevant	Aligned with functional need
T: Time-bound	Phased goals (e.g., 4-week, 12-week targets)

Q6. Explain the concepts of early versus delayed mobilization.

Source: MUHS 2020

Type: Short note

Early Mobilization

Initiating movement or ambulation **within 24–72 hours** post-injury/surgery.

Benefits

- Reduces stiffness, muscle wasting
- Enhances circulation → faster healing
- Reduces risk of DVT, pneumonia
- Psychological boost

Delayed Mobilization

Movement started **after a longer rest phase**, usually beyond **1–2 weeks**, especially in unstable injuries.

Indications

- Spinal instability
- Non-compliant fracture fixation
- Neurological deficits
- Severe pain/swelling

Clinical Decision Depends On

- Type of injury
- Surgical method
- Patient's general health
- Stability of fixation

Rehabilitation After Fracture and Trauma

Q7. Rehabilitation after femoral shaft fracture fixation.

Source: DNB 2021, RGUHS 2020

Type: Short essay

Rehabilitation Goals

- Restore **full range of motion**, **quadriceps strength**, **normal gait**
- Prevent **complications** like knee stiffness, DVT, muscle wasting

Phases of Rehabilitation

Phase	*Timeline*	*Goals and activities*
Immediate post-operative	0–2 weeks	Pain control, isometrics, passive ROM, ankle pumps
Early phase	2–6 weeks	Active ROM, assisted gait (walker/crutches)
Intermediate phase	6–12 weeks	Full weight-bearing (if union seen), strengthening
Late phase	3–6 months	Gait training, stair climbing, return to ADLs
Return to sport/work	>6 months	High-demand functional activities

Monitoring

- **Serial X-rays** for union
- Gait analysis
- Functional scores (e.g., LEFS—lower extremity functional scale)

Q8. Describe rehabilitation protocol following intertrochanteric fracture surgery.

Source: MUHS 2022

Type: Short essay

Unique Considerations

- Elderly patients
- Risk of DVT, pressure sores
- Early weight-bearing is often possible (especially with DHS/PFN)

Rehabilitation Timeline

Phase	*Activities*
Day 1–3	Breathing exercises, ankle pumps, quadriceps and gluteal sets
Day 3–7	Sitting, bedside mobility, walking with walker (as tolerated)
Week 2–6	Gait training, hip ROM exercises (avoiding hip flexion >90° initially)
Week 6–12	Progressive resistance training, balance training
After 3 months	Full functional rehabilitation and stair training

Precautions

- Avoid **external rotation and adduction** in unstable fractures
- Prevent **flexion contractures** with prone lying or hip extension exercises

Q9. Physiotherapy following fracture shaft humerus—outline a protocol.

Source: TNMGRMU 2021

Type: Short essay

Objectives

- Restore **shoulder and elbow ROM**
- Maintain **muscle strength** and prevent stiffness
- Protect radial nerve (if involved)

Phase-wise Rehabilitation

Phase	*Management*
Immobilization phase (0–3 weeks)	Shoulder pendulum exercises, wrist/finger mobilization
Mobilization phase (3–6 weeks)	Gentle passive → active-assisted ROM at shoulder and elbow
Strengthening phase (6–12 weeks)	Resisted exercises, isometrics for deltoid/biceps
Return to function (>12 weeks)	Functional and occupational training

Special Tips

- Prevent **shoulder-hand syndrome**
- **Sling weaning** based on radiological healing
- Monitor for **radial nerve recovery** (if injured)

Q10. Rehabilitation following Colles' fracture—phases and goals.

Source: RGUHS 2022, DNB 2020

Type: Short note

Goals

- Restore **wrist and hand function**
- Prevent **finger stiffness, shoulder-hand syndrome**
- Regain **fine motor skills**

Rehabilitation Protocol

Phase	*Timeline*	*Key focus*
Immobilization	0–4/6 weeks	Finger ROM, shoulder exercises, tendon gliding
Post-cast removal	4/6–8 weeks	Wrist ROM, pronation/supination, grip strength
Advanced rehabilitation	8–12+ weeks	Full ROM, ADL training, dexterity exercises

Techniques

- Contrast baths for edema
- Putty/Grip exercises
- Supination/Pronation with hammer
- Functional tasks (buttoning, writing)

Q11. Role of physiotherapy in supracondylar fracture (child) post-fixation.

Source: MUHS 2021

Type: Short note

Goals
- Restore **elbow range of motion**
- Prevent **myositis ossificans**
- Monitor for **nerve recovery (median, radial, ulnar)**

Timeline-based Protocol

Phase	Approach
0–3 weeks (splinting)	Finger, shoulder ROM, isometric biceps/triceps
3–6 weeks (after K-wire removal)	Gentle elbow flexion/extension, pronation/supination
6–12 weeks	Full ROM, strengthening, play-based rehabilitation

Special Considerations
- Avoid **aggressive ROM** early (risk of myositis)
- Encourage **functional hand use**
- Use of **home exercise program** for compliance

Rehabilitation After Joint Replacement (THA, TKA, Shoulder, Hemiarthroplasty)

Q12. Physiotherapy after total knee replacement (TKR)—stages and precautions.

Source: RGUHS 2021, DNB 2020

Type: Long essay

Goals of TKR Rehabilitation
- Restore **pain-free ROM and function**
- Prevent **DVT, stiffness, and contractures**
- Enable **independent ambulation**

Rehabilitation Phases

Phase	Timeline	Key interventions
Immediate phase	POD 1–3	Ankle pumps, quadriceps sets, deep breathing, assisted ROM
Early phase	Week 1–2	Passive/active-assisted ROM, gait with walker/crutches
Intermediate	Week 2–6	Target ROM ≥ 0–90°, stair climbing, strengthening
Advanced phase	Week 6–12	Improve to 0–110°+, normal gait, cycling, balance drills
Return to ADLs	3–6 months	Full ROM, independence, light recreational activities

Precautions
- Avoid **pillow under knee** → causes flexion contracture
- Monitor for signs of **infection/DVT**
- Avoid **deep squatting, kneeling** in early recovery

Functional Milestones
- 90° flexion → chair use
- 105° → stairs
- 110°+ → cycling, low seats

Q13. Rehabilitation after total hip arthroplasty (THA)—phases and contraindications.

Source: MUHS 2021, DNB 2022

Type: Short essay

Goals
- Prevent dislocation
- Restore **hip ROM, gait, and independence**

Posterior Approach: Precautions for 6–12 weeks
Avoid:
- Hip **flexion >90°**
- **Adduction past midline**
- Internal rotation

Use abduction pillow, high toilet seats, walker

Rehabilitation Phases

Phase	*Focus*
POD 1–3	Bed mobility, ankle pumps, static quads, log rolling
Week 1–2	Assisted ambulation with walker, chair sitting
Week 3–6	Hip abduction, extension strengthening, stair practice
Week 6–12	Transition to cane, dynamic balance, endurance training
After 3 months	Return to work, driving, low-impact activities

Anterior Approach—Less risk of dislocation, faster mobilization

Q14. Write a note on rehabilitation after bipolar hemiarthroplasty.

Source: TNMGRMU 2021

Type: Short note

Population
Mostly performed in **elderly with neck of femur fractures**

Rehabilitation Focus
- Early mobilization to **reduce morbidity**
- Restore **sitting, standing, walking, toileting independence**

Protocol

Day 1–3	Ankle pumps, deep breathing, static quads/glutes
Day 4–7	Sitting in chair, walking with walker, bedside standing
Week 2–4	Gait training, hip strengthening, stair practice
Week 4–12	Endurance, balance, transition to cane if needed

Precautions (Posterior Approach)
- No hip flexion >90°, adduction, internal rotation
- High chairs, abduction pillow if needed

Q15. Outline protocol for ambulation after THA.

Source: RGUHS 2022

Type: Short note

Day-wise Ambulation Goals (Posterior Approach)

Day	*Activity*
Day 1–2	Transfer to chair, walker ambulation within room
Day 3–5	Corridor walking, sit-to-stand training
Week 2	Ambulate 50–100 m, transition to cane (as tolerated)
Week 4–6	Increase distance, start stairs, normal gait pattern
>6 weeks	Independent household ambulation, driving, etc.

Precautions
- Weight-bearing based on implant type (cemented: early WB; uncemented: partial WB)
- Avoid combined **flexion + adduction + internal rotation**

Rehabilitation After Spine Surgery and Spinal Cord Injury

Q16. Describe rehabilitation after spinal instrumentation.

Source: DNB 2021, RGUHS 2020

Type: Short essay

Goals
- Prevent complications (e.g., DVT, pulmonary issues)
- Promote **safe mobilization and spinal protection**
- Restore **functional independence**

Rehabilitation Phases

Phase	*Timeline*	*Key activities*
Acute phase	POD 0–3	Breathing exercises, ankle pumps, log rolling, TLSO if advised
Early phase	POD 3–7	Bed–chair transfers, ambulation with brace, pain management
Subacute phase	1–6 weeks	Walking, sitting tolerance, posture training, core strengthening
Reconditioning phase	6–12 weeks	Flexibility, endurance, functional tasks
Return to work phase	3+ months	Ergonomics, gradual activity resumption

Use of Orthosis
- TLSO/LSO depending on level and approach
- *Bracing duration*: Usually 6–12 weeks (as per surgeon)

Q17. Outline rehabilitation after lumbar discectomy.

Source: MUHS 2022, DNB 2020

Type: Short essay

Goals
- Reduce pain
- Protect surgical site
- Restore mobility and prevent recurrence

Phases of Rehabilitation

Timeline	*Intervention*
POD 0–2	Bed mobility, log rolling, ankle pumps, deep breathing
Week 1–2	Ambulation, core activation, gentle stretching
Week 2–6	Back extension, McKenzie exercises, pelvic tilt
Week 6–12	Core strengthening, ergonomics, activity modification
>12 weeks	Return to work/sports, posture correction

Precautions
- Avoid **bending, lifting, twisting (BLT)** for 6–8 weeks
- No prolonged sitting >30 min without break
- Proper **body mechanics training** essential

Q18. Explain rehabilitation in spinal cord injury.

Source: TNMGRMU 2021, DNB 2023

Type: Long essay

Goals
- Maximize functional independence
- *Prevent complications*: Pressure sores, DVT, contractures
- Restore ambulation (if possible)
- Psychological and vocational reintegration

Team Approach
- Orthopedic surgeon
- Physiotherapist
- Occupational therapist
- Urologist/Neurosurgeon
- Psychologist
- Social worker

Phase-wise Management

Phase	*Goals and activities*
Acute phase (0–1 week)	Spinal alignment, pressure sore prevention, bladder care
Subacute (1–6 weeks)	Passive ROM, chest physio, wheelchair training
Rehabilitation phase (6–12 weeks)	Mat training, transfer techniques, bowel/bladder management
Community phase (>3 months)	Vocational rehabilitation, home modifications, orthosis use

Orthotic Support (based on level)

Injury level	*Orthosis/Aid*
T12–L1	Reciprocating gait orthosis (RGO), KAFO
L2–L4	KAFO/AFO
Cervical/High thoracic	Wheelchair-dependent

Q19. Describe complications prevented by early spinal rehabilitation.

Source: RGUHS 2022

Type: Short note

Early rehabilitation helps prevent

1. *Pressure sores*: By repositioning and skin care
2. *Respiratory complications*: Chest physiotherapy
3. *DVT/PE*: Ankle pumps, compression devices, LMWH
4. *Urinary tract infections*: Bladder management
5. *Contractures*: Passive ROM, splinting
6. *Joint stiffness*: Mobilization
7. *Depression and isolation*: Psychological support
8. *Muscle wasting*: Isometrics, functional electrical stimulation

Q20. Describe bladder and bowel rehabilitation after spinal injury.

Source: MUHS 2021

Type: Short note

A. Bladder Rehabilitation

Management goals	*Methods*
Prevent infections	Clean intermittent catheterization (CIC)
Ensure complete emptying	Bladder training, anticholinergics
Reduce high pressures	Alpha-blockers (if detrusor-sphincter dyssynergia)
Prevent renal damage	Regular ultrasound, urodynamic studies

B. Bowel Rehabilitation

Goal	*Interventions*
Regular predictable evacuation	Timed suppositories, digital stimulation
Prevent constipation	High fiber diet, adequate hydration
Prevent accidents	Bowel routines, caregiver training

Rehabilitation After Amputation, Prosthesis Use, and Gait Training

Q21. Describe stages of rehabilitation after lower limb amputation.

Source: RGUHS 2021, DNB 2020

Type: Long essay

Stages of Rehabilitation

Stage	*Goals and activities*
Pre-operative (if elective)	Psychological preparation, patient education, strength building
Post-operative (0–3 weeks)	Pain control, wound care, edema management, positioning
Pre-prosthetic (3–6 weeks)	Shrinker application, ROM, stump shaping, mobility with walker/crutches
Prosthetic fitting (6–12 weeks)	Temporary prosthesis trial, gait training, balance training
Definitive prosthesis phase	Advanced gait training, ADLs, vocational reintegration
Long-term follow-up	Prosthesis maintenance, skin care, psychosocial support

Key Points

- Early rehabilitation **reduces phantom pain**, improves prosthetic tolerance
- Emphasis on **stump care**, **contracture prevention**, and **early mobility**

Q22. Describe the role of physiotherapy in amputee rehabilitation.

Source: MUHS 2021

Type: Short essay

Key Roles

1. *Prevention of complications*:
   - *Contractures*: Prone lying, ROM exercises
   - *Edema*: Compression bandaging/shrinkers
   - *Pressure ulcers*: Regular skin inspection
2. *Stump shaping and conditioning*:
   - Elevation and wrapping
   - Desensitization massage
   - Strengthening residual limb
3. *Gait and balance training*:
   - Use of **parallel bars → walker → cane**
   - Weight transfer exercises
   - Mirror feedback
4. *Prosthesis training*:
   - Donning/Doffing
   - Gait pattern correction
   - Obstacle navigation
5. *Psychological support*: Motivation, reintegration, peer support

Q23. Outline rehabilitation protocol following below-knee amputation.

Source: TNMGRMU 2021, DNB 2022

Type: Short essay

Key Rehabilitation Focus

- **Prevent knee flexion contracture**
- **Stump shaping** for prosthesis
- **Strengthen remaining limb**

Phase-wise Protocol

Phase	*Interventions*
Post-operative (day 1–7)	Pain control, stump elevation, isometrics, breathing exercises
Week 2–3	Shrinker bandage, passive ROM, sitting balance
Week 3–6	Strength training (quads, glutes), ambulation with walker
Week 6 onward	Temporary prosthesis trial, gait training
Long term	Vocational training, advanced mobility, endurance

Common Contracture to Avoid

- **Knee flexion** (keep knee extended in rest/splint)
- Encourage **prone lying**

Q24. Describe gait training after prosthesis fitting.

Source: RGUHS 2022

Type: Short note

Stages of Gait Training

1. *Parallel bar training*:
   - Static standing
   - Weight shifting side-to-side and forward-back
   - Short steps with mirror feedback
2. *Assistive devices*:
   - Progress from walker → cane → independent
   - Encourage symmetrical step length and cadence
3. *Surface and obstacle training*:
   - Stairs, ramps, uneven surfaces
   - Practice with socks, shoes
4. *Balance and endurance*:
   - Static/dynamic balance drills
   - Functional tasks (e.g., carrying, turning)

Training Cues

- Equal weight on both limbs
- Avoid vaulting/circumduction
- Use verbal and visual cues

Q25. Define phantom limb pain. How is it managed in rehabilitation?

Source: DNB 2021

Type: Short note

Definition

Phantom limb pain is a **painful sensation perceived in the missing limb**, usually following amputation. It is different from phantom sensation (non-painful).

Mechanism

- Peripheral nerve damage → neuroma
- Central sensitization in spinal cord and brain
- Psychological factors

Management in Rehabilitation

Type	*Examples*
Physical	Mirror therapy, massage, TENS, desensitization
Pharmacological	Gabapentin, amitriptyline, opioids
Psychological	Cognitive behavioral therapy (CBT), relaxation
Surgical (if severe)	Neuroma excision, spinal cord stimulation

Q26. Classify orthoses used in lower limb rehabilitation.

Source: RGUHS 2022, DNB 2021

Type: Short essay

Definition

An **orthosis** is an externally applied device used to **support, align, prevent or correct deformities**, or **improve function of a body segment**.

Classification by Region

Type of orthosis	*Abbreviation*	*Common use*
Foot orthosis	FO	Flat foot, plantar fasciitis
Ankle–foot orthosis	AFO	Foot drop, CP, post-polio
Knee–ankle–foot	KAFO	Quadriceps paralysis, polio, SCI
Hip–knee–ankle–foot	HKAFO	SCI, muscular dystrophy
Knee orthosis	KO	ACL injury, post-operative stabilization

Classification by Function
- *Supportive*: Foot insoles, arch supports
- *Corrective*: Clubfoot splints, Denis Browne bar
- *Protective*: Knee braces post-ACL reconstruction
- *Functional assist*: Dynamic AFOs, floor-reaction orthoses

Q27. Describe indications and functions of ankle–foot orthosis (AFO).

Source: MUHS 2021, DNB 2022

Type: Short note

Definition
Ankle-foot orthosis (AFO) is a brace worn on the lower leg and foot to control **ankle motion and position**, often made of plastic or carbon fiber.

Indications
- Foot drop (common peroneal nerve palsy)
- Post-stroke hemiparesis
- Cerebral palsy
- Post-polio residual paralysis
- SCI (incomplete paraplegia)

Functions
- Prevent **toe dragging** during swing phase
- Control **plantarflexion/knee hyperextension**
- Improve **stability during stance phase**
- Facilitate **energy-efficient gait**

Types
- *Solid AFO*: Rigid, maximum stability
- *Hinged AFO*: Allows dorsiflexion, restricts plantarflexion
- *Posterior leaf spring*: Flexible, stores kinetic energy

Q28. What is floor reaction orthosis (FRO)? When is it used?

Source: TNMGRMU 2022

Type: Short note

Definition
A **floor reaction orthosis (FRO)** is a specialized AFO that uses **ground reaction forces** to promote **knee extension during stance**.

Indications
- Quadriceps weakness (e.g., poliomyelitis)
- Crouch gait in spastic diplegia (CP)
- Mild knee instability with dorsiflexion control

Mechanism
- Anteriorly positioned shell restricts dorsiflexion
- Ground reaction force passes **anterior to knee** → promotes extension

Features
- Made of lightweight thermoplastics
- Usually custom-molded
- Used in ambulatory children or adults with weak knee extensors

Q29. Enumerate types of crutches and their gait patterns.

Source: RGUHS 2021, DNB 2020

Type: Short essay

Types of Crutches

Type	*Use case*
Axillary crutches	Short-term, non-weight-bearing injuries
Elbow crutches (Lofstrand)	Long-term use, polio, CP
Platform crutches	Wrist/hand weakness or deformity

Crutch Gait Patterns

Pattern	*Indication*
2-point gait	Partial weight-bearing; mimics natural gait
3-point gait	One leg non-weight-bearing (e.g., fracture)
4-point gait	Bilateral weakness (e.g., polio)
Swing-to gait	SCI, paraplegics with KAFO
Swing-through gait	More advanced than swing-to, faster progression

Q30. What is HKAFO? Indications and limitations.

Source: MUHS 2022, DNB 2021

Type: Short note

Definition

Hip–Knee–Ankle–Foot orthosis (HKAFO) is a long-leg orthosis that **spans from pelvis to foot**, stabilizing the hip, knee, and ankle.

Indications
- **Paraplegia** (T12–L1 level)
- **Spinal muscular atrophy**
- **Myelomeningocele**
- Post-polio patients with weak hip and knee control

Features
- Hip joint locks
- Pelvic band or waist strap
- KAFO components
- Often combined with **reciprocating gait orthosis (RGO)**

Limitations
- Bulky, energy-consuming
- Requires high motivation and training
- May not be practical for elderly or cognitively impaired

Rehabilitation in Neurological and Pediatric Orthopedic

Q31. Describe rehabilitation in cerebral palsy (CP).

Source: RGUHS 2022, DNB 2021

Type: Short essay

Goals of CP Rehabilitation
- Improve **functional mobility**
- Prevent **contractures and deformities**
- Enhance **independence in ADLs**

Multidisciplinary Approach

Team member	*Role*
Orthopedician	Corrective surgeries, bracing
Physiotherapist	Gait training, spasticity reduction
Occupational therapist	ADLs, fine motor skills
Speech therapist	Feeding, communication
Orthotist	AFOs, walkers, seating supports
Psychologist	Cognitive stimulation, family counseling

Key Components
- **Stretching and ROM** to prevent contractures
- **Strengthening** (especially trunk and proximal muscles)
- **Gait training** with orthoses (AFO, FRO)
- **Postural control** and balance training
- Use of Gross Motor Function Classification System (**GMFCS**) to track progress

Q32. Outline rehabilitation principles in poliomyelitis.

Source: MUHS 2021, DNB 2020

Type: Short essay

Overview
Polio leads to **asymmetric LMN paralysis**, commonly affecting **lower limbs** → foot drop, knee instability, limb length discrepancy.

Rehabilitation Principles

Focus area	*Rehabilitation strategy*
Weak muscles	Strengthening of residual motor units
Contractures	Stretching, splinting, corrective surgery if needed
Gait issues	Orthotic support (e.g., KAFO for knee instability)
Limb length inequality	Shoe raise, epiphysiodesis (in children)
Deformities	Serial casting, tendon transfers

Common Orthoses

- *AFO*: Foot drop
- *KAFO*: Quadriceps weakness
- *HKAFO*: Extensive limb involvement

Vocational and Community Reintegration are Essential in Adult Cases

Q33. Rehabilitation approach in Duchenne muscular dystrophy (DMD).

Source: TNMGRMU 2022

Type: Short note

Key Characteristics

- Progressive, X-linked disorder
- Proximal muscle weakness → Gower's sign
- Wheelchair-bound by adolescence

Rehabilitation Goals

- Delay contractures and scoliosis
- Preserve ambulation as long as possible
- Improve quality of life

Multimodal Plan

1. *Stretching and ROM*: To prevent Achilles, hip flexor contractures
2. *Low-resistance exercises*: Swimming, cycling
3. *Orthoses*: Night splints, ankle-foot supports
4. *Spinal support*: TLSO for scoliosis control
5. *Respiratory therapy*: Breathing exercises, cough assist
6. *Counseling and education*: For patient and family

Assistive Devices

- Power wheelchair
- Assistive communication (late stages)
- Adjustable furniture

Q34. Role of orthoses in spina bifida rehabilitation.

Source: DNB 2021

Type: Short note

Spina Bifida Overview

- Neural tube defect → lower limb weakness, deformities, bladder/bowel issues
- *Common*: **Myelomeningocele** (thoracic to sacral level involvement)

Orthoses by Lesion Level

Lesion level	*Expected motor involvement*	*Orthosis*
Thoracic	Paraplegia	HKAFO + walker/RGO
Upper lumbar	Hip/Knee weakness	KAFO + crutches
Lower lumbar	Ankle/Foot weakness	AFO
Sacral	Minimal lower limb involvement	Shoe inserts, SMO (sub-malleolar)

Goals of Orthotic Use
- Promote upright posture and walking
- Prevent deformities (e.g., clubfoot)
- Improve stability during stance

Q35. Rehabilitation strategies in pediatric osteogenesis imperfecta (OI).

Source: RGUHS 2021

Type: Short note

Key Issues in OI
- Fragile bones
- Frequent fractures
- Limb deformities
- Delayed motor milestones

Rehabilitation Principles
1. *Fracture prevention*: Caregiver training, padded environments
2. *Weight-bearing aids*: Standing frames to stimulate bone
3. *Hydrotherapy*: Low-impact strengthening
4. *Orthoses*: Prevent joint deformities (e.g., KAFO for knee valgus)
5. *Bisphosphonate therapy*: Improves bone mineral density
6. *Assistive devices*: Walkers, wheelchairs for safe mobility
7. *Parental counseling*: Realistic goals and gentle handling

Functional Outcome Measures, Pain Management, and Return-to-activity in Orthopedic Rehabilitation

Q36. Enumerate commonly used outcome measures in orthopedic rehabilitation.

Source: DNB 2022, RGUHS 2021

Type: Short essay

Importance

Outcome scores objectively assess:
- Pain
- Function
- Quality of life
- Progress during rehabilitation
- Effectiveness of surgical/rehabilitation interventions

Commonly Used Scores

Region/Condition	*Outcome score*
Hip	Harris Hip Score, Oxford Hip Score
Knee	Lysholm Score, WOMAC, KOOS
Shoulder	Constant-Murley Score, DASH
Hand/UE	DASH, PRWE (wrist), Michigan Hand Outcome
Foot/Ankle	AOFAS score, FAAM
Spine	Oswestry Disability Index, Neck Disability Index
General function/QoL	SF-36, WHO-DAS, Barthel Index

Types

- Region-specific (e.g., Harris Hip Score)
- Disease-specific (e.g., ODI for low back pain)
- Patient-reported (e.g., DASH, SF-36)

Q37. Describe pain management strategies in orthopedic rehabilitation.

Source: MUHS 2022, DNB 2021

Type: Short essay

Multimodal Pain Management

Modality	*Examples*
Pharmacological	NSAIDs, paracetamol, muscle relaxants
Topical agents	Capsaicin, diclofenac gel
Electrotherapy	TENS, IFT
Cryotherapy	Ice packs post-operative or during acute phase
Thermotherapy	Heat packs for chronic pain
Manual therapy	Soft tissue mobilization, myofascial release
Psychological	Cognitive-behavioral therapy, relaxation
Complementary	Acupuncture, yoga, mindfulness

Chronic Pain Considerations

- Avoid dependence on opioids
- Use **pain behavior modification** techniques
- Address **central sensitization** (especially post-SCI, amputation)

Q38. Explain return-to-work assessment in musculoskeletal rehabilitation .

Source: RGUHS 2022

Type: Short note

Purpose

To assess **when and how safely** a patient can **resume occupational duties**, minimizing reinjury risk and ensuring functional capacity.

Assessment Tools

Tool	*Use*
Functional capacity evaluation (FCE)	Measures lifting, standing, sitting tolerance
Ergonomic assessment	Postural and workplace stress analysis
Physical demand levels	Light/medium/heavy job categorization
Outcome scores	DASH, LEFS, SF-36

Factors Considered

- Type of work (sedentary, manual, dynamic)
- Nature of injury (acute/chronic, surgical)
- Physical capacity versus job demands
- Motivation, psychological readiness

Return-to-work planning involves

- **Workplace adaptations**
- **Graduated return** (light duty → full duty)
- **Counseling/employer liaison**

Q39. Guidelines for return to sports after ligament reconstruction.

Source: TNMGRMU 2022

Type: Short note

Return-to-sport (RTS) Criteria after ACL Reconstruction

Criteria	*Target*
Strength	≥90% quadriceps/hamstring strength of opposite limb
ROM	Full symmetrical range
Functional tests	Hop test, agility drills
Stability	Negative Lachman/pivot shift
Psychological readiness	Confidence, absence of fear
Time since surgery	Minimum 6 months (average 9–12 months for pivot sports)

Graded Return
Jogging → Running → Sport-specific drills → Competitive play

Geriatric and Community-based Rehabilitation in Orthopedics

Q40. Describe rehabilitation principles in geriatric orthopedic patients.

Source: DNB 2021, RGUHS 2020

Type: Short essay

Key Challenges in Elderly Rehabilitation
- Reduced physiological reserve
- Multiple comorbidities
- Cognitive issues (e.g., dementia)
- Polypharmacy risks
- Poor balance and fall risk

Core Principles

Focus area	*Rehabilitation strategy*
Early mobilization	Prevents DVT, pneumonia, deconditioning
Multidisciplinary care	Ortho + Physio + Geriatrician + Social worker
Pain management	Avoid narcotics; use safe analgesia
Balance and fall prevention	Gait training, grab bars, footwear advice
Nutritional support	Protein + calcium + vitamin D supplementation
Cognitive support	Orientation, family involvement, avoid restraints

Tools Used
- Timed up and go (TUG) test for balance
- Berg balance scale
- Mini mental state exam (MMSE) if cognitive decline suspected

Q41. Explain fall prevention strategies in the elderly.

Source: MUHS 2021

Type: Short note

Why It Matters?
Falls are the **leading cause of fracture-related morbidity and mortality** in older adults, especially **hip and vertebral fractures**.

Modifiable Risk Factors

Category	Examples
Intrinsic	Muscle weakness, poor vision, dizziness
Extrinsic	Slippery floors, poor lighting, clutter
Medication-related	Sedatives, antihypertensives, polypharmacy

Fall Prevention Strategies

1. *Home modifications*: Grab bars, ramps, anti-slip flooring
2. *Footwear assessment*: Non-skid, snug fit
3. *Exercise programs*: Balance and strength training (Tai Chi)
4. *Vision correction*: Regular eye checks
5. *Medication review*: Minimize CNS depressants
6. *Vitamin D and calcium*: For bone strength
7. *Assistive devices*: Canes, walkers, handrails

Q42. Describe rehabilitation approach in osteoporotic vertebral fractures.

Source: DNB 2020, RGUHS 2022

Type: Short essay

Challenges
- Pain
- Kyphosis
- Limited mobility
- Risk of future fractures

Rehabilitation Protocol

Stage	Intervention
Acute (0–2 weeks)	Analgesics, bracing (TLSO), gentle bed mobility
Subacute (2–6 weeks)	Core strengthening, postural training, pain control
Reconditioning (6–12 weeks)	Resistance bands, upright posture drills, safe walking

Other Support
- **Bisphosphonates or denosumab**
- **Calcium + Vitamin D**
- Fall prevention counseling
- Back extensor training to improve kyphosis

Bracing
TLSO (Jewett brace) for 6–8 weeks for pain control and support

Q43. What is community-based rehabilitation (CBR)? Explain its principles.

Source: TNMGRMU 2022

Type: Short essay

Definition

Community-based rehabilitation (CBR) is a strategy within general community development for **rehabilitation, equalization of opportunities, and social integration** of people with disabilities, using **locally available resources**.

Principles of CBR

Principle	*Explanation*
Inclusion	Persons with disabilities are part of mainstream society
Participation	Families and community involved in decision-making
Empowerment	Skills, education, and resources to live independently
Accessibility	Services brought close to rural/remote areas
Use of local resources	Leverages local health workers, NGOs, schools

CBR Workers

- Community health workers
- Local rehabilitation volunteers
- NGOs and social workers
- Orthopedic outreach teams

Q44. Rehabilitation plan for an elderly patient after fragility hip fracture.

Source: RGUHS 2021

Type: Short note

Immediate Post-operative Goals

- Pain control
- Early weight-bearing (if fixation allows)
- Prevent DVT, pneumonia, pressure sores

Rehabilitation Components

Domain	*Plan*
Mobility	Walker-assisted ambulation from POD-1 (if stable fixation)
Physio	ROM, strengthening, breathing exercises
Fall prevention	Home safety, balance training
Bone health	Start anti-osteoporotic therapy (bisphosphonates, vitamin D)
Nutrition	High-protein diet, monitor calcium intake
Family training	Assist with transfers, compliance, support

Disability Assessment, Certification, and Legal Aspects in Orthopedic Rehabilitation

Q45. Define locomotor disability. How is it quantified in India?

Source: DNB 2022, RGUHS 2021

Type: Short essay

Definition (as per RPWD Act, 2016)

Locomotor disability means a person's **inability to execute distinctive activities associated with movement**, due to affliction of bones, joints, muscles, or nerves.

Includes

- Amputation
- Polio
- Cerebral palsy
- Post-fracture deformities
- Muscular dystrophies
- Spinal cord injuries

Quantification in India

1. Based on **Guidelines by Government of India (Gazette Notification, June 2001)**
2. Updated as per **RPWD Act, 2016 and 2018 rules**
3. Uses a **point-based percentage system** (0–100%) based on:
   - Joint involvement
   - Range of motion
   - Muscle strength
   - Amputation level
   - Neurological level (SCI)
4. If more than one limb affected → **combined disability formula**:

$$\mathbf{a + [b \times (90 - a)/90]}$$

Certificate Issued is If

Disability ≥ 40% (benchmark disability)

Q46. Describe procedure and authorities for issuing disability certificate.

Source: TNMGRMU 2021

Type: Short note

Authorities

- Government-designated hospitals (district or tertiary)
- Certified **Medical Boards** (usually three members including orthopedic surgeon, physiatrist, and medical officer)
- Valid across India if **UDID (Unique Disability ID)** issued

Procedure

1. Application via hospital or **online UDID portal** (www.swavlambancard.gov.in)
2. Clinical and functional assessment
3. Document review (diagnostic reports, imaging)
4. Disability % calculated using **GOI guidelines**
5. Certificate issued in **Form V/VI/VII** as per RPWD rules, 2017
6. Validity:
   - *Permanent*: For non-progressive cases (e.g., amputation)
   - *Temporary*: Progressive diseases (e.g., DMD)

Benefits

- Reservation in education, jobs
- Disability pension
- Tax exemption
- Concessions in transport

Q47. How is permanent physical impairment assessed in orthopedics?

Source: MUHS 2021

Type: Short essay

Based On

- Manual for evaluation of permanent physical impairment (DGHS, Government of India, 2001)
- Used for medico-legal, compensation, insurance, pension, and benefits

Common Parameters

Injury	*Assessment method*
Joint stiffness	ROM-based % for each movement compared to normal
Muscle weakness	Based on MRC grading (Grade 0 to 5)
Amputation	Level-specific % (e.g., above knee = 70%, below = 60%)
Spinal injury	Based on neurological level and functional limitation
Deformity	Angular deformities assessed by functional loss

Combining Impairments

Use formula:

$$\mathbf{a + [b \times (90 - a)/90]}$$

Where:

- a = higher %
- b = lower %

Ensures total never exceeds 100%

Q48. Write a note on role of orthopedic surgeon in disability management.

Source: DNB 2021

Type: Short note

Roles Include

1. **Diagnosis** and documentation of impairments
2. **Assessment of disability %** using standard guidelines
3. **Certification** and coordination with board
4. **Prescribing orthoses/prostheses**
5. **Surgical correction** where possible (e.g., tendon transfers, deformity correction)
6. **Rehabilitation referral** (physiotherapy, vocational training)
7. **Legal and ethical reporting** in injury, medico-legal cases

Q49. What is the significance of benchmark disability in India?

Source: RGUHS 2022

Type: Short note

Definition (as per RPWD Act, 2016)

Benchmark disability means disability of **40% or more**, as certified by the competent authority.

Significance

Persons with benchmark disability are **eligible for**:

- Reservation in jobs and education
- Concessions in public transport
- Income tax deduction (Section 80U)
- Govt schemes (e.g., Deendayal Disabled Rehabilitation Scheme)
- Free assistive devices (ADIP scheme)

Summary Table: Disability in Ortho Rehabilitation

Aspect	*Key points*
Legal framework	RPWD Act 2016, GOI guidelines 2001 (updated 2018)
Certification body	Govt Medical Board, UDID portal
Threshold (benchmark)	≥40% disability
Assessment tools	ROM, muscle power, amputation charts
Combined disability	a + [b × (90 – a)/90]
Surgeon's role	Certify, rehabilitate, refer, support access to entitlements

CHAPTER 19

Biomaterials and Bone Healing in Orthopedics

Irfan Andleeb Gul, Aakash Deep, Kanav Mahajan

Q1. Define biomaterials. Classify and describe their ideal properties.

Source: DNB 2021, RGUHS 2020
Type: Long essay

Definition of Biomaterial

A **biomaterial** is any **natural or synthetic material** used to **replace, augment, or repair** a tissue or function in the human body, without causing harm or rejection.

In orthopedics, biomaterials are widely used in **implants, joint replacements, fracture fixation devices, bone graft substitutes**, and **spacers**.

Classification of Biomaterials

Category	*Examples*
Metallic	Stainless steel, titanium alloys, cobalt–chrome
Ceramics	Alumina, zirconia, hydroxyapatite
Polymers	PMMA, UHMWPE, silicone
Composite	Carbon fiber-reinforced polymers
Biological	Bone grafts, collagen, cartilage
Biodegradable	PLA, PGA, bioresorbable screws

Ideal Properties of Biomaterials (Orthopedic Focus)

- *Mechanical*:
  - High **strength-to-weight ratio**
  - **Elastic modulus** matching host tissue (e.g., cortical bone = 10–20 GPa)
  - Good **fatigue and wear resistance**
- *Biological*:
  - *Biocompatibility*: Should not induce immune reaction
  - *Bioinert/Bioactive*: Inert in body or promote osseointegration
  - **Corrosion resistance** in physiological environment
- *Chemical*:
  - Non-toxic degradation products
  - **Sterilizability** without degradation
- *Surgical/Handling:*
  - Machinable, moldable
  - Radiolucent (for polymers/ceramics) or radiopaque (metals)

Q2. Classify biomaterials used in orthopedics.

Source: MUHS 2021, TNMGRMU 2022
Type: Short Essay

A. Based on Composition

Category	*Examples*
Metals	Stainless steel (316L), Titanium alloys, Cobalt–chrome
Ceramics	Alumina, Zirconia, Hydroxyapatite
Polymers	PMMA, UHMWPE, Silicone
Composites	Carbon fiber–reinforced polymers
Biologics	Bone, cartilage, collagen scaffolds
Biodegradable	PLA, PGA, bioresorbable screws

B. Based on Interaction with Tissue

Type	*Definition*	*Examples*
Bioinert	No interaction with tissue	Titanium, UHMWPE
Bioactive	Bonds with tissue	Hydroxyapatite
Bioresorbable	Degraded and replaced by tissue	PLA screws, collagen

C. Based on Application in Orthopedics

Application	*Material used*
Joint replacement	Titanium alloy, cobalt–chrome, UHMWPE
Fracture fixation	Stainless steel plates, screws
Bone graft substitute	Ceramic blocks, bioactive glass
Cement and spacers	PMMA with antibiotics

Q3. Describe various metallic biomaterials used in orthopedics.

Source: DNB 2022, RGUHS 2023
Type: Short essay

Importance

Metallic biomaterials are widely used in **load-bearing orthopedic applications** due to their **strength, durability, and machinability**.

Key Metallic Biomaterials

Material	*Properties*	*Applications*
Stainless steel (316L)	Corrosion-resistant, inexpensive, high strength	Plates, nails, screws
Titanium and alloys	Light, biocompatible, osseointegrative, corrosion-resistant	THA stems, spinal implants
Cobalt–chrome alloy	Very hard, wear-resistant, corrosion-resistant	Femoral heads in THA/TKA
Tantalum	Highly porous, promotes bone ingrowth	Porous acetabular cups, bone graft substitutes

Issues with Metals

- Corrosion (especially in modular implants)
- Stress shielding due to high stiffness (especially Cobalt–chrome)
- Metal sensitivity (Nickel in SS, cobalt allergy)

Q4. Discuss UHMWPE—properties, uses, and complications.

Source: MUHS 2022, DNB 2021
Type: Short note

Full Form
UHMWPE: Ultra-high molecular weight polyethylene
A commonly used **polymeric biomaterial** in **arthroplasty bearings**.

Properties
- High wear resistance
- Low friction coefficient
- Good biocompatibility
- Easily moldable
- Radiolucent

Uses
- **Acetabular liners** in THA
- **Tibial inserts** in TKA
- **Spacers** in infected joint revisions
- **Prosthetic intervertebral discs**

Complications
- **Wear debris** generation → osteolysis
- **Creep deformation** (under constant stress)
- **Oxidation** after gamma sterilization
- **Delamination** with long-term use

Q5. Write a note on ceramics in orthopedics.

Source: RGUHS 2022, DNB 2020
Type: Short Essay

Definition
Ceramics are **inorganic, non-metallic materials** that are **hard, wear-resistant**, and often **bioinert or bioactive**.

Common Ceramics in Orthopedics

Material	*Type*	*Applications*
Alumina (Al_2O_3)	Bioinert	Femoral heads, dental implants
Zirconia (ZrO_2)	Bioinert	Femoral heads
Hydroxyapatite (HA)	Bioactive	Coating for implants, bone grafts
Bio-glass	Bioactive	Bone graft substitute, cranial implants

Advantages
- High compressive strength
- Good wear resistance
- Promote bone ingrowth (for bioactive types)
- *Inert*: Low immune reaction

Limitations
- *Brittle*: Can fracture under tensile stress
- Difficult to machine or customize
- Expensive

Bone Grafts and Substitutes in Orthopedics

Q6. Classify bone grafts and substitutes. Describe uses of autograft and allograft.

Source: RGUHS 2021, DNB 2022
Type: Long essay

Classification of Bone Grafts

- *Based on source:*

Type	*Definition*	*Example*
Autograft	From same individual	Iliac crest, fibula
Allograft	From another human donor	Femoral head, freeze-dried bone
Xenograft	From other species	Bovine bone
Synthetic	Man-made substitutes	Hydroxyapatite, β-TCP, bioglass

- *Based on functionality:*

Property	*Definition*
Osteogenesis	Provides living osteoblasts (autograft only)
Osteoinduction	Induces differentiation of stem cells to bone
Osteoconduction	Provides scaffold for new bone

Uses of Bone Grafts

- *Autografts (gold standard):*
  - Spine fusion
  - Non-unions
  - Bone defects after tumor curettage
  - Arthrodesis procedures

Advantages: Osteogenic, osteoinductive, osteoconductive
Drawbacks: Limited quantity, donor site morbidity (e.g., iliac crest pain):

- *Allografts:*
  - Large structural defects
  - Revision arthroplasty (e.g., femoral head graft)
  - Tumor resections

Advantages: Abundant, no donor site issues
Drawbacks: No osteogenesis, risk of disease transmission, immune response

Q7. Classify bone grafts. Discuss osteoconduction versus osteoinduction.

Source: MUHS 2021
Type: Short essay

Refer to Q7 for Classification.

Compare: Osteoconduction versus Osteoinduction

Property	*Osteoconduction*	*Osteoinduction*
Definition	Passive scaffold for bone in-growth	Active recruitment of host stem cells to form bone
Mechanism	Bone grows along graft surface	Growth factors stimulate differentiation
Materials	Hydroxyapatite, β-TCP, coral	DBM, BMPs
Clinical role	Fills defects	Stimulates healing in non-union, spinal fusion

Q8. Write a note on synthetic bone graft substitutes.

Source: TNMGRMU 2020, DNB 2023
Type: Short essay

Definition
Synthetic bone graft substitutes are **engineered materials** that **mimic bone matrix** and serve as **osteoconductive scaffolds**.

Types of Synthetic Substitutes

Type	*Examples*
Ceramics	Hydroxyapatite, β-TCP, calcium sulfate
Composites	HA + collagen, HA + PLA
Bioactive glass	Silicate-based materials
Polymers	PLGA, PMMA (space filling only)

Properties
- Osteoconductive
- Bioresorbable (e.g., β-TCP) or bioinert
- Moldable into putty, blocks, or granules

Indications
- Filling bone voids after trauma or tumor
- Spinal fusion
- Non-unions or pseudoarthrosis

Limitations
- Lack of osteoinductive or osteogenic capacity
- Brittle (especially ceramics)
- Slower integration compared to autograft

Q9. What are bone graft substitutes? Classify them with examples.

Source: RGUHS 2021, TNMGRMU 2022
Type: Short essay

Definition
Bone graft substitutes are **synthetic or biological materials** used to **replace or augment bone**, especially in defects or non-unions.

Classification

Type	*Examples*	*Properties*
Ceramics	Hydroxyapatite, β-TCP	Osteoconductive
Polymers	PMMA, polylactic acid	Scaffold, drug delivery
Bioactive glasses	Bioglass	Osteoconductive + stimulatory
Growth factor-based	BMPs (e.g., BMP-2, BMP-7)	Osteoinductive
Demineralized bone matrix (DBM)	Commercial DBM gels	Osteoinductive (some forms)

Ideal Properties
- Osteoconductive scaffold
- Osteoinductive potential
- Biocompatible and biodegradable
- Mechanical support (if needed)

Q10. What are bone morphogenetic proteins (BMPs)? Mention their use in orthopedics.

Source: DNB 2021
Type: Short note

Definition
BMPs are a group of **growth factors from the TGF-β family** that stimulate **mesenchymal cell differentiation into osteoblasts**, promoting bone formation.

BMP-2 and BMP-7 (OP-1)
Most commonly used in orthopedics.

Uses
- Spinal fusion (e.g., ALIF)
- Non-unions
- Large bone defects
- Open tibial fractures (INFUSE® system)

Advantages
- Eliminates need for autograft
- Promotes faster bone healing
- Useful in compromised biology

Limitations
- High cost
- Risk of ectopic bone formation
- Controversies in spinal use (e.g., swelling, inflammation)

Q11. What is calcium phosphate cement (CPC)? Write its orthopedic applications.

Source: MUHS 2022
Type: Short note

Definition
CPC is a **biocompatible, injectable bone substitute** made of **calcium phosphate**, which hardens in vivo and integrates with bone.

Properties
- Osteoconductive
- Injectable and moldable
- Sets at body temperature
- Resorbable over months
- Radiopaque

Applications
- Filling metaphyseal voids (e.g., tibial plateau fractures)
- Spine surgery (vertebroplasty)
- Benign bone tumor curettage cavities
- Osteoporotic fracture augmentation

Advantages
- Easy to handle
- Good mechanical strength
- Avoids donor site morbidity

Q12. What is DBM? Write its composition and role in bone healing.

Source: MUHS 2022, RGUHS 2020
Type: Short note

DBM—Demineralized Bone Matrix
Allograft bone processed to remove mineral content, **retaining collagen and growth factors** like BMPs.

Composition
- **Type I collagen**
- **Non-collagenous proteins**
- *Growth factors:* BMPs, TGF-β, IGFs
- No viable osteoblasts (no osteogenesis)

Properties
- **Osteoinductive** (due to BMPs)
- Weakly osteoconductive
- Available as powder, putty, sheets

Indications in Orthopedics
- Spinal fusion
- Non-unions
- Filling cystic defects or cavities
- Revision arthroplasty

Summary Table: Bone Graft Types and Properties

Type	*Source*	*Osteogenesis*	*Osteoinduction*	*Osteoconduction*
Autograft	Same patient	✓	✓	✓
Allograft	Donor	✗	✗/✓	✓
DBM	Processed bone	✗	✓	Slight
Synthetic (HA)	Lab-made	✗	✗	✓
BMPs	Recombinant	✗	✓✓	✗

Implant–Tissue Interaction, Bioengineering, and Surface Phenomena

Q13. Describe host response to orthopedic implants.

Source: RGUHS 2021
Type: Short essay

Phases of Host Response to Implants
1. *Immediate (minutes to hours):*
   - Protein adsorption (fibrinogen, albumin) on implant surface
   - Neutrophils recruited
2. *Acute inflammatory phase (hours to days):*
   - Macrophages, monocytes accumulate
   - Cytokine release begins
3. *Chronic inflammation (days to weeks):*
   - Foreign body giant cells may form
   - Fibrous encapsulation may begin

4. *Tissue remodeling:*
    - **Osseointegration** (desired), or
    - **Fibrous encapsulation** (undesired)

Outcomes

Favorable	*Unfavorable*
Osseointegration (e.g., titanium implants)	Fibrous tissue interface (e.g., poor fixation)
Bone ongrowth or ingrowth	Chronic inflammation or foreign body response

Conclusion

The host response depends on **implant material**, **surface properties**, **sterility**, and **surgical technique**. Ideal implants promote **biocompatible integration** with minimal immune response.

Q14. Define biofilm. Explain its significance in implant infections.

Source: DNB 2022, MUHS 2021
Type: Short essay

Definition

A **biofilm** is a **structured community of microorganisms** encased in a **self-produced polymeric matrix** adhering to surfaces such as orthopedic implants.

Key Features

- Begins with **bacterial adhesion** (within hours of contamination)
- Organisms like *Staphylococcus aureus, epidermidis* commonly involved
- Biofilm protects bacteria from **host immune response** and **antibiotics**

Consequences in Orthopedics

Challenge	*Implication*
Antibiotic resistance	Organisms in biofilm up to 1,000× more resistant
Recurrent infections	Persistent low-grade infection even after debridement
Implant loosening	Due to chronic inflammation

Management

- **Implant removal** often required
- **Prolonged antibiotics (6–12 weeks)**
- Use of **antibiotic-loaded cement/spacers**
- *Prevention is key*: Aseptic technique, short or time, prophylactic antibiotics

Q15. Describe stress shielding and its role in implant loosening.

Source: RGUHS 2022, DNB 2021
Type: Short note

Definition

Stress shielding occurs when an implant **bears more load than the adjacent bone**, leading to **bone resorption due to disuse**.

Mechanism

- According to **Wolff's Law**, bone remodels in response to stress
- Implants (especially **stiff metals** like cobalt–chrome) shield bone from stress
- Results in **thinning and weakening of adjacent bone**

Sites commonly affected

- **Proximal femur** after cementless THA
- **Tibial plateau** under metal baseplate in TKA

Implications

- **Aseptic loosening**
- Periprosthetic fractures
- Reduced implant longevity

Solutions

- Use of **lower modulus materials** (e.g., titanium instead of stainless steel)
- **Porous coating** to enhance load transfer and bone ingrowth
- Modular stems with varying stiffness

Q16. Explain corrosion of orthopedic implants and its prevention.

Source: TNMGRMU 2022, DNB 2020
Type: Short note

Definition
Corrosion is the **electrochemical degradation** of metals in the body's **physiological (saline) environment**.

Types of Corrosion

Type	*Description*
Pitting	Localized corrosion in protective oxide layer
Crevice	Occurs in narrow spaces (e.g., under screws)
Fretting	From micromotion between implant components
Galvanic	Between dissimilar metals in contact

Consequences

- Metal ion release → **local inflammation or hypersensitivity**
- Surface roughness → **reduced fatigue strength**
- **Implant loosening or breakage**

Prevention

- *Use corrosion-resistant alloys:* Titanium, Co–Cr
- **Avoid mixing dissimilar metals**
- **Polished surfaces** to reduce crevices
- *Passivation:* Formation of stable oxide layer

Q17. What is galvanic corrosion?

Source: MUHS 2020
Type: Short note

Definition
Galvanic corrosion occurs when **two dissimilar metals** are in electrical contact within an **electrolytic (saline) environment**, like the human body.

Mechanism

- The **more active metal** (anode) corrodes preferentially
- The **noble metal** (cathode) is protected

Example in Orthopedics

- **Titanium femoral stem + cobalt–chrome head**
- **Stainless steel screw + titanium plate**

Consequences

- Accelerated corrosion
- **Implant failure** due to weakened interfaces
- Increased **metal ion release**

Prevention

- Avoid dissimilar metals in the same implant
- Use **coated interfaces**
- Prefer **modular systems made of same alloy**

Summary Table: Surface-related Complications and Phenomena

Phenomenon	*Cause*	*Consequence*	*Prevention*
Biofilm	Bacterial colonization	Persistent infection	Asepsis, early antibiotics
Stress shielding	Rigid implants reduce bone loading	Bone loss, loosening	Lower modulus materials (e.g., titanium)
Corrosion	Electrochemical breakdown	Metal ion release, breakage	Alloy selection, polishing, passivation
Galvanic corrosion	Dissimilar metals in contact	Accelerated corrosion	Use of single-metal systems or insulation

Tissue Engineering, Growth Factors, and Bone Biology in Orthopedics

Q18. What is tissue engineering? Describe its role in bone healing.

Source: DNB 2021, RGUHS 2020
Type: Short essay

Definition

Tissue engineering is an interdisciplinary field that combines **cells**, **biomaterials**, and **biological signals** to create or regenerate **functional tissues** to replace damaged or lost structures.

Key components

1. *Cells*: For example, mesenchymal stem cells (MSCs)
2. *Scaffolds:* For example, hydroxyapatite, collagen, PLGA
3. *Signaling molecules:* For example, BMPs, VEGF
4. *Mechanical stimulation:* For example, loading in bioreactors

Role in Bone Healing

Mechanism	*Effect*
Scaffold provides osteoconduction	Framework for new bone to grow
Growth factors (BMPs)	Stimulate osteoinduction
Stem cells	Differentiate into osteoblasts (osteogenesis)
Bioactive environment	Promotes vascularization and remodeling

Clinical Applications

- Segmental bone defects
- Large post-tumor resection voids
- Spinal fusion
- Trauma non-unions
- Customized implants with cell-seeded scaffolds

Q19. Describe osteoconduction, osteoinduction, and osteogenesis.

Source: MUHS 2022, TNMGRMU 2021
Type: Short essay

Definitions

Term	*Definition*
Osteoconduction	Passive scaffold allowing bone growth along surface
Osteoinduction	Active recruitment and differentiation of stem cells into osteoblasts
Osteogenesis	Formation of new bone by living cells present in the graft (only in autograft)

Examples:

Property	*Materials*
Osteoconduction	Hydroxyapatite, β-TCP, coral, allograft matrix
Osteoinduction	BMPs, demineralized bone matrix (DBM)
Osteogenesis	Autogenous cancellous graft (e.g., iliac crest)

Clinical significance

- Ideal bone graft substitute should have **all three properties**
- Most synthetic materials only offer **osteoconduction**
- Combining materials (e.g., scaffold + BMP + cells) enhances results

Q20. Enumerate growth factors involved in bone healing.

Source: DNB 2023, MUHS 2020
Type: Short note

Key Growth Factors in Bone Healing

Growth factor	*Role*
BMPs (2, 4, 7)	Induce mesenchymal cell differentiation into osteoblasts
TGF-β	Stimulates matrix production, inhibits osteoclasts
VEGF	Promotes angiogenesis (vessel growth)
IGF-1 and 2	Stimulate osteoblast proliferation
FGF	Enhances angiogenesis and fibroblast activity
PDGF	Attracts fibroblasts, enhances collagen formation

Application

- Used in **orthobiologics**, bone substitutes, and **tissue engineering scaffolds**
- Applied locally in **non-unions**, **spinal fusions**, and **joint reconstructions**

Q21. Role of mesenchymal stem cells (MSCs) in fracture healing.

Source: RGUHS 2022, DNB 2021
Type: Short essay

Definition

Mesenchymal stem cells (MSCs) are multipotent stromal cells capable of differentiating into **osteoblasts, chondrocytes, and fibroblasts**.

Sources of MSCs

- Bone marrow (most common)
- Adipose tissue

- Periosteum
- Umbilical cord
- Synovium

Mechanism in Fracture Healing

Stage	Role of MSCs
Inflammatory phase	Recruited by cytokines (e.g., IL-1, TNF-α)
Reparative phase	Differentiate into chondrocytes and osteoblasts
Remodeling phase	Aid in restoring mature lamellar bone

Clinical Applications
- MSCs used in **injectables for non-unions**
- **Loaded on scaffolds** for bone defect repair
- Potential use in **osteonecrosis, cartilage repair, and tendon healing**

Challenges
- Harvesting and expansion
- Regulatory approval for clinical use
- Cost and long-term outcome data

Summary Table: Bone Healing Biology and Tissue Engineering

Factor	Function in healing	Example in practice
BMPs	Induce osteoblast differentiation	BMP-2 in spinal fusion
DBM	Osteoinductive matrix	Used in non-unions and bone defects
MSCs	Osteogenesis via stem cell differentiation	MSC + scaffold in segmental bone loss
Scaffold (e.g., HA)	Osteoconductive structure	Bone void fillers
VEGF	Angiogenesis, vascular supply	Used in tissue-engineered constructs

CHAPTER 20

Recent Advances in Orthopedics

Ashish Jaiman, Harsh Chauhan, Sukhil Raina

Implants, Fixation Techniques, and Materials

Q1. What are bioabsorbable implants? Mention indications and limitations.

Source: DNB 2022, TNMGRMU 2021

Type: Short Note

Definition

Bioabsorbable implants are made of **polymers (e.g., PGA, PLA, PDS)** that gradually degrade in the body and are **replaced by tissue over time**.

Indications

- **Pediatric fractures** (avoiding second surgery)
- Small bone fixation (hand, foot)
- Ligament reconstruction (interference screws in ACL)
- Maxillofacial surgery
- *Arthroscopy*: **Meniscal arrows**, suture anchors

Advantages

- Avoids second surgery
- Biocompatible
- Minimal imaging interference (MRI-safe)

Limitations

- Low mechanical strength
- Foreign body reaction
- Expensive
- May degrade unpredictably in some cases

Q2. Describe features and benefits of titanium implants.

Source: MUHS 2022

Type: Short Note

Material Properties

- **Lightweight** (density ~4.5 g/cm^3)
- **High strength-to-weight ratio**

- Excellent **biocompatibility**
- **Corrosion resistant**
- MRI-compatible

Orthopedic Applications
- Plates, screws, intramedullary nails
- Spinal instrumentation
- Dental and maxillofacial implants
- Uncemented prosthesis stems (THA, TKA)

Advantages
- Promotes **osseointegration** (due to oxide layer)
- Less stress shielding (lower modulus than stainless steel)
- Hypoallergenic (safer for patients with nickel allergy)

Limitations
- Costlier than stainless steel
- More elastic (not always ideal in high load-bearing applications)

Q3. Write a note on hydroxyapatite (HA) coating in orthopedic implants.

Source: RGUHS 2021

Type: Short Note

Definition
Hydroxyapatite is a **bioactive ceramic** [$Ca_{10}(PO_4)_6(OH)_2$], chemically similar to bone mineral, used to **coat implants** to promote **osseointegration.**

Use in Orthopedics
- Coated on **uncemented THA stems and cups**
- **Dental implants**
- **Screw augmentation** in osteoporotic bone
- Coating on porous metal implants

Advantages
- Faster and stronger bone ingrowth
- Shortens **time to biological fixation**
- Enhanced bond between implant and bone

Limitations
- High cost
- Debonding risk over long term
- Degrades in acidic environment (infections)

Q4. What are antibiotic-coated orthopedic implants? Indications.

Source: DNB 2021

Type: Short Note

Definition
These are **implants coated with antibiotics (e.g., gentamicin, vancomycin)**, which elute the drug locally to reduce **post-operative infection risk.**

Examples
- **Gentamicin-coated tibial nails**
- PMMA cement-coated rods for temporary fixation
- Silver-coated mega-prosthesis (oncology)

Indications
- Open fractures (e.g., Gustilo and Anderson III)
- Revision surgery with infection history
- Immunocompromised patients
- Megaprostheses in tumor surgery
- Temporary spacers in 2-stage revisions

Advantages
- High local concentration of antibiotics
- Minimal systemic side effects
- Effective against **biofilm formation**

Limitations
- Drug-specific toxicity
- May delay bone healing (with silver or high antibiotic dose)
- Limited to specific bacteria

Joint Preservation, Biologics, and Regenerative Therapies

Q5. What is autologous chondrocyte implantation (ACI)? Mention indications and steps.

Source: DNB 2022, RGUHS 2021

Type: Short Essay

Definition
Autologous chondrocyte implantation (ACI) is a **two-stage surgical technique** that involves harvesting **autologous chondrocytes**, culturing them in a lab, and then re-implanting them into a cartilage defect to regenerate **hyaline-like cartilage**.

Indications
- Isolated full-thickness cartilage defects
- *Size*: 2–10 cm^2
- Age < 50 years
- High-demand patients with no OA

Steps
- *Stage 1*: Arthroscopy to harvest cartilage from non-weight-bearing area (intercondylar notch)
- Chondrocytes cultured in lab (~4–6 weeks)
- *Stage 2*: Re-implantation of cells under a periosteal flap or collagen membrane into the defect site

Generations
- *1st generation*: Cells under periosteal patch
- *2nd generation*: Collagen-covered (MACI)
- *3rd generation*: Matrix-associated ACI (cells pre-seeded in scaffold)

Q6. Write a note on platelet-rich plasma (PRP) in orthopedics.

Source: TNMGRMU 2021, DNB 2020

Type: Short Note

Definition

Platelet-rich plasma (PRP) is a concentration of platelets **derived from autologous blood**, rich in **growth factors** like PDGF, TGF-β, VEGF, IGF, etc., used to **promote tissue healing**.

Mechanism

Stimulates:

- Angiogenesis
- Cell proliferation
- Collagen synthesis
- Cartilage matrix regeneration

Orthopedic Uses

Indication	***Benefit***
Early knee OA	Pain relief, functional improvement
Tendinopathies (e.g., tennis elbow, plantar fasciitis)	Tissue healing
Muscle injuries	Faster recovery
Non-unions/fracture healing	Enhanced callus formation
Arthroscopic augmentation	Meniscus and rotator cuff repair

Limitations

- Mixed evidence in meta-analyses
- Short-term benefit in OA
- Operator-dependent
- No standard protocol for preparation

Q7. Discuss stem cell therapy in orthopedics—types, indications, and challenges.

Source: RGUHS 2022, DNB 2021

Type: Short Essay

Types of Stem Cells

Type	***Source***
Mesenchymal (MSC)	Bone marrow, adipose tissue
Hematopoietic	Bone marrow
Amniotic	Placenta, umbilical cord
iPSC (induced)	Lab-generated from adult cells

Orthopedic Indications

- Osteoarthritis
- Avascular necrosis (early stages)
- Tendon/ligament repair (e.g., rotator cuff)
- Cartilage regeneration
- Bone defects/non-unions

Challenges

- Regulatory issues (ICMR, FDA approvals)
- Expensive and logistically demanding

- Risk of tumorigenesis [in induced pluri-potent stem cell (iPSC)]
- No long-term data for most indications

Q8. Matrix-induced chondrogenesis—principle and applications.

Source: MUHS 2022

Type: Short Note

Definition

Matrix-induced autologous chondrogenesis (AMIC) combines **microfracture with collagen scaffold** to **stimulate cartilage regeneration**.

Steps

1. Debridement of cartilage defect
2. Microfracture to expose bone marrow
3. Collagen scaffold applied (e.g., Chondro-Gide®)
4. Fibrin glue seals construct

Applications

- Focal chondral defects (e.g., femoral condyle)
- Alternative to ACI in settings where cell culture is not feasible

Advantages

- Single-stage procedure
- No lab/culture requirement
- Less expensive than ACI

Limitations

- Smaller defect size only
- Fibrocartilage > hyaline cartilage
- Long-term durability under study

Q9. What is gene therapy in orthopedics? Mention potential applications.

Source: DNB 2021

Type: Short Note

Definition

Gene therapy introduces **genetic material (DNA/RNA)** into cells to **modulate or correct disease processes**.

Types

- *In vivo*: Direct injection of gene vectors
- *Ex vivo*: Cells modified in lab and re-injected

Vectors Used

- Viral (adenovirus, retrovirus)
- Non-viral (liposomes, plasmids)

Applications in Orthopedics (Experimental/Research)

Condition	*Gene targeted*
OA	Anti-inflammatory cytokines (IL-1Ra, TNF-α blockers)
Fracture healing	*BMPs*, *VEGF* genes
Tendon/ligament repair	Collagen synthesis genes
AVN/Bone defects	Runx2, osteocalcin genes

Challenges
- Safety and ethical concerns
- Limited clinical trials
- Cost and regulation barriers

Summary Table: Joint Preservation and Biologics

Technique	*Use*	*Stage of use*
ACI/MACI	Full-thickness cartilage defects	Clinical (early-mid OA)
PRP	OA, tendinopathy, muscle injury	Clinical, outpatient use
Stem cells (MSC)	OA, AVN, cartilage/bone healing	Investigational/clinical
AMIC	Microfracture + matrix (cartilage defect)	Clinical (cost-effective)
Gene therapy	OA, AVN, bone healing	Preclinical/limited trials

Navigation, Robotics, and Smart Technologies

Q10. Define computer-assisted orthopedic surgery (CAOS). What are its advantages?

Source: RGUHS 2022, DNB 2021

Type: Short Essay

Definition
Computer-assisted orthopedic surgery (CAOS) refers to the use of **real-time computer systems, sensors, and imaging** to guide and enhance **precision in bone and joint surgeries**.

Components of CAOS
- Optical trackers (infrared cameras)
- Navigated tools/instruments
- Reference arrays fixed to bone
- Real-time 3D visualization on a screen
- Software for planning and guidance

Applications
- Total knee and hip arthroplasty
- High tibial osteotomy
- Spinal instrumentation
- Deformity correction
- Tumor surgery (resection margins)

Advantages
- Precise component alignment
- Minimizes outliers in TKA/THA
- Improves ligament balancing
- Reduced soft tissue dissection
- Better reproducibility

Q11. What is robotic-assisted surgery in orthopedics? Advantages and limitations.

Source: DNB 2022, TNMGRMU 2021

Type: Short Essay

Definition
Robotic-assisted surgery uses a **robotic arm or platform**, integrated with imaging and navigation systems, to help perform **precise bone preparation and implant positioning**.

Types of Robotic Systems

Type	*Function*
Passive	Guidance only (surgeon operates fully)
Semi-active	Surgeon operates with robot feedback
Active	Robot executes with pre-set parameters

Popular Systems
- MAKO (Stryker)
- ROSA (Zimmer-Biomet)
- NAVIO/CORI (Smith and Nephew)

Advantages
- High accuracy of bone cuts
- Consistent implant alignment
- Reduced soft tissue damage
- May reduce early revision rates
- Individualized surgical planning

Limitations
- High cost (setup and disposables)
- Longer operative time (learning curve)
- Not suitable for severe deformities or infection
- Technical issues → intraoperative delays

Q12. Short note on 3D printing in orthopedics.

Source: RGUHS 2021, DNB 2020

Type: Short Note

Definition
3D printing (additive manufacturing) involves **layer-by-layer fabrication of objects** from a digital model, used to create **implants, guides, and models** in orthopedics.

Applications

Use	*Examples*
Pre-operative planning	Patient-specific bone models for complex trauma
Custom implants	Pelvic/acetabular recon, revision THA
Cutting guides	Patient-specific jigs for osteotomy
Education	Training models for residents/students

Materials Used
- Titanium alloys
- PEEK
- Polylactic acid (PLA) for models

Advantages
- Customization for unique anatomy
- Reduced intra-operative time in complex surgeries
- Enhances surgical precision
- Helps in patient counseling and simulation

Limitations
- Time and cost-intensive
- Regulatory and sterilization issues
- Requires imaging + computer aided design (CAD) expertise

Q13. What are smart implants? Mention potential benefits.

Source: DNB 2022

Type: Short Note

Definition

Smart implants are those embedded with **sensors or electronics** that can monitor parameters like **load, strain, temperature, or infection markers** in real time.

Examples

- Sensor-enabled TKA implants (e.g., Persona IQ®)
- Instrumented spinal rods (monitor fusion load)
- Pressure-sensing insoles for gait training
- Temperature-sensing implants for infection detection

Benefits

- Real-time feedback on implant performance
- Early detection of loosening or infection
- Tailored rehabilitation protocols
- Patient engagement and remote monitoring

Challenges

- Cost and power source issues
- Long-term biocompatibility
- Data integration and privacy concerns

Q14. Virtual reality (VR) and augmented reality (AR) in orthopedic training and surgery.

Source: MUHS 2022

Type: Short Note

Definitions

Virtual reality (VR)	Fully immersive environment (simulated surgeries/training)
Augmented reality (AR)	Overlays digital images on real-world surgical field

Applications in Orthopedics

- Resident training modules (fracture fixation simulation)
- Preoperative rehearsal of complex surgeries
- AR-assisted navigation during joint replacements
- Remote surgical mentoring

Benefits

- Enhanced understanding of 3D anatomy
- Reduces learning curve for residents
- Improves surgical precision in real-time
- Useful in low-resource or training centers

Limitations

- Expensive hardware/software
- Technical complexity
- Not yet mainstream in live surgery

Summary Table: Smart Technologies in Orthopedics

Technology	*Application*	*Key benefit*
Computer navigation	Arthroplasty, deformity correction	Alignment accuracy
Robotics	TKA, THA, spinal surgery	Personalized precision
3D printing	Models, custom implants, guides	Patient-specific, surgical planning
Smart implants	TKA, spine, infection detection	Real-time feedback, early failure detection
VR/AR	Education, simulation, live assistance	Safer training, enhanced intra-operative visualization

Trauma Fixation, Fracture Healing, and Bone Substitutes

Q15. What is minimally invasive percutaneous plate osteosynthesis (MIPPO)? Describe principles and advantages.

Source: RGUHS 2022, DNB 2021

Type: Short Essay

Definition

Minimally invasive percutaneous plate osteosynthesis (MIPPO) is a technique of fracture fixation where plates are inserted **through small incisions without exposing the fracture site**, preserving **soft tissue and fracture hematoma**.

Principles of MIPPO

- Indirect fracture reduction
- Bridge plating across fracture site
- Soft tissue and periosteum preservation
- Use of pre-contoured locking plates
- Fluoroscopic guidance

Advantages

Biological	*Mechanical*
Preserves blood supply	Strong bridging fixation
Promotes callus formation	Less implant stress (load sharing)
Reduces infection risk	Maintains bone length and alignment

Common Sites

- Distal femur
- Proximal and distal tibia
- Humerus (anterolateral approach)

Q16. Explain the concept of biological osteosynthesis.

Source: DNB 2022, MUHS 2021

Type: Short Note

Definition

Biological osteosynthesis emphasizes **preservation of the natural biology** (blood supply, soft tissues, fracture hematoma) to facilitate **natural healing**.

Core Concepts
- Limited periosteal stripping
- Indirect fracture reduction
- Stable fixation without rigid compression
- Use of bridging plates or intramedullary nails
- Avoidance of excessive hardware or exposure

Techniques Used
- MIPPO
- External fixators (especially in open fractures)
- Elastic IM nailing (pediatric)

Benefits
- Enhanced callus formation
- Reduced infection and non-union risk
- Faster rehabilitation

Spine Surgery, Tumor Reconstruction, and Custom Implants

Q17. Write a note on recent advances in spinal instrumentation.

Source: DNB 2021, RGUHS 2022

Type: Short Essay

Advances in Spinal Fixation

Innovation	*Benefit*
Polyaxial pedicle screws	Improved screw angulation and easier rod placement
Expandable cages	Vertebral body replacement with height adjustability
Navigation-guided fixation	Real-time, accurate screw placement
Robotic spine systems	For example, Mazor X, Excelsius GPS—precise
MIS spine systems	Tubular retractors, percutaneous screw systems

Materials
- *Titanium alloy*: MRI-compatible, corrosion-resistant
- *Carbon fiber-reinforced PEEK*: Radiolucent, used in tumor/cancer patients

Outcome Benefits
- Lower complication rates
- Better alignment in deformity correction
- Minimally invasive options for elderly and revision spine surgery

Q18. Discuss advances in orthopedic oncology reconstruction.

Source: TNMGRMU 2021

Type: Short Essay

Surgical Goals
- Wide tumor resection
- Limb salvage (instead of amputation)
- Immediate reconstruction
- Durable mechanical and biological function

Reconstruction Techniques

Method	Examples
Modular megaprosthesis	Distal femur, proximal tibia, humerus
Allografts	Osteoarticular or intercalary segment
Autograft recycling	Tumor bone treated via liquid nitrogen, radiation, or pasteurization and reimplanted
3D-printed custom implants	Pelvic/sacral defects, complex bone loss
Expandable prosthesis	Pediatric limb-sparing growing prosthesis

Benefits of Modular Systems

- Shorter surgical time
- Immediate weight-bearing
- Oncologic safety with functional restoration

Q19. What is an expandable megaprosthesis? Indications and mechanism.

Source: DNB 2022

Type: Short Note

Definition

Expandable megaprostheses are **growing joint replacements** used in **skeletally immature children** to compensate for **future limb length discrepancies** after tumor resection.

Indications

- Pediatric osteosarcoma/Ewing's sarcoma
- Resection near physes (e.g., distal femur, proximal tibia)

Mechanism

Type	Expansion method
Invasive	Requires repeat surgery to lengthen
Non-invasive	Uses magnetic drive (e.g., Stanmore® system)

Advantages

- Maintains limb length equality
- Avoids amputation
- Multiple expansions possible

Challenges

- Cost
- Mechanical failure
- Limited longevity—may need revision

Q20. What are 3D-printed custom implants in orthopedic oncology?

Source: RGUHS 2021

Type: Short Note

Definition

3D-printed implants are **patient-specific, CAD-designed prostheses**, manufactured to reconstruct **complex skeletal defects** after tumor resection.

Indications

- Pelvic and sacral resections
- Proximal femur with acetabular involvement

- Spine tumors (custom cages)
- Intercalary defects with unique geometry

Advantages
- Perfect anatomical fit
- Reduced intraoperative time
- May include screw holes, porous zones for ingrowth
- Enhanced stability and aesthetics

Materials
- Titanium alloy
- Carbon fiber
- PEEK (rare)

Q21. Role of carbon fiber implants in orthopedic oncology.

Source: DNB 2021

Type: Short Note

Definition
Carbon fiber–reinforced PEEK implants are **radiolucent, strong, and biocompatible alternatives** to metal used in **tumor reconstruction and spine surgery**.

Advantages
- Radiolucency → excellent post-operative MRI and CT surveillance
- Reduced imaging artifacts
- Lightweight but strong
- Less stress shielding

Indications
- Spinal stabilization after tumor resection
- Metaphyseal or diaphyseal defect fixation
- Pediatric tumor reconstructions
- Cases requiring frequent follow-up imaging

Limitations
- Expensive
- Not ideal in heavy load-bearing bones
- Fewer screw options and sizes compared to metal

Outcome Measures and Evidence-based Orthopedics

Q22. Enumerate and describe outcome scores used in total hip and total knee arthroplasty.

Source: RGUHS 2022, DNB 2021

Type: Short Essay

Hip Arthroplasty Scores

Score	*Domains assessed*
Harris hip score	Pain, function, absence of deformity, ROM
Oxford hip score	12-item patient-reported function/pain
Hip disability and osteoarthritis outcome score (HOOS)	ADLs, sport, QOL

Knee Arthroplasty Scores

Score	*Domains assessed*
Knee society score (KSS)	Knee (pain, ROM, stability) + function score
Oxford knee score	12-item patient satisfaction and pain
Knee injury and osteoarthritis outcome score (KOOS)	Includes symptoms, sport, QOL

Q23. Describe the DASH and AOFAS scoring systems.

Source: TNMGRMU 2022, DNB 2020

Type: Short Note

Disabilities of Arm, Shoulder, and Hand (DASH) Score

- 30-item patient-reported questionnaire
- Scored 0 (no disability) to 100 (maximum disability)
- *Covers*: Physical function, symptoms, social/psychological impact
- *Used in*: Brachial plexus injuries, distal radius, shoulder disorders

American Orthopedic Foot and Ankle Society (AOFAS) Score

- Physician-based scoring system
- *Evaluates*: Pain (40 pts), Function (50), Alignment (10)
- Specific versions for hindfoot, midfoot, hallux
- Score out of 100
- *Used in*: Plantar fasciitis, ankle arthritis, hallux valgus

Q24. What is the SF-36 score? How is it useful in orthopedics?

Source: DNB 2022

Type: Short Note

Definition

The SF-36 (Short Form-36) is a **generic health-related quality of life tool**, used across specialties, including orthopedics.

8 Domains Covered

1. Physical functioning
2. Role limitations (physical)
3. Role limitations (emotional)
4. Vitality
5. Emotional well-being
6. Social functioning
7. Bodily pain
8. General health perception

Orthopedic Use

- Compare surgical versus conservative outcomes
- Track long-term QOL post-arthroplasty, spine surgery, trauma
- Often used in multicentre trials and meta-analyses

Q25. Describe the levels of evidence and grades of recommendation.

Source: MUHS 2022, DNB 2021

Type: Short Essay

Levels of Evidence (Oxford Centre for Evidence-based Medicine)

Level	*Type of study*
I	High-quality RCTs, meta-analyses of RCTs
II	Lesser-quality RCTs, prospective cohort studies
III	Case-control or retrospective studies
IV	Case series
V	Expert opinion, mechanism-based reasoning

Grades of Recommendation

Grade	*Basis*
A	Consistent Level I evidence
B	Level II or III studies
C	Level IV studies
D	Level V (expert opinion)

Q26. What are PROMs? How are they useful in orthopedic research?

Source: RGUHS 2021

Type: Short Note

Definition

Patient-Reported Outcome Measures (PROMs) are **tools or questionnaires** that measure a patient's perception of their **health, function, and quality of life**, without clinician interpretation.

Examples in Orthopedics

- DASH
- HOOS, KOOS
- SF-36
- Oxford hip/knee score
- EQ-5D

Use in Research and Practice

- Outcome comparison after different surgeries
- Valid endpoints for trials
- Helps in shared decision-making
- Measures what matters most to the patient

Summary Table: Outcome Measures and Evidence Tools

Tool/Score	*Use case*	*Type*
Harris Hip/KSS	Hip/Knee arthroplasty outcomes	Clinician-reported
DASH/AOFAS	Upper limb/Foot outcomes	Patient or mixed
SF-36/EQ-5D	General health-related QoL	PROMs
KOOS/HOOS	OA-specific joint scores	Patient-reported
Evidence levels	Study evaluation in research/literature	Research hierarchy

CHAPTER 21

Basic Research and Publication Methodology

Asif Nazir Baba, Waseem Ahmad Sheikh, Nikhil Gupta

Section 1: General Research Methodology in Orthopedics

Q1. Define research. Enumerate types of research designs used in orthopedics.

Source: RGUHS 2022, DNB 2021

Type: Long essay

Definition of Research

"Research is a systematic and scientific process of collecting, analyzing, and interpreting data to answer a specific question or solve a problem."

In orthopedics, research improves patient care, treatment protocols, and contributes to evidence-based medicine.

Types of Research Designs in Orthopedics

A. *Based on nature of research*:
  1. *Basic (fundamental) research*: For example, stem cell studies on bone regeneration
  2. *Applied research*: For example, clinical trials of a new implant

B. *Based on approach*:
  1. *Quantitative research*: Numerical data (e.g., RCT measuring outcome scores)
  2. *Qualitative research*: Non-numerical (e.g., patient satisfaction interviews)

C. *Based on study design*:

Design type	***Examples***
Descriptive	Case reports, case series, cross-sectional studies
Analytical	Case-control, cohort studies
Experimental	Randomized controlled trials (RCTs)
Quasi-experimental	Non-randomized interventional studies
Systematic review/meta-analysis	Summarizing existing research

Q2. What is hypothesis? Differentiate between null and alternative hypothesis.

Source: MUHS 2021, DNB 2023

Type: Short essay

Definition

A **hypothesis** is a testable prediction or an assumption made about the relationship between variables in a study.

Types of Hypotheses

Type	*Explanation*
Null hypothesis (H_0)	States no difference or no association exists between variables
Alternative hypothesis (H_1)	States that a difference or association does exist

Example (Orthopedic Context)

Suppose a study is testing a new plate design for fracture healing.

- *H_0 (null)*: There is **no difference** in union rates between the new plate and standard plate.
- *H_1 (alternative)*: The new plate results in **better union rates** compared to the standard plate.

Conclusion

Hypotheses are the **backbone of clinical research**, guiding study design, data analysis, and interpretation of results.

Q3. Define evidence-based medicine (EBM). Write its steps and importance in orthopedics.

Source: RGUHS 2021, TNMGRMU 2020

Type: Short essay

Definition

"Evidence-based medicine (EBM) is the integration of best current clinical evidence, clinical expertise, and patient values in decision-making."

Five Steps of EBM

1. *Ask*: Frame a focused, answerable clinical question (e.g., using PICO format)
2. *Acquire*: Search the best available evidence (e.g., PubMed, Cochrane)
3. *Appraise*: Critically evaluate the evidence for validity and applicability
4. *Apply*: Integrate evidence with clinical expertise and patient needs
5. *Assess*: Evaluate the outcome and improve future practice

Importance in Orthopedics

- Guides **treatment choices** (e.g., when to choose arthroplasty vs. arthrodesis)
- Supports **clinical guidelines** and protocols
- Encourages **rational use of implants and medications**
- Improves **patient outcomes and resource utilization**

Q4. Enumerate levels of evidence in orthopedic literature.

Source: DNB 2022, MUHS 2022

Type: Short note

Definition

Levels of evidence classify the **strength of a research study** based on its methodology and design, used widely in orthopedic journals and guidelines (e.g., JBJS, AAOS).

Oxford Centre for Evidence-based Medicine (CEBM) Levels

Level	*Type of study*
I	High-quality RCTs, systematic reviews, meta-analyses
II	Lesser-quality RCTs, prospective cohort studies
III	Retrospective cohort or case-control studies
IV	Case series, poor-quality cohort or case-control studies
V	Expert opinion, bench research, personal experience

Use in Practice
- Helps determine **guideline strength**
- Influences **treatment protocols** and **funding decisions**

Section 2: Study Design and Ethics in Orthopedics

Q1. Classify study designs. Compare observational versus experimental studies.

Source: RGUHS 2021, MUHS 2022

Type: Long essay

Classification of Study Designs
Study designs are broadly classified into:

A. *Observational studies (No researcher intervention):*
   1. *Descriptive*:
      - Case reports
      - Case series
      - Cross-sectional studies
   2. *Analytical*:
      - Case-control
      - Cohort (prospective/retrospective)

B. *Experimental (interventional) studies:*
   1. Randomized controlled trials (RCTs)
   2. Non-randomized interventional studies
   3. Community trials

C. *Review-based*:
   - Systematic review
   - Meta-analysis

Comparison Table: Observational versus Experimental Studies

Feature	*Observational study*	*Experimental study*
Intervention by researcher	No	Yes
Example	Case-control, cohort	RCTs, drug trials
Bias control	Limited	High (through randomization/blinding)
Evidence strength	Moderate	Strongest (especially RCTs)

Q2. Explain Cohort and case-control studies with examples.

Source: DNB 2023, TNMGRMU 2020

Type: Short essay

A. *Cohort study*:
   - *Definition*: Prospective or retrospective study where groups are followed over time based on **exposure** (e.g., treatment).
   - *Example in ortho*: Comparing outcomes of patients receiving cemented versus uncemented hip arthroplasty.

Pros	*Cons*
Measures incidence and risk	Time-consuming
Good for rare exposures	Loss to follow-up

B. *Case-control study*:
- *Definition*: Retrospective study where subjects are selected based on **outcome**, and their prior exposures are compared.
- *Example in ortho*: Comparing prior steroid use in patients with versus without avascular necrosis (AVN).

Pros	*Cons*
Quick and cost-effective	Prone to recall bias
Useful for rare diseases	Cannot calculate incidence

Q3. Cross-sectional study—define, uses, and limitations in orthopedics.

Source: DNB 2021

Type: Short essay

Definition
A **cross-sectional study** is an observational study that assesses **both exposure and outcome at a single point in time** (a "snapshot").

Applications in Orthopedics
- Estimating **prevalence** of osteoporosis in postmenopausal women.
- Surveying practice patterns among orthopedic surgeons.
- Functional outcome studies using scores (e.g., DASH, Harris Hip Score).

Advantages
- Quick and economical
- Useful for **prevalence data**
- Hypothesis generation

Limitations
- Cannot establish causality
- Temporal ambiguity (which came first: Exposure or disease?)
- Not suitable for rare conditions

Q4. Define informed consent. Why is it important in research?

Source: MUHS 2021, RGUHS 2020

Type: Short note

Definition
Informed consent is a process by which a participant voluntarily confirms their willingness to participate in a study after being informed of all aspects relevant to the decision.

Components of Valid Informed Consent
1. *Disclosure*: Of study purpose, risks, benefits
2. *Comprehension*: Understandable language used
3. *Voluntariness*: Free from coercion or undue influence
4. *Competence*: Mentally and legally capable
5. *Documentation*: Signed consent form (and witnessed)

Importance in Orthopedic Research
- Upholds **autonomy and patient rights**
- Prevents **legal and ethical violations**

- Required by **ethics committees and legal frameworks**
- Ensures **transparency and trust** between researcher and participant

Q5. Discuss ethical issues in clinical research in orthopedics.

Source: DNB 2022

Type: Short essay

Key Ethical Principles

1. *Autonomy*: Right to make an informed decision
2. *Beneficence*: Maximize benefits
3. *Non-maleficence*: Avoid harm
4. *Justice*: Fair participant selection

Common Ethical Concerns

- Inadequate informed consent
- Unjust participant selection (e.g., poor or vulnerable groups)
- Conflict of interest (financial bias)
- Privacy and confidentiality violations
- Plagiarism and data manipulation
- Use of unregistered or unsafe implants

Safeguards

- Institutional ethics committee (IEC) review
- Trial registration (e.g., CTRI, ClinicalTrials.gov)
- Adherence to good clinical practice (GCP) guidelines

Q6. Institutional Ethics Committee (IEC)—functions and composition.

Source: TNMGRMU 2022

Type: Short essay

Functions of IEC

- Review and approve research proposals
- Ensure **ethical standards** are met
- Monitor **ongoing studies**
- Ensure **participant safety and informed consent**
- Investigate **protocol violations or misconduct**

Typical Composition

Member type	***Role***
Chairperson (external)	Oversight
Member Secretary	Coordination
Clinicians (2–3)	Scientific review
Legal expert	Legal compliance
Layperson	Community representation
Social scientist/ethicist	Ethical viewpoint

Minimum: 7 members
At least one **external and non-medical** member is mandatory

Section 3: Biostatistics in Orthopedics

Q1. Define mean, median, and mode. Explain with examples.

Source: MUHS 2020, DNB 2021

Type: Short note

Definitions

Term	*Definition*	*Example (e.g., fracture healing time in weeks)*
Mean	Arithmetic average of a set of values	(4 + 5 + 6 + 5 + 10)/5 = 6 weeks
Median	Middle value in an ordered dataset	Ordered: 4, 5, 5, 6, 10 → Median = 5 weeks
Mode	Most frequently occurring value	5 occurs twice → Mode = 5 weeks

Clinical Relevance in Orthopedics

- **Mean** healing time of tibial fractures in a study
- **Median** age of patients with hip fracture
- **Mode** for most common implant failure mode

Q2. What is standard deviation? Explain its relevance in clinical studies.

Source: RGUHS 2022, DNB 2023

Type: Short note

Definition

Standard deviation (SD) measures the **spread or variability** of a dataset around its mean.

A **low SD** indicates that data points are **close to the mean**, while a **high SD** indicates **greater variability**.

Formula

$$SD = \sqrt{\frac{\sum_{i=1}^{N}(x_i - \bar{x})^2}{n}} = SD = \frac{1}{n-1}\sum_{i=1}^{N}(x_i - \bar{x})^2$$

where: x_i is each data point,
$\bar{x}$ is each data point
n is number of data points

Example (Orthopedics Context)

- In a study on femoral fracture healing times:
  - *Mean*: 12 weeks
  - *SD*: 2 weeks

Most patients healed between **10–14 weeks** (Mean ± SD)

Importance

- Helps interpret **treatment consistency**
- Required for **calculating sample size, confidence intervals, and p-values**

Q3. Define *p*-value. What is statistical significance?

Source: DNB 2021, MUHS 2021

Type: Short essay

Definition

***p*-value** is the probability that the **observed result (or more extreme)** could occur **by chance** if the **null hypothesis is true**.

Interpretation

- If $p < 0.05$ → **Statistically significant** → Reject null hypothesis
- If $p \geq 0.05$ → **Not significant**

Example (Ortho)

In a trial comparing two plating techniques:

- $p = 0.03$ for union rate difference

→ Suggests **significant difference** in effectiveness

Clinical Relevance

- Helps **validate research results**
- Ensures that observed differences are **not due to random error**
- Widely used in **clinical trials and outcomes research**

Q4. Explain sensitivity and specificity in diagnostic tests.

Source: RGUHS 2020, DNB 2022

Type: Short essay

Definitions

Term	*Definition*
Sensitivity	Ability of a test to correctly identify patients with the disease (true positive rate)
Specificity	Ability of a test to correctly identify patients without the disease (true negative rate)

Formulas

- Sensitivity = TP/(TP + FN)
- Specificity = TN/(TN + FP)

Example (In Ortho – TB Spine Diagnosis)

- **MRI** has high **sensitivity** → Picks up most patients with TB
- **Histopathology** has high **specificity** → Confirms TB accurately

Clinical Use

- *High sensitivity*: **Screening tests** (few false negatives)
- *High specificity*: **Confirmatory tests** (few false positives)

Q5. What is a confidence interval? Discuss its interpretation.

Source: TNMGRMU 2021

Type: Short note

Definition

A **confidence interval (CI)** is the **range of values** within which the **true population parameter** is likely to lie, with a given level of confidence (typically 95%).

Example

- *Mean healing time*: 12 weeks
- *95% CI*: 10 to 14 weeks

→We are 95% confident that the **true average healing time lies between 10–14 weeks.**

Importance in Orthopedics
- Describes **precision** of study results
- *Narrow CI*: High precision
- Used in **clinical trials**, meta-analyses

Q6. Describe types of data and appropriate statistical tests.

Source: DNB 2022, MUHS 2022

Type: Short essay

Types of Data

Type	*Examples*	*Test Type*
Nominal	Gender, implant type	Chi-square test
Ordinal	Pain scale, functional grading	Mann–Whitney U, Kruskal–Wallis
Interval/Ratio	Range of motion (ROM), healing time, VAS score	t-test, ANOVA

Common Statistical Tests

Test	*Use*
Chi-square test	Association between categorical variables
t-test	Compare means between two groups
ANOVA	Compare means across ≥3 groups
Mann–Whitney U	Non-parametric test for 2 groups
Pearson's correlation	Correlation between continuous variables

Conclusion
Understanding **data types** and selecting the **appropriate statistical test** is key to conducting and interpreting research in orthopedics.

Q7. What is a meta-analysis? Describe its steps and clinical utility.

Source: RGUHS 2023, DNB 2023

Type: Short essay

Definition
Meta-analysis is a **statistical method** to combine results from multiple studies to arrive at a **pooled estimate of effect**.

Steps in Meta-analysis
1. **Define a clear research question**
2. **Systematic literature search**
3. **Select studies** based on inclusion criteria
4. **Extract and pool data**
5. Perform **statistical analysis (fixed or random effect models)**
6. Interpret results and assess **publication bias** (e.g., funnel plot)

Clinical Relevance in Orthopedics
- Summarizes evidence from multiple RCTs (e.g., for implant types, ACL techniques)
- Guides **clinical guidelines and protocols**
- Increases **statistical power**

Summary Table: Must-know Statistical Terms for Ortho Exams

Term	Definition	Clinical use
Mean/Median/Mode	Central tendency	Healing time, functional scores
Standard deviation	Data variability	Interpretation of range of outcomes
p-value	Statistical significance	Comparing treatment outcomes
Sensitivity/Specificity	Diagnostic test accuracy	Infections, tumors
Confidence interval	Precision of estimate	Research conclusions
Meta-analysis	Combining multiple studies	Guidelines and treatment algorithms

Section 4: Thesis Writing and Scientific Publication

Q1. Describe structure of a scientific research paper.

Source: DNB 2021, MUHS 2022

Type: Short essay

Standard Structure of a Scientific Paper – IMRAD Format
IMRAD stands for **Introduction, Methods, Results, and Discussion**

Section	Contents
Title and abstract	Clear, concise; summary of aims, methods, results, conclusion
Introduction	Background, research gap, aims/objectives, hypothesis
Methods	Study design, inclusion/exclusion criteria, interventions, outcome measures
Results	Data presentation (tables/figures), statistical analysis
Discussion	Interpretation, comparison with literature, strengths/limitations
Conclusion	Final summary and clinical relevance
References	Cited using standardized format (e.g. Vancouver)
Acknowledgements and conflict of interest	Optional but essential for transparency

Q2. IMRAD format—explain with components.

Source: RGUHS 2022

Type: Short note

IMRAD: Introduction, Methods, Results, and Discussion

Section	Purpose
I – Introduction	What is the problem and why is it important?
M – Methods	How was the problem studied? (design, tools, analysis)
R – Results	What was found? (without interpretation)
A and D – Discussion	What do the results mean? (compare with literature)

Most clinical orthopedic research papers in journals like JBJS, IJO, and CORR follow this format.

Conclusion
IMRAD provides a **logical structure** that enhances the **scientific quality and readability** of research papers.

Q3. Explain how to write an abstract and its components.

Source: MUHS 2021

Type: Short note

Definition

An **abstract** is a brief summary of a research article or thesis, usually **150–300 words**, giving a snapshot of the entire study.

Components of a Structured Abstract

1. *Background*: Why the study was done?
2. *Objectives*: Specific aims/hypotheses
3. *Methods*: Design, sample size, techniques used
4. *Results*: Key findings with data/statistics
5. *Conclusion*: Final interpretation or clinical relevance
6. *Keywords*: 4–6 words for indexing

Example (in Orthopedics)

"We conducted a prospective study on 60 patients with distal radius fractures to compare volar plating versus external fixation. Results showed significantly faster union and better DASH scores with volar plating..."

Q4. Describe steps in writing a thesis protocol in orthopedics.

Source: DNB 2023

Type: Short essay

Thesis Protocol Writing: Step-by-step Format

1. *Title*: Clear, concise, focused on one topic
2. *Introduction/Background*: Current knowledge + research gap
3. *Objectives*: Primary and secondary
4. Hypothesis/Research Question
5. *Review of literature*: Summary of existing work (at least 5–10 key studies)
6. *Methodology*:
   - Study design (RCT, cohort, etc.)
   - Sample size (with justification)
   - Inclusion/exclusion criteria
   - Data collection and tools (e.g., scoring systems like DASH, VAS)
   - Statistical analysis plan
7. *Ethical considerations*: IEC approval, informed consent
8. Timeline and Work Plan
9. Budget (if applicable)
10. *References*: Vancouver style

Q5. What is plagiarism? How can it be prevented in academic writing?

Source: TNMGRMU 2022, DNB 2021

Type: Short essay

Definition

Plagiarism is **presenting someone else's work, ideas, or data as your own**, without proper acknowledgment.

Types
- *Direct plagiarism*: Copy-pasting text without citation
- *Self-plagiarism*: Reusing own previously published work
- *Mosaic plagiarism*: Paraphrasing with identical structure
- *Accidental plagiarism*: Unintentional failure to cite

Prevention
- Use **original language and paraphrasing**
- Always **cite sources** properly (Vancouver/APA style)
- *Use plagiarism detection tools*: **Turnitin, iThenticate, Urkund**
- Learn and follow **institutional guidelines**
- Seek **ethical committee clearance**

Penalties
Academic suspension, thesis rejection, legal action in extreme cases

Q6. What is referencing? Describe Vancouver style of referencing.

Source: RGUHS 2021, DNB 2022

Type: Short essay

Definition
Referencing is the process of **acknowledging the sources** of information, ideas, or data used in a research work.

Common Referencing Styles in Medicine
- **Vancouver** (most common in orthopedics)
- APA, MLA, Harvard (less common in clinical work)

Vancouver Style
- **Numbered format**, references arranged in order of appearance
- In-text citation: Superscript or bracketed number (e.g., Smith et al[1] or [1])
- **Reference list** at the end with full details

Example (Journal Article)
Babhulkar S, Pande K. Tuberculosis of hip. Clin Orthop Relat Res. 2002;398:93–99.

Tools for Referencing
EndNote, Zotero, Mendeley, PubMed citation manager

Section 5: Critical Appraisal and Evidence-based Practice in Orthopedics

Q1. Define critical appraisal. Discuss steps in assessing a clinical research paper.

Source: DNB 2022

Type: Short essay

Definition
Critical appraisal is the process of **systematically evaluating a research article** to determine its **validity, reliability, relevance, and applicability** to clinical practice.

Why It's Important in Orthopedics?
- Prevents **adoption of flawed techniques**
- Ensures **evidence-based clinical decisions**
- Guides **implant/device selection**

Steps in Critical Appraisal (CASP-based framework)

1. *Assess validity*:
   - Was the study design appropriate?
   - Was it randomized/blinded?
   - Were biases minimized?
2. *Evaluate results:*
   - Are results statistically and clinically significant?
   - Were outcome measures appropriate?
3. *Relevance and applicability:*
   - Are the results applicable to your patient population?
   - Are benefits worth the risks/cost?
4. Consider conflicts of interest/funding sources

Tools for Appraisal

- CASP (Critical Appraisal Skills Programme) checklists
- CONSORT guidelines (for RCTs)
- STROBE checklist (for observational studies)

Q2. Levels of evidence and grades of recommendation—describe.

Source: MUHS 2021, RGUHS 2020

Type: Short essay

A. **Levels of Evidence (Oxford CEBM)**

Level	*Type of evidence*
I	High-quality RCTs, meta-analysis of RCTs
II	Lesser-quality RCTs, prospective cohort studies
III	Retrospective cohort or case-control studies
IV	Case series, poor cohort studies
V	Expert opinion, bench research

B. **Grades of Recommendation**

Grade	*Basis*
A	Consistent level I evidence
B	Level II or III studies
C	Level IV studies or expert opinion
D	Inconsistent or insufficient evidence

Example (Ortho Context)

- *Grade A*: THA versus hemiarthroplasty for elderly NOF → supported by RCTs
- *Grade C*: Use of vitamin D for fracture healing → limited case series

Q3. Discuss PICO format in research question framing.

Source: DNB 2023, TNMGRMU 2021

Type: Short note

PICO Framework
Used to formulate **structured clinical questions** in evidence-based orthopedics.

PICO component	*Definition*	*Example—ACL reconstruction*
P: Patient	Specific patient group	Young athletes with ACL tear
I: Intervention	Proposed treatment	Arthroscopic ACL reconstruction
C: Comparison	Alternative intervention (if applicable)	Conservative treatment
O: Outcome	What is being measured	Time to return to sport, stability scores

Benefits of PICO
- Helps create **focused, answerable questions**
- Guides **literature search**
- Aids **critical appraisal and synthesis**

Q4. Describe systematic review versus meta-analysis—differences and applications.

Source: RGUHS 2022, MUHS 2021

Type: Short essay

Systematic Review
A **comprehensive summary of literature** on a specific clinical question using **predefined methods and inclusion criteria**.
- Focuses on **qualitative synthesis**
- Follows **PRISMA guidelines**

Meta-analysis
A **quantitative statistical method** to **combine results from multiple studies** (usually RCTs).
- Pooled analysis provides **effect size and confidence interval**
- Often part of a systematic review

Key Differences

Feature	*Systematic review*	*Meta-analysis*
Nature	Qualitative	Quantitative
Statistics used	No	Yes
Output	Summary of literature	Single pooled effect measure

Example
- **Systematic review** of volar plating versus dorsal plating for distal radius fractures
- **Meta-analysis** gives pooled odds ratio for complication rate

Q5. Explain bias in clinical studies. How to reduce it?

(RUHS 2021)

Source: DNB 2021

Type: Short essay

Definition
Bias is a **systematic error** that results in **incorrect estimation** of the association between exposure and outcome in a study.

Types of Bias

Type	*Description*
Selection bias	Improper selection of participants
Recall bias	Inaccurate memory of exposure (especially case-control studies)
Observer bias	Investigator's expectations influence outcome
Publication bias	Studies with positive results more likely to be published

Methods to Minimize Bias

- **Randomization** → avoids selection bias
- **Blinding (single/double)** → reduces observer bias
- **Standardized protocols** → uniform data collection
- **Pre-registered protocols** → reduce publication bias
- Use validated tools (e.g., DASH score)

Summary Table: Key Concepts in Evidence-based Practice

Concept	*Use in orthopedics*
Critical appraisal	Evaluate quality of literature
Levels of evidence	Rank study reliability (RCT > cohort > case series)
PICO	Frame focused clinical questions
Systematic review	Summarize research on a topic
Meta-analysis	Combine data from studies for pooled result
Bias	Systematic error to be minimized by good design

Section 6: Tools and Software in Orthopedic Research

Q1. Role of SPSS in orthopedic research.

Source: MUHS 2022

Type: Short note

Statistical Package for the Social Sciences (SPSS)
A user-friendly statistical software used for **data analysis in medical research**, including orthopedics.

Uses in Orthopedic Research

- *Descriptive statistics*: Mean, SD, median, mode
- *Inferential tests*:
  - t-test, Chi-square, ANOVA
  - Correlation, regression analysis
- *Data visualization*: Graphs, histograms, scatter plots
- **Handling large datasets** from multicentric studies
- ***P*-value and confidence intervals** calculation
- Facilitates **randomization and stratification** in trials

Q2. Software used for reference management—name and uses.

Source: DNB 2022

Type: Short note

Reference Management Tools

Tool	*Use*
EndNote	Automatically format references in journals' preferred styles
Mendeley	Store, organize, cite, and share references and PDFs
Zotero	Free tool; integrates with browsers for web citation
BibTeX	Reference tool for LaTeX users

Features

- Automatically generate **bibliographies** (e.g., Vancouver format)
- Store and **organize citations** and full-text PDFs
- Insert in-text citations using **Word plugins**

Q3. Plagiarism detection tools—list and describe.

Source: RGUHS 2021

Type: Short note

What is Plagiarism Detection?

Software tools that **scan written content** and **compare it** with existing literature/databases to detect **duplicate content.**

Common Tools

Tool	*Features*
Turnitin	Widely used in academics; provides detailed similarity index
iThenticate	Preferred by journals for research articles
Urkund	Used by Indian universities and regulatory bodies
Grammarly premium	Offers basic plagiarism detection

Uses in Orthopedics

- Thesis checking (required by most universities)
- Journal submission compliance
- Avoiding unintentional duplication

Q4. Online databases for literature search—PubMed, Scopus, Cochrane – discuss.

Source: DNB 2021

Type: Short essay

PubMed

- Maintained by **US National Library of Medicine**
- Contains **30M+ citations** for biomedical literature
- **Free access**, uses **MeSH terms** for precise searches
- Key for **evidence-based orthopedics**

Scopus

- A **commercial** database by Elsevier
- Covers **journals + conference proceedings**
- Provides **citation tracking and author metrics**

Cochrane Library

- Gold standard for **systematic reviews and meta-analyses**
- Maintains **Cochrane reviews** for EBM
- Subscription-based but summaries are **publicly available**

Search Tips for PGs

- Use **Boolean operators** (AND, OR, NOT)
- Use **filters** for RCTs, free full text
- Apply **date limits** and **article type**

Summary Table: Research Tools for Orthopedic PGs

Tool/Resource	*Function*
SPSS	Data analysis and statistics
EndNote/Mendeley	Referencing and bibliography
Turnitin/iThenticate	Plagiarism check
PubMed	Biomedical literature search
Cochrane library	Evidence-based reviews
Zotero	Free citation manager

Q5. What are predatory journals, and how do they differ from indexed journals?

Predatory journals also are also called fraudulent, deceptive, or pseudo-journals. The term was coined by Jeffrey Beall, a librarian at the University of Colorado, Denver. He describes them as "organizations that publish counterfeit journals to exploit the open-access model in which the author pays. These predatory publishers are dishonest and lack transparency. They aim to dupe researchers, especially those inexperienced in scholarly communication."

Features differentiating predatory journals differ from indexed journals

a. Claim to be peer-reviewed but do not provide adequate peer review.
b. The impact factor given is incorrect and cannot be verified
c. Promise to publish article sin days or a couple of weeks
d. Published articles have grammatical mistakes
e. Editorial board members cannot be verified or lack credentials
f. Target authors through emails or phone calls
g. Publish articles even before authors have signed the publishing agreement
h. The name of journal may mimic well established journals

Q6. What is the peer-review process, and why is it important?

Peer review is an important step in the publication of scientific research. In this process the study is independently assessed by experts in the given field and based upon the comments of the experts the editor may accept, reject or send the paper back to authors for necessary changes. The peer review determines whether the research is suitable for publication.

Peer review is important as it gives feedback and suggestions to improve the overall quality of research and identifies the lacunae and gaps in methodology

Q7. Define the impact factor and its significance in journal ranking.

(Kashmir University 2017)

Impact factor is the ratio between the number of citations received in that year for publications in that journal that were published in the two preceding years and the total number of "citable items" published in that journal during the two preceding years. Impact factor is calculated when all the issues for the year have been completed. If a journal gets an impact factor of 15 in year 2024 it is for the year 2023. This means that its articles published in the preceding two years (2021 and 2022) have received average 15 citations in year 2023. Impact factor can thus be calculated only after a journal has been published for 3 consecutive years.

Impact factor shows the relative importance of the journal in its field and how commonly the article published in that journal get cited. Although initially used by libraries to determine which journals to subscribe to, nowadays it is used by researchers to show academic success and by publishers to **garner more research articles.**

2023 impact factor of JBJS is 5.3 while that of Indian Journal of Orthopedics is 1.1. A Cancer journal for clinicians had the highest impact factor of 268.3.

Q8. What is the declaration of Helsinki?

Declaration of Helsinki is a set of ethical principles regarding human experimentation. It was developed originally in 1964 by the World Medical Association (WMA). Initially adopted in June 1964 in Helsinki, Finland it has since undergone eight revisions till now. It is the cornerstone document regarding ethics involving human subjects and human research ethics. Although meant for physicians it should be upheld by everyone involved in medical research.

Q9. What are the principles of declaration of Helsenki?

The main principles on which the declaration of Helaenki is based are:

- *Respect for persons*: Respecting the autonomy and dignity of research participants.
- *Informed consent*: Participants should be provided with sufficient information about the research to make an informed decision about whether to participate
- *Beneficence*: Maximize potential benefits and minimize risks to participants.
- *Non-maleficence*: Avoid causing harm to participants.
- *Justice*: Research should be conducted in a way that ensures equitable access to benefits and risks for all participants.
- *Vulnerable populations*: Special considerations should be given to research involving vulnerable populations, such as children, individuals with disabilities, or those in dependent relationships.
- *Confidentiality*: Participants' personal information should be protected and kept confidential.
- *Withdrawal*: Participants should have the right to withdraw from the research at any time, without penalty.
- *Research integrity*: Research should be conducted with integrity and objectivity.

Q10. What is Nuremberg Code and what are its main features?

To promote the concept of racial hygiene and promote pure Aryan race, German physicians conducted many unethical practices from 1920 onwards. To prevent such attemopts in future the **Nuremberg Code** was drafted. It is a set of ethical research principles for human experimentation .

Its main principles are:

a. Voluntary consent
b. Scientific benefit
c. Benefits outweigh risks
d. Animal experiments first
e. Avoid suffering
f. No intentional death or disability
g. Protection from harm
h. Qualified investigator
i. Subject ability to withdraw
j. Stop if harm occurs.

Q11. Define conflict of interest in research and its implications.

Conflict of interest is said to occur when an investigator in a research study has personal, financial, institutional or other interests pertaining to the institution and/or the individual, their family members, friends, or their former, current or prospective professional associates from which they can benefit.

Q12. Explain scientific misconduct (fabrication, falsification, and plagiarism).

Researchers are expected to adhere to ethical, legal, and professional guidelines that structure how research is conducted. The consequences that research misconduct can have are considerable and potentially disastrous. For one, misconduct can irreparably erode trust among colleagues. It can erode trust between researchers and funding agencies, which may make it more difficult for colleagues at the same institution to receive grants. More importantly, research misconduct can cause the public to lose confidence in the ability and integrity of researchers. Scientific misconduct encompasses intentional actions that violate standards of scholarly conduct and behaviour in research.

The important types of research misconduct are:

a. *Plagiarism*: It is the appropriation of another person's ideas, thoughts or language without giving credit to the original source and presenting it as one's own original work.
b. *Falsification*: It is the manipulation of research materials, equipment, or processes, or changing or omitting data or results. As a result the research is not accurately represented in the research record.
c. *Fabrication*: It involves making up data or results without actually having performed the relevant research and recording or reporting them.
d. *Misappropriation of the ideas of others*: While reviewing grants of articles the reviewer may come across a novel idea. Improper use of such information is also a misconduct.
e. *Improprieties of authorship*: Improper assignment of credit, such as excluding others, misrepresentation of the same material as original in more than one publication, inclusion of individuals as authors who have not made a definite contribution to the work published; or submission of multi-authored publications without the concurrence of all authors.

CHAPTER 22

General and Non-specific Orthopedic

Shubhranshu Choudhary, Abdul Maajid Bhat, Shubham Pandoh

Q1. Write the commonly used absorbable sutures in orthopedics and compare their properties.

(PGI Chandigarh 2011)

Suture type	*Material*	*Absorption time*	*Tensile strength retention*	*Features*
Vicryl	Polyglactin 910	~60–90 days	50% at 2–3 weeks	Braided, good handling
PDS	Polydioxanone	~180 days	70% at 2 weeks	Monofilament, slow absorption
Monocryl	Poliglecaprone	~90–120 days	60–70% at 1 week	Monofilament, soft tissues
Chromic catgut	Treated collagen	~60–90 days	Variable	Natural, inflammatory reaction

Uses

Tendon repair (PDS), soft tissue approximation (vicryl), subcuticular (monocryl).

Q2. What are different types of tourniquets in orthopedics? Discuss their uses, complications and safety guidelines.

Types

- Pneumatic (most common)
- Esmarch bandage (rubber)
- Silicone ring tourniquets

Uses

- Bloodless surgical field
- Improved visualization and precision
- Used in extremity surgeries (e.g., limb trauma, TKA)

Complications

- Nerve injury (e.g., radial/fibular nerve palsy)
- Muscle damage (ischemia >2 hours)
- DVT/Thrombosis
- Tourniquet pain
- Skin burns/blisters

Safety Guidelines

- Inflate 100–150 mmHg above SBP (upper limb: ~250 mmHg, lower limb: ~300 mmHg)
- Maximum duration: ≤2 hours
- Deflate gradually after use
- Document inflation/deflation time
- Use limb padding and proper cuff size

Q3. Write the composition of bone cement. What are the different generations of cementing techniques in arthroplasty?

Composition of PMMA Bone Cement

- *Powder*: PMMA, benzoyl peroxide (initiator), radio-opacifier ($BaSO_4$)
- *Liquid*: Methylmethacrylate monomer, N,N-dimethyl-p-toluidine (activator), hydroquinone (stabilizer)

Generations of Cementing Technique

1. *First generation*: Manual mixing, no medullary plug, finger-packing
2. *Second generation*: Retrograde cement gun, cement restrictor, pulsatile lavage
3. *Third generation*: Vacuum mixing, pressurization, canal drying
4. *Fourth generation*: Improved viscosity control, antibiotic-loaded cement, modern instrumentation

Q4. What are orthobiologicals?

Definition

Orthobiologics are substances that promote healing of bones, joints, and soft tissues, derived from natural sources.

Examples

- Platelet-rich plasma (PRP)
- Bone morphogenetic proteins (BMPs)
- Stem cells (e.g., mesenchymal)
- Demineralized bone matrix (DBM)
- Autologous conditioned serum
- Hyaluronic acid injections

Uses in Orthopedics

- Non-union fracture healing
- Tendon/Ligament repair
- Osteoarthritis (intra-articular PRP)
- Cartilage regeneration

Q5. Describe shortwave diathermy (SWD).

[All India Institute of Medical Sciences (AIIMS) Jodhpur Rajasthan 2017]

Definition

Shortwave diathermy (SWD) is a physical therapy modality using high-frequency electromagnetic energy (27.12 MHz) to produce deep tissue heating.

Mechanism

- Causes molecular vibration → friction → heat
- Promotes vasodilation, tissue extensibility, and pain relief

Indications

- Muscle spasms
- Chronic joint stiffness
- Soft tissue injuries

Contraindications

- Metal implants, pacemakers
- Pregnancy
- Open wounds/infection
- Malignancy

Q6. Describe transcutaneous electrical nerve stimulation (TENS).

Definition

Transcutaneous electrical nerve stimulation (TENS) is a non-invasive technique delivering low-voltage electrical currents via skin electrodes to relieve pain.

Mechanism

- Stimulates large diameter Aβ fibers
- Inhibits transmission from nociceptive C fibers via gate control theory

Indications

- Neuropathic pain
- Post-operative pain
- Tendinopathies, arthritis

Contraindications

- Pacemakers
- Over carotid sinus or uterus in pregnancy
- Broken skin or infected areas

Q7. What are the types of exercises? Describe the benefits of each.

Type of exercise	*Description*	*Benefits*
Isometric	Muscle contracts without joint movement	Maintains strength during immobilization
Isotonic	Muscle contracts with movement (concentric/eccentric)	Builds muscle strength and endurance
Isokinetic	Muscle contracts at constant speed using special equipment	Measures muscle power; rehabilitation in controlled setting
Passive ROM	Movement done by therapist/device without patient effort	Prevents stiffness, contractures
Active ROM	Patient moves joint voluntarily	Improves coordination, strength
Resistive exercises	Against resistance (e.g., weights, bands)	Strengthening muscles post-injury/surgery

Q8. Write a short note on thermoplastic splints.

Thermoplastic Splints

- Made from materials that become moldable when heated (~60–70°C)
- Custom-fitted to patient contours
- *Types*:
  - Low-temperature thermoplastics (e.g., orthoplast, aquaplast)
  - High-temperature thermplastics (e.g. Orfitrans)

Advantages

- Lightweight, moldable, reusable
- Good patient compliance
- Allows dynamic or static splinting

Uses in Orthopedics

- Hand and wrist immobilization
- Tendon injuries
- Post-burn contractures
- Spasticity management

Q9. What is crush injury? Describe reperfusion injury.

(GGMC 2021)

Crush Injury

- Results from prolonged compression of muscle mass
- Leads to muscle necrosis, edema, and release of myoglobin, potassium, phosphate, creatinine kinase (CK)

Reperfusion Injury

- Occurs after revascularization of ischemic tissue
- *Mechanisms*:
  - Free radical generation → lipid peroxidation
  - Calcium overload in myocytes
  - Neutrophil infiltration → inflammation
- *Leads to*:
  - Local tissue damage
  - Systemic effects: renal failure (due to myoglobin), ARDS

Q10. What is dynamization? How will you achieve this in various implants?

Definition

Technique to stimulate fracture healing by controlled micro-movement at fracture site

In Nails

- Removal of static locking screws (usually proximal or distal)
- Allows controlled axial loading

In External Fixators

- Reducing frame stiffness (e.g., removing rods or pins)
- Using dynamic modules

Benefits

- Promotes callus formation via mechanical stimulation
- Speeds up union in delayed healing

Q11. Write a short note on limb length equalization.

[All India Institute of Medical Sciences (AIIMS) Jodhpur Rajasthan 2019}

Indications

- LLD >2–2.5 cm is clinically significant
- *Causes*: Congenital, post-traumatic, infection, tumors

Methods

1. *Shortening the longer limb*:
   - Epiphysiodesis (growth modulation)
   - Bone resection (rarely used now)
2. *Lengthening the shorter limb*:
   - Ilizarov external fixator
   - PRECICE nail (magnetically controlled)
   - LON (lengthening over nail)

Complications

- Joint contractures
- Infection (external fixator)
- Non-union
- Neurovascular compromise

Q12. What is a critical bone defect? Explain induced membrane formation to cover bone defect.

Critical Bone Defect

A bone gap (>2.5–3 cm or >50% of the bone circumference) unlikely to heal without intervention

Induced Membrane Technique (Masquelet Technique)

- *Stage 1*: Debridement and placement of cement spacer → forms vascularized membrane
- *Stage 2 (after 6–8 weeks)*:
  - Remove cement
  - Bone grafting within the membrane

Advantages

- Membrane promotes revascularization and osteoinduction
- Prevents graft resorption
- Useful in infected/non-union cases

Q13. What are the clinical applications of distraction osteogenesis?

Definition

Distraction osteogenesis (DO) is the process of bone lengthening by gradual mechanical distraction after corticotomy.

Clinical Applications

- Limb lengthening (e.g., congenital short femur, post-traumatic shortening)
- Correction of angular deformities (e.g., genu varum/valgum)
- Bone transport in segmental defects (trauma, tumor resection)
- Maxillofacial reconstruction (craniofacial DO)
- Joint contracture release (e.g., knee or elbow)
- Pseudoarthrosis correction
- Cosmetic height increase (controversial)

Q14. Describe DEXA scan.

Full Form

DEXA: Dual-energy X-ray absorptiometry

Principle

Uses two X-ray beams with different energy levels to assess bone mineral density (BMD).

Sites Assessed

- Lumbar spine
- Hip (femoral neck, total hip)
- Forearm (distal radius)

T-score Interpretation

- *Normal*: ≥ –1.0
- *Osteopenia*: –1.0 to –2.5
- *Osteoporosis*: ≤ –2.5

Uses in Orthopedics

- Diagnosis of osteoporosis
- Monitoring response to treatment
- Fracture risk prediction (FRAX score)

Q15. Write a short note on haptic robotic system.

Definition

Haptic systems provide tactile feedback to surgeons during robotic or computer-assisted orthopedic procedures.

Applications

- Robotic-assisted joint arthroplasty (e.g., MAKO for knee/hip)
- Precision in bone resection and implant placement
- Training simulators for orthopedic residents
- Reduces human error and improves outcomes

Advantages

- Enhanced control and feedback
- Increased surgical accuracy
- Reduced soft tissue trauma

Q16. What is myositis ossificans? How will you diagnose? Describe its management.

(Amrita Institute of Medical Sciences Kochi Kerala 2019)

Definition

Formation of heterotopic bone within muscle or soft tissue, commonly after trauma.

Common Sites

Quadriceps, brachialis, adductors

Diagnosis

- *Clinical*: Painful swelling, restricted motion
- *Radiology*:
    - *X-ray*: Peripheral ossification pattern (zoning phenomenon)
    - *CT/MRI*: Clarifies location and extent
    - *Bone scan*: Early uptake

Management

- *Conservative*: Rest, NSAIDs (e.g., indomethacin), physical therapy
- *Surgical*: Excision after maturation (>6 months) if functional limitation persists

Q17. Write a short note on skin grafts.

(GMCJ 2019)

Definition

Transplantation of skin from a donor site to a recipient area lacking skin cover.

Types

- *Split thickness skin graft (STSG)*: Epidermis + part dermis
- *Full thickness skin graft (FTSG)*: Entire dermis and epidermis

Indications

- Raw areas post-trauma, burns, ulcers
- Post-tumor excision

Limitations

- No vascular structures (depends on recipient site for revascularization)
- Not suitable over exposed tendon, bone without periosteum

Q18. What are flaps? Write its classification. Describe different free flaps.

Definition

Flaps are vascularized tissues transferred from donor to recipient site to cover defects.

Classification

1. *Based on blood supply*:
   - Random pattern
   - Axial pattern
2. *Based on tissue components*:
   - Fasciocutaneous
   - Myocutaneous
   - Bone-containing (osteocutaneous)
3. *Based on transfer*:
   - Local flap
   - Regional flap
   - Free flap (microsurgical)

Common Free Flaps

- Latissimus dorsi
- Fibular flap (for long bone defects)
- Radial forearm flap
- Anterolateral thigh flap (ALT)

Uses: Large soft tissue defects, limb salvage surgeries

Q19. Describe the principles of wound debridement.

Definition

Removal of devitalized, infected, or contaminated tissue to promote wound healing.

Principles (5 D's)

1. *D*ead tissue removal
2. *D*rainage of pus
3. *D*ebulking infection
4. *D*elivery of antibiotics
5. *D*efinitive closure later

Types

- Surgical (sharp dissection)
- Mechanical (wet-to-dry dressings)
- Enzymatic (collagenase)
- Autolytic (moisture-retaining dressings)

Timing

Early and repeated if needed (serial debridement).

Q20. What are different bleeding disorders? Describe hemophilic arthropathy.

Common Bleeding Disorders

- Hemophilia A (factor VIII deficiency)
- Hemophilia B (factor IX deficiency)
- von Willebrand disease
- Platelet function disorders

- Vitamin K deficiency
- Liver disease

Hemophilic Arthropathy
- Repeated hemarthroses → chronic synovitis → joint destruction
- *Most commonly affects*: Knees, elbows, ankles

Clinical Features
- Pain, swelling
- Decreased ROM
- Joint deformity

Management
- Factor replacement therapy
- Synoviorthesis (chemical/radioactive)
- Arthroscopic synovectomy
- Physiotherapy
- Arthroplasty in late stages

Q21. Describe the principles and implications of blood transfusion in orthopedic trauma.

(AIIMS May 2020)

Indications in Ortho Trauma
- Polytrauma with blood loss
- Open fractures
- Pelvic fractures
- Spine trauma with hypotension

Transfusion Principles
- Crossmatch, group-compatible
- Transfuse only when necessary (restrictive protocols)

Types
- Packed RBCs
- FFP (coagulopathy)
- Platelets (thrombocytopenia)
- Cryoprecipitate (low fibrinogen)

Hazards
- Hemolytic reactions
- Transfusion-related infections (HIV, hepatitis)
- Febrile non-hemolytic reactions
- Iron overload
- Transfusion-related acute lung injury (TRALI)

Q22. Discuss the role and techniques of autologous blood transfusion in orthopedic surgery.

(MUHS Maharashtra 2020)

Definition
Reinfusion of the patient's own blood to avoid allogenic transfusion.

Types
1. *Preoperative donation*: Weeks before surgery.
2. *Intraoperative hemodilution*: Draw blood and replace with crystalloids.
3. *Cell salvage*: Blood lost intra/post-operatively collected, filtered, reinfused.

Advantages

- Eliminates transfusion reactions and disease transmission.
- Useful in elective joint arthroplasty, scoliosis surgery.

Limitations

- Not useful in infection/malignancy.
- Requires planning, equipment.

Q23. What is massive blood transfusion? What are the hazards of blood transfusion?

Definition

10 units of packed RBCs within 24 hours or >1 blood volume within 24 hours.

Hazards

- *Immediate*:
  - Hemolytic reaction
  - Febrile non-hemolytic
  - Allergic reaction
  - Air embolism
- *Delayed*:
  - Infections (HIV, HCV, HBV)
  - Iron overload
  - Graft-versus-host disease
  - Hypocalcemia (due to citrate)
  - Hypothermia

Q24. Describe battered baby syndrome.

Definition

A form of non-accidental trauma (child abuse) presenting with unexplained injuries in infants/young children.

Clinical Features

- Multiple fractures in different healing stages
- Posterior rib fractures
- Metaphyseal corner fractures
- Subdural hematomas
- Retinal hemorrhages

Orthopedic Role

- Radiographic documentation
- Skeletal survey
- Reporting to child protection authorities

Q25. Describe flail chest and its management.

Definition

Segmental fracture of ≥3 consecutive ribs in ≥2 places leading to paradoxical chest wall movement.

Clinical Features

- Chest pain
- Paradoxical movement
- Respiratory distress
- Associated pulmonary contusion

Management
- *Initial*: Oxygenation, analgesia, respiratory support
- *Definitive*: Surgical fixation (indicated in severe cases)
- Chest physiotherapy

Q26. Describe the causes, clinical features, and management of disseminated intravascular coagulation (DIC).

(Madras Medical College Chennai Tamil Nadu 2017)

Causes
- Sepsis
- Trauma
- Malignancy
- Obstetric complications

Pathophysiology
Widespread clotting → consumption of clotting factors → bleeding

Clinical Features
- Bleeding from venipuncture sites
- Petechiae, ecchymosis
- Organ failure

Management
- Treat underlying cause
- Fresh frozen plasma, platelet transfusion
- Heparin in chronic DIC

Q27. Write different acid-base disorders. Discuss the management of metabolic acidosis.

Acid-base Disorders
- Metabolic acidosis
- Metabolic alkalosis
- Respiratory acidosis
- Respiratory alkalosis

Metabolic Acidosis
$\downarrow$ pH, $\downarrow$ HCO_3^-

Causes
- Renal failure
- Diabetic ketoacidosis
- Lactic acidosis
- Diarrhea

Management
- Treat underlying cause
- Sodium bicarbonate (if pH <7.1)
- IV fluids and electrolyte correction

Q28. What is Volkmann's contracture? Describe its etiopathogenesis, clinical features, classification, and management.

Volkmann's Sign
Flexion contracture of the wrist/fingers due to ischemic injury to forearm flexor muscles. **Volkmann's sign** is a clinical sign indicating **Volkmann's ischemic contracture**, which is caused by **compartment syndrome**—usually in the forearm due to injury, tight casts, or vascular compromise.

Brief Description
- *Sign*: Fingers are flexed at the interphalangeal joints and cannot be fully extended.
- *Cause*: Ischemic damage to the forearm flexor muscles and nerves (especially the median and ulnar nerves).
- *Common scenario*: Seen after supracondylar fractures of the humerus in children.

Key Point
Volkmann's sign suggests **permanent muscle and nerve damage** due to prolonged lack of blood supply, requiring urgent intervention if recognized early.

Etiopathogenesis
Compartment syndrome → ischemia of flexor muscles → fibrosis → contracture

Clinical Features
- Pain, pallor, pulselessness
- Passive finger extension pain
- *Later*: Fixed flexion deformity

Classification (Tsuge)
- *Mild*: Only fingers
- *Moderate*: Fingers + some wrist
- *Severe*: Fingers, wrist, elbow

Management
- *Acute stage*: Fasciotomy
- *Late stage*: Tendon lengthening, muscle slide, free functional muscle transfer

Q29. John Charnley's contributions to orthopedics.

(Madras Medical College Chennai Tamil Nadu 2011)

Sir John Charnley (1911–1982) was a British orthopedic surgeon known as the *father of modern hip replacement*.

Major Contributions
- Low friction arthroplasty (LFA)
- *Introduced in the 1960s using*:
  - High-density polyethylene (acetabular cup)
  - Stainless steel femoral component
  - Acrylic bone cement (PMMA)
- *Concept of low friction torque*: Reduced wear and improved implant longevity.
- *Clean air operating theatre*: Introduced laminar airflow system to reduce post-operative infection rates.
- *Charnley hip prosthesis*: A model for modern THR design; still widely referenced.
- *Charnley compression arthrodesis frame*: Used for arthrodesis in TB hips and knees.

GA Ilizarov

Q30. Write a note on contribution of GA Ilizarov to orthopedics.

Gavriil Abramovich Ilizarov (1921–1992) was a Russian orthopedic surgeon and inventor of the Ilizarov apparatus.

Key Contributions
- *Ilizarov technique (distraction osteogenesis)*:
  - Used for bone lengthening, deformity correction, and non-unions.
  - Based on the principle of tension-stress stimulating bone and soft tissue regeneration.
- *Ilizarov external fixator:*
  - Circular fixator with wires and rings allowing multidirectional stability and dynamization.
  - Widely used in limb lengthening and complex deformity corrections.

- *Applications:*
  - Congenital limb deficiencies
  - Post-traumatic bone loss
  - Osteomyelitis
  - Pseudoarthrosis (e.g., tibia)

Global Influence
Though initially confined to the Soviet Union, his work gained global recognition post-1980s.

Q31. Marius Smith-Petersen contribution to orthopedics (1886–1953).

Pioneer in hip surgery and orthopedic innovation.

Key Contributions
1. *Smith-Petersen nail (1925–1931)*:
   - Triflanged nail for internal fixation of **femoral neck fractures**.
   - Marked a major advancement in operative fracture care.
   - Introduced the concept of **open reduction and internal fixation** (ORIF) for hip fractures.
2. *Mold arthroplasty (1938)*:
   - Developed **vitallium mold arthroplasty** for hip arthritis.
   - One of the **earliest forms of hemiarthroplasty**, paved the way for modern hip replacements.
3. *Surgical approaches*:
   - **Smith-Petersen anterior approach to the hip joint**, still used today.
     - *Interval*: Sartorius–TFL
     - Safe for preserving abductors and ideal for arthroplasty
4. *Other innovations*:
   - Early advocate for **open treatment of fractures**.
   - *Work on ankylosing spondylitis*: Performed osteotomy of spine to restore erect posture.

Legacy
- Laid the foundation for modern hip arthroplasty.
- His anterior approach is widely used in **minimally invasive hip surgeries** today.

Q32. Electrocautery.

Definition
Use of heat or electrical energy to coagulate or cut tissue.

Types
- *Monopolar*: Requires grounding pad; used for cutting/coagulation
- *Bipolar*: Safer near nerves; current passes between forceps tips

Uses in Orthopedics
- Hemostasis
- Dissection and exposure
- Tumor ablation (radiofrequency cautery)

Risks
- Thermal burns
- Delayed wound healing
- Interference with pacemakers

Q33. Use of drains.

(KGMU 2018)

Purpose

To evacuate fluid or blood from surgical sites and prevent hematoma/seroma.

Types

- *Passive*: Penrose drain (uses gravity)
- *Active*: Closed suction (e.g., Romovac, Jackson-Pratt)

Indications

- Joint replacements (selectively used)
- Tumor excision
- Spine surgery
- Extensive soft tissue dissection

Complications

- Infection
- Drain blockage
- Premature dislodgement

Q34. Describe the principles and setup of a bone bank.

(RGUHS Karnataka 2021)

Definition

A bone bank is a facility where bone grafts (usually allografts) are collected, processed, stored, and distributed for clinical use.

Setup and Principles

- *Donor selection*: From living donors (e.g., femoral heads post-THR) or cadaveric donors.
- *Screening*: Medical history, blood tests (HIV, hepatitis B/C, syphilis).
- *Harvesting*: Under sterile conditions.
- *Processing*: Removal of soft tissue, fat; antibiotic washing.
- *Preservation*: Freeze-dried or fresh frozen; stored at –80°C.
- *Sterilization*: Gamma radiation or ethylene oxide.
- *Record keeping*: Traceability, expiry, donor-recipient linkage.

Clinical Uses

Non-union, tumor reconstruction, arthroplasty, spinal fusion.

Q35. Define and classify pressure sores. Discuss prevention and management.

(NTRUHS Andhra Pradesh 2022)

Definition

Localized injury to skin and/or underlying tissue over a bony prominence due to pressure.

Common Sites

Sacrum, heels, elbows

Stages

- *Stage I*: Non-blanchable erythema
- *Stage II*: Partial thickness skin loss

- *Stage III*: Full thickness skin loss
- *Stage IV*: Exposed bone/tendon

Prevention
- Frequent repositioning (every hours)
- Pressure-relieving surfaces
- Skin inspection, nutrition

Management
- Debridement
- Dressings (hydrocolloids, alginates)
- Antibiotics if infected
- Flap cover (Stage III/IV)

Q36. Write a short note on medico-legal issues in orthopedic trauma.

(Frequently asked)

Common Medico-legal Issues
- Failure to obtain **informed consent**
- Delay in diagnosis or surgery
- Negligence in trauma care (missed injuries)
- Documentation lapses
- Death in casualty → medicolegal case
- Fractures due to assault/accident → reporting required

Legal Documentation
- Maintain detailed records
- MLC reporting to police
- Consent for surgery, transfusion, amputation
- Consent from guardian for minors

Role of Orthopedician
- Document injury pattern
- Assist in medico-legal certification
- Adhere to protocols to avoid litigation

Q37. Discuss occupational and industrial hazards related to orthopedic practice.

(RGUHS Karnataka 2023)

Hazards Faced by Orthopedic Surgeons
1. *Musculoskeletal injuries*:
    - Repetitive strain injuries (RSI), back and neck pain
    - Long-standing during surgeries → disc issues
2. *Radiation exposure*:
    - C-arm/fluoroscopy in trauma/spine surgeries
    - Risk of malignancy, cataracts
3. *Sharps injuries and infections*: Risk of bloodborne infections (HIV, hepatitis B/C)
4. *Mental health and stress*: Burnout, depression, sleep deprivation
5. *Noise and ergonomic issues*: Drill/saw use → noise-induced hearing loss

Prevention
- Use of lead aprons, dosimeters
- Proper posture, ergonomic design

- Adherence to WHO surgical safety checklist
- Work-life balance and mental health awareness

Q38. Discuss the radiation hazard and its preventive measures in orthopedics.

Radiation Hazards

- *Stochastic effects*: Long-term risks including malignancy (e.g., leukemia, thyroid, skin cancer)
- *Deterministic effects*: Skin erythema, cataracts, infertility, bone marrow suppression

Sources in Orthopedics

- C-arm fluoroscopy in trauma and spine surgery
- CT-guided interventions

Preventive Measures

- Use of **lead aprons**, thyroid shields, lead gloves
- **Minimize exposure time**
- **Maximize distance** from radiation source (inverse square law)
- Use of **pulsed fluoroscopy** and **low-dose settings**
- Proper **collimation and beam direction**
- **Dosimeter badges** to monitor cumulative exposure
- **Barriers/screens** between staff and source

Q39. Discuss challenges and opportunities in rural orthopedic practice.

(NMC/NBE recommended general topic)

Challenges

- Lack of infrastructure and implants
- Limited access to diagnostic tools
- Scarcity of trained personnel
- Delayed presentation and treatment
- Patient education barriers

Opportunities

- High clinical exposure
- Broad spectrum of cases
- Community impact and satisfaction
- Scope for low-cost innovation
- Opportunities for outreach and preventive care

Solutions

- Mobile clinics and camps
- Telemedicine
- Rural surgeon training programs

Q40. Describe the economic burden and cost-effectiveness of orthopedic procedures.

(RGUHS Karnataka 2020)

Economic Burden

- Implants (THR, TKR, spine fixation)
- Long hospital stays
- Revision surgeries
- Post-operative rehabilitation costs

Cost-effectiveness

- TKR/THR improve quality-adjusted life years (QALY)
- Day-care surgeries and MIS reduce hospital stay
- Government schemes (PMJAY) improve affordability

Tools

- Health economic analysis (cost/benefit, cost/QALY)
- Use of indigenous implants
- Judicious implant selection based on outcome

Q41. Describe the principles of mass casualty management in orthopedics.

Definition

A mass casualty event (MCE) is when the number of patients exceeds the capacity of available medical resources.

Principles

- *Triage*: Prioritize treatment using color-coded tags
    - *Red*: Immediate
    - *Yellow*: Delayed
    - *Green*: Minor
    - *Black*: Deceased/Expectant
- *Damage control orthopedics (DCO)*:
    - Temporary stabilization (external fixators, splints) over definitive surgery
    - Delay major procedures until patient is hemodynamically stable
- *Team organization*: Division of zones (triage, treatment, evacuation)
- *Communication*: Rapid coordination with emergency, surgical, and ICU teams
- Documentation and identification

Orthopedic Role

- Rapid assessment and stabilization of fractures
- Focus on life and limb-saving interventions

Q42. Describe principles of disaster preparedness and triage in orthopedic trauma.

(JIPMER 2020)

Disaster Preparedness Principles

- *Planning*: Protocols for natural and man-made disasters
- *Resource allocation*: Inventory of orthopedic supplies, splints, fixators
- *Team formation*: Trauma teams and defined roles
- *Communication*: Coordination with EMS, disaster response agencies
- *Training*: Regular mock drills and courses (ATLS, MCI)

Triage System

- *Red (immediate)*: Life-threatening but treatable
- *Yellow (delayed)*: Serious but not immediately life-threatening
- *Green (minor)*: Walking wounded
- *Black (expectant)*: Dead or non-survivable injuries

Orthopedic Role

- Early stabilization
- Prioritize damage control
- Referral to definitive care centers

Q43. Principles of disaster preparedness and triage in orthopedic trauma.

- *Preparedness*: Involves institutional planning, identification of disaster-prone areas, resource mapping, and readiness of personnel. Includes regular simulation drills, stocking essential orthopedic implants and splints, and creating communication protocols.
- *Triage*: A dynamic process of categorizing patients based on urgency:
  - *Red (immediate)*: Life or limb-threatening injuries requiring urgent attention (e.g., open fractures with vascular compromise).
  - *Yellow (delayed)*: Serious but non-life-threatening injuries (e.g., closed long bone fractures).
  - *Green (minimal)*: Minor injuries (e.g., sprains).
  - *Black (expectant)*: Unsurvivable injuries.
- *Principles*: Optimize outcomes using limited resources, team-based approach, continuous reassessment, documentation.

Q44. Discuss the ethics of informed consent in orthopedic surgery.

(RGUHS Karnataka 2022)

Definition

Informed consent is the voluntary agreement of a patient to undergo a medical procedure after understanding its risks, benefits, and alternatives.

Key Elements

1. Competence (patient is of sound mind)
2. Disclosure (clear explanation of procedure and risks)
3. Comprehension (patient understands the information)
4. Voluntariness (no coercion)
5. Consent (documented approval)

Ethical Relevance

- Ensures respect for patient autonomy
- Reduces medicolegal liability

Orthopedic Specifics

- Consent for blood transfusion, implants, anesthesia
- Discuss alternatives like conservative management
- High-risk procedures like spine surgery require detailed documentation

Q45. What is the role of simulation-based training in orthopedic education?

Definition

Simulation-based training uses models, mannequins, VR, and AR platforms to replicate clinical scenarios for educational purposes.

Advantages

- Safe environment to practice surgical skills
- Enhances hand-eye coordination
- Standardized learning opportunities
- Feedback-driven improvement
- Reduces patient risk during the learning curve

Tools Used

- Arthroscopy simulators (e.g., Sawbones, VR arthro-skills)
- Fracture fixation practice modules
- CPR and trauma response mannequins

Limitations
- Cost, limited availability
- May not perfectly replicate tissue handling

Future
- Integration into residency curricula
- Objective skill assessment before OT entry

Q46. Describe rehabilitation and social reintegration of amputees.

(MUHS Maharashtra 2019)

Goals
- Restore function and independence
- Prevent complications (contractures, depression)

Components
1. *Physical rehabilitation*:
   - Stump shaping, desensitization
   - Strengthening, balance training
   - Gait training with prosthesis
2. *Prosthetic fitting*:
   - Based on level of amputation and needs
   - Regular review and adjustment
3. *Psychosocial support*:
   - Counseling for grief, body image
   - Vocational training and support
4. *Social reintegration*:
   - Return to work
   - Home/workplace modifications

Q47. Describe the importance of clinical audits in orthopedic departments.

(NBE DNB 2022)

Definition

A systematic review of clinical practices to improve patient care and outcomes.

Importance
- Monitors adherence to standards
- Identifies gaps in treatment protocols
- Improves resource utilization
- Enhances patient safety
- Supports research and teaching

Steps in Clinical Audit
1. Select topic (e.g., infection control)
2. Set standard (e.g., SSI <2%)
3. Data collection
4. Analysis
5. Action and re-audit

Examples in Orthopedics
- Post-operative infection rates

- Implant usage and cost analysis
- Reoperation rates

Q48. Approach to management of a limping child.

- *History*: Age (guides likely diagnosis), trauma, infection, systemic illness, congenital disorders.
- *Physical examination*: Observe gait, limb length, joint mobility, tenderness, swelling, systemic signs (fever, rash).
- *Common conditions by age*:
  - *Toddler*: DDH, toddler's fracture
  - *4–10 years*: Perthes disease, transient synovitis
  - *Adolescents*: SCFE, infections, neoplasms
- *Investigations*: CBC, ESR, CRP, X-ray, USG, MRI as needed.
- *Management*: Urgent in septic arthritis/SCFE; otherwise tailored to diagnosis.

Q49. Wrist arthrodesis.

- *Indications*: Painful wrist arthritis (RA, TB), post-traumatic instability, failed surgeries.
- *Types*:
  - *Total arthrodesis*: Complete fusion; indicated in severe pain with gross instability.
  - *Partial arthrodesis*: Preserves some motion; used selectively.
- *Surgical techniques*: Dorsal plate fixation, use of iliac crest bone graft.
- *Complications*: Non-union, malunion, hardware prominence, loss of wrist motion.

Q50. Obstetric palsy. Brachial plexus injury during birth, due to shoulder dystocia.

Obstetric Palsy

Brachial plexus injury during birth, due to shoulder dystocia.

Types

- *Erb's palsy (C5–C6)*: Waiter's tip posture.
- *Klumpke's palsy (C8–T1)*: Claw hand, Horner's syndrome.

Management

Physiotherapy, neurosurgical repair if no recovery by 3–6 months.

1. *PTB cast*: A weight-bearing cast used for mid-to-distal tibial fractures. Transfers weight to patellar tendon, tibial flares. Allows ambulation during healing. Contraindicated in proximal tibial fractures.
2. *Skull traction*: Used for reduction and stabilization of cervical spine fractures/dislocations. Applied via tongs (Gardner–Wells) or halo. Indicated in cervical spine trauma, cervical spondylotic myelopathy (pre-operative), and TB spine.

Q51. Implant removal—indications, contraindications, dos and don'ts.

(RIMS 2018)

- *Indications*:
  - Symptomatic implants (pain, infection)
  - Prominent hardware
  - Pediatric patients (to avoid growth interference)
  - Prior to joint replacement
  - Implant-related allergies
- *Contraindications*:
  - Asymptomatic implants

- Elderly patients with poor bone quality
- Osteoporotic bone
- High surgical risk
- *Dos*:
  - Pre-operative imaging and planning
  - Informed consent including risks
  - Ensure aseptic technique
  - Availability of implant system-specific tools
- *Don'ts*:
  - Do not remove for routine practice if asymptomatic
  - Avoid in areas with risk of fracture
  - Avoid in patients with poor healing
  - Do not underestimate surgical time and blood loss

Q52. Write a short note on pain management strategies in orthopedic patients.

(TNMGRMU Tamil Nadu 2021)

Acute Pain Management
- *Oral analgesics*: NSAIDs, paracetamol
- *IV analgesics*: Tramadol, diclofenac, opioids
- *Regional blocks*: Brachial plexus, femoral nerve block
- *Epidural analgesia*: Especially in spine/lower limb surgeries

Chronic Pain Management
- Physiotherapy and rehabilitation
- *Neuropathic pain agents*: Gabapentin, pregabalin
- *Multimodal approach*: Physical + psychological support
- Pain clinics/referrals in complex cases

Principles
- WHO pain ladder
- Individualized plan
- Multimodal analgesia to minimize opioid use

Q53. Describe analgesics and anti-inflammatory agents in musculoskeletal disorders.

Introduction
Musculoskeletal disorders (MSDs) like arthritis, fractures, soft tissue injuries, and degenerative conditions cause pain and inflammation that significantly impair function. Pharmacologic management involves **analgesics** and **anti-inflammatory drugs** to relieve pain, reduce inflammation, and improve mobility.

1. Classification

A. *Analgesics*:
- *Non-opioid analgesics*: Paracetamol (acetaminophen)
- *Opioid analgesics*:
  - Tramadol
  - Morphine
  - Fentanyl
- *Adjuvant analgesics*:
  - Gabapentin, pregabalin (neuropathic pain)
  - Antidepressants (amitriptyline)

B. *Anti-inflammatory drugs*:
   - *Non-steroidal anti-inflammatory drugs (NSAIDs)*:
     - *Non-selective*: Ibuprofen, diclofenac, indomethacin, naproxen
     - *COX-2 selective*: Etoricoxib, celecoxib
   - *Steroids*:
     - Prednisolone, methylprednisolone
     - *Intra-articular*: Triamcinolone, dexamethasone

2. Mechanism of Action
- *NSAIDs*: Inhibit cyclooxygenase (COX-1 and COX-2), reducing prostaglandin synthesis.
- *Paracetamol*: Central COX inhibition with minimal peripheral anti-inflammatory action.
- *Opioids*: Act on μ-opioid receptors to block pain transmission.
- *Steroids*: Suppress the entire arachidonic acid pathway and reduce cytokine production.

3. Indications in Orthopedics
- *NSAIDs*: Acute injury pain, arthritis (OA, RA), post-operative pain, low back pain.
- *Paracetamol*: Mild-to-moderate pain, osteoarthritis (first-line).
- *Opioids*: Severe pain, post-operative pain, terminal cancer pain.
- *Steroids*:
  - *Systemic*: Rheumatoid arthritis, autoimmune arthropathies.
  - *Local*: Intra-articular injections for inflammatory arthropathies and bursitis.

4. Adverse Effects
- *NSAIDs*: Gastritis, GI bleed, nephrotoxicity, cardiovascular risks.
- *COX-2 inhibitors*: Lower GI risk but may increase CV events.
- *Steroids*: Immunosuppression, osteoporosis, hyperglycemia.
- *Opioids*: Constipation, respiratory depression, dependency.

5. Recent Advances
- *Topical NSAIDs (diclofenac gel)*: Effective in soft tissue pain.
- *Transdermal patches*: Fentanyl patches in chronic pain.
- *Biologic agents (anti-TNF)*: Indirectly reduce inflammation in RA.

Short Notes

Q54. Skeletal muscle relaxants.

(GMCJ 2018)

used to relieve muscle spasm and reduce muscle tone in musculoskeletal disorders.

Classification
- *Centrally acting*:
  - Baclofen
  - Tizanidine
  - Diazepam
  - Cyclobenzaprine
- *Peripherally acting*: Dantrolene

Indications
- Acute low back pain
- Muscle spasm post-injury
- Cerebral palsy/spasticity (e.g., baclofen)
- Tetanus (diazepam)

Adverse Effects

- Sedation
- Dizziness
- Weakness

Q55. Antibiotics in orthopedics.

Introduction

Antibiotics play a pivotal role in orthopedics, particularly in the **prevention and treatment of infections** associated with trauma, surgical procedures, open fractures, prosthetic joints, and chronic osteomyelitis. Judicious use is vital to minimize complications such as **antibiotic resistance**, delayed healing, and implant failure.

Classification of Antibiotics Used in Orthopedics

1. *Beta-lactams*:
    - *Penicillins*: Ampicillin, amoxicillin, and piperacillin
    - *Cephalosporins*:
        - *First generation*: Cefazolin (preferred in prophylaxis)
        - *Second generation*: Cefuroxime
        - *Third generation*: Ceftriaxone, ceftazidime
    - *Carbapenems*: Meropenem, imipenem
2. *Glycopeptides*: **Vancomycin, teicoplanin**—effective against MRSA, used when beta-lactams are contraindicated
3. *Lincosamides*: **Clindamycin**—effective against anaerobes and Gram-positive cocci; used in penicillin-allergic patients
4. *Fluoroquinolones*: **Ciprofloxacin, levofloxacin, moxifloxacin**—broad-spectrum, good bone penetration
5. *Aminoglycosides*: **Gentamicin, amikacin**—used in combination for synergy, especially in Gram-negative infections
6. *Tetracyclines*: **Doxycycline**—used in chronic osteomyelitis and some atypical infections
7. *Others*:
    - *Linezolid*: MRSA and VRE
    - *Rifampicin*: Used in prosthetic joint infections (in combination due to rapid resistance)
    - *Metronidazole*: Anaerobic coverage
    - *Sulfonamides*: TMP-SMX in chronic infections like *Nocardia*, actinomycosis

Clinical Uses of Antibiotics in Orthopedics

1. *Prophylactic use in surgery*:
    - *Goal*: Prevent surgical site infection (SSI)
    - *Timing*: Ideally within 60 minutes before incision
    - *Drug of choice*: Cefazolin 1–2 g IV (or vancomycin in MRSA-prone or allergic cases)
    - *Duration*: Usually not >24 hours post-operative unless prolonged surgery or implants involved
2. *Open fractures*:
    - *According to Gustilo–Anderson classification*:
        - *Type I and II*: First generation cephalosporin (cefazolin)
        - *Type III*: Add aminoglycoside (e.g., gentamicin)
        - *Farm injuries/high contamination*: Add penicillin or metronidazole for anaerobic coverage
3. *Chronic osteomyelitis*:
    - Requires long-term antibiotic therapy (6–12 weeks)
    - **Culture-guided therapy** is essential
    - Surgical debridement + IV antibiotics initially, followed by oral antibiotics
4. *Septic arthritis*:
    - Emergency requiring prompt empiric therapy followed by culture-specific antibiotics
    - *Empiric*: Ceftriaxone + Vancomycin until culture reports

5. *Implant-associated infections (periprosthetic joint infection—PJI)*:
   - **Biofilm formation** is a key concern
   - **Debridement, antibiotics, and implant retention (DAIR)** protocol may be used
   - Rifampicin-based combinations are effective due to anti-biofilm properties
   - Long-term suppressive therapy may be required in some cases

Antibiotic Delivery Methods

1. *Systemic (oral/IV)*:
   - Primary route in acute infections
   - IV route preferred in severe cases initially
2. *Local delivery*:
   - **Antibiotic-impregnated PMMA cement beads/spacers**
     - Common in osteomyelitis, PJI
     - Allows high local concentration with low systemic toxicity
   - **Coated implants (e.g., silver-coated nails)**—emerging area

Antibiotic Stewardship in Orthopedics

- **Avoid overuse** to prevent resistance and secondary complications
- Use **narrow-spectrum antibiotics** when possible
- Monitor therapeutic levels (especially aminoglycosides, vancomycin)
- Follow **institutional guidelines** and update based on local antibiograms

Complications of Antibiotic Use

- Resistance (e.g., MRSA, ESBL organisms)
- Nephrotoxicity (aminoglycosides, vancomycin)
- Ototoxicity (aminoglycosides)
- Allergic reactions, including anaphylaxis
- *Clostridium difficile*-associated colitis
- Drug interactions (especially rifampicin)

Recent Advances

- Antibiotic-loaded hydrogels and coatings
- Biodegradable antibiotic carriers
- Bacteriophage therapy (experimental)
- Targeted nano-delivery systems in infected bone

Conclusion

Antibiotics are an indispensable tool in orthopedic practice. Their rational and evidence-based use is crucial to treat infections effectively while minimizing adverse effects and resistance. A multidisciplinary approach involving microbiologists, orthopedic surgeons, and infection specialists ensures optimal outcomes, especially in complex infections like osteomyelitis and PJI.

Q56. Fondaparinux.

- *Type*: Synthetic pentasaccharide; selective Factor Xa inhibitor
- *Use*: DVT prophylaxis post-orthopedic surgery (e.g., hip/knee replacement)
- *Advantage*: Once daily SC injection, no need for routine monitoring
- *Contraindications*: Renal impairment, bleeding disorders

Q57. Warfarin.

- *Type*: Vitamin K antagonist; inhibits factors II, VII, IX, X
- *Use*: Long-term anticoagulation—DVT, PE prevention

- *Monitoring*: INR (target 2.0–3.0)
- *Reversal*: Vitamin K, fresh frozen plasma
- *Interactions*: Many drugs and dietary restrictions
- *Onset*: Slow, overlap with heparin needed initially

Q58. Low molecular weight heparin (LMWH).

(JIPMER 2016)

- *Drugs*: Enoxaparin, dalteparin
- *Mechanism*: Inhibits Factor Xa > IIa
- *Use*: DVT prophylaxis after orthopedic surgery
- *Advantages*:
  - Predictable response
  - No need for aPTT monitoring
- *Complications*: Bleeding, heparin-induced thrombocytopenia (less than UFH)

Q59. Calcitonin.

- *Source*: Hormone from parafollicular cells (or synthetic)
- *Mechanism*: Inhibits osteoclast activity, reduces bone resorption
- *Uses*:
  - Osteoporosis
  - Paget's disease
  - Hypercalcemia
  - Pain relief in vertebral fractures
- *Routes*: Nasal spray, IM, SC
- *Side effects*: Nausea, flushing, nasal irritation

Q60. Parathormone (PTH analogues).

- *Drugs*: Teriparatide (recombinant PTH 1-34)
- *Mechanism*: Intermittent dosing stimulates osteoblasts → bone formation
- *Use*: Severe osteoporosis, especially postmenopausal and steroid-induced
- *Route*: Daily SC injection
- *Duration*: Up to 2 years (anabolic window)
- *Caution*: Contraindicated in bone metastases, Paget's disease (osteosarcoma risk in animals)

Q61. Glucocorticoids.

Definition

Synthetic analogues of cortisol used for their **anti-inflammatory and immunosuppressive effects.**

Mechanism

- Inhibit phospholipase A2 → reduce prostaglandins and leukotrienes
- Suppress cytokine production and immune cell function

Uses in Orthopedics

- **Rheumatoid arthritis**, autoimmune arthropathies
- **Polymyalgia rheumatica**
- **Acute gout** (if NSAIDs contraindicated)
- Intra-articular injections in **synovitis** and **bursitis**

Common Drugs
Prednisolone, dexamethasone, methylprednisolone

Side Effects
- Osteoporosis
- Hyperglycemia
- Avascular necrosis (especially femoral head)
- Immunosuppression

Q62. Colchicine.

Mechanism
Inhibits microtubule polymerization → prevents neutrophil chemotaxis and inflammation

Use
- Acute gout (if started within 24 hours)
- Prophylaxis when starting urate-lowering therapy

Dosage
Low dose: 0.5 mg bid/tid

Adverse Effects
- GI upset (nausea, diarrhea)
- Myopathy, especially with statins
- Bone marrow suppression (rare)

Q63. Allopurinol.

Mechanism
Xanthine oxidase inhibitor → ↓ uric acid production

Use
- Chronic gout
- Prevention of **tumor lysis syndrome**

Precautions
- Start **after** acute attack subsides
- Use with colchicine initially to prevent flares

Adverse Effects
- Rash, hypersensitivity
- Allopurinol hypersensitivity syndrome (especially in renal failure)

Q64. What are Bisphosphonates? Write their classification and uses in various orthopedic disorders.

(AIMS Kochi 2019)

Definition
Synthetic analogues of pyrophosphate that inhibit osteoclast-mediated bone resorption.

Classification
- *Non-nitrogenous*: Etidronate, clodronate
- *Nitrogenous (more potent)*: Alendronate, risedronate, zoledronic acid

Mechanism
- Induce osteoclast apoptosis
- Reduce bone turnover

Uses
- Osteoporosis (postmenopausal, steroid-induced)
- Paget's disease
- Osteogenesis imperfecta
- Bone metastases (reduce skeletal-related events)
- Avascular necrosis (controversial, adjunct)

Adverse Effects
- GI upset
- Osteonecrosis of jaw
- Atypical femoral fractures (long-term use)

Q65. Nanotechnology in orthopedics.

Definition
Application of materials and technologies at nanoscale (1–100 nm) to improve diagnosis, drug delivery, implant design, and tissue regeneration.

Applications
- *Nano-coated implants*: Improved osseointegration and infection resistance
- **Nanocarriers** for targeted drug delivery in bone tumors or infections
- *Bone grafts with nano-hydroxyapatite*: Mimic natural bone
- **Scaffolds** for cartilage/bone regeneration in tissue engineering

Q66. Cup and stem design of cemented versus uncemented THR.

(DYPU Pune 2017)

Feature	*Cemented THR*	*Uncemented THR*
Cup design	All-polyethylene or metal-backed	Porous-coated or hydroxyapatite-coated for bone ingrowth
Fixation	Bone cement (PMMA)	Biological fixation (press-fit, bone ingrowth)
Stem design	Polished or roughened stem with taper	Grit-blasted or porous-coated titanium or cobalt-chrome
Indications	Elderly, low-demand, osteoporotic bone	Young, high-demand patients with good bone stock

Newer Trends
- Modular stems and acetabular components
- Dual-mobility cups in unstable hips

Q67. How to reduce recurrence rate in giant cell tumor (GCT).

(Goa Medical College 2018)

Strategies
1. **Extended curettage** using high-speed burr
2. *Use of adjuvants*:
   - Phenol, hydrogen peroxide
   - Cryotherapy or argon beam
   - Polymethylmethacrylate (PMMA) cement

3. **En bloc excision** in expendable bones or recurrent cases
4. **Denosumab therapy** (RANKL inhibitor) to reduce tumor size pre-operative
5. **Careful follow-up** with imaging

Q68. Articular tissue engineering.

Goal

Regenerate damaged **cartilage** and **subchondral bone** using biological and material sciences.

Components

1. *Cells*: Autologous chondrocytes, stem cells (MSCs)
2. *Scaffolds*: Biodegradable polymers (collagen, PGA, PLA)
3. *Growth factors*: TGF-β, BMPs, IGF
4. *Techniques*:
   - Autologous chondrocyte implantation (ACI)
   - Matrix-assisted chondrocyte implantation (MACI)
   - 3D bioprinting of cartilage

Clinical Use

- Focal cartilage defects (e.g., knee)
- Early OA (limited role)
- Pediatric osteochondral lesions

Index

Page numbers followed by *fc* refer to flowchart.

A

B

C

D

G

I

J

K

N

O

P

T

W

X

Z